Continuous Pharmaceutical Processing and Process Analytical Technology

Continuous manufacturing of pharmaceuticals, including aspects of modern process development, is highlighted in this book with both the 'why' and the 'how', emphasizing process modeling and process analytical technologies. Presenting specific case studies and drawing upon extensive experience from industry and academic opinion leaders, this book focuses on the practical aspects of continuous manufacturing. It gives the readers the strategic perspective and technical depth needed to adopt and implement these technologies, where appropriate, in order to gain the competitive edge in speed, agility, and reliability.

Drugs and the Pharmaceutical Sciences

A Series of Textbooks and Monographs
Series Editor
Anthony J. Hickey
RTI International, Research Triangle Park, USA

The Drugs and Pharmaceutical Sciences series is designed to enable the pharmaceutical scientist to stay abreast of the changing trends, advances and innovations associated with therapeutic drugs and that area of expertise and interest that has come to be known as the pharmaceutical sciences. The body of knowledge that those working in the pharmaceutical environment have to work with, and master, has been, and continues, to expand at a rapid pace as new scientific approaches, technologies, instrumentations, clinical advances, economic factors and social needs arise and influence the discovery, development, manufacture, commercialization and clinical use of new agents and devices.

Recent Titles in Series

Pharmaceutical Extrusion Technology, Second Edition
Isaac Ghebre-Sellassie, Charles E. Martin, Feng Zhang, and James Dinunzio

Biosimilar Drug Product Development
Laszlo Endrenyi, Paul Declerck, and Shein-Chung Chow

High Throughput Screening in Drug Discovery
Amancio Carnero

Generic Drug Product Development: International Regulatory Requirements for Bioequivalence, Second Edition
Isadore Kanfer and Leon Shargel

Aqueous Polymeric Coatings for Pharmaceutical Dosage Forms, Fourth Edition
Linda A. Felton

Good Design Practices for GMP Pharmaceutical Facilities, Second Edition
Terry Jacobs and Andrew A. Signore

Handbook of Bioequivalence Testing, Second Edition
Sarfaraz K. Niazi

FDA Good Laboratory Practice Requirements, First Edition
Graham Bunn

Continuous Pharmaceutical Processing and Process Analytical Technology
Ajit S. Narang and Atul Dubey

Project Management for Drug Developers
Joseph P. Stalder

For more information about this series, please visit: www.crcpress.com/Drugs-and-the-Pharmaceutical-Sciences/book-series/IHCDRUPHASCI

Continuous Pharmaceutical Processing and Process Analytical Technology

Edited by

Ajit S. Narang
Department of Pharmaceutical Sciences,
ORIC Pharmaceuticals, Inc., South San Francisco, CA

Atul Dubey
Pharmaceutical Continuous Manufacturing,
US Pharmacopeial Convention, Rockville, MD

CRC Press
Taylor & Francis Group
Boca Raton London New York

CRC Press is an imprint of the
Taylor & Francis Group, an **informa** business

Cover image: The cover image is produced with kind permission of Lyndra Therapeutics. We also acknowledge the help from Louis Garguilo, Chief Editor, *Outsourced Pharma* in this regard.

First edition published 2023
by CRC Press
6000 Broken Sound Parkway NW, Suite 300, Boca Raton, FL 33487-2742

and by CRC Press
4 Park Square, Milton Park, Abingdon, Oxon, OX14 4RN

CRC Press is an imprint of Taylor & Francis Group, LLC

© 2023 selection and editorial matter, **Ajit S. Narang, Atul Dubey**; individual chapters, the contributors

Library of Congress Cataloging-in-Publication Data
Names: Narang, Ajit S., editor. | Dubey, Atul, editor.
Title: Continuous pharmaceutical processing and process analytical
   technology / edited by Ajit S. Narang, Atul Dubey.
Other titles: Drugs and the pharmaceutical sciences 0360-2583
Description: First edition. | Boca Raton : CRC Press, 2023. | Series: Drugs
   and the pharmaceutical sciences | Includes bibliographical references
   and index.
Identifiers: LCCN 2022029286 (print) | LCCN 2022029287 (ebook) | ISBN
   9780367707668 (hardback) | ISBN 9780367712150 (paperback) | ISBN
   9781003149835 (ebook)
Subjects: MESH: Technology, Pharmaceutical | Drug Industry | Chemistry,
   Pharmaceutical | Pharmaceutical Preparations
Classification: LCC RS403 (print) | LCC RS403 (ebook) | NLM QV 778 | DDC
   615.1/9--dc23/eng/20220919
LC record available at https://lccn.loc.gov/2022029286
LC ebook record available at https://lccn.loc.gov/2022029287

ISBN: 978-0-367-70766-8 (hbk)
ISBN: 978-0-367-71215-0 (pbk)
ISBN: 978-1-003-14983-5 (ebk)

DOI: 10.1201/9781003149835

Typeset in Times
by SPi Technologies India Pvt Ltd (Straive)

To my Dad, Tirath Singh, the loquacious warrior.
Ajit S. Narang

To my dear family, for shaping me and putting up with me.
Atul Dubey

Contents

Part I   Design and Control: Continuous Manufacturing of <u>Small</u> Molecule Drug Substances and Products

Part II   Design and Control: Continuous Manufacturing of <u>Large</u> Molecule Drug Substances and Products

Part III   Process Analytical Technologies

Part IV   Modeling, Design Space, and Future Outlook

Preface

Continuous manufacturing is an established modality in several industries, such as fine chemicals, food ingredients, and oil and gas industry. Its adoption in pharmaceutical industry has picked up pace in the last 20 years. The early part of this period saw the development of fundamental methods in solid oral drug product manufacturing. With a fresh perspective, innovative adaptations, introduction of novel equipment, and more importantly, coming together of various stakeholders, new approaches involving continuous direct compression were developed.

In the years following these developments, techniques like residence time distribution measurements and process analytical technology (PAT) tools such as near- and mid-infrared and Raman spectroscopies became widely used. A confluence of disciplines in chemistry and chemical engineering came about resulting in reimagined manufacturing approaches. The efforts in drug substance manufacturing, utilizing flow chemistry, resulted in novel chemistries, processes, and products with higher production flexibility, safety, and environmental friendliness. The successes in small molecules inspired developments in the therapeutic proteins or biologics arena. While the upstream–downstream integration remains a challenge to date, continuous manufacturing in biologics is growing fast.

As of today, there are several products in the market that utilize continuous processing. The continuous direct compression methodology is no longer considered an 'emerging' modality and is instead considered at par with established batch methods in terms of maturity. In this book, we provide a broad perspective of continuous manufacturing in pharmaceuticals and present practical knowledge gathered over decades of research done by our authors and others.

The book is organized into four parts. Part I focuses on design and control aspects of continuous manufacturing of small molecules covering both drug substance and drug products. We begin with a broad survey of continuous API syntheses and show various synthetic routes, specific reactions, and the lessons learned over the years. This, we believe, is a great starting point for someone looking to make a beginning in continuous small molecule drug product synthesis. This is followed by an in-depth look at the emerging field of continuous crystallization. Residence time distribution finds applications in all type of continuous processes and is discussed in depth with the latest learnings, which will be useful not only to a beginner but also to experienced practitioners. A more challenging topic of electrostatics and its impact on powder-based processes is covered in Chapter 4. Newer topics like continuous impregnation and mini-batch modality are also covered. A detailed discussion of practically applicable approaches for predictive in vitro dissolution for real-time release rounds off Part I of the book.

Part II introduces the challenges and describes the current understanding in continuous manufacturing of biologics, including cGMP considerations. Applications of lyophilization are also covered in Chapter 9 by Pisano and team. The all-important PAT area is covered in detail in Part III starting with the near-infrared spectroscopy and its applications. The applications in biologics are covered in Chapter 11. Finally, Chapter 12 is a compilation of knowledge distilled from decades of research from Prof. Rodolfo Romanach who has championed process analytical technologies throughout his academic career. These 'lessons learned' are an invaluable resource for anyone looking to choose the right technology, equipment, and process design approaches.

Finally, Part IV covers modeling and process control techniques, including introduction to key topics such as design space, hybrid modeling approaches, and control strategy development. All these are essential to the success of any modern manufacturing process. Modeling is becoming a key to increased process understanding, process design, and troubleshooting. Increasingly, model-generated data are finding their way into regulatory submissions. The framework for validation of models developed by Valente et al., utilizing their practical experience of developing several commercial processes, will serve as a guide to aspiring process modelers. We round off this text with a broad outlook by industry veteran Ian Leavesley, covering the historical developments in continuous manufacturing out-side the pharmaceutical industry and how such developments may shape the future of pharmaceutical manufacturing.

We are confident that this book will be equally useful to industry personnel, researchers, and scientists aspiring to adopt continuous manufacturing.

Editor Biographies

Dr. Ajit S. Narang works for the Department of Pharmaceutical Sciences of ORIC Pharmaceuticals, Inc., in South San Francisco, CA, responsible for the pharmaceutical development of new chemical entities through preclinical and early clinical stages.

He holds about two decades of pharmaceutical industry experience in the development and commercialization of oral and parenteral dosage forms and drug delivery platforms across preclinical through commercialization stages for both small and large molecule drugs. In addition to Genentech, he has worked for Bristol-Myers Squibb, Co., in New Brunswick, NJ; Ranbaxy Research Labs (currently a subsidiary of Daiichi Sankyo, Japan) in Gurgaon, India; and Morton Grove Pharmaceuticals (currently, Wockhardt USA) in Gurnee, IL.

He holds an undergraduate Pharmacy degree from the University of Delhi, India, and graduate degrees in Pharmaceutics from the Banaras Hindu University, India, and the University of Tennessee Health Science Center (UTHSC) in Memphis, TN. Ajit has contributed to several preclinical, clinical, and commercialized drug products including NDAs, ANDAs, and 505B2s.

He is credited with 54 peer-reviewed articles; 22 editorial contributions; 5 books; 10 patent applications; 47 invited talks; and 85 presentations at various scientific meetings. His current research interests are translation from preclinical to clinical and commercial drug product design; incorporation of QbD elements in drug product development; and mechanistic understanding of the role of material properties on product performance.

Dr. Atul Dubey is the Senior Principal Scientist, Documentary Standards, Pharmaceutical Continuous Manufacturing (PCM) at the United States Pharmacopeial Convention (USP). Headquartered in Rockville, MD, USA, USP is committed to global public health and quality of medicines for 200 years.

At USP, his group is focused on supporting the ongoing adoption of CM through education programs, public standards, and collaborative work for standardization and harmonization. Atul is involved in the development of a training curriculum for industry personnel to bring about technological awareness about CM. He is also a part of the expert working group (EWG) for drafting the ICH Q13 guideline for CM. He collaborates with various stakeholders to carry out scientific research in various aspects of CM.

After earning his PhD degree in Mechanical Engineering, he carried out research in pharmaceutical manufacturing processes using modeling and simulation to understand and optimize unit operations such as continuous mixing, granulation, and pan coating. He has authored several journal articles and book chapters in the domain.

After his stint at the C-SOPS (Rutgers University), he moved to India where he worked as a consultant to pharmaceutical companies, as well as a Sr. Scientist in the Aditya Birla Group in India. With a strong motivation to facilitate access to quality medicines worldwide, he is interested in applied R&D toward the development of new standards, training, and guidelines for CM.

Contributors

Merve B. Adali
Molecular Engineering Laboratory (molE)
Department of Applied Science and
    Technology
Politecnico di Torino
Torino, Italy

Stan Altan
Janssen Pharmaceutical LLC.
Spring House, PA

James Angelo
Global Product Development & Supply, Bristol
    Myers Squibb
New Brunswick, NJ
Devens, MA

Sherif Badawy
Bristol Myers Squibb Company
New Brunswick, NJ

Dwaine Banton
Janssen Pharmaceutical LLC
Spring House, PA

Michela Beretta
Research Center Pharmaceutical Engineering
    GmbH
Graz, Austria
Institute of Process and Particle
    Engineering
Graz University of Technology
Graz, Austria

Pooja Bhalode
Department of Chemical and Biochemical
    Engineering
Rutgers University
Piscataway, NJ

Sayantan Chattoraj, Ph.D.
Pharmaceutical Development
GlaxoSmithKline Pharmaceuticals R&D
Collegeville, PA

Yingjie Chen
Department of Chemical and Biomolecular
    Engineering
University of Delaware
Newark, DE

Prof. Dr. Thomas De Beer
Laboratory of Pharmaceutical Process Analytical
    Technology
Department of Pharmaceutical Analysis
Ghent University
Ghent, Belgium

Atul Dubey
Pharmaceutical Continuous Manufacturing
US Pharmacopeial Convention
Rockville, MD

Luís Eça
Instituto FarmaCiência Técnico
Lisbon, Portugal

Aaron Garrett
Global Quality Laboratory, Eli Lilly and
    Company
Indianapolis, IN

Junbo Gong
School of Chemical Engineering and
    Technology
State Key Laboratory of Chemical
    Engineering
Tianjin University
Tianjin, People's Republic of China

B. Frank Gupton
Virginia Commonwealth University
Richmond, VA

Marianthi Ierapetritou
Department of Chemical and Biomolecular
    Engineering
University of Delaware
Newark, DE

Prof. Dr. Ashish Kumar
Laboratory of Pharmaceutical Engineering
Ghent University
Ghent, Belgium

Ian M. Leavesley
Modern Pharma Consulting LLC
Eliot, ME

Yiming Ma
School of Chemical Engineering and Technology
State Key Laboratory of Chemical Engineering
Tianjin University
Tianjin, People's Republic of China

Nuno Matos
Corporate Quality, Hovione FarmaCiência
Lisbon, Portugal

Reto Maurer
Pharmaceutical R&D, F. Hoffmann-La Roche AG
Basel, Switzerland

Fernando J. Muzzio
Chemical and Biochemical Engineering
Rutgers University
New Brunswick, NJ

Sarah Nielsen
Janssen Supply Chain
Spring House, PA

Thamer A. Omar
Rutgers University
New Brunswick, NJ

Martin Otava
Janssen-Cilag s.r.o. Janssen Pharmaceutical
   Companies of Johnson & Johnson
Praha, Czechia

Bhumit A. Patel, Ph.D.
Analytical Research and Development
Merck & Co., Inc
Kenilworth, NJ

Amrit Paudel
Research Center Pharmaceutical Engineering
   GmbH
Graz, Austria
Institute of Process and Particle Engineering
Graz University of Technology, Graz, Austria

Michiel Peeters
Laboratory of Pharmaceutical Process Analytical
   Technology
Department of Pharmaceutical Analysis
Ghent University
Ghent, Belgium

Patrick M. Piccione
Pharmaceutical R&D, F. Hoffmann-La
   Roche AG
Basel, Switzerland

Joana T. Pinto
Research Center Pharmaceutical Engineering
   GmbH
Graz, Austria

Roberto Pisano
Molecular Engineering Laboratory (molE)
Department of Applied Science and Technology
Politecnico di Torino
Torino, Italy

Sonia M. Razavi
Rutgers University
New Brunswick, NJ

Dylan D. Rodene
Virginia Commonwealth University
Richmond, VA

Rodolfo J. Romañach
Department of Chemistry, Ph.D.
University of Puerto Rico, Mayagüez Campus
Mayaguez, Puerto Rico

Erinc Sahin
Global Product Development and Supply,
   Bristol Myers Squibb
New Brunswick, NJ, USA

Zhenqi Shi
Small Molecule Pharmaceutical Sciences,
   Genentech
South San Francisco, CA

Lorenzo Stratta
Molecular Engineering Laboratory (molE)
Department of Applied Science and Technology
Politecnico di Torino
Torino, Italy

John W. Tomlin
Virginia Commonwealth University
Richmond, VA

Pedro Valente
Research & Development, Hovione
   FarmaCiência
Lisbon, Portugal

Aditya Vanarase
Bristol Myers Squibb Company
New Brunswick, NJ

Matthew Walworth
Small Molecule Design and Development
Eli Lilly and Company
Indianapolis, IN

Martin Warman
University of Strathclyde
Glasgow, UK

Dhanuka P. Wasalathanthri, Ph.D.
Global Process Analytical Science
Bristol-Myers Squibb Company
Devens, MA

Jay West
Global Product Development & Supply,
   Bristol Myers Squibb
New Brunswick, NJ
Devens, MA

Songgu Wu
School of Chemical Engineering and Technology
State Key Laboratory of Chemical Engineering
Tianjin University
Tianjin, People's Republic of China

Xuankuo Xu
Global Product Development & Supply,
   Bristol Myers Squibb
New Brunswick, NJ
Devens, MA

Part I

Design and Control

Continuous Manufacturing of Small Molecule Drug Substances and Products

1

A Survey of Continuous API Syntheses: Insights at the Interface of Chemistry and Chemical Engineering

John W. Tomlin, Dylan D. Rodene, and B. Frank Gupton
Virginia Commonwealth University

CONTENTS

DOI: 10.1201/9781003149835-2

1.1 Introduction

Continuous manufacturing platforms offer numerous advantages in the development of greener and more cost-effective routes toward active pharmaceutical ingredient (API) drug targets (Wiles and Watts 2014; Baumann et al. 2020; López et al. 2020; Jas and Kirschning 2003; Alcázar 2017). Continuous chemical manufacturing operations have been practiced routinely in the commodity chemical sector for many years, but only recently has it been applied to pharmaceutical operations (Poechlauer et al. 2013; Dumarey et al. 2019; Poechlauer et al. 2012). In many ways, these continuous systems incorporate the overall principles of process intensification, where an increased output of APIs can be achieved through significant reductions of the operational complexity, leading to a substantially smaller, cleaner, safer, and more energy-efficient technology. This holistic approach requires a detailed examination of the chemistry, solvent systems, equipment requirements, and raw material needs for a specific process. Herein, we have provided some insights into the strategies and examples of processes that embrace this approach.

One of the best and earliest examples of continuous manufacturing operations is that of Henry Ford and his advancements in the development of assembly line technology (Mead and Brinkley 2003). This approach highlights the dramatic and beneficial impact that continuous operations can have on both labor and product quality. In contrast, API production is an event-driven platform that has a well-defined beginning and end to each step of the synthetic process. In addition, batch processes typically incur greater operating and capital costs, often at the expense of process reproducibility (Wiles and Watts 2014).

Implementation of a continuous chemical process often requires the employment of a multidisciplinary approach, which is at the interface of chemistry and chemical engineering. Numerous examples of atom-economical chemical transformations that are precluded from use in batch processes due to safety concerns, arising from dangerous exothermic reactions and excessive equivalents of hazardous reagents, have effectively been applied to continuous platforms (Mcquade and Seeberger 2013; Poechlauer et al. 2012; Dumarey et al. 2019). The improved heat transfer and mixing offered by flow reactors promote higher yields and invite innovative engineering solutions to accommodate improved reaction conditions. Examples of unique reactor systems that mitigate safety concerns and facilitate challenging chemical transformations will also be highlighted throughout this text.

An important element to consider when establishing a continuous synthetic strategy is the ability to mitigate the use of separation methods that lead to increased waste generation and operational complexity (Van Aken et al. 2006). These separation operations are employed when high-yielding chemical transformations cannot be achieved, thus requiring an overall increase in the number of unit operations to purge side products from the crude reaction mixture. Two alternative methods have been routinely used to quantify the impact of waste produced from chemical processes. The method developed by Rodger Sheldon, commonly referred to as E Factors, is based on the mass of waste generated per mass of product isolated (Dach et al. 2012). Alternatively, process mass intensity (PMI) is defined as 'the total mass of materials used to produce a specified mass of product, where materials include reactants, reagents, solvent media, and catalysts' (Jimenez-Gonzalez et al. 2011; Dicks and Hent 2015).

Batch API Plant

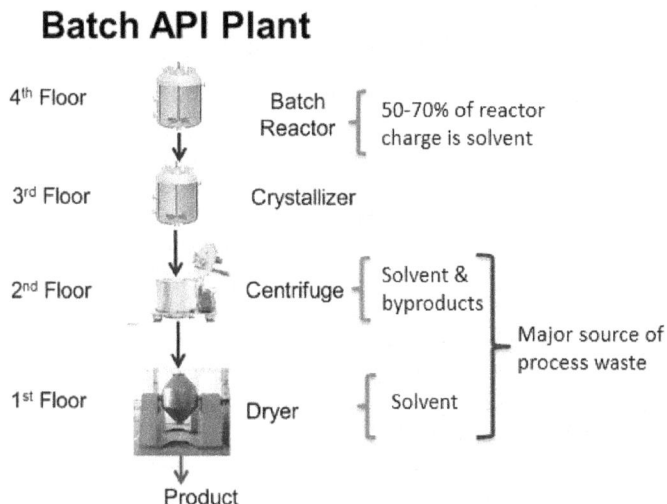

FIGURE 1.1 Generalized industrial process depicting the unit operations involved for a non-optimized batch process.

A single step in a typical pharmaceutical process typically requires large volumes of solvent that can account for 60–75% of the overall charged mass (Jimenez-Gonzalez et al. 2011). It is a general practice for the products of the individual reaction steps to be crystalized, isolated, and then dried as discrete intermediates in the overall process, as shown in Figure 1.1. In doing so, the solvent mass is removed and is rarely recycled in order to avoid re-introduction of byproduct impurities into the process. The need for these intermediate isolations can be greatly minimized when high-yielding chemical transformations can be achieved.

A practical example of this approach is a comparative analysis of a commercial process for the production of nevirapine, a widely prescribed HIV drug (Verghese et al. 2017). The original process developed by Boehringer Ingelheim Pharmaceuticals gave an overall yield of 56% while requiring multiple isolation steps throughout the process in order to remove byproduct impurities. The resulting PMI was 56 kg of input per 1 kg of product. In contrast, the streamline process developed by Verghese et al., not only increased the overall process yield to 92%, but eliminated multiple isolation steps, resulting in a PMI of less than 5. The revised process is currently being carried out in both batch and continuous commercial operations. This example, along with highly energetic reactions in flow, continuous catalytic reactions, continuous flow API syntheses and process refinement techniques are highlighted throughout this book chapter (Figure 1.2).

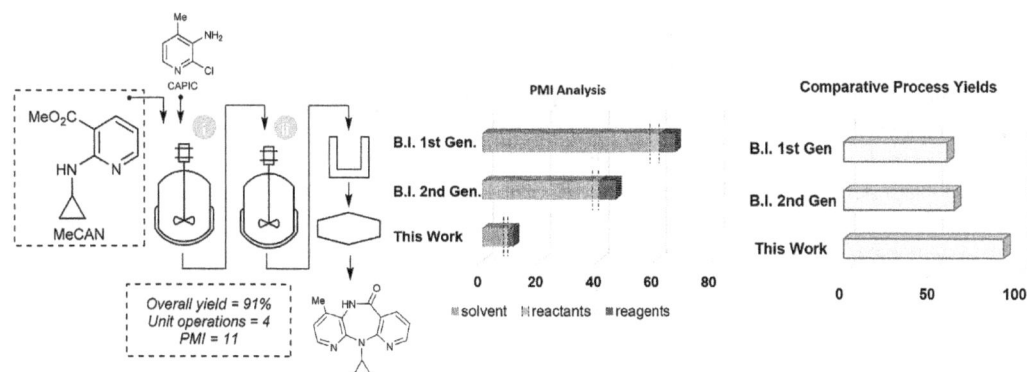

FIGURE 1.2 Comparative metrics of the Medicines for All Nevirapine process with B.I. processes, taking into account yield, PMI, and unit operations. (From Green Chemistry, "Increasing global access to the high-volume HIV drug nevirapine through process intensification", Verghese, J. et al, 2017. – Adapted with permission of The Royal Society of Chemistry.)

1.2 Reaction Types That Lend Themselves for Continuous Processing

Flow chemistry also offers a safer means to adapt highly exothermic reactions, and makes highly endo-thermic reactions achievable in order to accommodate exceedingly low temperatures. The fine temper-ature control, residence time manipulation, and facile parameterization offered by continuous platforms also allow for improved selectivity (Plutschack et al. 2017). Specific applications of these innovations in terms of pharmaceutical-relevant syntheses will be disclosed within this text.

1.2.1 Highly Energetic Reactions

The range of chemical reactions carried out in batch operations have historically been constrained by the inability to effectively manage and control the application of highly reactive reagents such as diazometh-ane, azides, oxidizing agents, and a variety of organo-metallic species. However, the risks associated with these materials can be greatly mitigated by the judicious application of continuous methodologies that limit the instantaneous amounts of these materials within the reaction medium. Equally important, the enhanced surface-to-volume ratio of continuous reactor systems provides the ability to efficiently remove heat from these types of reactions (Plutschack et al. 2017). Several novel examples of flow processes that have effectively implemented this approach are provided in this section.

1.2.2 Diazomethane

There are numerous organic building blocks essential in API production that are traditionally formed from toxic reagents. One example is diazoketones, traditionally prepared from hazardous acyl chlorides and toxic diazomethane. While diazoketones are important motifs for the preparation of quinoxalines, a key skeletal fragment in a number of antibiotics, the required handling of these potentially explosive starting materials is a problem for large-scale manufacturers (Doyle et al. 1998). It is for this reason that Martin and other researchers at Novartis developed a continuous flow protocol for the safe and scalable preparation of diazomethane in which polymer-supported Diazald was used to generate the diazomethane and then transform them to diazoketones *in situ* (Martin et al. 2011). They further demonstrated how these prepared diazoketones could be used to prepare quinoxalines while minimizing the amount of catalyst required and avoiding strong oxidizing reagents or excessive workup and purification while enhancing the overall safety of preparation as well (Figure 1.3).

The Novartis team tested the feasibility of forming diazomethane by first attempting methylation of benzoic acid in order to attempt the reaction conditions with a safer substrate. Using a Vapourtec R2+/R4 combination reactor, their team used two independent injection loops, one loaded with a solution of ben-zoic acid in methanol, the other with TMSCHN$_2$ in diethyl ether, which were mixed at a T-piece junction and then flowed into a convection flow coil for 25 minutes. Evaporation of the solvent removed excess TMSCHN$_2$ and provided a quantitative yield of the methyl ester product. A simple swap of acyl chloride in place of benzoic acid and the introduction of a packed bed of PS-fluoride at the end of the exiting flow stream allowed for various alkyl and aryl-substituted diazoketones to be isolated in 2 hours total run time in purities above 95%.

These materials were then telescoped in another flow reactor and mixed with toxic phenylenediamine and solid-supported copper triflate catalyst to produce quinoxalines. It was found that electron-with-drawing and donating groups were well-tolerated. Adding a plug of PS-thiourea, PS-isocyanate, and PS-tosylhydrazine to the end of the flow-stream allowed for in-line separation of reactions salts and impu-rities to allow for highly pure (>95%) quinoxalines to be collected after simple evaporation of the solvent.

The safe production and instantaneous consumption of diazomethane have been carried out in a num-ber of other laboratory and commercial applications. Continuous commercial production of diazometh-ane has been demonstrated by Aerojet General and Phoenix Chemicals, Ltd. (Archibald et al. 2020; Malik et al. 2016; Proctor and Warr 2001). The Aerojet process produces diazomethane from NaOH and N-methyl-N-nitrosamine in an ethereal solution within a reactor coil. This method allows for up to 60

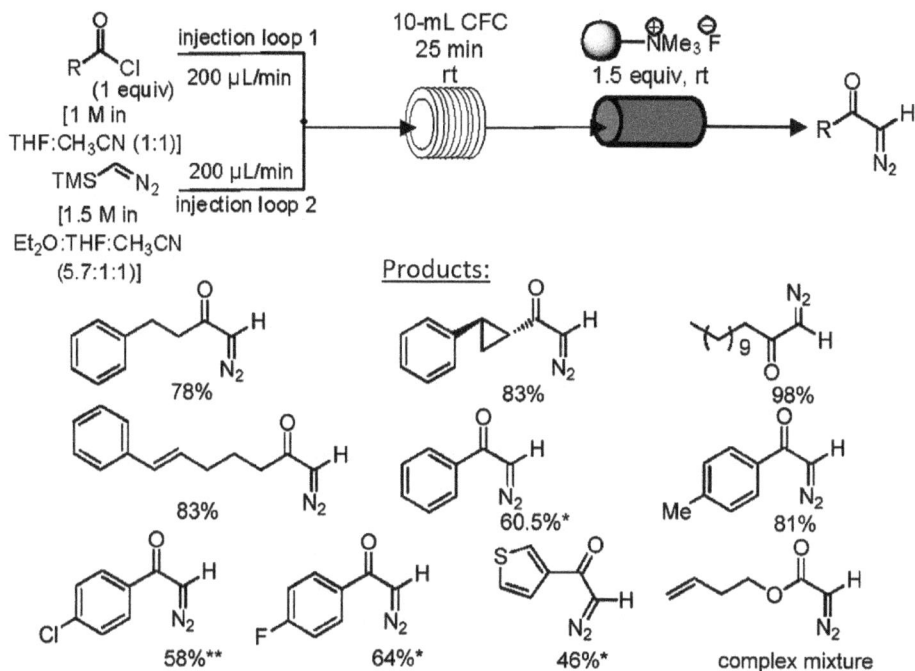

FIGURE 1.3 Synthesis of diazoketones in flow. (Reprinted with permission from "Safe and Reliable Synthesis of Diazoketones and Quinoxalines in a Continuous Flow Reactor", Martin, L.J et al, Organic Letters, 2011. Copyright 2010 American Chemical Society.)

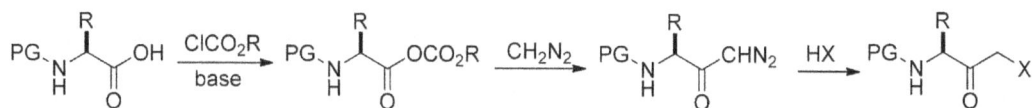

FIGURE 1.4 Synthesis of *a*-Halo ketones from diazomethane compounds. (Reprinted from https://pubs.acs.org/doi/full/10.1021/jo402849z. All further use and permissions should be directed to ACS.)

metric tons of diazomethane production annually. In addition, DSM Pharmaceutical Products reported a flow synthesis of diazomethane where the N-methyl-N-nitroso-p-toluenesulfonamide (Diazald) starting material was generated in organic solvent and then hydrolyzed in an aqueous base, with the diazomethane separated from the aqueous phase by using a semi-permeable, microporous hydrophobic membrane.

In later work, the Kappe group applied the use of a Teflon AF-2400 reactor to continuously generate, separate, and react diazomethane with a tube-in-tube continuous reactor system similar to the DSM process (Mastronardi et al. 2013) (Figure 1.4).

This tube-in-tube reactor system had been previously applied by the Ley group for ozonolysis reactions, catalytic hydrogenations, and oxygen-mediated gas-liquid transformations (O'Brien et al. 2010; Brzozowski et al. 2015). This methodology used a semi-permeable, microporous hydrophobic membrane and ran the reaction neat so that the hydrolyzed diazomethane could be collected as an anhydrous gas while still directing the waste stream out of the reactor as an aqueous mixture. The collected gas was then immediately flowed through in the next chamber to react with the prepared amino acid derivative for the preparation of α-halo ketones, a motif present in the synthesis of HIV protease inhibitor drugs such as darunavir and atazanavir (Pinho et al. 2014). The three-step continuous flow synthesis thus proceeds as outlined in Figure 1.5 below.

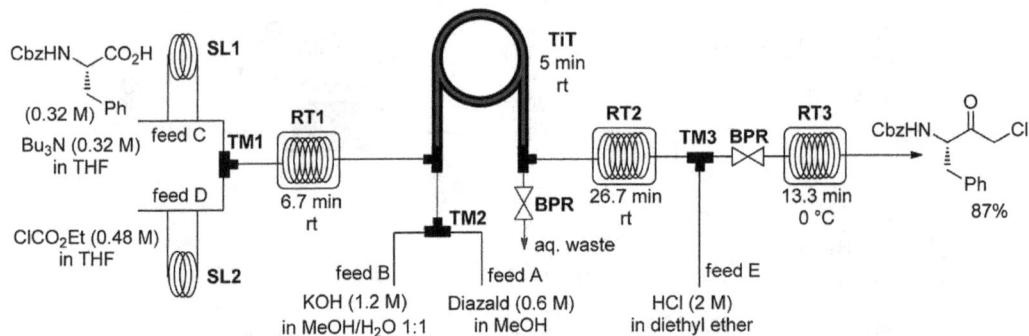

FIGURE 1.5   Synthesis of *a*-chloro ketones via a three-step continuous flow process. (Reprinted from https://pubs.acs.org/doi/full/10.1021/jo402849z. All further use and permissions should be directed to ACS.)

1.2.3 Nitration Reactions

The ability to carry out nitration reactions in a safe and controlled manner has been of significant importance not only in the preparation of APIs, but also in the production of munitions and explosives. Continuous reactor systems are uniquely suited to control the stoichiometry and heat of reaction while minimizing the reactor residence time (Plutschack et al. 2017). There are numerous examples of continuous nitration reactions that have been carried out in both laboratory and commercial applications, a few specific examples of both are provided in this section (Levin 2014; Kulkarni 2014).

The production of multikilogram quantities of nitropyridines in a continuous coiled reactor system was reported by Gage and co-workers at Asymchem Life Science (Gage et al. 2012). The group used a jacketed 304 stainless steel coil reactor shown in Figure 1.6 along with metering pumps to accurately control the rate of addition as well as the reaction stoichiometry. This careful tuning of addition rate from the two feed solutions of N-(5-bromo-4-methylpyridin-2-yl)acetamide and fuming nitric (1/12 HNO_3/H_2SO_4) proved critical to achieving yields >97% and improved operator safety by eliminating the formation of harmful side products.

The Kappe group reported a similar approach to the synthesis of a key intermediate in the preparation of 1,4-benzoxazinone ABO, a motif found in herbicides (Cantillo et al. 2017). Beginning from FPAA, the group sought to form the dinitro intermediate and convert this explosive transient intermediate to the desired diamine through a tandem nitration/catalytic hydrogenation as depicted in Figure 1.7.

The researchers used a coiled reactor system to conduct the di-nitration at 1mmole/min rate and extracted the product in organic solvent using a continuous liquid-liquid extractor. The compound

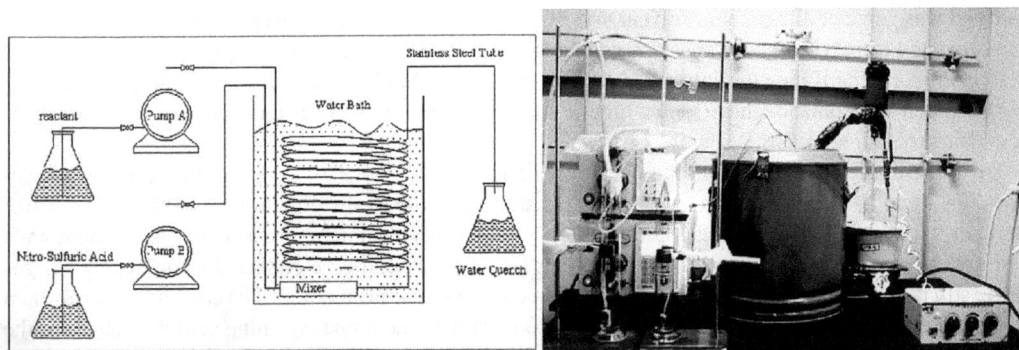

FIGURE 1.6   Depiction of nitration apparatus and image of reactor setup inside fume hood. (Reprinted with permission from Organic Process Research & Development, "High Output Continuous Nitration", Gage, J.R. et al, 2012. Copyright 2012 American Chemical Society.)

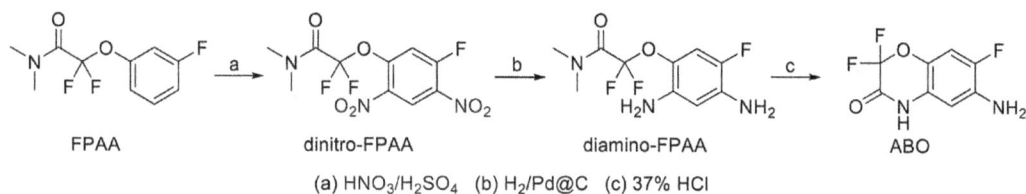

FIGURE 1.7 Synthetic sequence for the preparation of ABO Benzooxazinone from FPAA. (Reprinted with permission from Organic Process Research & Development, "Continuous Flow Synthesis of a Key 1,4-Benzooxazinone Intermediate via a Nitration/Hydrogenation/Cyclization Sequence", Cantillo, D. et al, 2017. Copyright 2017 American Chemical Society.)

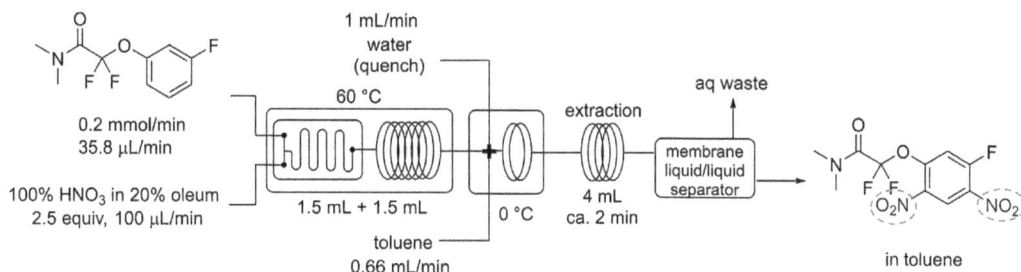

FIGURE 1.8 Continuous Flow diagram for the combined dinitration/liquid-liquid extraction via membrane separator. (Reprinted with permission from Organic Process Research & Development, "Continuous Flow Synthesis of a Key 1,4-Benzooxazinone Intermediate via a Nitration/Hydrogenation/Cyclization Sequence", Cantillo, D. et al, 2017. Copyright 2017 American Chemical Society.)

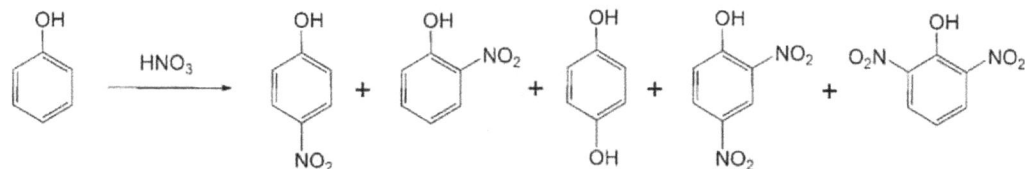

FIGURE 1.9 Nitration of phenol to afford various nitration major products and polymeric side-products. (Reprinted with permission from Angewandte Chemie – International Edition, "Controlled Autocatalytic Nitration of Phenol in a Microreactor", Laurent Ducry and Dominique M. Roberge, 2005. Copyright 2005 WILEY-VCH Verlag GmbH & Co. KGaA, Weinheim.)

was then transported to the downstream hydrogenation chamber where it was readily converted to the hydroquinone product without the need for handling or purification of the reactive nitrated intermediate (Figure 1.8).

On a laboratory scale, microfluidic reactors were used to carry out nitrations in a safe and efficient manner. Ducry and Roberge employed a glass microreactor to carry out the continuous nitration of phenol as provided in (Ducry and Roberge 2005). The reaction was further optimized under continuous flow in order to maximize the formation of the desired mono-nitration products (Figure 1.9).

1.2.4 Oxidations

Attenuating exotherms in order to avoid cryogenic conditions represents another area where continuous flow processes offer a significant advantage over batch processes (Levin 2014). Bleie et al. demonstrated a continuous flow process for the highly versatile Moffatt–Swern oxidation (MSO) reaction, a reaction typically ran at prohibitively low temperatures and that generates highly reactive trifluoroacetoxydimethylsulfonium and alkoxydimethylsulfonium salt intermediates (Bleie et al. 2015). The use of

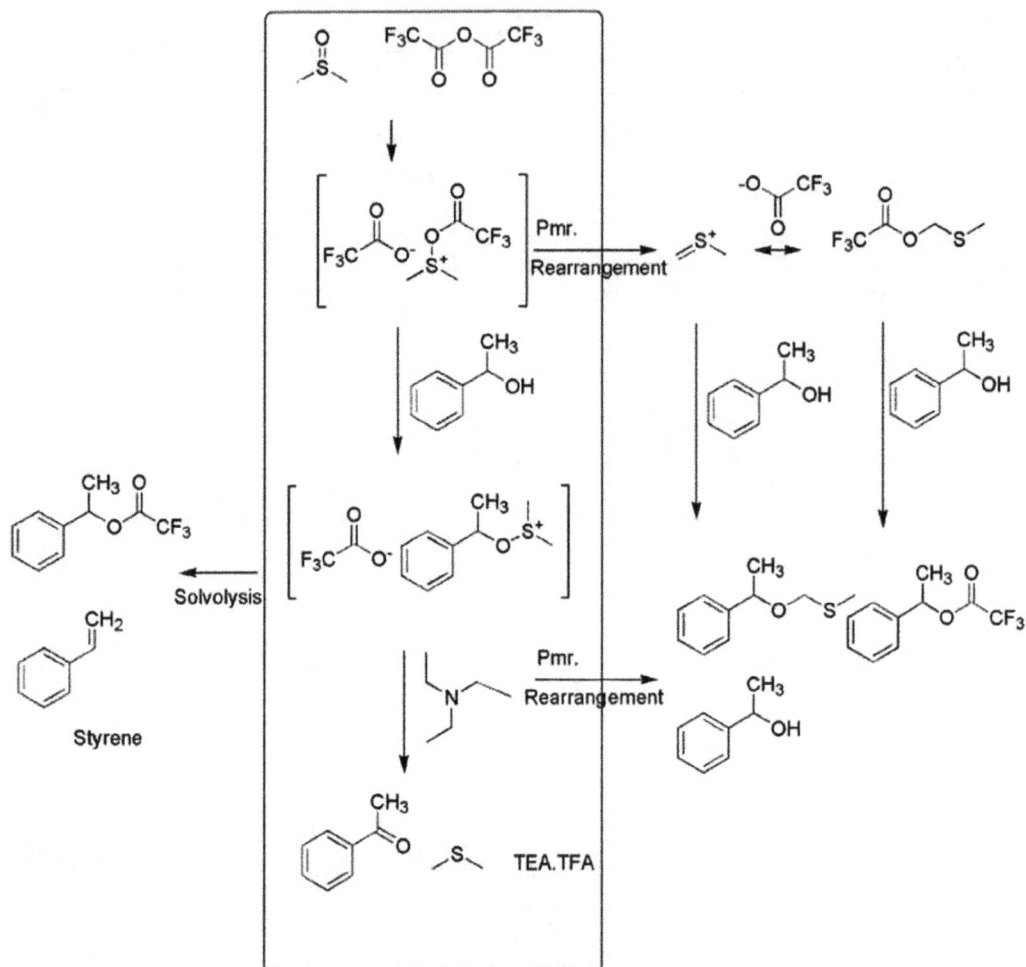

FIGURE 1.10 The desired chemical path for Swern oxidation, depicted inside the box, with chemical pathways for side-product formation depicted outside the box. (Reprinted by permission from Akadémiai Kiadó: Springer Nature, Journal of Flow Chemistry. Moffat-Swern Oxidation of Alcohols: Translating a Batch Reaction to a Continuous-Flow Reaction, Olav Bleie et al., Copyright © 2015.)

real-time monitoring techniques with Raman spectroscopy was used to validate mechanistic pathways, quantify yield in 15-second intervals in order to optimize the reaction, and provide proof of concept for the potential scalability of these reactions (Figure 1.10).

The Raman analysis of batch MSO reactions proved critical to the optimization of the flow process, as it made possible the real-time tracking of byproduct and intermediate formation under each set of conditions screened. Determining reaction rate through this method enabled the researchers to optimize existing batch procedures, such as pre-stir time and thermal control during reagent addition. Adaptation as a continuous process further improved yield due to preventing potential thermal runaway by instead forming both sulfonium salt intermediates in rapid succession. It was hypothesized based on the Raman analysis that shortening the residence time of the intermediate forming steps would allow for the higher yielding high-temperature conditions to be operated without concern of thermal runaway (Figure 1.11).

This hypothesis was tested by building two continuous flow reactors, one operating under the normal batch process order of addition and residence time, and another using the mechanistic insight gleaned from the Raman PAT to maximize conversion (Figure 1.12).

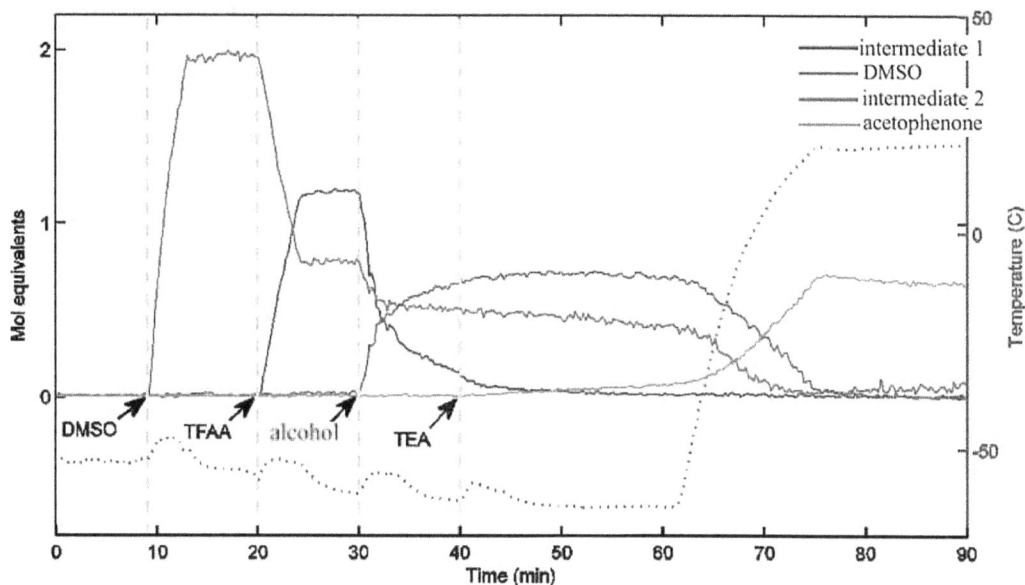

FIGURE 1.11   Raman spectroscopy tracking reaction progression over time. (Reprinted by permission from Akadémiai Kiadó: Springer Nature, Journal of Flow Chemistry. Moffat-Swern Oxidation of Alcohols: Translating a Batch Reaction to a Continuous-Flow Reaction, Olav Bleie et al., Copyright © 2015.)

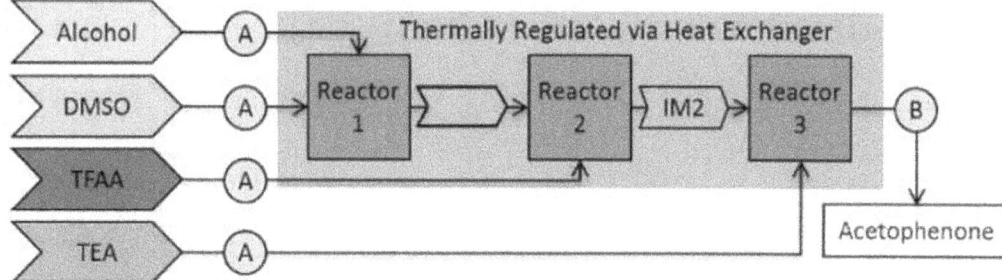

FIGURE 1.12   Depiction of 2 distinct CFR set-ups for the Moffat-Swern oxidation reaction following direct translation of batch conditions (Configuration 1) and modified conditions reflecting mechanistic insight (Configuration 2). (Reprinted by permission from Akadémiai Kiadó: Springer Nature, Journal of Flow Chemistry. Moffat-Swern Oxidation of Alcohols: Translating a Batch Reaction to a Continuous-Flow Reaction, Olav Bleie et al., Copyright © 2015.)

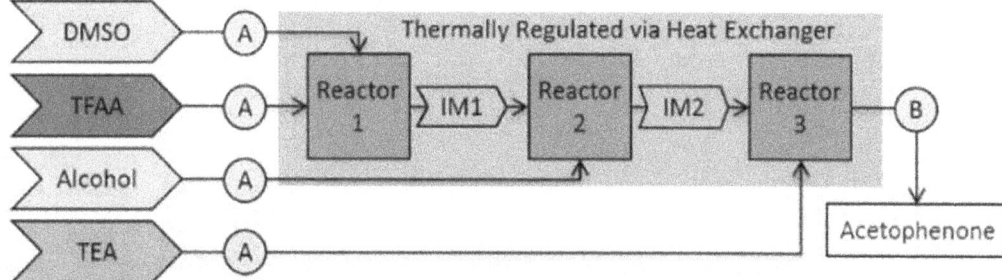

The short residence time for intermediate 1 (IM1) allows for the rapid consumption of the intermediate in the next step before it can decompose at the elevated temperature. This configuration provided similar yields to traditional SMO reactions at −20°C but continued to produce good yields of up to 79% and 67% at 0 and 20°C respectively at a fast flow rate of 10 mL/min. This model proved to be much higher yielding than traditional SMO reaction conditions and provided faster throughput as well, providing a significant leap in both safety, scalability, and production value of SMO reactions compared to batch processes.

1.2.5 Azides

The ability to produce multifunctional triazoles using "click" chemistry has highlighted the need to safely and efficiently produce and consume azides (Smith et al. 2007; Hein et al. 2008; Cintas et al. 2010; NRC 2007; Murrey et al. 2015). Ley and co-workers prepared a wide variety of triazoles continuously from substituted alkynes and azides with a copper catalyst (Smith et al. 2007). This seminal demonstration of the copper(I)-catalyzed alkyne-azide cycloaddition (CuAAC) "click" reaction utilized a modular flow reactor fitted with copper immobilized on solid Amberlyst A-21 resin and a Quadrapure TU (QP-TU) metal-scavenging resin to prevent catalyst leaching (Figure 1.13).

This reactor design was further refined by efforts from Fülöp's group using a packed bed reactor (PBR) filled with copper powder as provided in Figure 1.14 (Ötvös and Fülöp 2015).

Delville et al. reported a continuous method for the preparation of benzyl azide from benzylamine using imidazole-1-sulfonyl azide hydrochloride as a diazo transfer agent, as shown in Figure 1.15 (Delville et al. 2011). This diazotransfer unit, first reported in 2007 by Goddard-Borger and Stick, is non-explosive and able to be produced at a large scale (Goddard-borger and Stick 2007, 2011). Delville et al. used a microreactor system depicted in Figure 1.16 to effectively control the residence time and stoichiometry of the reaction, employing a zinc catalyst to achieve high conversions towards benzyl azide. This work provides an excellent example of the use of continuous platforms to rapidly carry out process optimizations using the factorial design of experiments.

In related work, Mata and co-workers demonstrated a continuous method for the synthesis of dipeptides from acyl azides (Mata et al. 2020). The acyl azides were prepared *in situ* by treatment of the corresponding hydrazide with aqueous nitrous acid followed by coupling with the desired amino acid

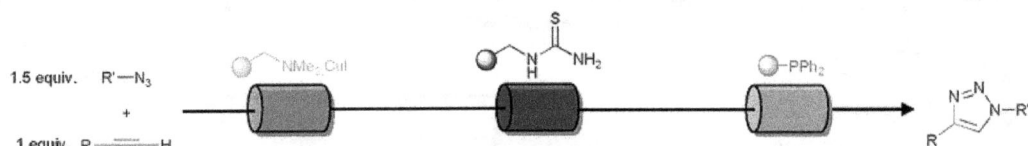

FIGURE 1.13 Diagram of continuous flow setup for safe formation of triazoles from various azides. (C.D. Smith, I.R. Baxendale, S. Lanners, J.J. Hayward, S.C. Smith and S.V. Ley, *Org. Biomol. Chem.*, 2007, **5**, 1559 DOI: 10.1039/B702995K – Reproduced by permission of The Royal Society of Chemistry.)

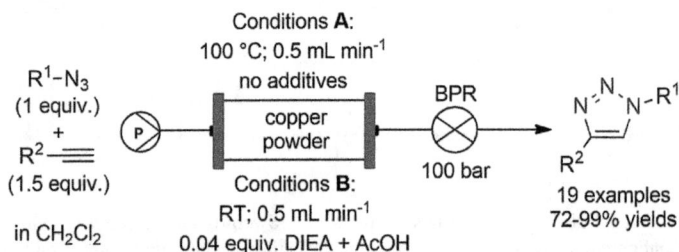

FIGURE 1.14 Continuous flow diagram of triazole synthesis with copper powder using various azide starting materials. (S.B. Ötvös and F. Fülöp, *Catal. Sci. Technol.*, 2015, **5**, 4926 DOI: 10.1039/C5CY00523J – Reproduced by permission of The Royal Society of Chemistry.)

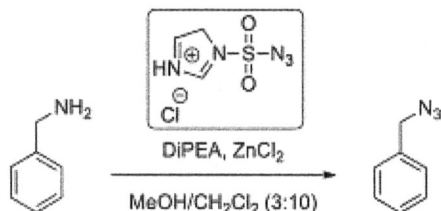

FIGURE 1.15 Diazotransfer reaction from benzylamine. (Copyright 2010 Elsevier B.V.)

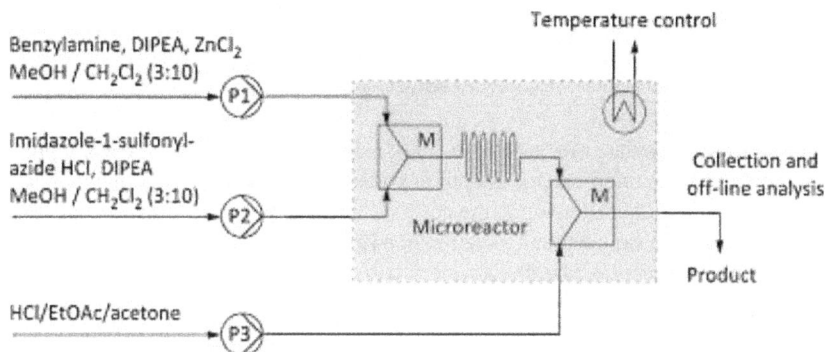

FIGURE 1.16 Continuous flow benzyl azide formation from benzylamine featuring microreactors. (Copyright 2010 Elsevier B.V.)

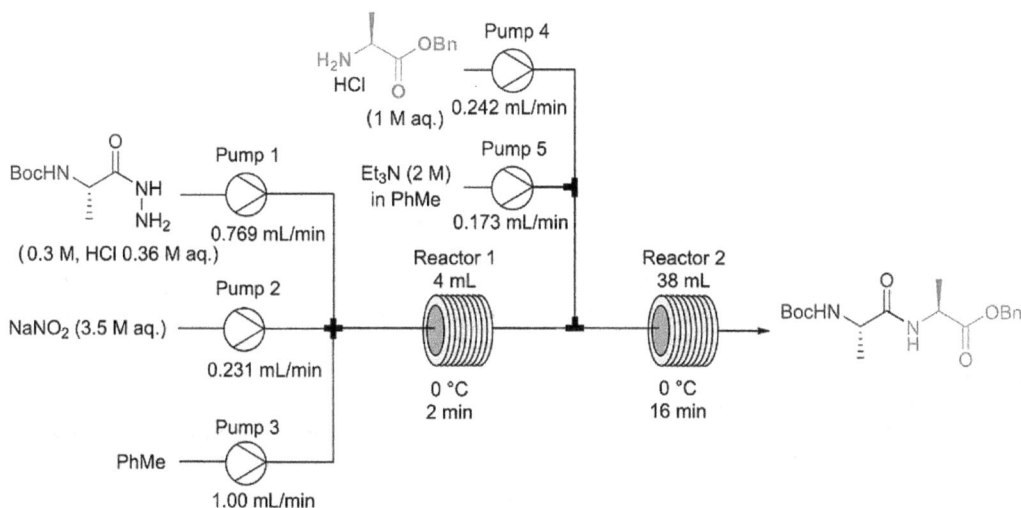

FIGURE 1.17 Diagram of the continuous flow preparation of acyl azides and subsequent amide couplings. (A. Mata, U. Weigl, O. Flögel, P. Baur, C.A. Hone and C.O. Kappe, *React. Chem. Eng.*, 2020, **5**, 645 DOI: 10.1039/D0RE00034E – Published by The Royal Society of Chemistry.)

using PEEK tubing (0.5mm id), as shown in Figure 1.17. This azide coupling proceeded with retention of configuration for chiral substrates, demonstrating an ideal platform for enantiospecific syntheses.

Sagandira and Watts also employed a continuous approach in the preparation of oseltamivir (Tamiflu), in which azide chemistry was used to prepare a key acyl azide intermediate in high yield as depicted in Figure 1.18 (Sagandira and Watts 2019). Aqueous sodium azide was used as the azide source for

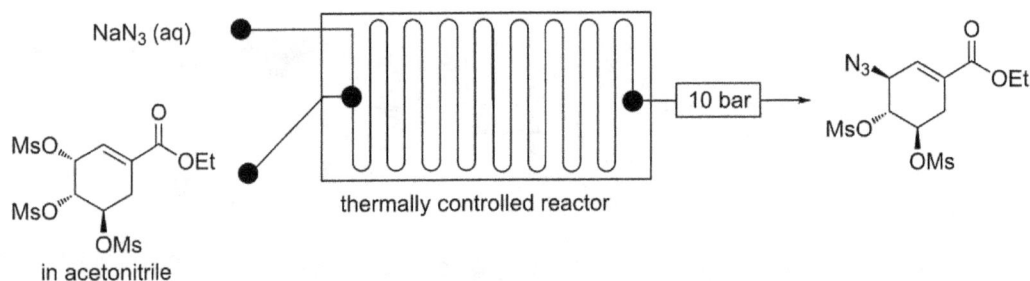

FIGURE 1.18 Continuous flow system for C-3 azidation of mesyl shikimate using aqueous sodium azide. (Sagandira, C.R.; Watts, P. *Beilstein J. Org. Chem.* 2019, *15*, 2577–2589. doi:10.3762/bjoc.15.251 – Reprinted from https://www.beilstein-journals.org/bjoc/articles/15/251. All further use and permissions should be directed to the license and the Beilstein Journal of Organic Chemistry terms and conditions: (https://www.beilstein-journals.org/bjoc). Copyright 2019.)

substitution at one of the mesylate moieties on the mesyl shikimate. The group found the precise temperature control afforded by the microreactor system provided improved selectivity and a drastic reduction in reaction time, affording full conversion to the desired C-3 azide product. The subsequent Curtius rearrangement was telescoped in flow without isolation in 84% yield.

1.2.6 Organometallic Reactions

Grignard reactions represent one of the most synthetically versatile C-C bond transformations in an organic chemist's toolbox (Peltzer et al. 2020; Kiso et al. 1973; Terao and Kambe 2008; Wang et al. 2005; Murai and Asai 2007). One of the preferred methods for preparing Grignard reagents is through halogen insertion via an atom economical and cost-effective organomagnesium reagent (Heinz et al. 2020; Hatano et al. 2005). Scaling these reactions up in traditional batch processes presents an issue as these reactions can be highly exothermic and are typically both air and moisture-sensitive. Huck et al. at Janssen developed a continuous process for the production of Grignard reagents using a packed magnesium column which tolerated a broad range of functional groups for simple on-column initiation of continuous Grignard reactions without the need for purification or handling of intermediates (Huck et al. 2017).

Magnesium particles were packed at the ideal particle size (20–230 µm) for flow systems to prevent an increase in system pressure while maintaining high available surface area for binding between the metal and halogenated compound. The Grignard was activated in a 1:1 ratio of THF and toluene and then extracted from the reaction solvent by addition of LiCl in THF solution at 50°C. Concentration of the formed organomagnesium was determined through colourimetric titration, allowing for varied concentrations of the Grignard reagent to be prepared with ease from the same protocol. Huck et al. further demonstrated that a variety of organomagnesium products could be formed at any desired concentration and telescoped to the desired reaction with an array of electrophiles as shown in Figure 1.19.

On a commercial scale, Wong and co-workers at Eli Lilly developed a process for the production of edivoxetine·HCl in which a key intermediate was prepared via Grignard reaction using a continuous stirred tank reactor (CSTR) (Kopach et al. 2015). A kinetic model was developed to optimize the mass transfer rates of a batch Grignard reaction in order to effectively scale the reaction into the CSTR (Changi and Wong 2016) (Figure 1.20).

Implementation of the CSTR in the flow system allowed for more facile mass transfer and fine control of residence time. This enabled the team to obtain kinetic data for the Grignard reaction without relying solely on mass-transfer parameterization and instead model their kinetic data plot on magnesium loading, speed of agitation, temperature, and other parameters. This translated to a highly optimized, high-yielding continuous process with a robust understanding of reaction parameters, greatly expediting scale-up of this platform (Figure 1.21).

Organozinc reagents also serve as useful building blocks in organic synthesis (Knochel and Singer 1993). However, these materials typically represent significant safety issues related to their instability (Tamura and Kodama 2014). Berton et al. developed a continuous method for the preparation of these

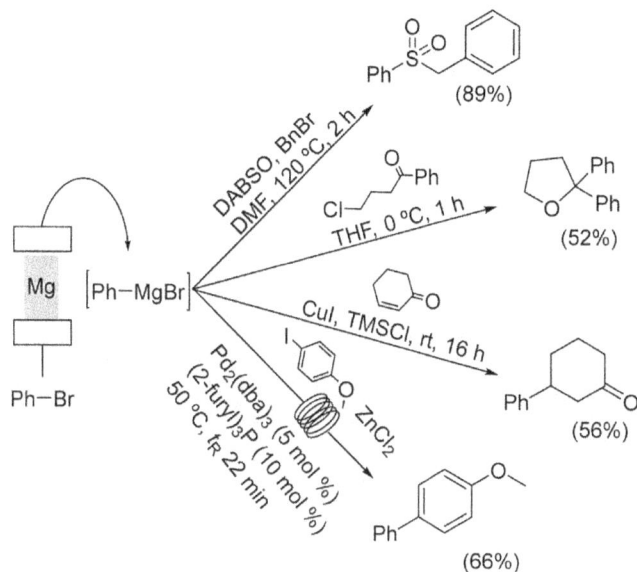

FIGURE 1.19 The synthesis of Grignard reagents for immediate use in batch and flow reactions. (Reprinted with permission from "Grignard Reagents on a Tab: Direct Magnesium Insertion under Flow Conditions", Huck, L. et al, Organic Letters 2017. Copyright 2017 American Chemical Society.)

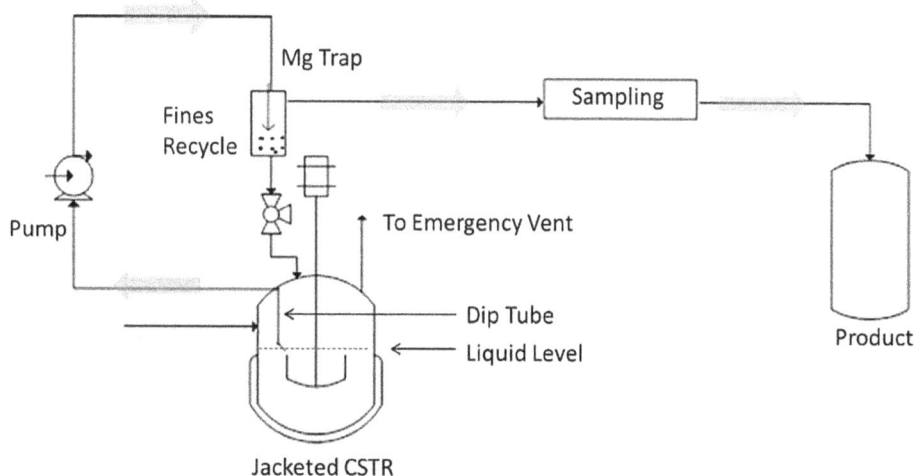

FIGURE 1.20 Depiction of continuous flow CSTR setup for continuous Grignard reaction. (Reprinted with permission from Organic Process Research & Development, "Kinetics Model for Designing Grignard Reactions in Batch or Flow Operations", Shujauddin M. Changi and Sze-Wing Wong, 2016. Copyright 2016 American Chemical Society.)

materials using zinc cartridges to prepare these materials in situ (Berton et al. 2018). This approach was used to prepare ethyl zinc bromoacetate which was then employed in a downstream tandem Reformatsky reaction and Negishi coupling, both in flow (Figure 1.22).

1.2.6.1 Fluconazole

The continuous Grignard reaction has been demonstrated en route to the preparation of Fluconazole, an API in several HIV and anti-fungal drugs, from Korwar and others at Medicines for All (Korwar et al.

operation	scale (mL)	variable change	range	goal
batch	500	temperature	0 and 30 °C	E_a dependency on T
CSTR	250	R_{ini}	12:1 and 6:1	effect of ζ and Mg loading
CSTR	250	agitation	400 and 600 rpm	confirm mass transfer free regime
batch	250	agitation	300 and 500 rpm	correlate k_{SL} to rpm

FIGURE 1.21 Experimental design for estimating model parameters for the efficiency of a continuous Grignard reaction compared to batch conditions. (Reprinted with permission from Organic Process Research & Development, "Kinetics Model for Designing Grignard Reactions in Batch or Flow Operations", Shujauddin M. Changi and Sze-Wing Wong, 2016. Copyright 2016 American Chemical Society.)

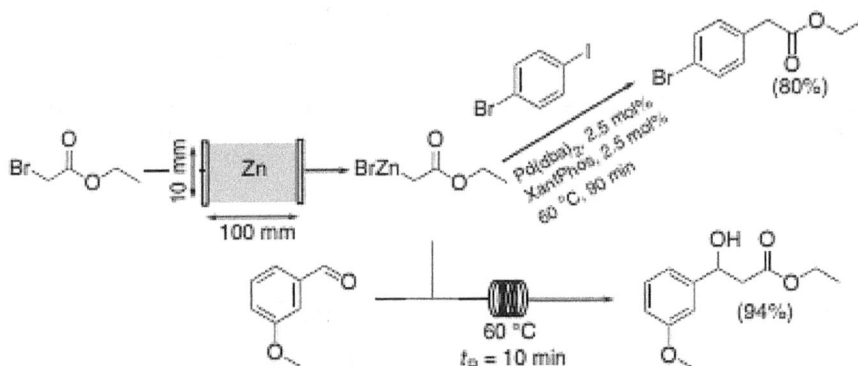

FIGURE 1.22 Continuous flow preparation of ethyl zincbromoacetate using packed zinc cartridges for subsequent Reformatsky and Negishi reactions. (Reprinted by permission from Nature Publishing Group: Macmillan Publishers Limited. Nature Protocols. On-demand synthesis of organozinc halides under continuous flow conditions, Mateo Berton et al., Copyright © 2018.)

2017). This cost-effective synthesis sought to improve upon existing processes in terms of yield, cost, and safety by replacing the expensive organolanthanoid-based reagents from the commercial process with a turbo-Grignard to install the fluorinated aromatic onto abundantly available 1,3-chloroacetone. Superior mass transfer and fine temperature control allowed for avoidance of undesired side reactions common in Grignard reactions involving 1,3-chloroacetone, allowing for a 90% yield of the alkyl alcohol product after addition of the isolated turbo-Grignard reagent. It was further found that combining the ideal flow rate established in the turbo-Grignard formation with a CSTR to maximize available volume allowed for a telescoped procedure from 2,4-difluorobromobenzene to the alkyl alcohol in 87% overall yield (Figure 1.23).

From this key intermediate, the final base-mediated amination step with 1, 2, 4-triazole was attempted, utilizing Na_2CO_3 in a 10% solution of methanol in water. This process provided Fluconazole in 74% yield for an overall yield of 64% across two semi-continuous steps. The utilization of continuous flow processes developed by Alcázar and further refined to suit the Medicines for All team's desired synthetic route helped overcome the key hurdle in cutting production costs while avoiding additional step counts or negatively impacting the yield. The turbo-Grignard formation performs with such efficiency that the overall yield improvements contributed significantly towards the cost-reduction aspects of this continuous process (Figure 1.24).

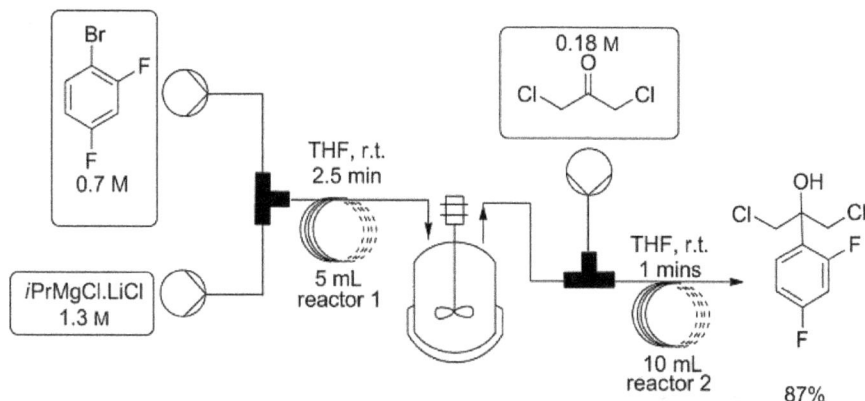

FIGURE 1.23 Flow process for turbo-Grignard reaction from 2,4-difluorobromobenzene. (Reprinted with permission from the European Journal of Organic Chemistry, "The Application of a Continuous Grignard Reaction in the Preparation of Fluconazole", Gupton, Frank B., et al, 2017.)

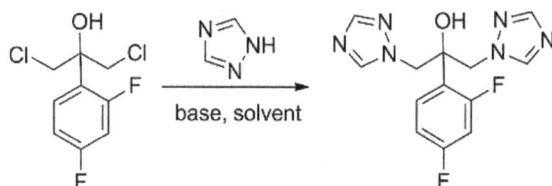

FIGURE 1.24 Base-mediated amination to form fluconazole. (Reprinted with permission from the European Journal of Organic Chemistry, "The Application of a Continuous Grignard Reaction in the Preparation of Fluconazole", Gupton, Frank B., et al. 2017.)

1.2.6.2 Goniothalamin

Another implementation of the continuous Grignard reaction can be found in the Ley group's works on a semi-continuous route towards goniothalamin, a natural product identified as a promising chemical platform for new anti-tumor drug candidates (Pastre et al. 2020). This natural product is the starting point for several studies concerning the preparation of goniothalamin drug derivatives, but there are few examples of gram-scale syntheses of the natural product itself (Pastre et al. 2020). Their effort to develop a cost-effective initial semi-continuous process hinged upon a critical *in situ* Grignard formation and reaction in a single reactor. This reaction motif was presented in routes towards both the *rac*-goniothalamin and its enantiopure variants, which are both described in the text.

The three-step process described begins from allylmagnesium chloride as the Grignard source coupled with cinnamaldehyde to form the alkyl-olefin secondary alcohol product and set up for esterification downstream. Telescoping this process required finding a solution to the eventual magnesium salt precipitation from the Grignard reaction, as an in-line aqueous purification was incompatible with both the product solubility and downstream process. Since swapping halogens did not prevent this salt precipitation from occurring, utilization of a symmetric anhydride trans-crotonic anhydride instead allowed for the magnesium byproduct to form an acetate salt that did not clump up or cause blockage. This material was gratifyingly able to be carried through the acylation step and esterification without issue (Figure 1.25).

Byproduct formation was not the only issue present, however, as the use of peristaltic pumps proved to be insufficient in the telescoped procedure. This was likely due to the presence of remaining allyl chloride starting material in the allylmagnesium chloride solution negatively impacting reactivity. An external piston pump purged with argon from an attached gas line was added as depicted in Figure 1.26 below to overcome the flow-rate issues and prevent exposure of the Grignard reagent to air, resulting in quantitative conversion towards allylmagnesium chloride.

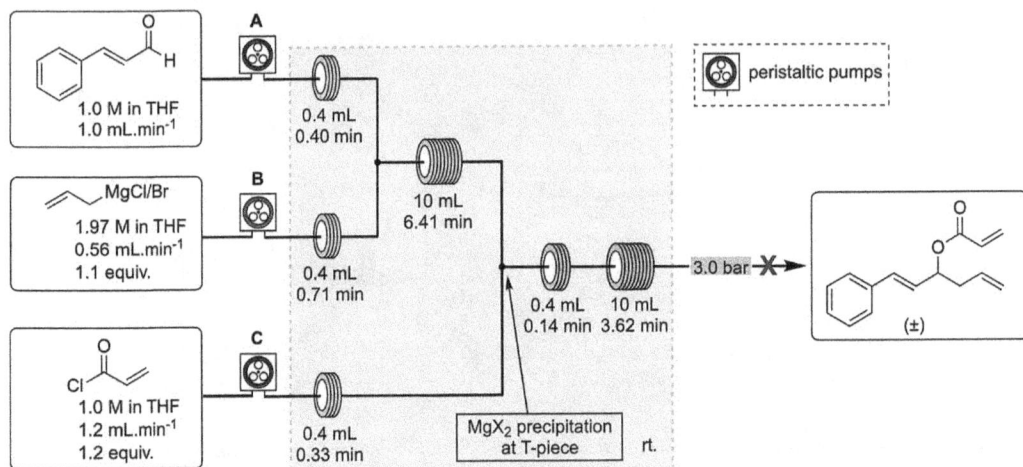

FIGURE 1.25 Scheme for the unsuccessful addition of allylmagnesium chloride/bromide to the aldehyde starting material, followed by acylation in flow en route towards goniothalamin. (Reprinted from https://pubs.acs.org/doi/10.1021/acsomega.0c02390. All further use and permissions should be directed to ACS.)

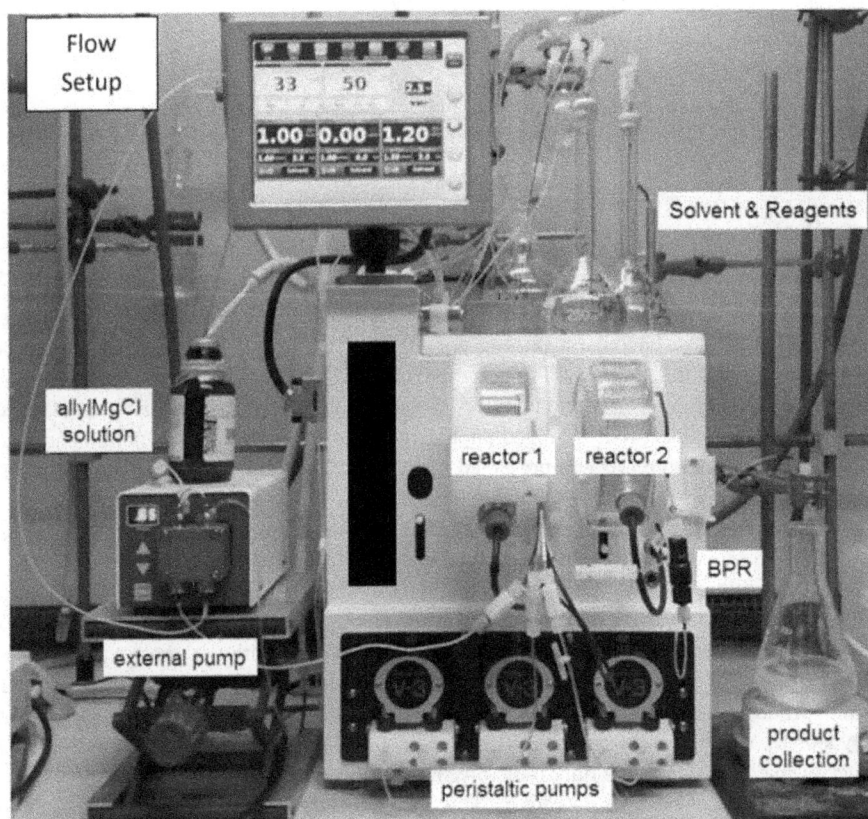

FIGURE 1.26 Vapourtek flow platform for the synthesis of goniothalamin. (Reprinted from https://pubs.acs.org/doi/10.1021/acsomega.0c02390. All further use and permissions should be directed to ACS.)

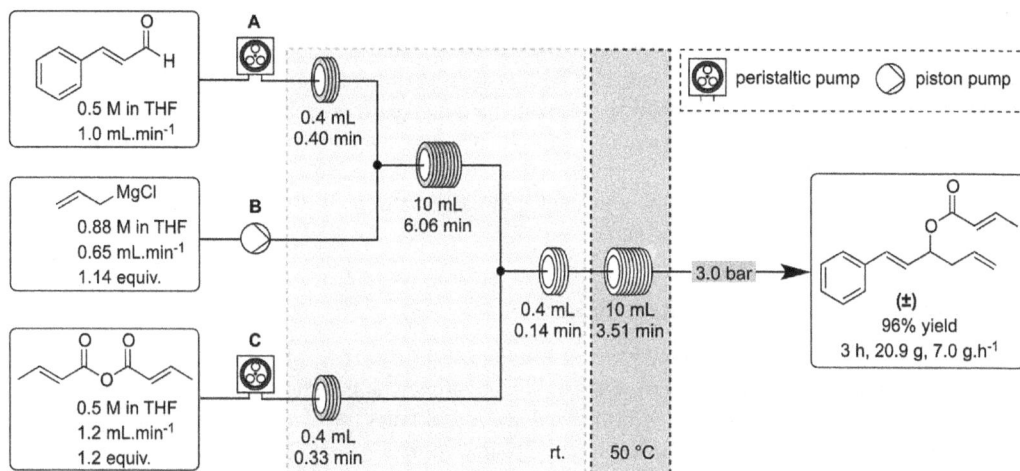

FIGURE 1.27 Scheme for the successful adaptation of a continuous Grignard reaction followed by acylation by symmetric anhydride en route towards goniothalamin. (Reprinted from https://pubs.acs.org/doi/10.1021/acsomega.0c02390. All further use and permissions should be directed to ACS.)

These reaction engineering protocols allowed for the implementation of the racemic and asymmetric protocols detailed in the corresponding Figure 1.27 to proceed quickly with 20+ grams of the pre-ring closed material produced above 90% overall yield in 3 hours. While the group was unable to translate the final Grubbs catalyst olefin metathesis reaction into a continuous process, their reported efforts may provide insight to future teams interested in adapting a similar technique.

1.3 Continuous Catalytic Reactions

The upside to performing catalyzed reactions is the added boost in kinetics (and therefore reduced reaction times), increased yields, improved selectivity, and access to previously unattainable transformations (Ishitani et al. 2020). However, applying catalyzed reactions to industrial processes comes with some inherent drawbacks. Both homogeneous and heterogeneous metal catalysts can leave behind impurities and residues. In addition, the catalysts themselves have associated costs, as the active metals are typically precious in nature such as palladium-based catalysts. These catalysts are also frequently unable to be recycled, with some notable exceptions (Molnár 2011; Zeng et al. 2011; Moore et al. 2013; Kwon et al. 2017; Afewerki et al. 2020; Fantoni et al. 2021). Therefore, it is of great importance to perform catalyzed reactions while minimizing catalyst loading in order to significantly reduce the catalyst costs and removal efforts. Additionally, there are also policies and regulation to consider that affect the tolerable limits for impurities of specific drug targets as dictated by both the ICH and FDA (Dicks and Hent 2015; Dach et al. 2012; ICH Consensus 2021). Final targets should be synthesized with no metal impurities present from catalysts used.

If catalyst recovery or separation is desirable; distillation, adsorption, extraction, or crystallization can be attempted to separate the catalytic residues from the target compounds (Garrett and Prasad 2004). Unfortunately, these additional unit operations serve to further reduce the value gained by implementing metal-catalyzed reactions. A catalyzed process can instead be modified to reduce metal impurities by selecting a specific order for unit operations to be performed. For example, running catalytic reactions early on can lower the probability that metal residues are carried all the way through the process. Developing a method to effectively recycle the catalyst material is another effective method (Molnár 2011). Often catalyst recyclability, like solvent recyclability, is underutilized in industrial processes due to issues of reproducibility and the increased likelihood of introducing impurities into the APIs.

To this end, continuous flow methodologies have adapted catalyzed reaction motifs with reduced catalyst loading, improved regeneration/recyclability of the metal catalyst, improved tolerance and longevity of the catalyst, and reduced catalyst leaching (Teoh et al. 2017; Mandoli 2019). Flow provides a unique advantage in that numerous reactor platforms provide increased surface area interactions, a key aspect of mass transfer that facilitates catalytic reaction's rate of reaction and conversion. Implementation of flow reactor motifs such as PBRs filled with immobilized catalysts provides an excellent platform for reducing catalyst leaching as well. Several notable examples of catalytic transformations in continuous flow are discussed herein.

1.3.1 Catalytic Hydrogenation Reactions

Hydrogenation reactions are extremely prominent in industrial syntheses of API, representing over 13% of all reaction motifs (Carey et al. 2006). Gas phase H_2 hydrogenation methodology is an ideal candidate for implementation in a PBR due to the enhanced gas-liquid mass transfer. Selective hydrogenation of alkynes, alkenes, and heteroatoms such as nitro groups, nitriles, esters, aldehydes, and ketones have been demonstrated under continuous flow (Yu et al. 2020). Herein we will highlight traditional catalytic hydrogenation and transfer hydrogenation reaction motifs that have been successfully implemented in the continuous preparations of APIs. Key aspects of this innovation are the efficient use of homogenous and heterogeneous catalysts, improved biphasic mixing in flow reactors, and increased scalability.

1.3.1.1 Thebaine (Hydrocodone)

Many APIs have been natural product derivatives or feature a common skeletal element found in a natural product. As many natural products feature numerous isomers and derivatives of their own, there are often numerous potential synthetic strategies in the preparation of APIs that have come from natural products. Hydrocodone is one such example, a common narcotic drug that can be prepared from a variety of synthetic pathways starting from poppy plant (*Papaver somniferum*) alkaloids morphine, codeine, or thebaine (Pieber et al. 2016). Pieber et al. demonstrated that a continuous flow preparation of hydrocodone from abundant thebaine starting material could be achieved under atom economic conditions through effective implementation of catalytic transfer hydrogenation in a two-step selective olefin reduction – hydrolysis strategy (Figure 1.28).

The key transformation involved formation of an *in situ* diimide through oxidation of hydrazine hydrate, a highly explosive reaction made safe and scalable through a high-temperature/high-pressure continuous flow reactor (Figure 1.29).

The synthetic strategy envisaged in this process replaces the current state of the art where *p*-toluenesulfonyl hydrazide is used with weak base to generate the transfer hydrogenation material. Oxidation of hydrazine with O_2 gas to form a diimide transfer hydrogenation agent had been previously reported, and while this reaction design drastically cuts down on waste generation and cost, the potential explosive nature of this gaseous mixture and the need for stoichiometric amounts of toxic hydrazine preclude

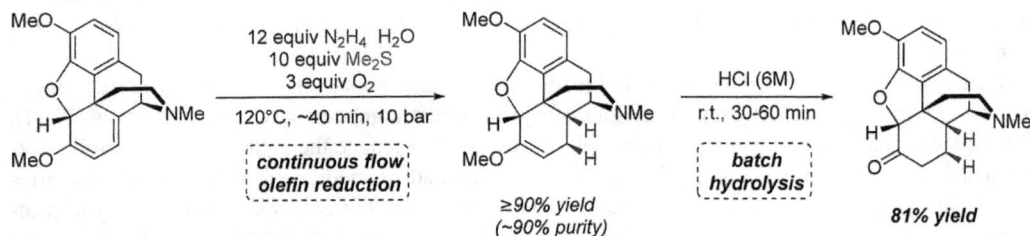

FIGURE 1.28   A synthesis scheme utilizing transfer hydrogenation in continuous flow and batch hydrolysis for the preparation of hydrocodone from thebaine. (Reprinted with permission from Organic Process Research & Development, "Selective Olefin Reduction in Thebaine Using Hydrazine Hydrate and O_2 under Intensified Continuous Flow Conditions", Pieber, B. et al, 2015. Copyright 2016 American Chemical Society.)

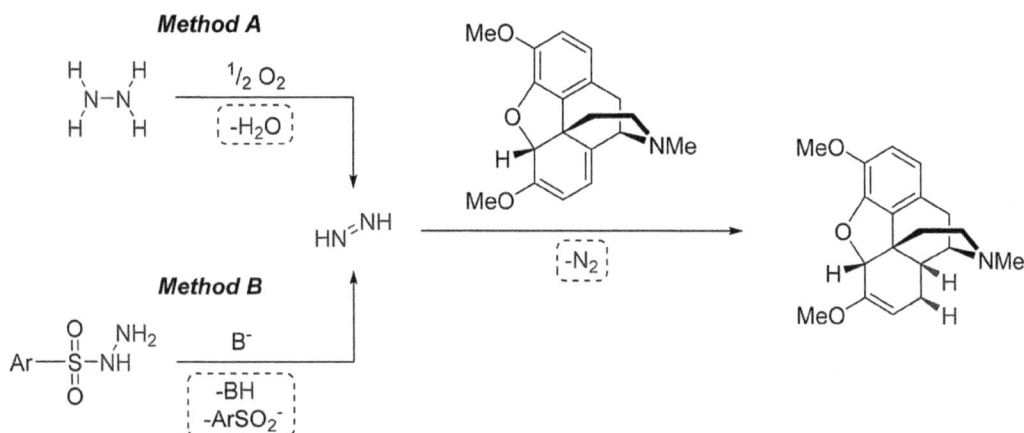

FIGURE 1.29 Scheme depicting two methods to generate the chiral diimide in situ towards the synthesis of thebaine. (Reprinted with permission from Organic Process Research & Development, "Selective Olefin Reduction in Thebaine Using Hydrazine Hydrate and O_2 under Intensified Continuous Flow Conditions", Pieber, B. et al, 2015. Copyright 2016 American Chemical Society.)

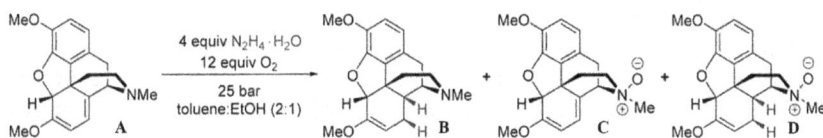

entry	T (°C)	coil^b (mL)	t_{res} (min)	A (%)	B (%)	C (%)	D (%)
1	50	PFA (13)	10	81	9	<1	<1
2	100	PFA (13)	12	18	26	32	26
3	120	PFA (13)	14	<1	2	38	58
4	140	PFA (13)	16	<1	<1	23	73
5	120	SS (20)	10	44	49	<1	<1
6	140	SS (20)	10	40	54	<1	<1

^{a}Reactions were carried out using 0.5 mmol of **A** and 2 mmol of $N_2H_4 \cdot H_2O$ in 1.5 mL of toluene:EtOH (2:1) at a liquid flow rate of 0.4 mL min^{-1} and an O_2 flow rate of 40 mL$_N$ min^{-1}. ^{b}PFA = perfluoroakoxy, SS = stainless steel. ^{c}Determined as HPLC peak area percent at 215 nm.

FIGURE 1.30 Flow reactor conditions for the selective reduction of thebaine. (Reprinted with permission from Organic Process Research & Development, "Selective Olefin Reduction in Thebaine Using Hydrazine Hydrate and O_2 under Intensified Continuous Flow Conditions", Pieber, B. et al, 2015. Copyright 2016 American Chemical Society.)

commercial adoption of the process (Grew and Roberston 1974). Pieber et al. sought to translate this reaction design to a continuous flow methodology by developing suitable segmented flow of the biphasic mixture without exposing excess hydrazine hydrate to the oxygen gas feed line. It was found that pre-heating the sample loop of hydrazine hydrate in a 2:1 toluene/ethanol mixture allowed for introduction of the material to the reactor coil as a homogenous solution, increasing the likelihood of developing ideal segmented flow conditions between a purely liquid-gas phase chemical feedstock. The use of stainless-steel coils for the reactor made high-temperature/high-pressure conditions tenable but unfortunately corrosion of the coil surface led to reduced yields that would presumably hamper scalability and throughput (Figure 1.30).

Therefore, a multi-injection strategy combined with addition of an excess antioxidant (Me_2S) to trap the formed hydrogen peroxide was attempted and found to provide 5 in >90% yield and purity. Subsequent acid-promoted hydrolysis afforded hydrocodone in 81% yield in a two-step telescoped continuous process. Use of the multi-injection strategy allowed for greater conversion of starting material while avoiding potential thermal decomposition, and control of the flow rate and pressure build-up in the flow reactor prevented excess hydrazine exposure to molecular oxygen. In this way, the risk of explosive side reactions was eliminated and the atom-economic key reaction step was successfully implemented to provide an

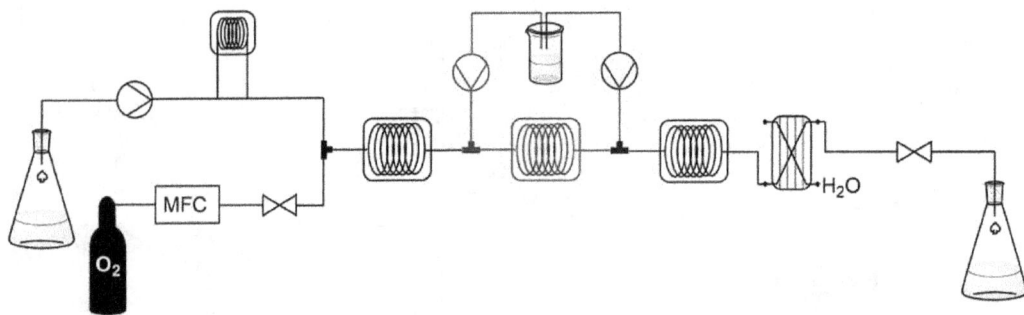

FIGURE 1.31 Scheme for the expansion of a multi-injection continuous flow process by the additional feeds (second and third loops). (Reprinted with permission from Organic Process Research & Development, "Selective Olefin Reduction in Thebaine Using Hydrazine Hydrate and O_2 under Intensified Continuous Flow Conditions", Pieber, B. et al, 2015. Copyright 2016 American Chemical Society.)

alternative, safe, and scalable cost-effective synthesis of hydrocodone from an abundant natural product starting material (Figure 1.31).

1.3.1.2 Mepivacaine

Kappe's group demonstrated the preparation of mepivacaine and other amino amide-based local anaesthetics through catalytic reductive amination in flow, improving the yield, processing time, and material goods cost without compromising scalability (Suveges et al. 2017). The key transformations in this route involve the hydrogenation of the α-picolinic acid and amidation of the resultant terminal carboxylic acid, with the order of these steps being inconsequential as both motifs have been reported in similar yields (Sandberg 1989; Tullar and Bolen 1969) (Figure 1.32).

However, a commonality in previously reported syntheses was that N-alkylation to produce the desired anaesthetic drug molecule always occurred separately from the two preceding steps. This transformation additionally faces issues of amine-selectivity and poor PMI, as most approaches rely on stoichiometric amount of bulky reducing agents such as $NaBH_3CN$ or $NaBH(OAc)_3$, in addition to lengthy workup protocols (Shankaraiah et al. 2008). By utilizing high-pressure continuous flow technology in an H-Cube Pro, Suveges et al. developed a tandem ring-hydrogenation/reductive amination reaction that cut down on step count and improved atom-economy while eliminating the need for a lengthy workup procedure.

1.3.1.3 API 1 (JAK2 Kinase Inhibitor by AstraZeneca) – Augustine Method

As many APIs feature optically active moieties, there is a significant need for an industrially relevant asymmetric hydrogenation protocol. Augustine et al. developed a method referred to as the "Augustine method" where a commercially available chiral catalyst (Rh/ (S,S)-EthylDuphos) immobilized on a solid support was used for a single-pass asymmetric hydrogenation with high enantioselectivity (Augustine et al. 1999). Key features of this method include the use of non-covalent immobilization of the catalyst

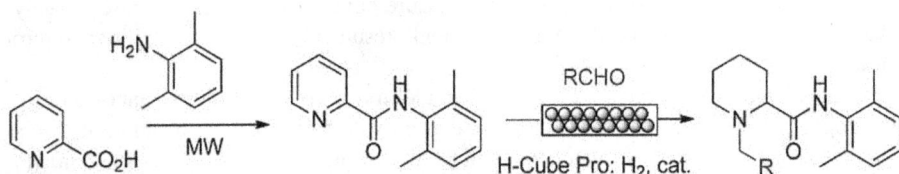

FIGURE 1.32 Synthetic scheme for continuous hydrogenation/reductive amination preparation of mepivacaine. (Reprinted with permission from the European Journal of Organic Chemistry, "Synthesis of Mepivacaine and its Analogues by a Continuous Flow Tandem Hydrogenation-Reductive Amination Strategy", Suveges, N.S. et al, 2017.)

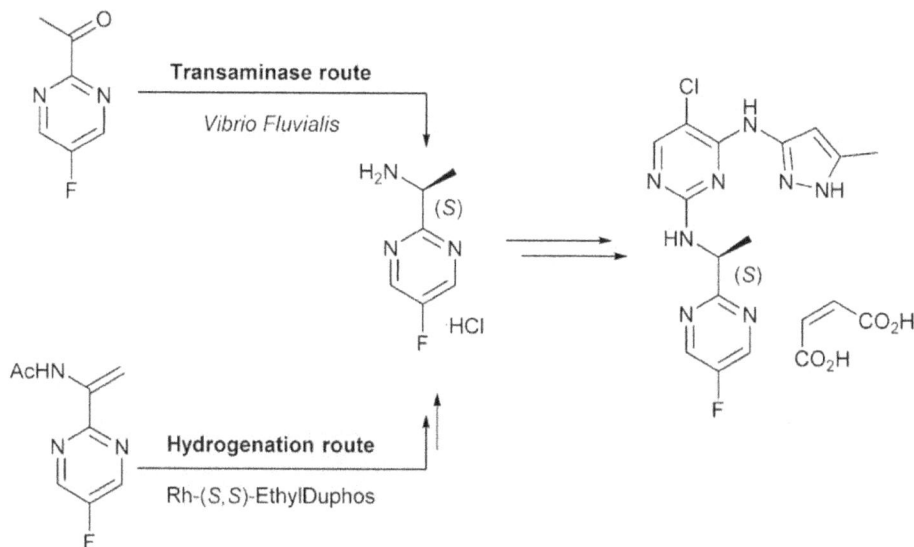

FIGURE 1.33 Scheme depicting two synthetic routes for an API from Astraeneca. (Reprinted from https://pubs.acs.org/doi/10.1021/acs.oprd.6b00143. All further use and permissions should be directed to ACS.)

on a heteropolyacid anchor dispersed on a metal oxide surface. The strong interactions between the catalyst center and the pi-electrons of the oxygen atoms in the heteropolyacid result in strong affinity of the catalyst to the support and prevents catalyst leaching. This Augustine method was then used to prepare the chiral enamide API 1 on the kilogram scale in collaboration with AstraZeneca (Amara et al. 2016; Ioannidis et al. 2011) (Figure 1.33).

AstraZeneca had reported two routes towards API 1: a transamination reaction from the ketone starting material and an asymmetric hydrogenation from the enamide. As the transamination route required a protecting group strategy to isolate the amine salt product, a cost-effective method for the asymmetric hydrogenation with increased conversion to avoid the protecting group strategy was needed. Due to their prior success with the Augustine method, Amara et al. developed a catalyst support consisting of phosphotungstic acid and aluminum oxide (PTA/Alox) to trap their chiral catalyst through induced required electroneutrality. Attenuation of the moisture sensitivity of the system was accomplished by incorporating a high-vacuum pump with in-line argon purge (Figure 1.34).

Catalyst activity with a turnover number (TON) of 935 was achieved using this setup, enabling selective asymmetric hydrogenation of the enamide to give the chiral amine product an average yield of 98% with 99% ee. Throughput of up to 400 grams/liter per hour was achieved where the catalyst did not lose its initial activity over an 18-hour period, with less than 1 ppm Rh present in the isolated product. This demonstration provides significant implications of the utility the Augustine method holds in realizing sustainable, efficient, and scalable catalytic asymmetric hydrogenations of APIs that meet strict product specification limits.

1.3.1.4 N-4-Nitrophenyl Nicotinamide

Due to the relative ease less reactive species such as nitriles or nitro groups can be carried through downstream applications, late-stage reductive formation of amines is an appealing synthetic strategy for API production (Afanasyev et al. 2019; Moir et al. 2019). Catalytic hydrogenation is an ideal reaction platform for the formation of amines from nitro starting materials as it offers atom economy from an abundant cost-effective source. The use of a continuous flow strategy to further reduce required catalyst loading and improve conversion and selectivity for the catalytic hydrogenation of N-4-nitrophenyl nicotinamide to the primary amine product was demonstrated by Yang et al. in collaboration with Novartis (Yang et al. 2018) (Figure 1.35).

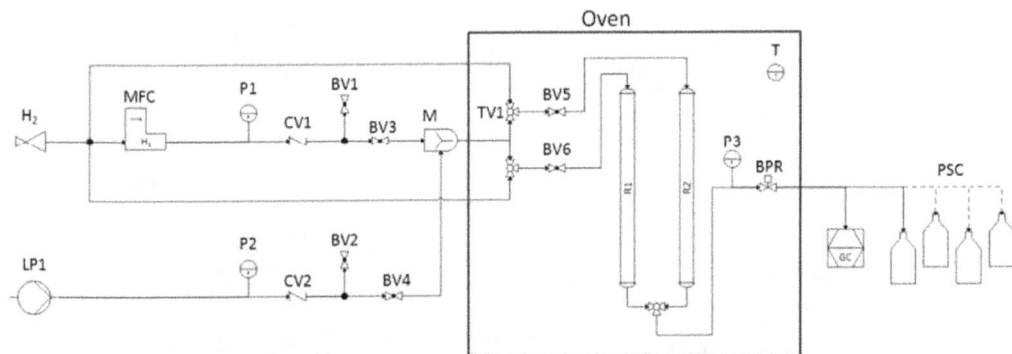

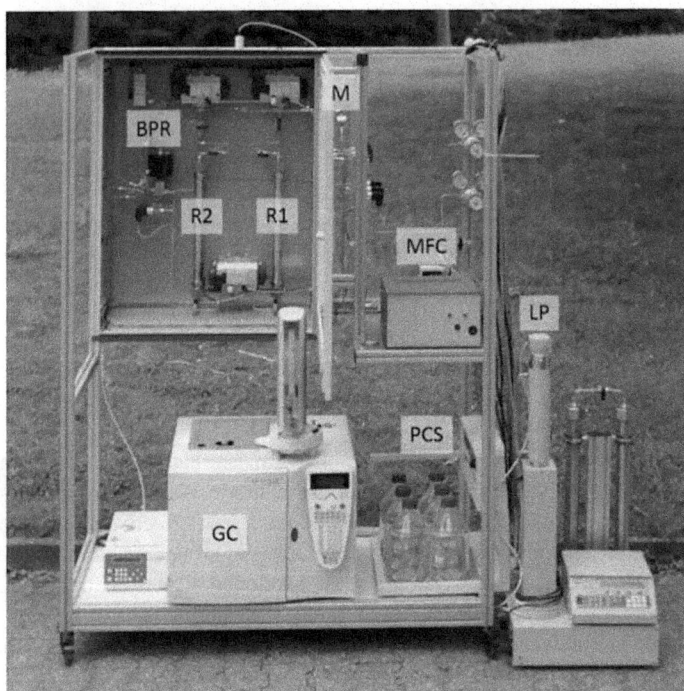

FIGURE 1.34 Scheme of the continuous flow process with visual representation of the reactor set-up. (Reprinted from https://pubs.acs.org/doi/10.1021/acs.oprd.6b00143. All further use and permissions should be directed to ACS.)

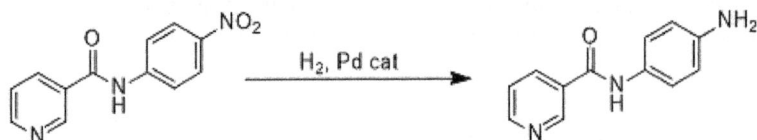

FIGURE 1.35   Jensen N-4-nitrophenyl nicotinamide continuous hydrogenation.

A packed bed design fitted with a hydrogen-specific thermal mass flow controller (MFC) and fitted with check valves to attenuate backflow was utilized for the reaction. N-4-nitrophenyl nicotinamide was prepared as a molar stock solution in dimethyl acetamide (DMAc). DMAc flowed through the PBR filled with Pd on silica (Silicycle) with H_2 gas entering after solvent to prevent channeling and ensure ideal diffusion on the wet catalyst surface. The reaction was able to reach steady state and the Pd catalyst was able to be regenerated *in situ* after each run through simple adjustment of H_2/ambient air flow rate to control

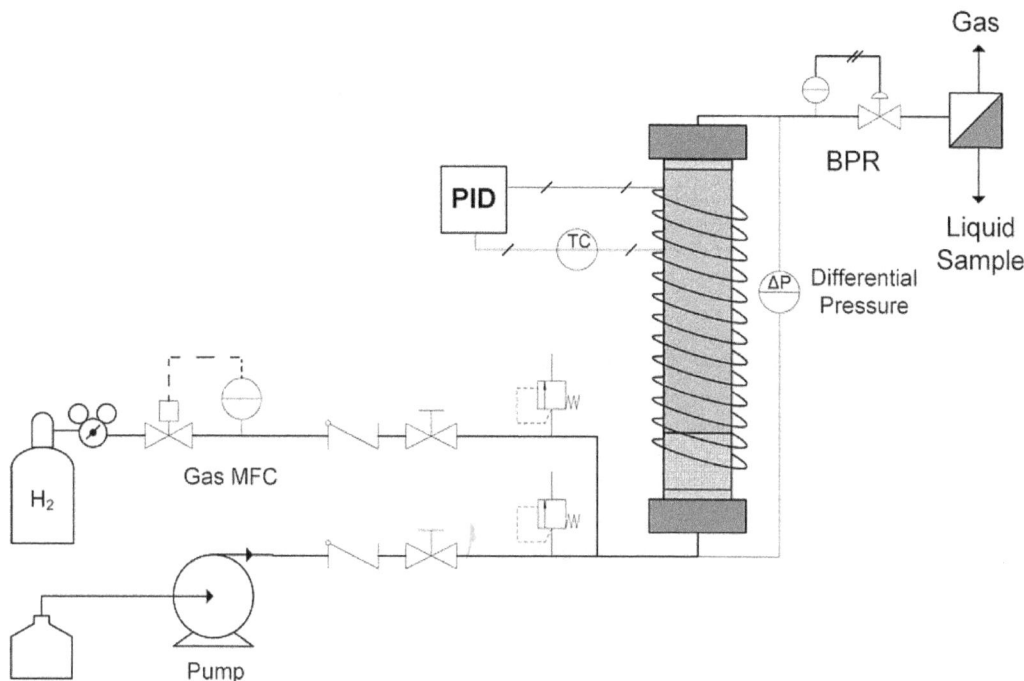

FIGURE 1.36 Continuous biphasic flow reactor for a gas and liquid fed micro-packed bed reactor followed by an effluent fractionation isolation. ("Catalytic Hydrogenation of N-4-nitrophenyl Nicotinamide in a Micro-Packed Bed Reactor", Yang, C. et al, Green Chemistry, 2018. Published by The Royal Society of Chemistry.)

for screening ideal operating parameters. It was found that the reaction was largely pressure and flow rate dependent. Increasing the gas-to-liquid flow rate ratio to 4:1 enabled high conversion and selectivity at an elevated pressure of 75 psi. Ultimately this design enabled quantitative yield of the desired primary amine under continuous flow conditions, where 24-hour operation with operator-induced catalyst regeneration enabled throughput in excess of 1 kg per day. This catalytic hydrogenation notably proceeds with excellent PMI as no excess reducing agents or homogenous catalysts were required (Figure 1.36).

1.3.1.5 Linezolid (Zyvox)

Another example of the continuous catalytic hydrogenation of a nitro group to the corresponding primary amine was developed by a team of researchers at CSIRO Manufacturing in Australia (Gardiner et al. 2018). They demonstrated nitro-chemoselectivity for the hydrogenation of a nitrobenzene used in the preparation of the oxazolidinone Linezolid (Zyvox), an FDA-approved pneumonia and MRSA treatment drug. Gardiner et al. demonstrated a key innovation in the implementation of heterogeneous catalysts in flow by using catalytic static mixers (CSM) designed to cut down on retention time and boost flow rate. This novel reactor design cuts costs and was able to provide a highly pure product without any catalyst leaching, boosting PMI by eliminating the need for purification.

The CSM was designed so that the immobilized solid catalyst used would act as both flow guide and mixer inside a series of tubes within the reactor. The CSM was 3D printed in house with the immobilizing charcoal and then had Pd adhered to the surface using electroplating. As the design was made in house as well, channel distribution, size, and designed irregularities intended to increase exposed surface area were easily implemented (Figure 1.37).

Each CSM was prepared so that roughly 200 mg Pd(0) was adhered onto each mixer, with a set of 12 total mixers distributed evenly throughout the stainless-steel reactor shell. In contrast to PBR designs, the CSM reactor allows for a simple homogenous solvent stream with little to no attenuation of pressure or

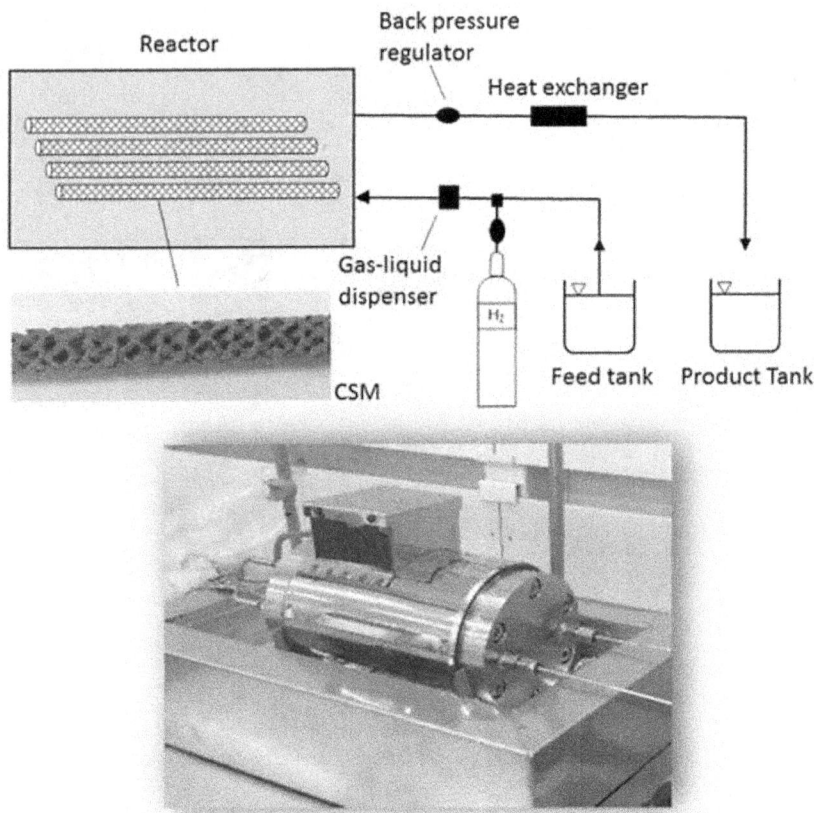

FIGURE 1.37 Catalytic static mixer reactor scheme and reactor. (Reprinted with permission from Organic Process Research & Development, "Catalytic Static Mixers for the continuous Flow Hydrogenation of a Key Intermediate of Linezolid (Zyvox)", Gardiner, J. et al, 2018. Copyright 2018 American Chemical Society.)

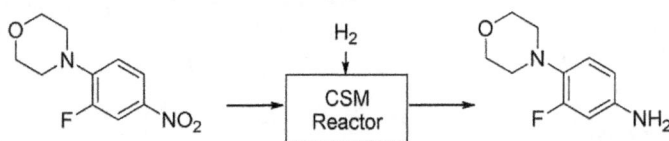

FIGURE 1.38 Implementation of a CSM for the continuous hydrogenation of the nitro-functional group en route towards Linezolid. (Reprinted with permission from Organic Process Research & Development, "Catalytic Static Mixers for the continuous Flow Hydrogenation of a Key Intermediate of Linezolid (Zyvox)", Gardiner, J. et al, 2018. Copyright 2018 American Chemical Society.)

phase diffusion effects on reactivity. Additionally, the electroplating deposition of the catalyst onto the 3D printed CSM surface is so robust that catalyst leaching is not observed at all, removing the need for any post-process workup or purification. Thus, near quantitative yield (>99%) was achieved for the hydrogenation of the nitrobenzene starting material to the desired aniline with the use of simple pumps, cheaply prepared and easily replaced CSM that served the dual role of catalyst and mixer, and cut in relative PMI through elimination of purification solvent (Figure 1.38).

1.3.2 Cross-Coupling Reactions

Catalyzed cross-coupling reactions for C-C, C-H, C-N, and C-O coupling reactions are routinely employed to synthesize pharmaceutical intermediates and APIs (King and Yasuda 2004; Beller and

Noe 2011; Colacot, and Johnson Matthey, and Chiral Technologies 2016; Ruiz-castillo and Buchwald 2016). Cross-coupling reactions are useful to synthesize many biaryl, heteroatom, and heterobiaryl compounds found in APIs. Like the organometallic reactions described in the previous section, cross-coupling reactions require a transmetallation step within the reaction scheme. There are also a wide variety of cross-coupling reactions defined by the reactants mediating the reaction, that is, boronic acid-mediated (Suzuki-Miyaura), organozinc-mediated (Negishi), olefin-mediated (Heck), and magnesium-mediated cross-coupling reactions (Kumada) (Miyaura et al. 1979; Negishi et al. 2005; Heck 1982; Kiso et al. 1973). Many cross-couplings like these offer access to a wide array of complex building blocks in a single-step transformation from a library of functionalized organohalides and other substrates. Given the robust nature of these reactions, there is significant interest in developing strategies for implementing cross-couplings in continuous flow.

1.3.2.1 Suzuki-Miyaura Cross-Coupling

The Suzuki-Miyaura reaction represents a powerful tool within organic synthesis and is one of the most popular cross-coupling reactions owing to practical applications within the fine chemical and pharmaceutical industries (Beller and Noe 2011). The typical Suzuki-Miyaura reaction is a palladium-catalyzed cross-coupling between an organoboronic acid and an aryl halide, though the scope has been expanded to include alkyl, alkenyl, and alkynyl halides as well. This reaction has been implemented at the multikilogram scale numerous times. For example, Jacks et al. utilized a Suzuki-Miyaura reaction between boronic acid and an aromatic sulfonate ester at an 80-kilogram scale in route towards the synthesis of CI-1034, a potent endothelin receptor antagonist (Jacks et al. 2004).

Noel and Musacchio developed a continuous flow protocol for the Suzuki-Miyaura cross-coupling of heteroaryl halides and (hetero)arylboronic acids featuring reduced catalyst loading (Noël and Musacchio 2011). Like other processes reported within this chapter, the Suzuki-Miyaura cross-coupling reactions reported by Noel and Musacchio were conducted in batches prior to adaptation as a continuous process. The reaction conditions were studied in batch to optimize PMI and ideal reaction temperature. It should be noted that for this reaction, higher temperatures (90°C) lead to lower conversion due to the instability of the reagents during the cross-coupling reaction. Therefore, a temperature of 60°C was determined to perform the experiments moving forward. The batch reactions were able to determine an optimal ratio of solvents (NMP: Toluene: H_2O, 4:1:5) so that all of the reagents and products remained soluble within a biphasic system. This prevented clogging issues in the reactor tubing for the continuous process. Addition of tetrabutylammonium bromide (TBAB) as phase transfer catalyst allowed for this multisolvent solution to be employed without impacting reactivity (Figure 1.39).

Pd-catalyzed Suzuki-Miyaura cross-coupling reactions were reported in flow with low catalyst loadings (0.05–1.5 mol% Pd) and short residence times (< 5 min) to produce a wide range of heterobiaryl components in high yields (87–99%) Solutions of various heteroaryl halides, (hetero)arylboronic acids, and a formed XPhos second-generation palladium catalyst were combined with aqueous streams of TBAB and K_3PO_4. The microfluidic system was also able to successfully couple unstable five-membered 2-heteroarylboronic acid reactants, which are known to have issues with protodeboronation at elevated temperatures in aqueous bases (Kinzel et al. 2010). At the time of publication, this work reported the lowest known palladium loading for the Suzuki-Miyaura reaction in flow.

For this study, the flow process initially had an issue of blockage due to precipitation from the reactant stream. This was overcome by changing the solvent system to create two distinct phases. For a biphasic system in batch, the efficiency of the batch reactor is limited by the mixing capabilities of the system. To scale up such a system would require a specialized reactor design to increase mixing by the incorporation of baffles and agitator blades within the batch reactor. A continuous microfluidic system was implemented to increase the mixing efficiency of the system by utilizing a packed-bed reactor loaded with stainless steel spheres. Such a system improves the interfacial contact of the immiscible phases while providing uniform heating. In addition, the microfluidic system was able to be run continuously to increase the reaction scale by extending the operating time of the reactor (5 h) to obtain heterobiaryl products in excellent yields (2.77 grams, 97% isolated yield) with low catalyst loadings (0.5 mol%).

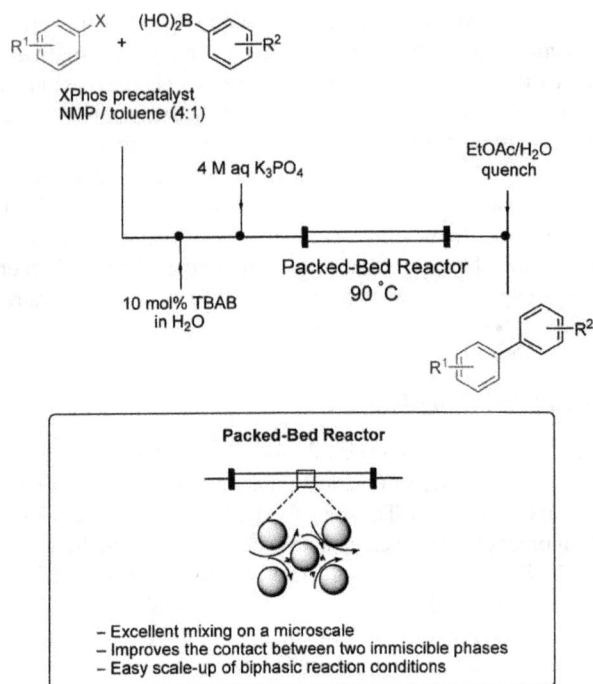

FIGURE 1.39 Continuous flow diagram of the microreactor setup for continuous flow Suzuki-Miyaura cross-coupling reactions. (Reprinted with permission from Organic Letters, "Suzuki-Miyaura Cross-Coupling of Heteroaryl Halides and Arylboronic Acids in Continuous Flow", Timothy Noël and Andrew J. Musacchio, 2011. Copyright 2011 American Chemical Society.)

Continuous processes represent an appealing platform not only for cross-coupling reactions but also for the preparation of catalysts. This is due to the inherent increased catalyst throughput and more consistent reaction parameters which results in more consistent yields and catalyst quality (Plutschack et al. 2017). A continuous process for the preparation and immediate utilization of such a catalyst came from Brinkley et al. when they demonstrated a method for the continuous synthesis of palladium on graphene nanoparticles that was then immediately used for Suzuki-Miyaura cross-couplings in a packed bed flow reactor (Brinkley et al. 2015). This reproducible and scalable synthesis represents the first example of a continuous preparation of a solid-supported palladium catalyst.

The metal nanoparticle catalyst was prepared by reductive deposition of Pd(II) nitrate onto graphene oxide using an ArrheniusOne Wavecraft microwave flow reactor with an overall flow rate of 4 mL/min (internal reactor volume 1.4 mL, residence time 0.35 min). The collected solution was dried in an oven set to 70°C to afford a fine black powder catalyst. The Pd/G nanoparticles displayed a narrow particle size distribution with an average particle diameter of 9.37 nm as confirmed by TEM imaging, with a high concentration of 80% Pd(0) needed to initiate the Suzuki-Miyaura cross-coupling reaction as confirmed by XPS spectroscopy. With the continuously prepared catalyst in hand, Brinkley and co-workers sought to determine the optimal catalyst loadings, lot-to-lot variability of the catalyst's activity, and the recyclability of the catalyst by using two different aryl halide starting materials for the Suzuki reaction with phenylboronic acid. Complete conversion towards the desired coupled product was achieved with only 1 mole % catalyst loading, while smaller concentrations of catalyst provided less overall conversion. With the optimal standard conditions in hand, activity level was then tested and found to only vary by as much as 3% across eight different prepared lots of catalysts, and the catalyst was able to be recycled with a minimal 5% drop in conversion over three rounds of reactions with a calculated TON of 372 (Figure 1.40).

The final test of the Pd/G catalyst was to translate these batch conditions into a continuous Suzuki reaction using a packed bed flow reactor. Utilizing a ThalesNano X-Cube flow reactor fit with a catalyst

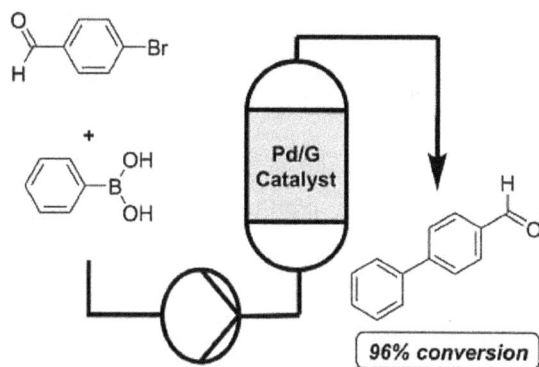

FIGURE 1.40 Continuous flow synthesis and application of Pd/GNP for Suzuki-Miyaura cross-coupling reactions. (Reprinted with permission from Green Processing and Synthesis, "The continuous synthesis and application of graphene supported palladium nanoparticles: a highly effective catalyst for Suzuki-Miyaura cross-coupling reactions", Brinkley, K.W. et al, 2015, De Gruyer.)

cartridge containing 100 mg of catalyst, a Suzuki-Miyaura cross-coupling between 4-bromobenzalde-hyde and phenylboronic acid was conducted at a flow rate of 0.2 mL/min for 2 hours, resulting in an over-all conversion of 96%. Notably, the collected product was found to contain only 347 ppb Pd, indicating that these non-equilibrium continuous conditions were able to provide low catalyst leaching. This result indicates that graphene is a reliable support for Pd and a potentially strong candidate for other cross-couplings to be conducted under continuous flow.

In addition to optimizing the reaction parameters for Suzuki reactions, unique reactor designs can be implemented in continuous manufacturing. Jas and Kirschning developed a chemically functionalized glass/polymer composite as a monolith contained inside of a PBR (Jas and Kirschning 2003). Multiple polymer-assisted solution-phase synthesis (PASSflow) reactors (110 mm L. × 5 mm dia.) were made with a unique design where ion exchange resins are adhered to the column wall to interact with the reagents as they pass through the solid support. Transfer hydrogenations, Suzuki-Miyaura and Heck reactions were able to be conducted within the PASSflow reactors comprised of immobilized palladium catalysts and ammonium cations bound within a polymer shown in Figure 1.41.

For the Suzuki reaction, the PASSflow reactor was run following two different methods: one where the boronic acid can be bound to a strong ion exchange resin and activated prior to the introduction of the aryl halide (1.0 equiv), and another where Pd catalyst (2 mol%) and boronic acid (1.5 equiv) can be pumped through the reactor simultaneously (Kunz et al. 2005). These methods were able to accommodate a wide variety of functionalized aryl halides and were able to achieve complete conversion by a recirculation of the reactants through the reactor. Similar yields and reaction times between the two methods were achieved, however the second method greatly reduced processing time by simplifying the reactor setup. Interestingly, the boron-based byproducts and excess boronic acids were found to remain immobilized within the ion exchange resin after reaction. The reactor was also easily regenerated without exhibiting clogging or other issues. This work showcases the robust nature of the PASSflow technique and suggests similar unique solutions are achievable to make continuous catalytic processes more industrially friendly.

1.3.3 Photochemical Organic Syntheses

Photochemistry provides one of the most sustainable continuous processing approaches available owing to the use of photoactive materials and reagents that are typically more benign than those of more com-monly implemented approaches (Aaron B. Beeler 2016; Rehm 2020). Therefore, photochemistry is one of the key technologies within organic synthesis to replace toxic chemicals and provides greener synthe-ses (Hoffmann 2008). Furthermore, photochemistry can offer additional fine control over reactivity with the ability to readily quench a reaction by turning off or removing the light source.

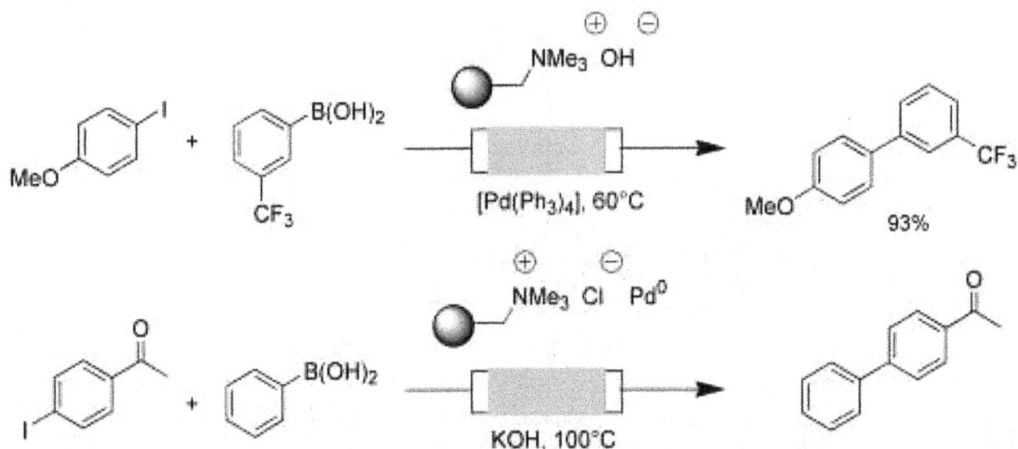

FIGURE 1.41   PASSflow columns in flow reactors for palladium-catalyzed Suzuki-Miyaura and Heck cross-coupling reactions. (Reprinted with permission from Chemistry – A European Journal, "Continuous Flow Techniques in Organic Synthesis", Gerhard Jas and Andreas Kirschning, 2003. Copyright 2003 WILEY-VCH Verlag GmbH & Co. KGaA, Weinheim.)

However, there are some inherent setbacks that need to be overcome and addressed for photochemical schemes to be implemented at a large scale within the pharmaceutical industry. For example, photochemical reactors are limited by the penetration depth of light into the reaction mixture. According to Beer–Lambert–Bouguer's law, there is a logarithmic decrease of light through a given solution (Plutschack et al. 2017). Even less usable light may be transmitted based upon the reaction mixture, such as in the presence of chromophores and excess catalysts. This is a significant issue that prevents the scaling of photochemical reactions and suggests why the pharmaceutical industry does not typically embrace photochemical routes for the routine synthesis of drug targets (Rehm 2020). Many inherent issues of photochemical reactors can be overcome by a continuous approach, building off of continuous advantages already mentioned in previous sections.

Continuous photoreactors have advantages of aspect ratios that allow more efficient light penetration, reaction time, and temperature control through variable-temperature flow photoreactors. These photoreactors are scale independent and can produce multikilogram scale quantities of a product without any necessary modifications to the reactor.

1.3.3.1 Practical Flow Reactor Designs for Continuous Organic Photochemistry

Photochemical reactors require light to pass through the reactor wall to facilitate chemical reactions. A dedicated light source is also required to perform photochemical reactions. An example of a sustainable light source is often considered as natural light through the Sun, however, mercury and xenon lamps, as well as LEDs are commonly implemented in practice. Immersion well batch reactors are commercially available and have been utilized in the past for synthetic organic photochemistry (Hook et al. 2005). Immersion well reactors are irradiated from the inside by a single lamp. Other types of photoreactors exist where one or more adjacent light sources are used to irradiate the reactor from the sides, such as a Rayonet-type reactor system.

Regardless of the irradiation configuration, batch photochemical reaction mixtures are inefficiently irradiated and therefore, inherently give low conversion and rates of reaction. Photochemical transformations are present in numerous preparations of drug molecules, however, due to the scale-dependent nature of these reactions, they are rarely implemented in industrial batch manufacturing. The issue of scaleup associated with organic photochemistry can be overcome by switching from conventional batch processes to continuous flow.

Elliot et al. developed a UV transparent single pass continuous flow photochemical reactor by coiling fluorinated ethylenepropylene (FEP) tubing around a traditional water-cooled immersion well reactor (Elliott et al. 2016; Hook et al. 2005). Simple changes to the initial configuration of this reactor design led to a drastic increase in photochemical conversion efficiencies. A [2+2] photocycloaddition of maleimide and 1-hexyne was used to assess the efficiencies of the photochemical reactor configurations.

Firstly, coil placement was studied and it was found that the reaction mixture should be placed as close to the lamp as possible. Next, the coil was wrapped around the reactor multiple times to utilize as much light as possible, provide a large surface area-to-volume ratio, and increase the reactor volume/residence time without exceeding the total size of the reactor of the batch immersion well. Furthermore, the reaction gave the maximum conversion efficiency when the reaction mixture flowed into the outer layers of coils first.

The intensity (i.e., power) and available wavelengths of the light source are critical for a given photochemical reaction and the rate of reaction. The lamp was upgraded from a 400 W medium-pressure Hg lamp to a 600 W lamp and conversion increased from 46% to 62% at 8 mL/min of 0.2 M maleimide reactants. The commercial immersion well reactors were made out of Pyrex. The Pyrex filtered the lower wavelengths of light necessary for the photocycloaddition (280–300 nm). Therefore, an immersion well made out of Vycor was produced and utilized to increase the efficiency of the reactor system. A [5 + 2] intramolecular photocycloaddition of 3,4-dimethyl-1-pent-4-enylpyrrole-2,5-dione was studied as a candidate to scale-up in the optimized FEP tubing reactor with a Vycor immersion well. A 24-hour reaction yielded 178 grams of the product, which was over four times greater than that of the same reaction filtered by the Pyrex immersion well. This clearly demonstrates the influence of light filtering and reactor selection on the synthesis.

Many photochemical reactions are able to undergo further photochemical transformations when left exposed to a light source indefinitely (Hoffmann 2008). In a batch reactor, the reaction must be stopped before significant product degradation occurs and the reaction repeated as required in order to acquire the desired quantity of product. Using a flow reactor, the residence time can be finely tuned by adjusting the volume of reactor and flow rate. In this way, problematic photochemical reactions can be performed continuously, achieving the highest possible yield of product and limiting byproduct formation.

For clean photochemical reactions, a maximum residence time and photo-energy (optimal UV transmission and light intensity) are ideal to give the greatest conversion efficiencies. However, maxima energy conditions may not be ideal for reactions that lead to byproducts. Therefore, the [5 + 2] intramolecular photocycloaddition of 3,4-dichloro-1-pent-4-enylpyrrole-2,5-dione (key reaction within the total synthesis of Stemona alkaloids) was performed (Booker-Milburn et al. 2003). For this batch reaction, the product is known to degrade after prolonged irradiation and is limited to 0.5–1 gram per batch. In the FEP photoreactor system, the prolonged exposure issue was accounted for by diluting the solution to 0.02 M and reducing the residence time by decreasing the reactor volume (amount of tubing) and increasing the flow rate to 10 mL/min. Furthermore, the Pyrex immersion well was utilized to obtain an isolated yield of 67% for the desired product and the reaction gave a product yield of 45 gram after 24 hours.

Building off of the FEP reactor design, the same team set out to design a photochemical reactor system capable of delivering ≥1 kg per day productivity, the same efficiency of light adsorption, small footprint, durability, and safety. They were able to create a modular parallel quartz tube flow reactor deemed the "Firefly" (Elliott et al. 2016). The quartz tubes of the reactor were arranged axially around a high-power UV source and linked in series to form one continuous reactor. The reactor also featured a metal reflective layer on the outside of the tube to contain the light and also amplify it back at the quartz reactors. The reflector layer significantly raised the temperature of the reactor and therefore two cooling methods were implemented.

The Firefly reactor was shown to be significantly more efficient than the previously described FEP-based reactors. The [2 + 2] cycloaddition of N-methyl maleimide and trichloroethene was carried out in both reactor types, where the FEP reactor at 400 W and the Firefly at 3 kW gave a yield of 2.85 g/hr (68%) and 28.8 g/hr (66%), respectively. Therefore, a 7.5x power increase for the Firefly gave 10.1 times increase in productivity between the reactor designs, indicating a 30% increase in power efficiency. This case emphasizes the importance of reactor design where improved cooling and efficient use of light lead to a significant improvement in synthesis (Figures 1.42 and 1.43).

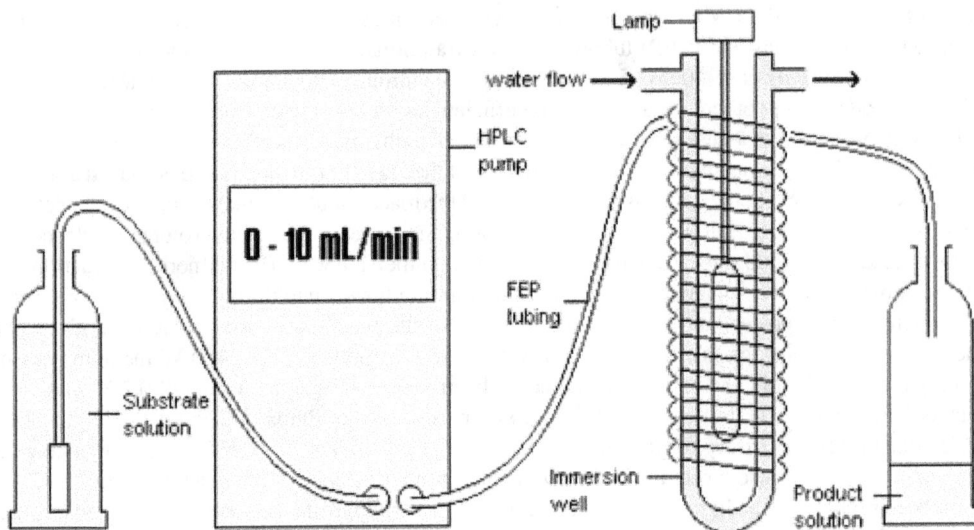

FIGURE 1.42   Depiction of a fluorinated polymer (FEP) tubing continuous flow photo-reactor. (Reprinted with permission from the Journal of Organic Chemistry, "A Practical Flow Reactor for Continuous Organic Photochemistry", Hook, B.D.A. et al, 2005. Copyright 2005 American Chemical Society.)

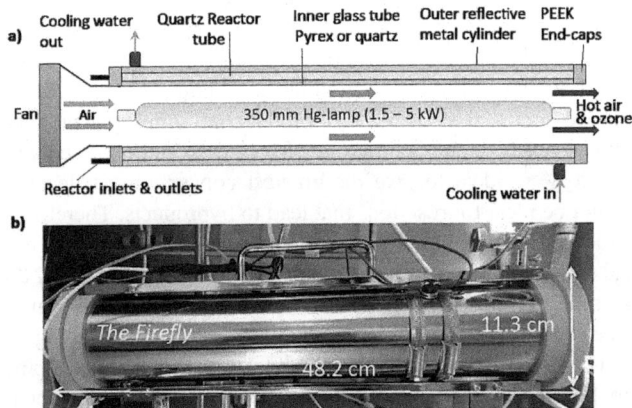

FIGURE 1.43   Scheme and image of an optimized parallel tube flow photo-reactor (PTFR) dubbed "The Firefly". (Reprinted from https://pubs.acs.org/doi/10.1021/acs.oprd.6b00277. All further use and permissions should be directed to ACS.)

1.3.3.2 Photochemical Flow Synthesis of Artemisinin

Continuous photochemical reactors were exceptionally useful in the preparation of artemisinin, a common malaria treatment API, from dihydroartemisinic acid (DHAA), a common intermediate that can be prepared in generous yields from artemisinic acid from yeast (Pieber et al. 2015). This biomimetic photochemical reaction was discovered nearly 40 years ago, but due to difficulties in the generation of singlet oxygen and in scale-up, failed to see industrial implementation until the early 2000s (Lévesque and Seeberger 2012; Kopetzki et al. 2013) (Figure 1.44).

A challenge in implementing this process from the telescoped preparation of DHAA lies in developing reaction conditions for the diastereoselective reduction that do not interfere with the photocatalyzed oxidation step, a challenging proposition as both reactions exhibit sensitivity to a variety of functionalized compounds and aerobic concentrations. For this reason, Pieber et al. were inspired to develop the multi-injection continuous protocol outlined in Figure 1.45.

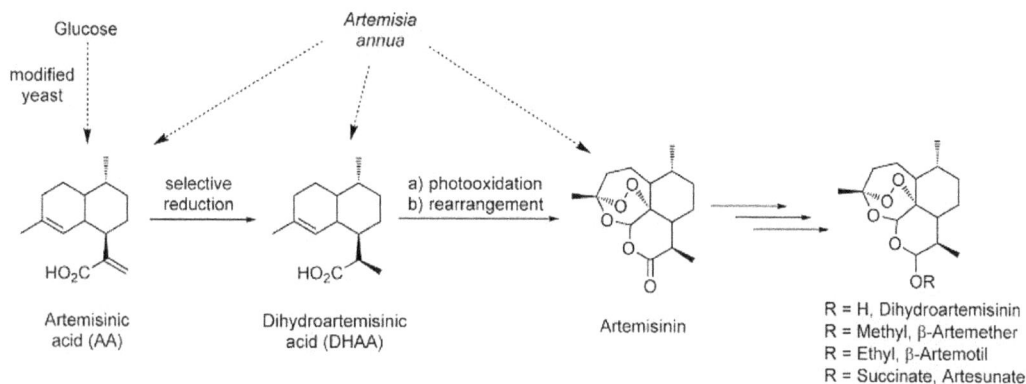

FIGURE 1.44 Natural product derived production routes towards Artemisinin and tis derivatives. (Reprinted with permission from Chemistry – A European Journal, "Continuous Flow Reduction of Artemisinic Acid Utilizing Multi-Injection Strategies – Closing the Gap Towards a Fully Continuous Synthesis of Antimalarial Drugs", Pieber, B. et al, 2015. Copyright 2015 WILEY-VCH Verlag GmbH & Co. KGaA, Weinheim.)

Implementing a catalyst-free continuous-flow protocol for the selective reduction of olefins published in their previous work, Kappe's group was able to demonstrate a mild reduction of artemisinic acid to DHAA with high dr and conversion of starting material up to 92% (Pieber et al. 2013). A drawback to this system was the disproportionation of the hydrazine hydrate as the reaction proceeded, though high yields could still be achieved by flowing excess oxygen gas through the reactor. However, these reactions conditions proved unsuitable for the downstream photochemical process due to leached oxygen poisoning as evidenced in earlier attempts towards the photochemical motif, so a need for an alternate synthetic strategy led researchers to explore a multi-injection process (Lévesque and Seeberger 2012).

This multi-injection strategy was intended to mimic traditional dropping funnel additions and drive the reaction to completion without the need for excess oxygen gas to be present in the reactor. Utilizing hydrazine hydrate as the injection reagent was theorized to help drive the reaction to completion by presenting fresh reagent for consumption *in situ* as the reaction proceeded, similar to trapping methodologies which introduce reagents in line with the formation of reactive intermediates. After optimization to prevent unwanted side-product reactions, Kappe's team developed a catalyst-free strategy that resulted in >99% conversion and an isolated yield of >93%, reducing both reaction time and temperature while attenuating both the oxygen content and artemisinic acid consumption through continuous flow process intensification. This work also highlights the potential advantages a telescoped photochemical transformation would carry (Figure 1.46).

Demonstration of this continuous photochemical reaction would come from Kong et al. in the Medicines for All lab in their route towards a continuous process for the preparation of artemisinin (Kong et al. 2017). Key features of this innovation are in switching from more common homogenous catalysis to heterogeneous catalysis for simplified purification procedures along with the use of cost-effective photocatalyst Rose Bengal immobilized on polystyrene. These milder reagents and elimination of a purification step from the photosensitizer allow for facile telescoping of the reaction. Efforts were also made to improve the photocatalyst's recyclability in order to improve long-term and large-scale production value for industrial implementation.

As shown in Figure 1.47, Kong et al. built a custom packed-bed photoreactor for the generation of singlet oxygen to then flow into a reaction coil for continuous photo-oxidation. Initial examination of the utility of this reactor was conducted on the [4 + 2] cycloaddition of α-terpinene to form the endoperoxide product in 94% yield, which matches literature precedent using alternate reaction conditions (Lévesque and Seeberger 2011). The setup was tested on numerous other polycyclic alkenes prior to testing of DHAA, which proceeded as well for an overall yield of 87% towards the hydroperoxide intermediate 1 (Figure 1.48).

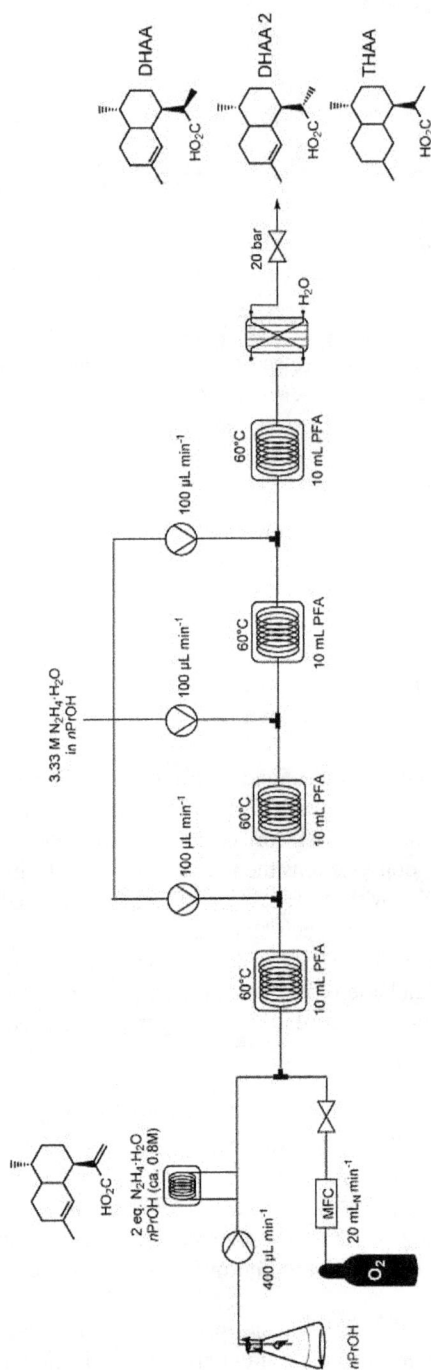

FIGURE 1.45 The optimized multi-injection setup for the reduction of artemisinic acid. (Reprinted with permission from Chemistry – A European Journal, "Continuous Flow Reduction of Artemisinic Acid Utilizing Multi-Injection Strategies – Closing the Gap Towards a Fully Continuous Synthesis of Antimalarial Drugs", Pieber, B. et al, 2015. Copyright 2015 WILEY-VCH Verlag GmbH & Co. KGaA, Weinheim.)

Table	Comparison of different strategies for the reduction of artemisinic acid.			
	Amyris[a]	Sanofi–Aventis[b]	Sanofi–Aventis[c]	This work
Technology	batch	Batch	batch	continuous flow
Reducing agent	H_2	H_2	N_2H_2	N_2H_2
Catalyst	[RhCl(PPh$_3$)$_3$] [0.05 mol%]	[RuCl$_2${(R)-dtbm-Segphos)](dmf)$_2$[e] [0.01 mol%]	–	–
T [°C]	80	25	40	60
P [bar]	47	22	atm.	20
t [h]	19	6	11	ca. 0.6
Yield [%]	quantitative (not isolated)	quantitative (not isolated)	>90	≥93
	Amyris[a]	Sanofi–Aventis[b]	Sanofi–Aventis[c]	This work
Technology	batch	Batch	batch	continuous flow
Reducing agent	H_2	H_2	N_2H_2	N_2H_2
Catalyst	[RhCl(PPh$_3$)$_3$] [0.05 mol%]	[RuCl$_2${(R)-dtbm-Segphos)](dmf)$_2$[e] [0.01 mol%]	–	–
T [°C]	80	25	40	60
P [bar]	47	22	atm.	20
t [h]	19	6	11	ca. 0.6
Yield [%]	quantitative (not isolated)	quantitative (not isolated)	>90	≥93
d.r.	94:6	95:5	≥97:3	≥97:3
Space–time yield [mmol L^{-1} h^{-1}]	0.023	–[d]	0.023	0.56

[a] Data taken from ref. [9b]. [b] Data taken from ref. [10]. [c] Data taken from ref. [13]. [d] Apace–time-yield cannot be calculated as no reactor volume was reported. [e] dtbm = (R)-dtbm-Segphos = (R)-(−)-5,5′-bis[di(3,5-di-*tert*-butyl-4-methoxyphenyl)phosphino]-4,4′-bi-1,3-benzodioxole.

FIGURE 1.46 Comparison of different strategies for the reduction of artemisinic acid. (Reprinted with permission from Chemistry – A European Journal, "Continuous Flow Reduction of Artemisinic Acid Utilizing Multi-Injection Strategies – Closing the Gap Towards a Fully Continuous Synthesis of Antimalarial Drugs", Pieber, B. et al, 2015. Copyright 2015 WILEY-VCH Verlag GmbH & Co. KGaA, Weinheim.)

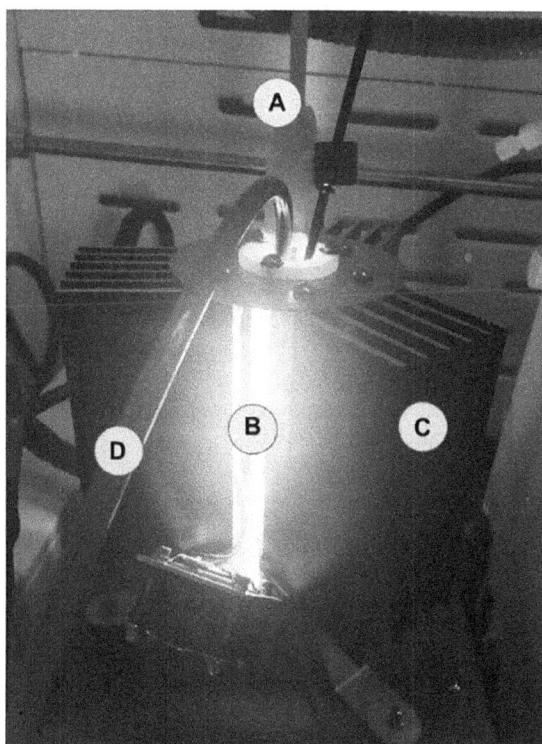

FIGURE 1.47 Visual representation of the LED based photoreactor. (Reprinted from Bioorganic & Medicinal Chemistry, "High throughput photo-oxidations in a packed bed reactor system", Vol 25, Iss 23, Caleb J. Kong et al., Pages 6203-6208, Copyright (2017), with permission from Elsevier.)

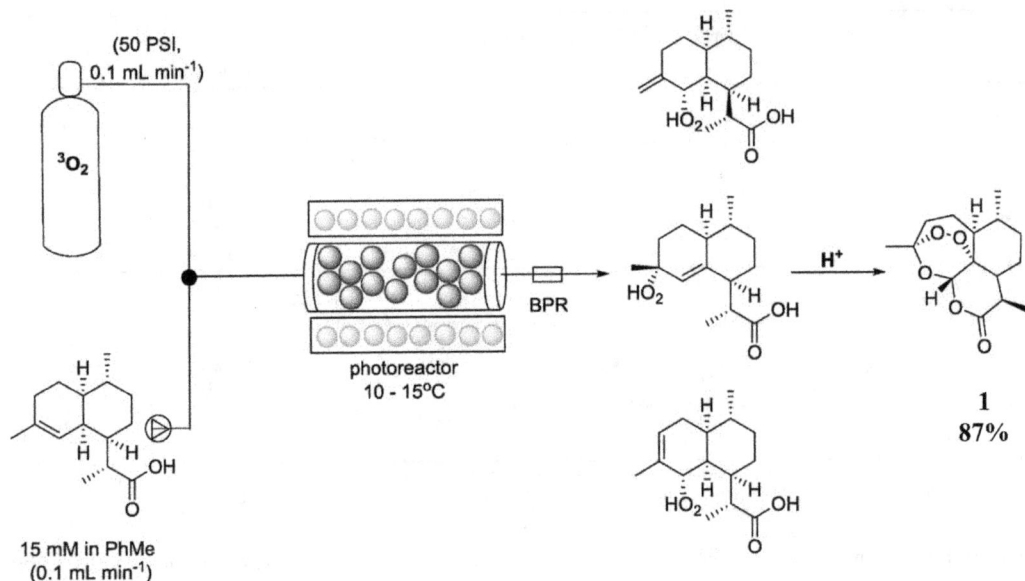

FIGURE 1.48 Continuous photo-oxidation of dihydroartemisinic acid to form 1. (Reprinted from Bioorganic & Medicinal Chemistry, "High throughput photo-oxidations in a packed bed reactor system", Vol 25, Iss 23, Caleb J. Kong et al., Pages 6203-6208, Copyright (2017), with permission from Elsevier.)

Chloroform was also substituted from the original process for the more pharmaceutically friendly green solvent toluene without negatively impacting the yield as well. Acid-promoted Hock-cleavage of 1 can afford artemisinin in isolated yields close to 40%, as demonstrated by Lévesque and Seeberger in their continuous preparation of the API (Lévesque and Seeberger 2012). This efficient methodology in tandem with the work detailed by Kappe's group demonstrates the potential for a true end-to-end continuous manufacturing process of artemisinin from the abundant artemisinic acid isolated from glucose yeast.

1.3.3.3 Photocatalysts as Alternatives to Precious Metal Catalysts

Cross-coupling reactions are desirable for the synthesis of many pharmaceutical drug targets which are typically enabled through Pd and Ni-based catalysts, as previously mentioned. The cost and relative toxicity of Pd and Ni catalysts give rise to the study of earth-abundant, cheaper, and non-toxic alternatives (Mandoli 2019). In this way, photocatalysts or photosensitizers can provide alternatives to traditional catalysts, which may prove to be cheaper and more effective alternatives to commonly implemented noble-metal-based catalysts (Hoffmann 2008).

For example, the Kumada reaction has limited examples for coupling electron-rich aryl chlorides with aliphatic Grignard reagents (Heravi et al. 2019). An Fe-based visible light photocatalyst was shown to facilitate Csp^2–Csp^3 bond formation in a continuous flow reactor (Wei et al. 2019). Chlorobenzene as a model substrate was able to react with cyclohexylmagnesium chloride (CyMgCl) by using $Fe(acac)_3$ (2 mol% catalyst loading) and 3-bis(2,6-diisopropylphenyl) imidazolinium chloride (SIPr · HCl) as ligand (2 mol%) under irradiation of blue LED (450 nm) to give full conversion after a residence time of 5 minutes at 25°C. Wei et al. further utilized this system to couple additional unfunctionalized and functionalized aryl chlorides with various Grignard reagents. Notably, the aryl halides with strongly electron-donating (–MeO) and strong electron- withdrawing groups (e.g., –NHMe) gave good to high yields of 61–93% and 82–96%, respectively. All of the reactions were studied in the dark as well, and the effect of irradiation on the aryl halide substituents was more significant for the electron-rich reactants. Most reactions displayed a significant increase in yield, accelerated by the presence of the blue light (Figure 1.49).

This methodology allows for the previously limited Kumada cross-coupling reaction of aryl chlorides to occur under very mild and scalable conditions in flow. Furthermore, this is a prime example of

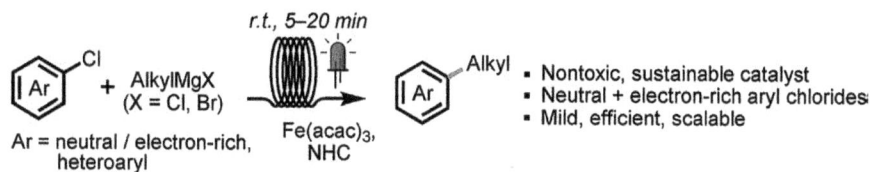

FIGURE 1.49 Light-promoted Fe-catalyzed Kumada cross-coupling reactions conducted under continuous flow. (Reprinted with permission from Angewandte Chemie – International Edition, "Visible light-promoted Fe-catalyzed Csp2-Csp3 Kumada cross-coupling in flow", Wei, X.J. et al., 2019. Copyright 2019 Angewandte. Published by Wiley-VCH Verlag GmbH & Co. KGaA.)

combining continuous photochemical processing with a continuous Grignard-based cross-coupling reaction to access large drug molecules through an efficient single-step transformation.

1.3.4 (R) and (S) Rolipram Paper

Heterogeneous catalysis offers single-step transformations at typically reduced conditions through the power of metal catalysts. A distinct advantage of heterogenous catalysis over homogenous catalysis is the potential to entirely avoid catalyst separation, streamlining the purification process, and offering no contamination of catalysts under ideal conditions (Dach et al. 2012). Tsubogo et al. developed a continuous flow process for the preparation of the GABA derivative drug (R) and (S)-rolipram using eight sequential steps using only packed columns of heterogeneous catalysts to achieve each chemical transformation (Tsubogo et al. 2015). This synthetic strategy represents a significant achievement in translating heterogeneous catalysis to continuous flow where no isolation steps or excess reagents are required, and the catalysts used were able to be recycled for continuous high throughput production of both enantiomers of rolipram.

Conversion of each starting material was envisaged to proceed through a catalytic method, so starting materials and reaction intermediates were selected during retrosynthetic mapping that would follow known literature precedent for the necessary transformations. As depicted in Figure 1.50, the team

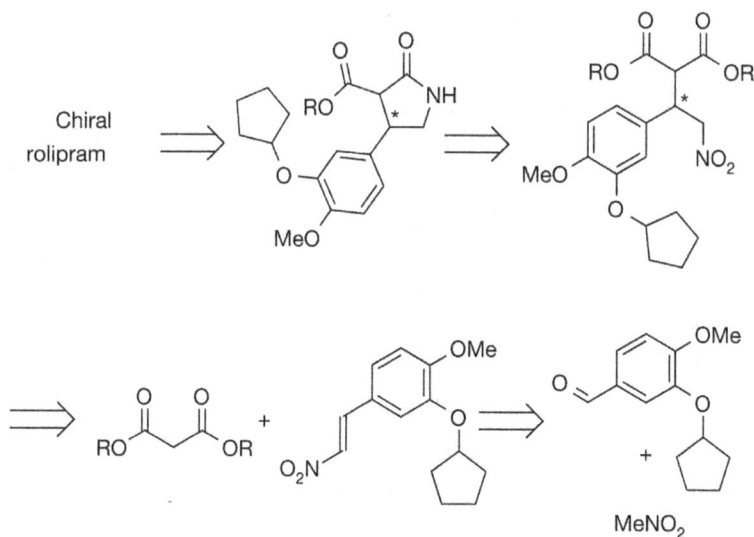

FIGURE 1.50 Retrosynthetic analysis of rolipram potential synthesis from commercially available aldehyde and nitromethane. (Reprinted/adapted by permission from Springer Nature: Nature Publishing Group, a division of Macmillan Publishers Limited. "Multistep continuous-flow synthesis of (R)- and (S)-rolipram using heterogeneous catalysts" by Tetsu Tsubogo et al. Copyright © 2015.)

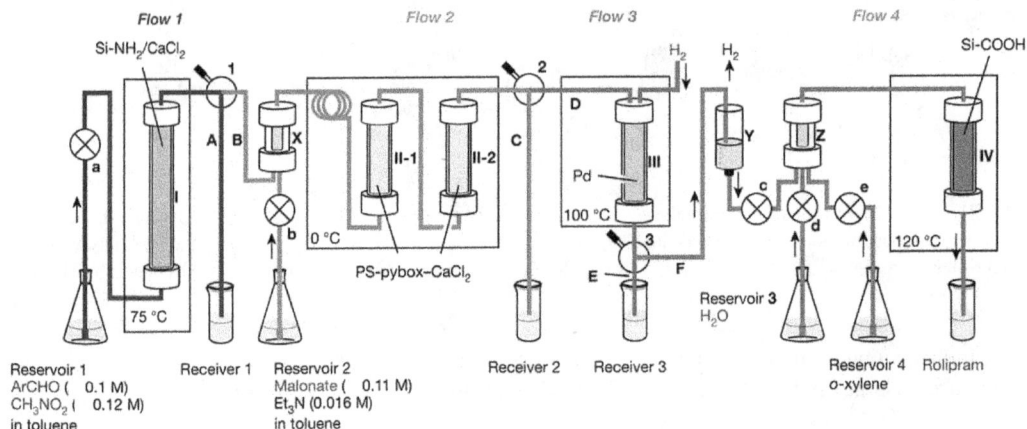

FIGURE 1.51 Continuous end-to-end continuous flow cross-coupling reactor diagram for the synthesis of both enantiomers of rolipram. (Reprinted/adapted by permission from Springer Nature: Nature Publishing Group, a division of Macmillan Publishers Limited. "Multistep continuous-flow synthesis of (R)- and (S)-rolipram using heterogeneous catalysts" by Tetsu Tsubogo et al. Copyright © 2015.)

selected a commercially available aldehyde building block to convert to a nitroalkene through base-promoted catalysis with nitromethane. This reaction proceeded nicely in >90% yield in toluene, the ideal reaction solvent for telescoping to the proceeding 1,4-asymmetric addition of the symmetric malonate. This flow output material is mixed with triethylamine and the malonate in toluene at matching flow rates through a built-in loop so as to enter the PBR and diffuse simultaneously upon the calcium catalyst. The loop also permitted the flow input to return to ambient temperature upon exiting the elevated thermal conditions in the preceding step.

The designed process began with selective nitro reduction through a polysilane-supported palladium on a carbon catalyst. This catalytic hydrogenation reaction required temperatures of 100°C and proceeded conveniently at normal H_2 gas pressure and without epimerization. With the formed γ-lactam in hand, the final catalyzed hydrolysis and decarboxylation step to form rolipram presented the final engineering challenge of removing the hydrogen gas from the system and introducing water along with the immiscible solvent xylenes. The incorporation of Amerblyst 15Dry and celite in a small column effectively purged hydrogen gas from the system. Attenuation of flow rates allowed for an even mixing of water and xylenes that increased surface-solvent interactions in the now well-partitioned layers, boosting product conversion. (S) and (R) rolipram were able to be obtained in 50% yield and >96% ee through this series of connected heterogeneous catalysts (Figure 1.51).

Due to the superior heat transfer and increased number of surface interactions offered in a packed bed continuous flow reactor, less moles of catalyst were required to activate each reaction when compared to a typical batch process. Columns could also be sustained off a single load of catalyst for up to a week before needing to be replaced. In the instance of the chiral calcium catalyst used in the malonate coupling, a single packed column could last upwards of 1 month before needing to be replaced. A throughput of just under 1 g/day was achieved, demonstrating that heterogeneous catalysts can be implemented in continuous processes as solid supports with robust effectiveness and longevity.

1.4 Total Syntheses of API

Consistency of reaction parameters is key in pharmaceutical production (Dach et al. 2012). Continuous flow processes demonstrate less amounts of variability due to improved control of key reaction parameters (temperature, residence time, pressure, mixing, etc.) (Plutschack et al. 2017; Dumarey et al. 2019). Since pharmaceutical production in particular requires simultaneous processing at multiple production scales, having well-defined reaction parameters in a flow reactor that can be scaled indefinitely drastically reduces optimization development time.

Improved conversion/selectivity in flow also allows for non-protecting group strategies to be implemented (Baumann et al. 2020). Avoidance of protecting groups is yet another example of an improvement in atom economy, cost, and waste generation. Additionally, many common protecting groups in synthetic organic chemistry implement bulky chains or potentially harmful counterions, and many of these same counterions also form salts which can interfere with product formation and purity in downstream operations.

Reducing the reaction time is not the only way in which flow operations cut down on plant processing time. Continuous flow allows for significantly easier telescoping of multistep syntheses, along with the ability to run parallel chain reactions that are then connected via T-junction or other means to allow for efficient streamlining of subsequent steps. It is also easier to achieve *in situ* quenching of reactive species in flow by employing this parallel processing technique. An existing drawback to telescoping reactions in this manner is that a greater excess of reagents may be required to afford similar conversion as found in a batch process that isolates after each stage. There are some examples in the literature where manipulation of the residence time (τ) or implementation of a recirculation pathway for these reactions allows for less material to be used (Dumarey et al. 2019; Ötvös and Fülöp 2015; Ishitani et al. 2020). This is especially prominent in flow chemistry that employs solid-supported reagents or catalysts.

Solid supports also offer a unique solution for the pharmaceutical industry in terms of meeting purification standards by allowing the crude solution to flow through a solid scavenger (Jimenez-Gonzalez et al. 2011). Trapping impurities on this solid scavenger allows for them to be easily removed from the waste stream and converting them to plug flow reactor-based systems, allowing for selective in-process purification at any step during a continuous flow route.

These innovations cut down on plant operation time by converting traditional pre-process and post-process concerns such as reaction timing/mapping and purification into in-process operations. This negates the need for material transfer and streamlines workflow and optimization testing for pilot plant operators as well. An examination of the continuous total syntheses of APIs and API skeletal fragments will be discussed in this section. Emphasis will be made on the improvements the flow process demonstrates over existing batch manufacturing processes, as well as highlighting the significant gains in terms of safety, PMI, yield, and cost.

1.4.1 Significant Jump from Batch to Flow

Batch processing traditionally addresses material transformation in single steps sequentially through a process, where parametrization and optimization are conducted on individual steps before progressing to the next step. In the context of large-scale API production, this can entail months being devoted to early steps in a process before poor reproducibility or parameter control in a late-stage reaction ultimately eliminates a manufacturing route from adaptation beyond the pilot plant (Wiles and Watts 2014; Poechlauer et al. 2013). The slower progress of batch processing results in higher overall costs for manufacturers, despite the low initial costs batch processes offer due to the ubiquitous nature of batch reactor setups.

Process intensification is made easier with flow chemistry, allowing for cost reduction by more easily hitting optimal parameters. This allows for higher-yielding reaction conditions to be adapted. Reduced lead times also result in an increase in overall productivity, allowing for process development and refinement to be accelerated as well. Because continuous flow processes invite examining the overall process in sequence, impurity formation and other process defects can frequently be identified more easily and earlier on (Baumann et al. 2020; Plutschack et al. 2017). Several demonstrations of the improved yields and cost-reducing nature of continuous flow processes over existing batch processes are discussed herein.

1.4.1.1 Dolutegravir

Medicines for All demonstrated a concise route to the API dolutegravir that made use of more abundant commodity chemical feedstock while improving the overall yield of the process compared to previously reported industry precedents (Ziegler et al. 2018). Dolutegravir is an HIV integrase inhibitor developed

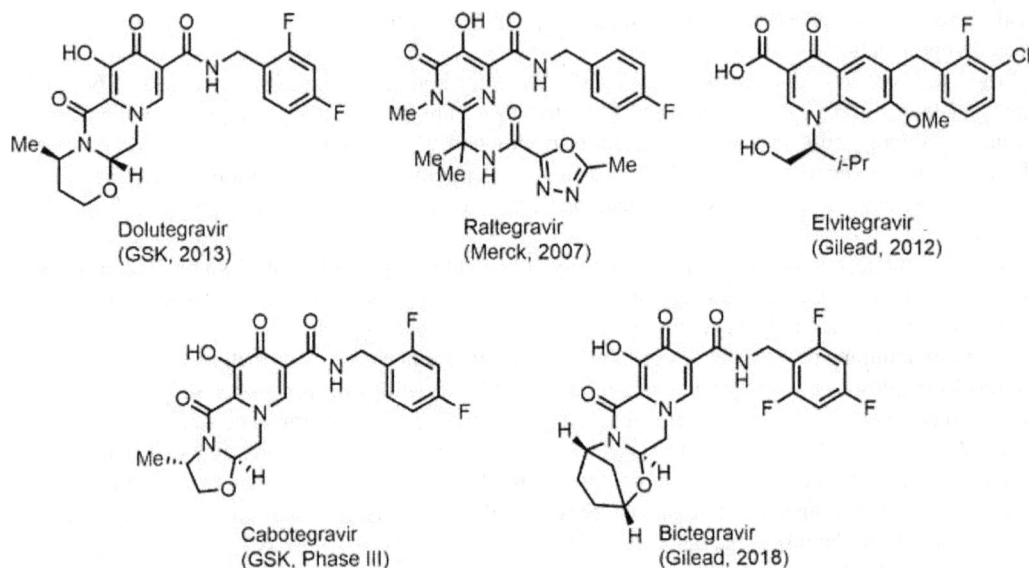

FIGURE 1.52 Examples of integrase inhibitors for HIV treatment, including Dolutegravir. (Reprinted with permission from Angewandte Chemie – International Edition, "7-Step Flow Synthesis of the HIV Integrase Inhibitor Dolutegravir", Ziegler, R.E. et al, 2018. Copyright 2018 Angewandte. Published by Wiley-VCH Verlag GmbH & Co. KGaA.)

by GlaxoSmithKline (GSK) and Shinogi which has numerous analogues in clinical trials. To better accommodate potential future routes to these analogues, preparations of dolutegravir should provide the opportunity to access these molecules through the same set of conditions (Figure 1.52).

Retrosynthetic analysis of the enamine intermediate 4 revealed that, where this reagent is synthesized *in situ* from a neat epimolar ratio of the corresponding reagents, it could be introduced in sequence to the dimethylacetal coupling partner to yield the GSK starting material 6 in higher yield and from more abundant chemical feedstock without increasing the number of unit operations. This reaction proceeded in quantitative yield at elevated temperature with a residence time of 10 minutes. Downstream introduction of the neat dimethylacetal 5 to the formed intermediate afforded intermediate 6 in 95% yield with a throughput of 43 g/hr (Figure 1.53).

Investigation of the pyridine forming step was conducted using isolated solid 6 in order to determine optimal solvent and concentration for the reaction, given the varying solubility profiles of the solid reagents 6 and 7. While optimal conditions were achieved in acetonitrile, a basic solution of methanol provided high conversion under high-pressure conditions (100 psi), inviting the possibility of telescoping all reactions under a single green solvent and boosting PMI by removing a purification step. An alternate flow-through strategy was devised that afforded 16 in 56% yield over three steps over a total reaction time of 74 minutes with a throughput of 3.4 g/hr. While throughput was reduced, the boost in PMI compensates for the drop in productivity. After testing solubility profiles to further reduce step count by implementing direct amidation on the terminal ester of 8, it was found that the introduction of amine 9 in toluene could produce this coupled product in 96% yield under the same basic medium present in the prior steps (Figure 1.54).

The cyclization to form DTG-OMe 10 presented a synthetic challenge where acid deprotection of the acetal moiety on the amine-coupled product could produce a ring-opening byproduct through the elimination of the intermediate hemiaminal ether. A two-stage flow reaction where acid mixed with the unpurified intermediate in one reactor and then met chiral amino alcohol 10 in a second reactor after full deprotection proved successful. This two-stage procedure could additionally be incorporated with the preceding step to create a three-step telescoped synthesis of 10 from 8 in 48% yield with a 7:1 dr. Simple demethylation using lithium bromide from the GSK state of the art afforded DTG in 89% yield with a residence time of 31 min, with optimal reaction conditions being held at 100°C as reaction temperatures

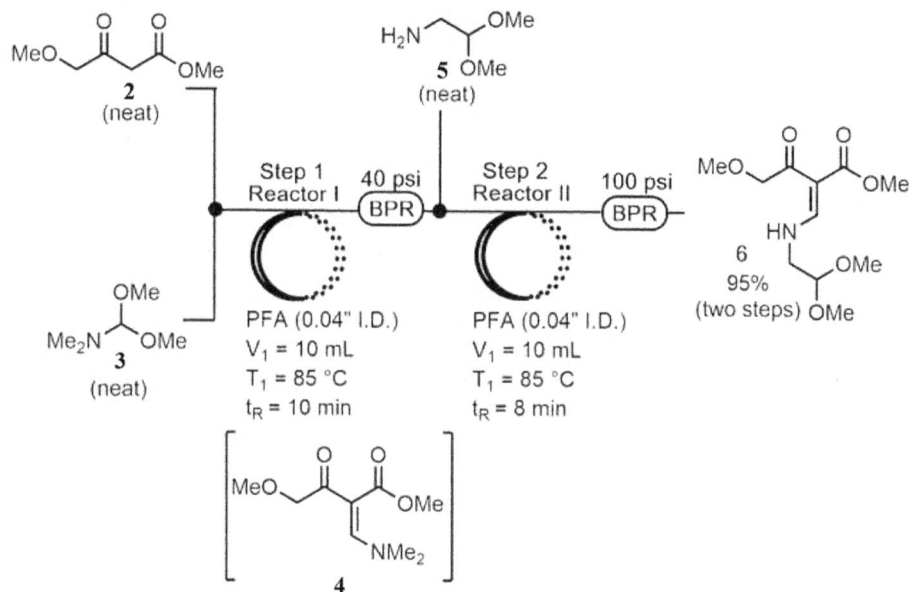

FIGURE 1.53 Telescoped synthesis of 6 from amine 3 and diester 2. PFA = perfluoroalkoxy, I.D. = inside diameter. (Reprinted with permission from Angewandte Chemie – International Edition, "7-Step Flow Synthesis of the HIV Integrase Inhibitor Dolutegravir", Ziegler, R.E. et al, 2018. Copyright 2018 Angewandte. Published by Wiley-VCH Verlag GmbH & Co. KGaA.)

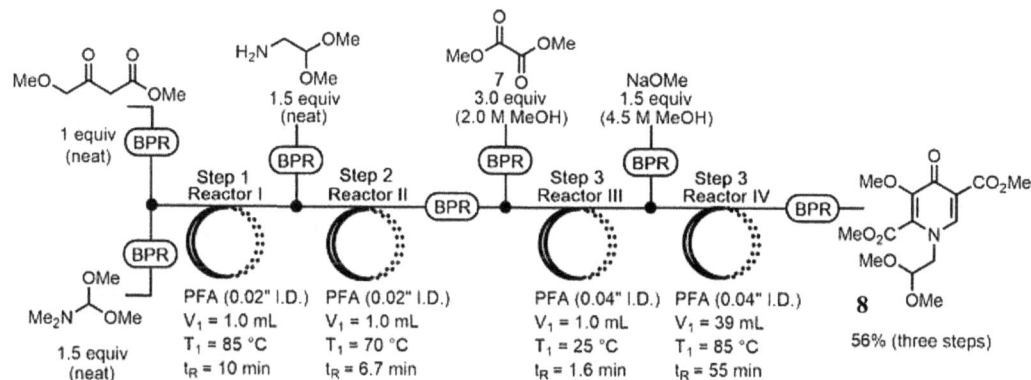

FIGURE 1.54 Three-step telescoped synthesis of pyridone 8. (Reprinted with permission from Angewandte Chemie – International Edition, "7-Step Flow Synthesis of the HIV Integrase Inhibitor Dolutegravir", Ziegler, R.E. et al, 2018. Copyright 2018 Angewandte. Published by Wiley-VCH Verlag GmbH & Co. KGaA.)

above 120°C resulted in the elimination product. This flow synthesis significantly improves the PMI of existing commercial processes while retaining functionality for the preparation of dolutegravir analogues through simple starting material swaps (Figure 1.55).

1.4.1.2 Noroxymorphone

Another advantage that continuous flow reactors offer over batch processes is the superior mixing of liquid-gas phase reactions. The biphasic slow-moving mixture known as slug flow frequently runs into the issue during scale-up in traditional batch reactors where heat transfer and gas-liquid phase surface interactions are reduced. Within thin-diameter tubing, the number of surface interactions increases, improving

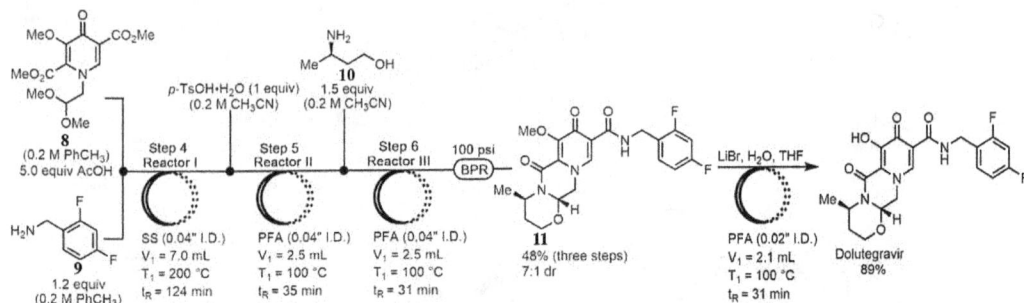

FIGURE 1.55 Fully telescoped synthesis of DTG-Ome 11 and demethylation to afford DTG. (Reprinted with permission from Angewandte Chemie – International Edition, "7-Step Flow Synthesis of the HIV Integrase Inhibitor Dolutegravir", Ziegler, R.E. et al, 2018. Copyright 2018 Angewandte. Published by Wiley-VCH Verlag GmbH & Co. KGaA.)

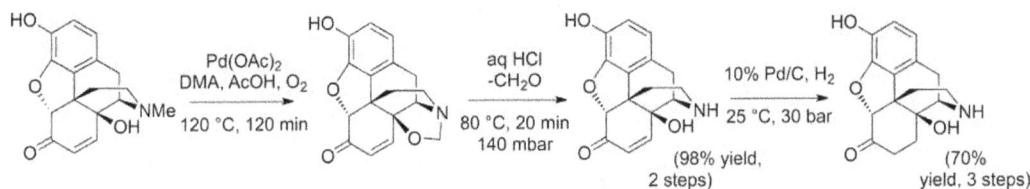

FIGURE 1.56 N-demethylation of 14-hydroxymorpinone and subsequent hydrogenation to afford noroxymorphone. (Reprinted with permission from Chemistry – A European Journal, "Batch- and Continuous-Flow Aerobic Oxidation of 14-Hydroxy Opiods to 1,3-Oxazolidines – A Concise Synthesis of Noroxymorphone", Gutmann, B. et al, 2016. Copyright 2016 WILEY-VCH Verlag GmbH & Co. KGaA, Weinheim.)

reaction rate. An example of this improved reaction motif can be found in the atom-efficient three-step continuous flow synthesis of Noroxymorphone by Gutmann et al. (2016). Noroxymorphone is a precursor molecule of opioid antagonists such as naltrexone and naloxone which are traditionally made under normal batch processes that incorporate large quantities of toxic reagents and waste (Endoma-Arias et al. 2013). Implementation of continuous flow reactors allowed for the more PMI-friendly aerobic oxidation of 14-hydroxynormorphinone, avoiding the use of toxic material and achieving the desired chemical transformation in fewer steps with reduced cost (Figure 1.56).

Incorporation of an MFC for fine control of the amount of oxygen gas fed into the reaction coil helped control reaction rate and concentration, while the use of a thick-walled, gastight fluoropolymer tube for the residence reactor tubing helped prevent precipitation of the formed oxazolidine intermediate and keep the flow output stream in the liquid phase. To prevent fouling of the system due to clogging from potential precipitation of the acetate salts, 1N HCl was fed into the reactor prior to flow through a back pressure regulator. The gas-liquid phase reaction was able to proceed as a homogenous slug flow mixture, featuring oxygen bubbles of diameter less than 2 mm and therefore likely too small for harmful autoignition to occur (Figure 1.57).

This reaction was telescoped into a facile precipitation with mixing in the presence of ammonia and subsequent filtration to afford crude 14-hydroxynormorphinone in 70% yield. Oxidation consuming O_2 in catalytic amounts represents a significant improvement in atom economy over traditional stoichiometric oxidations, with this reaction motif made tenable for large-scale manufacturing purposes through continuous process engineering.

1.4.1.3 Ciprofloxacin

Continuous processes can also offer novel innovations in routes towards APIs developed as long as 40 years ago, as demonstrated by work from the Gupton group at Medicines for All in developing an end-to-end continuous process for the synthesis of Ciprofloxacin (Tosso et al. 2019). As one of the most

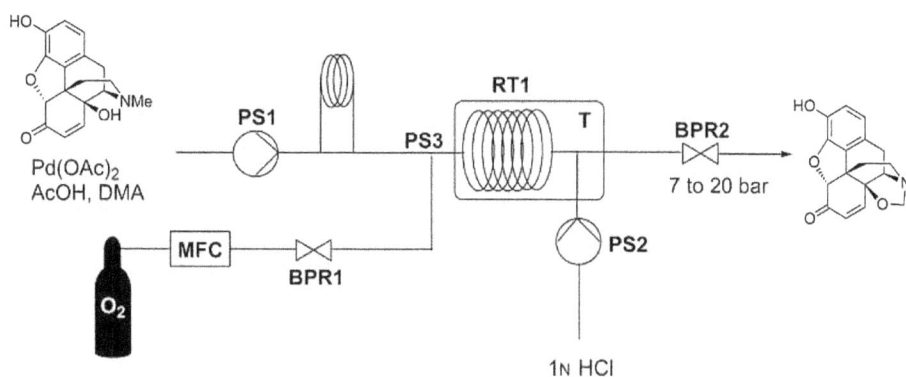

FIGURE 1.57 Diagram of the continuous flow reactor set-up for aerobic oxidation en route towards noroxymorphone. (Reprinted with permission from Chemistry – A European Journal, "Batch- and Continuous-Flow Aerobic Oxidation of 14-Hydroxy Opiods to 1,3-Oxazolidines – A Concise Synthesis of Noroxymorphone", Gutmann, B. et al, 2016. Copyright 2016 WILEY-VCH Verlag GmbH & Co. KGaA, Weinheim.)

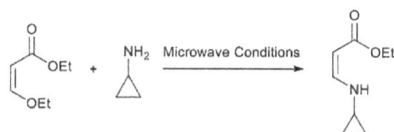

Entry	Solvent	Temp (°C)	Time (min)	Conv. (%)[b]
1	EtOH	78	90	35
2	-	60	30	0
3	Toluene	90	30	0
4	THF	90	30	0
5	ACN	140	60	38
6	DMF	150	30	87
7	DMF	150	60	100 (96)[c]
8	DMSO	150	60	99 (96)[c]

[a]Reaction conditions: **7** (1.0 equiv.), cyclopropylamine (3.0 equiv.). The aminations were carried out in a septum-sealed vial using the Biotage Initiator Microwave Reactor. [b]Conversions are determined by HPLC. [c]Isolated yield.

FIGURE 1.58 Synthesis of vinylogous amides in microwave conditions. (Reprinted with permission from The Journal of Organic Chemistry, "A Consolidated and Continuous Synthesis of Ciprofloxacin from a Vinylogous Cyclopropyl Amide", Tosso, N.P. et al, 2019. Copyright 2019 American Chemical Society.)

prescribed fluoroquinolone antibiotics, Ciprofloxacin has seen numerous groups take on its preparation, with the first continuous process reported by Lin et al. in 2017 (Lin et al. 2017). Tosso et al. demonstrated further modifications to the synthetic route to include a chemoselective C-acylation, avoid formation of an early side-product impurity, and telescope several multistep sequences to cut PMI.

Initial optimization included switching from the dimethylaminoacrylate material to the cheaper, more abundant ethyl ethoxyacrylate material and utilizing sealed vials in microwave to prepare the desired vinylogous amide in one step, as shown in Figure 1.58. Overcoming the barrier presented by the poor electrophilic nature of the ethoxyacrylate starting material was achieved by carrying the reaction under high temperature and pressure (120°C 25 PSI) to afford a 96% yield of the desired cyclopropyl amide. With the desired coupling partner in hand, the next hurdle to overcome presented itself as fixing the selectivity issue present between the coupling of the acyl chloride and the phenyl halide with the prepared

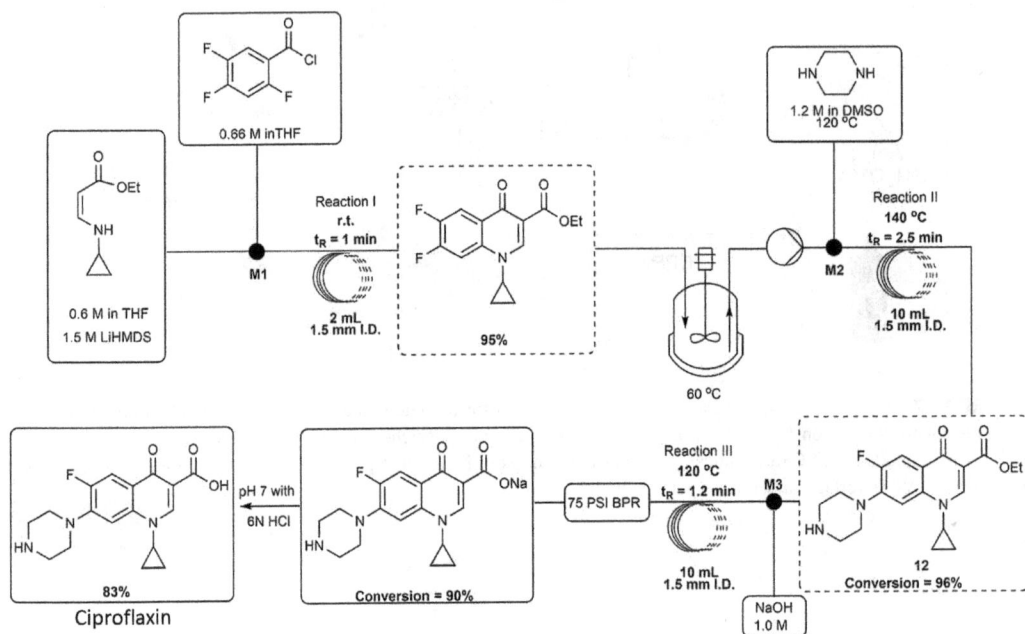

FIGURE 1.59 Diagram of the continuous synthesis of ciprofloxacin. (Reprinted with permission from The Journal of Organic Chemistry, "A Consolidated and Continuous Synthesis of Ciprofloxacin from a Vinylogous Cyclopropyl Amide", Tosso, N.P. et al, 2019. Copyright 2019 American Chemical Society.)

vinylogous amide. Selective C-acylation was observed when LiHMDS was used as base, which is readily soluble in THF allowing for an all-liquid phase reaction to be translated easily in flow (Figure 1.59).

Additionally, it was found that by using a slight excess of base the C-acylation and ring-closing S_NAr could be conducted in a single coil, reducing step count. Pre-heating piperazine in a separate coil before mixing with the ring-closed product output allowed for facile condensation to intermediate 12 which was hydrolyzed to form Ciprofloxacin in 83% overall yield. By preparing the cyclopropyl amine coupling partner in batch, Tosso et al. were able to implement this semi-continuous process providing 15.8g/hr throughput over only four unit operations with a single extraction. This work demonstrates the value in designing a continuous flow operation around a unique synthetic strategy to optimize PMI for chemistry conducted entirely in the liquid phase.

1.4.2 Greenness, Safety, PMI in Continuous Flow Processes

The inherent improved mass transfer offered by tube reactors allows for reduced equivalents of excess material to achieve high-yielding reactions. The increased mass transfer typically presents itself as a boost of overall yield, lowering the elevated molar ratios needed to achieve similar results in normal batch processing. Indeed, several syntheses of API have demonstrated epimolar concentrations of material when conducted under plug flow, normal liquid phase continuous flow, or packed bed flow reactors (Alcázar 2017; Plutschack et al. 2017). Improved atom economy carries with it a reduction in generated waste, as does an increase in overall yield as reaction parameters can be more closely controlled to direct towards product formation and away from non-productive pathways. This compounding impact on waste generation is exclusive to continuous flow operation's inherent qualities.

Continuous processes allow for reduced volume of solvents compared to batch processes, and with improved yields and eliminating the need for numerous extractions and chromatography, drastically reduce overall solvent use and waste production. In some cases, for all-liquid phase reactions, solvent use can be eliminated entirely as flow reactors allow for neat reaction conditions (Plutschack et al. 2017).

Solvent plays a big role in the environmental and safety considerations of a chemical process as well, causing a growing trend towards so-called "green solvents" in the pharmaceutical industry and elsewhere (Clarke et al. 2018). There are several notable examples in the literature where researchers have demonstrated how flow technology allows for a reduction in the use of undesirable solvents by allowing for biphasic reactions to work where they otherwise fail in batch conditions due in part to inferior mixing (Weeranoppanant 2019; Volk et al. 2021). Slug-flow improves yield in these biphasic systems by increasing the available surface area between each reactant in the separate phases. The use of two different solvents isn't limited to biphasic solutions as well, other examples take advantage of variance in solubility profiles of reaction intermediates by introducing solvent washes to both remove undesired reactive intermediates *in situ* or to prevent precipitation of a solid intermediate and telescope it directly into the next step without leaving the flow reactor.

The consideration of safety is well-addressed in continuous processes as well due to the smaller reactor size and superior thermal regulation (Jas and Kirschning 2003). Where a batch process may necessitate the handling of unstable reactive intermediates, telescoped continuous processes can avoid such conditions. Reaction conditions that necessitate the use of exceedingly high temperatures and pressure can also be adapted in continuous flow to lessen their environmental impact. Flow technology is remarkably versatile, allowing for a wide array of customization in both reactor technology and processing strategy to help mitigate exposure risk. Several examples of continuous processes developing safer, greener routes towards APIs are discussed within this section.

1.4.2.1 Nevirapine

Verghese et al. developed an end-to-end continuous flow process for the preparation of Nevirapine, an essential HIV medicine, which features reduced unit operations and PMI through a new strategy for the construction of the seven-membered central lactam ring (Verghese et al. 2017). A significant advantage offered by this strategy is the isocyanate intermediate present in a Hofmann rearrangement to generate coupling partner CAPIC in high yields over two telescoped steps, as seen in Figure 1.60. This drastically reduced step count and eliminated purification requirements while allowing water to be employed as solvent through the remaining downstream development. The developed reactions were then further optimized for a continuous flow method which featured further improvements in the Volume-Time Output (VTO), a measure of the throughput of product compared to the required reactor space. Key features of this process include limited solvent exchanges, vertical integration of advanced starting materials, and implementation of recycled solvent distillate made possible by reduced impurity formation.

Process intensification techniques were implemented to select high-yielding conditions as the primary goal, with second-stage optimization centered around identifying telescoped routes that could allow for parallel processing. With this strategy, a one-pot amination and subsequent nitrile hydrolysis were developed to provide 2-CAN in 91% yield, which was able to be telescoped to MeCAN in 95% yield with traditional batch processing. Prior work from the group was implemented successfully here in the preparation of CAPIC from acetone and malononitrile (Longstreet et al. 2013). Further improvements were made in regard to solvent volumes and the implementation of solvent recycles throughout the flow reactor. It was then discovered that these advanced starting materials could flow through two step-wise temperature gradients to undergo reductive coupling and subsequent ring closure towards nevirapine through two charges of NaH. Due to safety concerns surrounding the off-gassing of hydrogen gas and handling of pure, solid NaH, as well as a desire to further refine reaction parameters and minimize by-product and waste formation, this batch process was adapted to a continuous flow method (Figure 1.61).

The batch process for the preparation of CAPIC and MeCAN was adapted without significant change to the chemistry beyond reduction of equivalents and implementation of solvent recycling systems. A thin-film reactor was implemented in the first stage of the process for the formation of CYCLOR, where CAPIC and a suspension of NaH in Digylme were fed into the reactor at 95°C and then passed through to a CSTR charged with MeCAN. Upon full conversion to CYCLOR, the product was fed through a packed bed of NaH at 165°C to undergo ring closure. The use of the packed bed allowed for huge improvements in the concentration of solid-liquid phase reactions and provided higher conversion to nevirapine than

a. Preparation of MeCAN

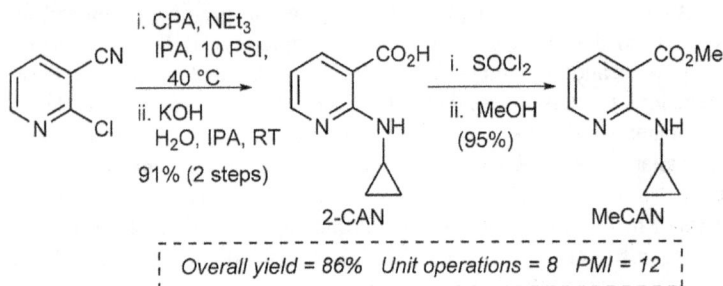

Overall yield = 86%   Unit operations = 8   PMI = 12

b. Preparation of CAPIC

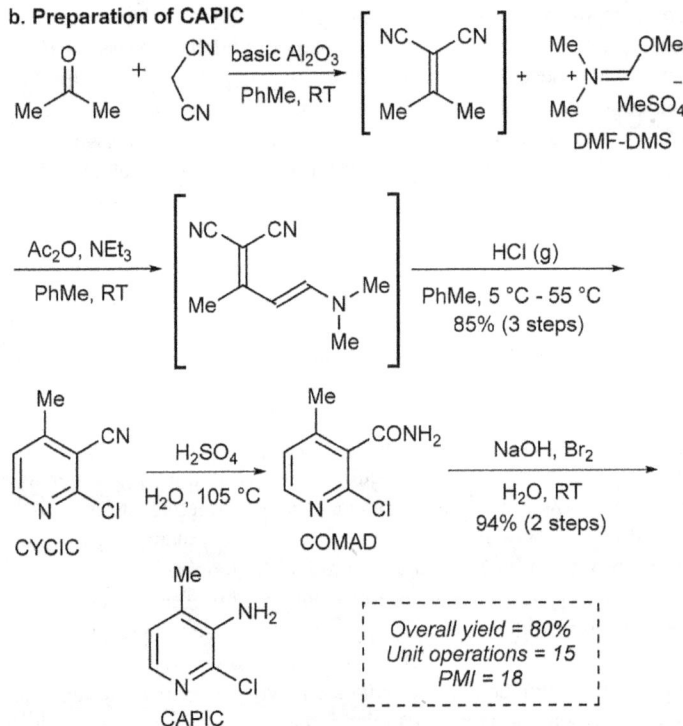

Overall yield = 80%
Unit operations = 15
PMI = 18

FIGURE 1.60 Optimized reaction conditions towards MeCAN and CAPIC en route towards nevirapine. (From Green Chemistry, "Increasing global access to the high-volume HIV drug nevirapine through process intensification", Verghese, J. et al, 2017. – Adapted with permission of The Royal Society of Chemistry.)

the batch method. The overall continuous process significantly improved the isolated yield of nevirapine from a reported 63% to 92% while also improving the VTO, PMI, and scalability. Improvements in safety also make this fully continuous process an appealing candidate for industrial adaptation.

1.4.2.2 1 H-4-Substituted Imidazoles

In an effort to develop a robust route towards common pharmacophore 1 *H*-4-substituted imidazoles, Scott May et al. at Eli Lilly developed two novel continuous processes utilizing plug flow tube reactors (PFR) that adhered to GMP guidelines (May et al. 2012). Their route features an early first-generation approach to forming a common intermediate, *N*-methyl imidazole 5, through a series of linear cyclization, alkylation, and deprotection steps that were later telescoped into a two-step high-temperature/high-pressure fully continuous process.

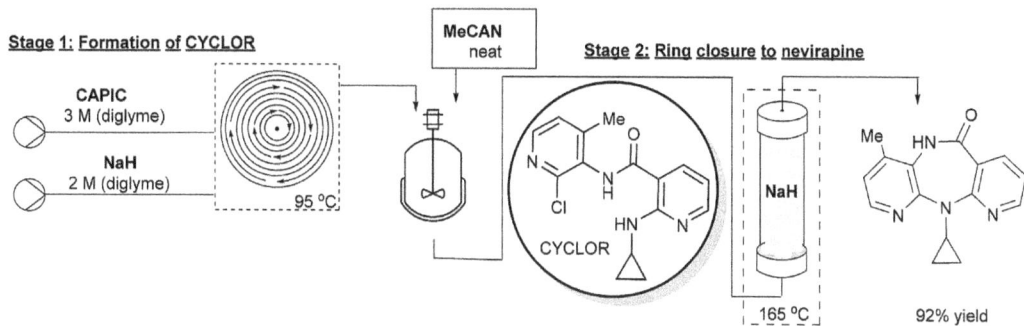

FIGURE 1.61 Continuous process for the coupling of CAPIC and MeCAN to form CYCLOR and nevirapine through NaH-mediated ring closure. (From Green Chemistry, "Increasing global access to the high-volume HIV drug nevirapine through process intensification", Verghese, J. et al, 2017. – Adapted with permission of The Royal Society of Chemistry.)

They demonstrated a 1 kg continuous process in PFR under manual and automated conditions, streamlining the process to include in-line analytical sampling and analysis to improve real-time optimization of the reaction parameters. Careful examination of kinetic data was made more efficient through the use of continuous reactors, accelerating the development of the optimized conditions and showcasing the significant opportunity continuous flow technology offers in decreasing pilot plant parameter processing time.

The initial small-scale attempts at cyclizing ketoamide to form the N-methyl imidazole precursor proceeded in butanol in a sealed tube over 24 hours with 87% yield upon workup with gaseous HCl. This first-generation cyclization reaction suffered under normal batch conditions due to loss of ammonia at elevated reaction temperatures and longer reaction times due to the necessary recharging of ammonium acetate. Translating the conditions to a PFR allowed for the high temperature and pressure reaction to proceed smoothly and with relatively short mean residence times in the range of 5–90 minutes. Implementation of the PFR also allowed for more precise temperature control, allowing for a more accurate temperature screening of the reaction conditions to be conducted for improved optimization. Subsequent acid deprotection afforded the desired N-methyl imidazole in >99% purity.

The results from this cyclization protocol led the team at Eli Lilly to seek a consolidated protocol from the parafluorinated material ketoamide, isolating the protected cyclized product while minimizing formation of the free amine or coupled byproducts. May et al. faced issues in scale-up such as unproductive, longer heating regimes that resulted in increased byproduct formation, and labor-intensive workup procedures.

Telescoping this reaction through a PFR after screening to determine the optimal reactor size allowed for cyclization protocols to be examined at an accelerated pace and with increased parameters for analysis. Through monitoring by-product formation and product stability in the presence of excess reagents, the team was able to identify multiple oligomerizations and decomposition pathways with reasonable rationale for their formation through rate studies (Figure 1.62).

These undesirable reaction pathways were addressed by running the reaction at an elevated temperature of 140°C. This thermodynamic manipulation of the lower activation energy barriers for side-chain reactions allowed the reaction to proceed more favorably (52% isolated yield) toward the product. With the Boc-protected material in hand, a 3-step alkylation, acidic deprotection, solvent transfer, and work-up of the resulting hydrochloride salt afforded the desired *N*-methyl imidazole in greater than 74% yield.

This semi-continuous process suffers from an early yield-hit in the cyclization step (84%) and extraneous unit operations for the removal of the Boc protecting group. For this reason, the team at Eli Lilly sought to develop a fully-continuous process that could leverage the fine temperature control offered in PFR to increase the yield in the cyclization step. Addition of 10 equivalents of acetic acid and a temperature screen above 100°C revealed that at 190°C and residence time above 15 minutes resulted in conversion of starting material but also interestingly proceeded to undergo thermal deprotection at a rate that increased linearly with residence time (Figure 1.63).

As this deprotection, unfortunately, coincided with impurity formation through an acylation side chain, a two-step continuous cyclization and deprotection process through precise thermal control and retention

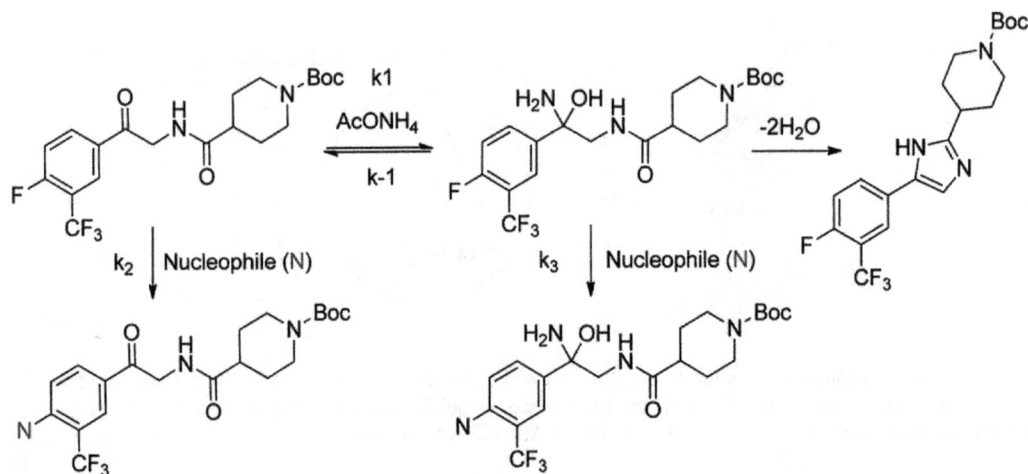

FIGURE 1.62 Examination of different reaction rates depicting a temperature-dependent degradation pathway. (Reprinted (adapted) with permission from Organic Process Research & Development, "Rapid Development and Scale-up of a 1*H*-4-Substituted Imidazole Intermediate Enabled by Chemistry in Continuous Plug Flow Reactors", May, S.A. et al, 2012. Copyright 2012 American Chemical Society.)

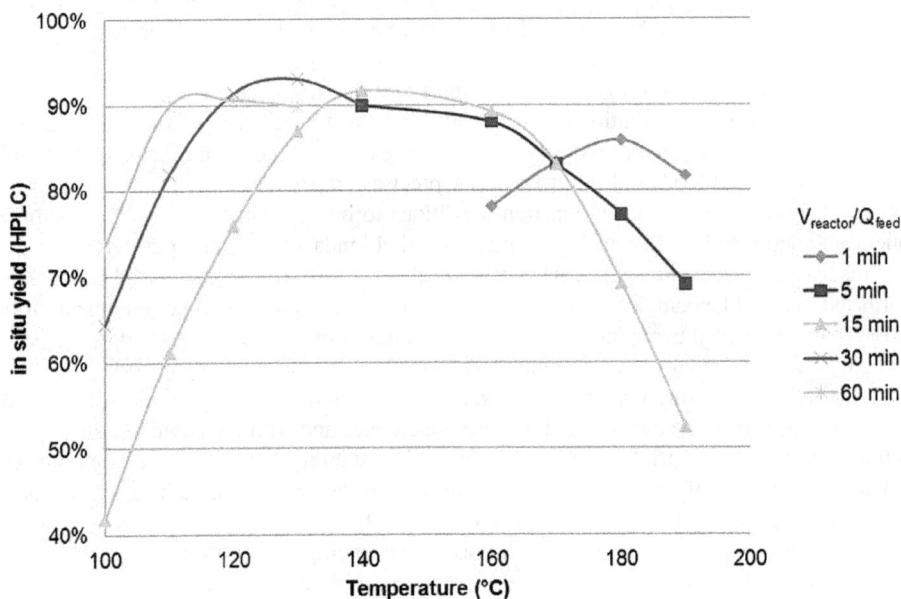

FIGURE 1.63 Cyclization in situ yield with respect to reactor size (volume) and the feed-rate of the reactor (Q_{feed}). (Reprinted (adapted) with permission from Organic Process Research & Development, "Rapid Development and Scale-up of a 1*H*-4-Substituted Imidazole Intermediate Enabled by Chemistry in Continuous Plug Flow Reactors", May, S.A. et al, 2012. Copyright 2012 American Chemical Society.)

time was envisaged. Through these efforts, a scaled-up 221 mL PFR was able to produce an 80% isolated yield of the desired cyclized *N*-methyl imidazole with a $\tau = 10.7$ min, which was then telescoped to another PFR for the thermal deprotection step. The deprotection protocol was also run in a 221 mL PFR and produced 1 kg of the desired deprotected *N*-methyl imidazole in quantitative yield upon evaporation of solvent with a $\tau = 9.4$ min. Additionally, this material was able to be crystallized to afford a 79% isolated yield of >99% purity.

The PFR was uniquely suited for this thermal deprotection as it provided a means for the reaction to be run under its optimal supercritical fluid conditions at 270°C and 1000 psig. While supercritical fluid conditions are considered unsafe for batch operations in plant scale manufacturing, PFR provides reduced reactor volume and improved heat transfer over a wider surface area per unit volume, leveraging these reactors as a viable industrial alternative.

1.4.2.3 Daclatasvir

Members of the Kappe group developed an alternate concise flow synthesis of 1*H*-4-substituted imidazoles that represents a significant improvement upon batch conditions in terms of energy, cost, and environmental impact (Carneiro et al. 2015). They further demonstrated how this motif could be used to prepare the API Daclatasvir, a prominent hepatitis C treatment drug. High reaction rates and the elimination of headspace in flow reactors keep volatile reagents in the liquid phase, improving safety of handling and preventing off-gassing of toxic material (Plutschack et al. 2017; Weeranoppanant 2019; Alcázar 2017). This also reduces PMI as excess material isn't lost to the gas phase. These inherent traits of continuous flow chemistry allowed for hazardous high-temperature/high-pressure gas-liquid phase conditions to be translated safely for the preparation of imidazoles from α-bromoacetophenones and carboxylic acids within stainless steel coiled reactors. Carneiro et al. cleverly demonstrated how once defunct chemistry from the 1930s can now be implemented successfully using modern technology and continuous flow synthetic techniques (Figure 1.64).

Reactions requiring high temperature and pressure can tend to slow upon scale up and present issues of parameter consistency. The increased reaction rate and fine temperature control in flow reactors resolve this problem. Since flow reactors allow for liquids to be heated beyond their boiling points without phase change, the need for a high boiling solvent was removed and acetonitrile, a comparatively green solvent, was implemented instead. This single solvent telescoped motif proceeded well with a yield of 81% for the desired imidazole 4b below, with demonstrations of other amino acid derivative carboxylic acids proceeding in good yield as well. Utilization of these common building blocks for the preparation of this 1 H-4-substituted imidazole motif provides an alternate route towards these highly sought reagents from an abundant pharmaceutical feedstock (Figure 1.65).

1.4.2.4 Iloperidone

Inductive heating has recently emerged as a continuous flow technique for bringing high temperature/high-pressure conditions into the realm of possibility for production scale (Ceylan et al. 2011; Coutable et al. 2013). Hartwig and Kirschning demonstrated an inductive heating continuous flow reactor design

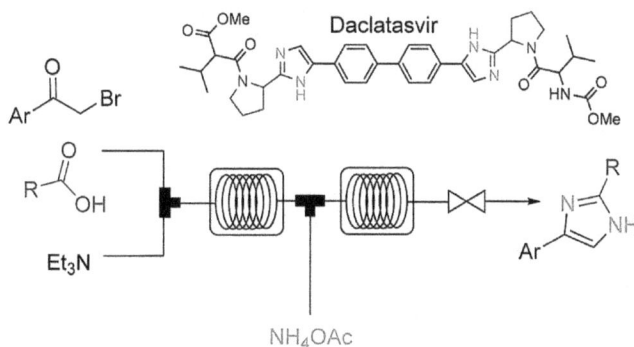

FIGURE 1.64 Continuous flow route for the formation of 1H-4-substituted imidazoles such as daclatasvir. (Reprinted with permission from ACS Sustainable Chemistry and Engineering, "A Process Intensified Flow Synthesis of 1H-4-Substituted Imidazoles – Towards the Continuous Production of Daclatasvir", Carneiro, P.F. et al. 2015. Copyright 2015 American Chemical Society.)

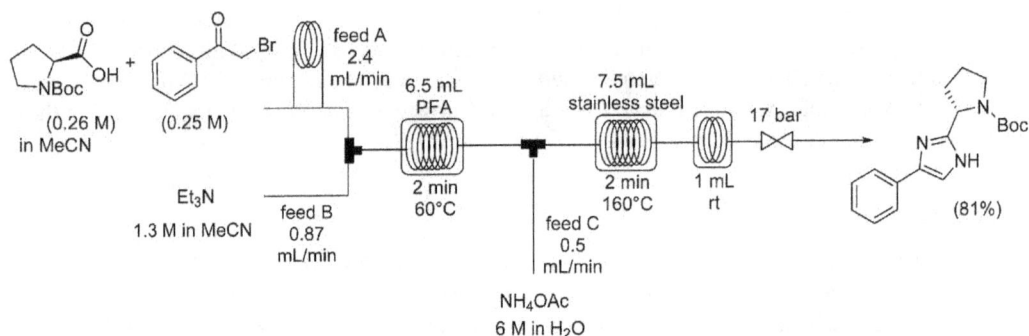

FIGURE 1.65 Two step flow synthesis of the desired imidazole en route towards daclatasvir. (Reprinted with permission from ACS Sustainable Chemistry and Engineering, "A Process Intensified Flow Synthesis of 1H-4-Substituted Imidazoles – Towards the Continuous Production of Daclatasvir", Carneiro, P.F. et al. 2015. Copyright 2015 American Chemical Society.)

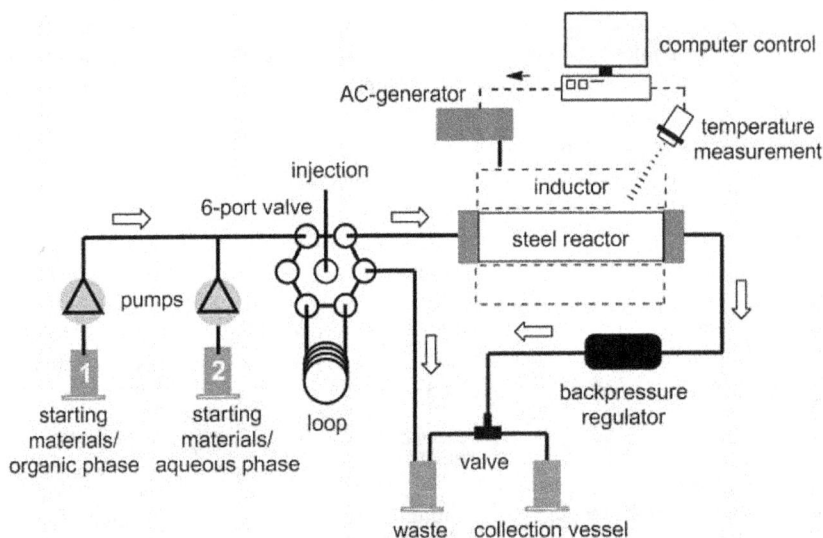

FIGURE 1.66 Depiction of continuous flow diagram complete with waste collection and inductive heating controllers. (Reprinted with permission from Chemistry – A European Journal, "Flow Synthesis in Hot Water: Synthesis of the Atypical Antipsychotic Iloperidone", Jan Hartwig and Andreas Kirschning, 2016. Copyright 2016 WILEY-VCH Verlag GmbH & Co. KGaA, Weinheim.)

in their route towards the antipsychotic Iloperidone (Hartwig and Kirschning 2016). This inductive heating element allowed for implementation of near supercritical water as solvent, providing a significant improvement in the yield, cost, and environmental impact of the key transformation step of this synthesis.

Supercritical water's inherent properties make it an appealing solvent for organic transformations in an industrial setting where waste reduction and cost are important considerations. At above 250°C, water displays similar organic solubility as methanol or acetonitrile while maintaining an elevated pK$_a$, allowing for the dual acid/base functionality of water to be retained. Combining high-temperature conditions with high pressure can improve phase boundary alignment between the supercritical solvent and reagents in solution, improving reaction rate by increasing the number of phase interactions between materials. While high temperature and pressure conditions are not ideal for scale up under normal batch processing, a continuous flow reactor can be modified to accommodate such conditions without impacting reaction rate or scalability (Figure 1.66).

Inductive heating involves the use of an external medium- to high-frequency electromagnetic field in order to induce heat inside a reactor coil. This technique heats at a faster rate than traditional thermocouple-mediated methods and, more specifically for flow reactions, allows for residence time to be controlled entirely by flow rate without extra consideration for a heating feedback loop. This reduces the time a reaction mixture spends at elevated temperature and is thus ideal for reactions or reagents with high-temperature sensitivity. A drawback to this method in continuous flow can be in accurately measuring internal reaction temperature due to interference from the external electromagnetic. Hartwig and Kirschning overcame this hurdle by building a direct temperature measurement into the flow reactor via T-joint. This protocol was able to heat the reaction mixture to 240°C from room temperature within 30 seconds, with a variance of temperature between the steel loop coil maintained below 1%. Continuous preparation of triacetyl benzene was carried out in 89% assay yield in 2 minutes where simple addition of toluene was able to extract the product while all byproducts remained in the aqueous phase.

This promising initial result in the optimization of inductive heating methods in continuous flow was then translated to adapting a continuous flow method for the synthesis of iloperidone (Figure 1.67).

The multistep synthesis envisaged took full advantage of the potential for near supercritical water solvents in altering existing precedent. The ketone was converted to the corresponding oxime through acid-promoted addition of hydroxylamine. This material was then telescoped through cyclization and chemoselective N-alkylation with 3-bromo-1-propane under inductive heating. The quick temperature ramp allowed for rapid rate of reaction to afford a 76% yield of the desired intermediate. The Fries rearrangement step to prepare downstream coupling partner 13 remained largely unchanged from existing commercial procedures beyond the implementation of inductive heating through steel beads packed in a pass-through polyether ether ketone (PEEK) reactor.

As this step was the only one that could not be conducted in aqueous media it was carried out independently for parallel stepwise processing. Combination of 13 with the prepared chlorinated coupling partner 14 formed iloperidone 15 in a separate stainless-steel reactor. The flow reactor was fitted with an in-line purification unit operating under "catch and release" methodology where a silica gel plug trapped iloperidone for selective removal with 2% MeOH, leaving impurities behind in the silica (Figure 1.68).

This work demonstrates the value supercritical water brings to acid-promoted reactions as a substitute for traditional organic solvents. Hartwig and Kirschning's inductive heating protocol in tandem with continuous flow provides a realistic method for bringing this cost-effective, environmental-friendly solution to large-scale pharmaceutical production.

1.4.3 Overcoming Challenges in Chemistry and Reaction Engineering with Flow

Several reaction motifs present challenges for commercial adaptation in terms of poor scalability, exceedingly long reaction times, or prohibitively long purification procedures (Dumarey et al. 2019; Mcquade and Seeberger 2013; Plutschack et al. 2017; Poechlauer et al. 2013; 2012; Jas and Kirschning 2003;

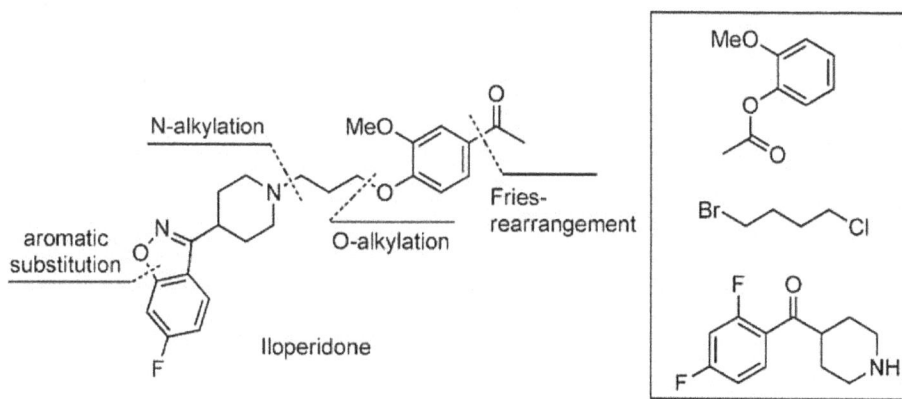

FIGURE 1.67 Synthetic plan for preparation of iloperidone. (Reprinted with permission from Chemistry – A European Journal, "Flow Synthesis in Hot Water: Synthesis of the Atypical Antipsychotic Iloperidone", Jan Hartwig and Andreas Kirschning, 2016. Copyright 2016 WILEY-VCH Verlag GmbH & Co. KGaA, Weinheim.)

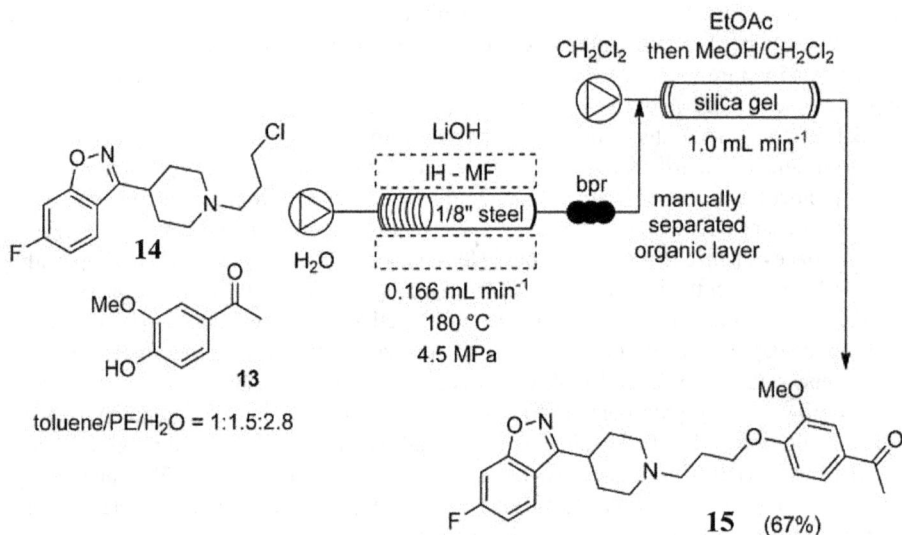

FIGURE 1.68 Catch and release protocol for preparation and in-line purification of iloperidone 15. (Reprinted with permission from Chemistry – A European Journal, "Flow Synthesis in Hot Water: Synthesis of the Atypical Antipsychotic Iloperidone", Jan Hartwig and Andreas Kirschning, 2016. Copyright 2016 WILEY-VCH Verlag GmbH & Co. KGaA, Weinheim.)

Alcázar 2017). Advances in continuous flow have been made to account for these issues present in traditional batch processes. While there are numerous examples where modification of the reactor platform can accommodate these issues, the inherent impact flow reactors have on kinetics has been exploited to great benefit as well.

Examples of modifications to the chemical processing techniques for the continuous flow production of APIs will be highlighted throughout this section. A further refinement of automated protocols to provide highly pure APIs will be discussed as well, further highlighting the union of novel chemistry and engineering techniques.

1.4.3.1 Ibuprofen

Important landmarks have been established in the past two decades to develop microreactors as continuous flow instruments for faster, safer, and more selective syntheses of API molecules (Hakke et al. 2021; Atobe et al. 2018; Cao et al. 2019; Fanelli et al. 2017). One of the first examples of implementing microreactors in parallel for a multistep end-to-end continuous synthesis comes from the McQuade group's 2009 continuous flow synthesis of ibuprofen (Bogdan et al. 2009). This three-step process was designed to tolerate the presence of both excess reagents and byproducts downstream so as to avoid purification procedures and the handling of transient intermediates.

The McQuade group's approach began with a Friedel-Crafts acylation at 150°C with a residence time of 5 minutes, carrying over notable excess reagents triflic acid and unreacted isobutylbenzene starting material. As depicted in Figure 1.69, 1,2 aryl migration was achieved through the implementation of once defunct reaction conditions that lend themselves readily to implementation under continuous flow due to improved mixing.

Careful stoichiometry in the initial Friedel-Crafts stage also allows for the correct amount of excess triflic acid to be used so as to permit the second stage 1, 2-aryl migration to proceed optimally. Saponification of the methyl ester afforded ibuprofen in 51% yield upon recrystallization from the flow stream. In-line quenching of the second stage flow output with a molar solution of KOH was amenable due to the superior heat transfer characteristic of flow tube reactors, minimizing the risk of dangerous exotherm and allowing for the base-mediated saponification to proceed uninhibited without the need for isolation.

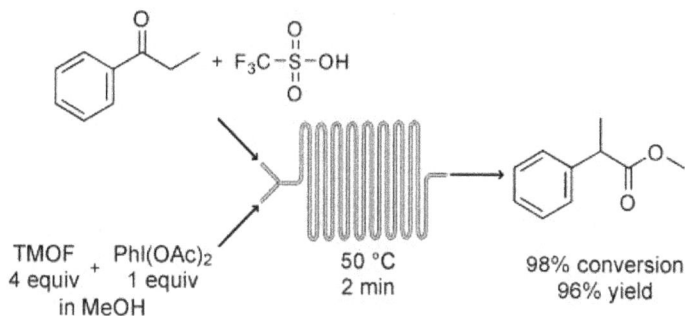

FIGURE 1.69 Optimized reaction conditions for the continuous flow 1,2-aryl migration. (Reprinted with permission from Angewandte Chemie – International Edition, "The Continuous-Flow Synthesis of Ibuprofen", Bogdan, A.R. et al, 2009. Copyright 2009 WILEY-VCH Verlag GmbH & Co. KGaA, Weinheim.)

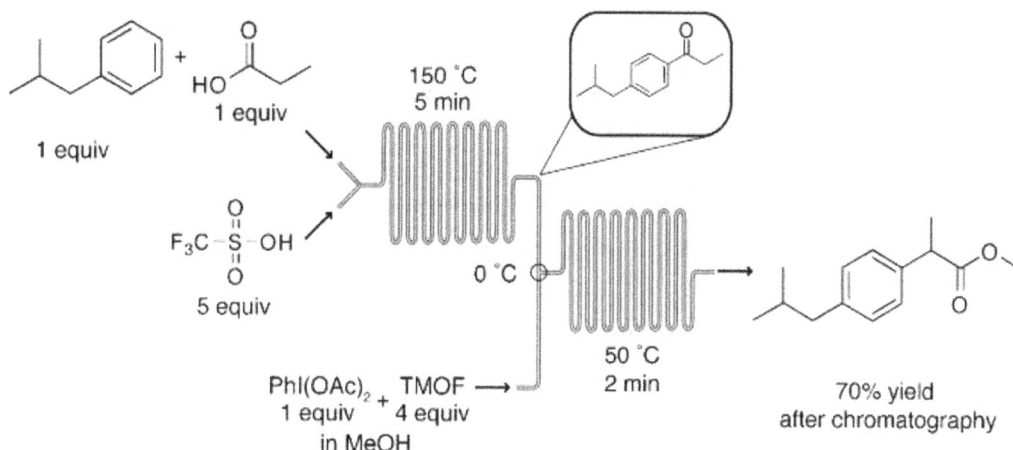

FIGURE 1.70 Diagram depicting the 3-step continuous flow of ibuprofen. (Reprinted with permission from Angewandte Chemie – International Edition, "The Continuous-Flow Synthesis of Ibuprofen", Bogdan, A.R. et al, 2009. Copyright 2009 WILEY-VCH Verlag GmbH & Co. KGaA, Weinheim.)

This continuous flow process represents an enormous stride for the successful implementation of Friedel Crafts acylations without the need for purification or handling of the reactive intermediate (Figure 1.70).

1.4.3.2 Benadryl

The HCl salt form of diphenhydramine is one of the most common APIs in circulation, present in Benadryl and Tylenol and other over-the-counter (OTC) medications (Snead and Jamison 2013). Snead et al. sought to refine the synthesis of this API through the implementation of end-to-end continuous preparation and purification of the salt form directly, featuring high atom economy and waste minimization through the elimination of solvent. This process features in-line purification and crystallization of diphenhydramine in high yields and purity at a reduced cost and number of unit operations, along with increased greenness and PMI due to the elimination of hazardous chlorobenzene as solvent (Figure 1.71).

It was found that chlorodiphenylmethane and the retrosynthetic amino alcohol coupling partner exhibited relatively high selectivity for product formation while also providing a means to access the HCl salt form directly from the resultant salt byproduct. About 80% conversion to diphenhydramine HCl was achieved in the presence of NMP as solvent and sufficient residence time of 20 minutes at 180°C. Believing the conversion to be lowered by side-product formation with NMP, the reaction was explored under neat conditions in an excess of the amino alcohol resulting in an increase of conversion

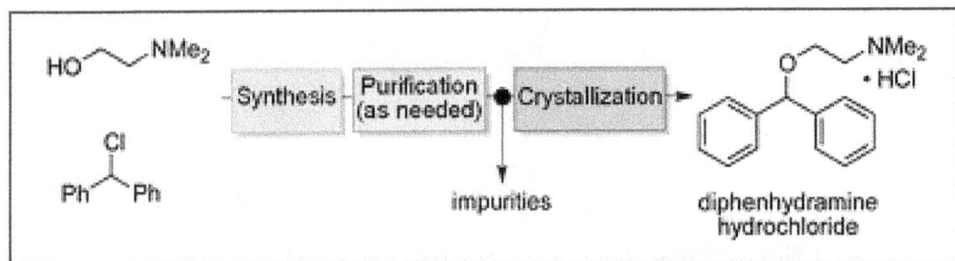

FIGURE 1.71 The continuous end-to-end synthesis, purification, and crystallization of diphenhydramine hydrochloride. (D.R. Snead and T.F. Jamison, *Chem. Sci.*, 2013, **4**, 2822 DOI: 10.1039/C3SC50859E – Reproduced by permission of The Royal Society of Chemistry.)

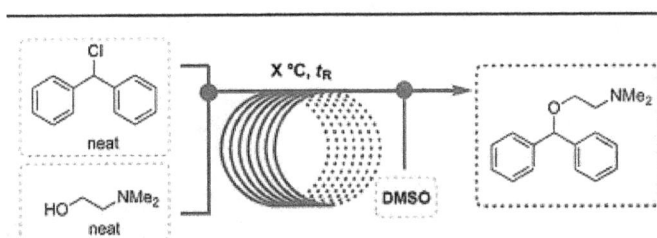

Entry	Equiv. 3	t_R (min)	Temp (°C)	1 : 6 : 7 : 4	Yield[b]
1	4	16	175	97 : 3 : 0 : 0	91%
2	3	16	175	98 : 2 : 0 : 0	92%
3	2	16	175	96 : 2 : 2 : 0	91%
4	1	16	175	92 : 4 : 4 : 0	86%
5	1	32	175	89 : 4 : 7 : 0	85%[c]
6	1	16	200	93 : 1 : 6 : 0	78%[c]

[a] See Experimental for details. [b] Average yield obtained in three runs (^{1}H NMR, external standard). [c] Single experiment.

FIGURE 1.72 Optimization towards solvent-free neat conditions. (D.R. Snead and T.F. Jamison, *Chem. Sci.*, 2013, **4**, 2822 DOI: 10.1039/C3SC50859E – Reproduced by permission of The Royal Society of Chemistry.)

and resultant 91% isolated yield after external crystallization of the product. Considering the operating temperature and significant disparity between the melting point of the HCl salt and the excess reagents, the API synthesis was explored as a flow output of an ionic liquid mixture of the crystalline product in a molten liquid mixture (Figure 1.72).

Thicker walled reactor tubing (0.02-inch ID) proved successful for the implementation of this molten flow strategy, from there an in-line quench with aqueous NaOH, organic extraction, and separation through a membrane provided the API as an organic salt mixture which could be crystallized to afford the product in 90% yield with 98% purity. Implementation of a continuous crystallizer further improved atom

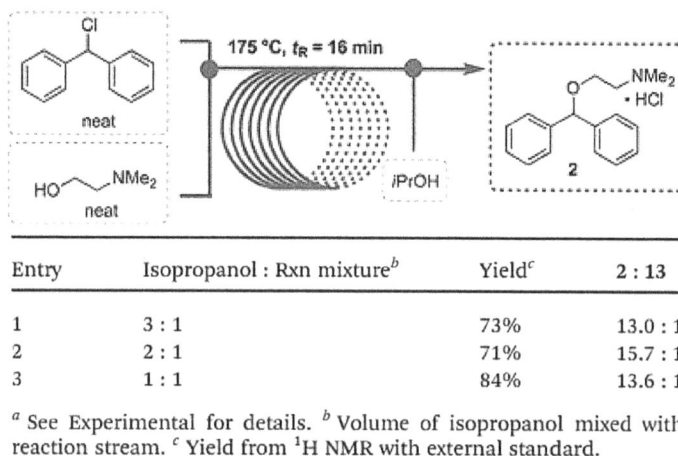

Entry	Isopropanol : Rxn mixture[b]	Yield[c]	2 : 13
1	3 : 1	73%	13.0 : 1
2	2 : 1	71%	15.7 : 1
3	1 : 1	84%	13.6 : 1

[a] See Experimental for details. [b] Volume of isopropanol mixed with reaction stream. [c] Yield from ^{1}H NMR with external standard.

FIGURE 1.73 Optimization of direct crystallization from isopropanol under continuous flow. (D.R. Snead and T.F. Jamison, *Chem. Sci.*, 2013, **4**, 2822 DOI: 10.1039/C3SC50859E – Reproduced by permission of The Royal Society of Chemistry.)

economy and waste output by providing a means to convert stoichiometric amino alcohol 3 and chlorodiphenylmethane to diphenhydramine HCl in up to 84% yield with the simple addition of isopropanol as crystallization solvent post reaction completion (Figure 1.73).

Total atom economy was achieved through this continuous crystallization set up with minimal impact on the overall yield of the process. This process has been implemented and further refined in terms of PMI and by Sonavane et al. through continuous process intensification at an industrial scale (Sonavane et al. 2017).

1.4.3.3 4,5-Disubstituted Oxazoles

An example of automated flow systems preparing medicinally relevant building blocks can be found in work by Baumann et al. out of the University of Cambridge in 2006 (Baumann et al. 2006). Their efforts to produce 4,5-disubstituted oxazoles completely autonomously represent one of the earliest examples in this ground-breaking use of continuous flow technology.

Despite their prevalence as skeletal fragments in numerous APIs, there were few reported methods for regioselective preparations of 4,5-substituted oxazoles (Maeda et al. 1984; Ohba et al. 1998). Thus, the desire to build a drug motif library in a simple, expedient manner was appealing. The group envisioned a synthetic route that proceeded with the addition of an alkyl isocyanoacetate to an acyl chloride via base-catalyzed intramolecular cyclization (Figure 1.74).

Use of this isocyanate intermediate is present in a number of process routes of oxazoles en route towards APIs due to the ideal atom economy and abundance of cyano starting materials (Nunes et al. 2013; Wu et al. 2009; Bloemendal et al. 2020; Porta et al. 2016). The process operated entirely autonomously to provide up to 10 grams scale preparations of a wide variety of oxazoles as depicted in Figure 1.75. This automated sequence was also one of the first to introduce the addition of solid-support scavenger QP-BZA to the end of continuous flow reactor setups in order to provide facile in-process purification (Figure 1.76).

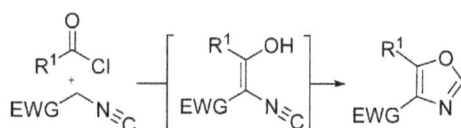

FIGURE 1.74 Model synthesis of 4,5-disubstituted oxazoles from alkyl isocyanates and acyl chlorides. (Reprinted (adapted) with permission from Organic Letters, "Fully Automated Continuous Flow Synthesis of 4,5-Disubstituted Oxazoles", Baumann, M. et al, 2006. Copyright 2006 American Chemical Society.)

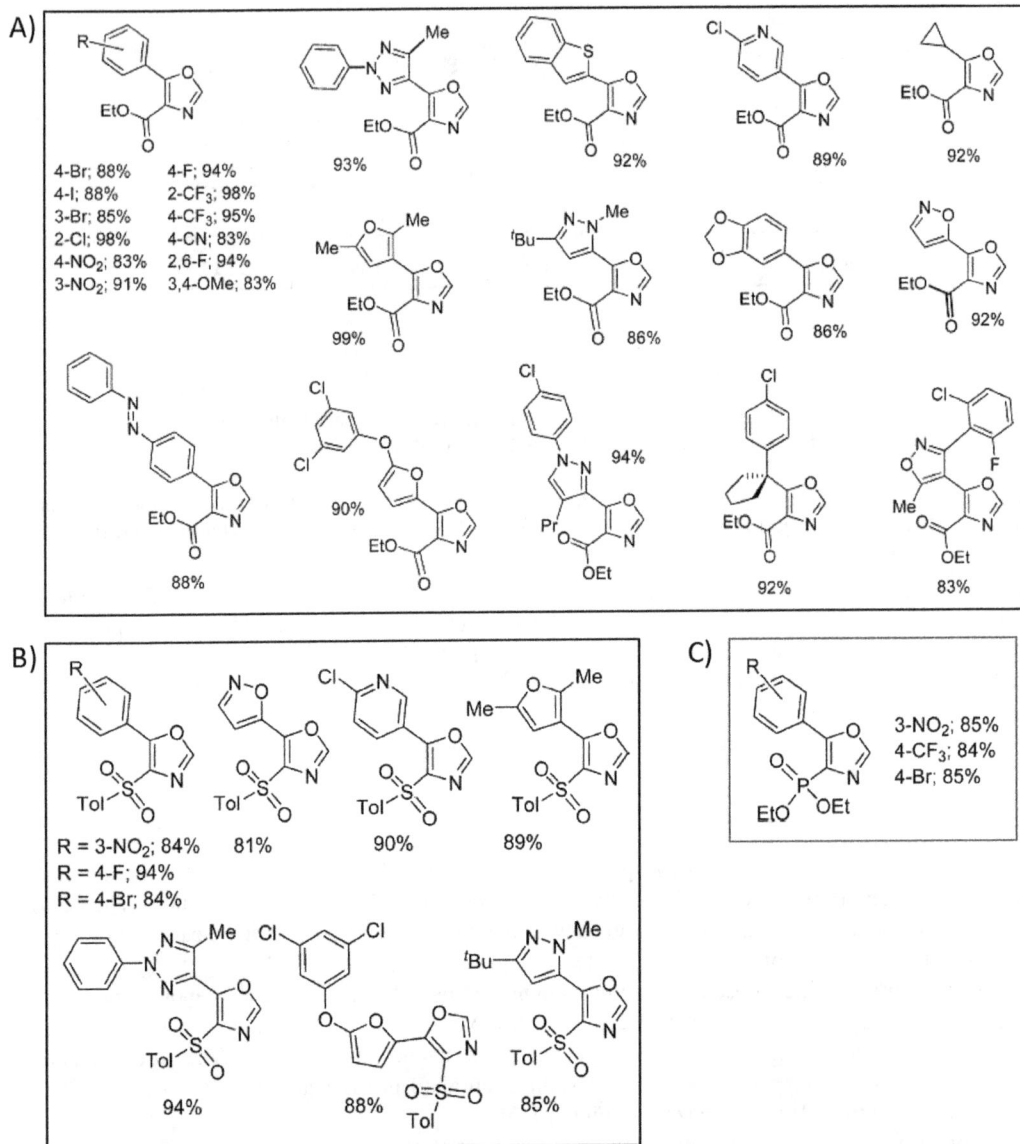

FIGURE 1.75 Scope of prepared 4,5-disubstited oxazoles. (Reprinted (adapted) with permission from Organic Letters, "Fully Automated Continuous Flow Synthesis of 4,5-Disubstituted Oxazoles", Baumann, M. et al, 2006. Copyright 2006 American Chemical Society.)

1.4.3.4 Efavirenz

The aforementioned isocyanate moiety is a common intermediate found in a number of API synthe- ses, a recent example being the flow synthesis of Efavirenz published in partnership by Seeberger and McQuade's groups in 2015 (Correia et al. 2015). With manufacturing routes published by Merck and Lonza, the bulk of the challenges present in the synthesis of this HIV drug present themselves in the installation and subsequent cyclization of the carbamate core. Toxic reagents and downstream purifi- cation protocols pose detrimental drawbacks towards potential scale-up of the existing manufacturing procedures. Careful manipulation of an *in-situ* formed isocyanate to deliver the *N*-aryl carbamate in a single step was employed in this work to achieve more ideal PMI and improve the overall process safety (Figure 1.77).

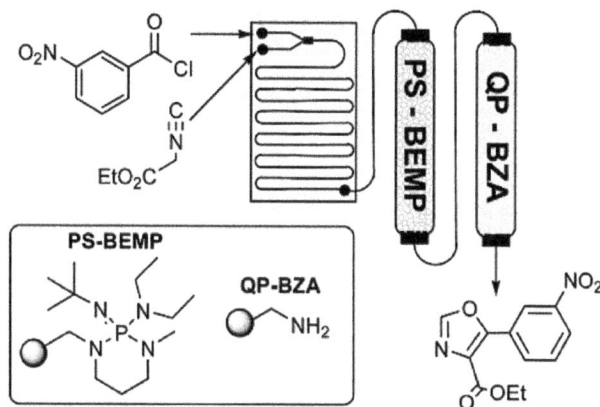

FIGURE 1.76 Reaction diagram featuring in-line purification with QP-BZA column. (Reprinted (adapted) with permission from Organic Letters, "Fully Automated Continuous Flow Synthesis of 4,5-Disubstituted Oxazoles", Baumann, M. et al, 2006. Copyright 2006 American Chemical Society.)

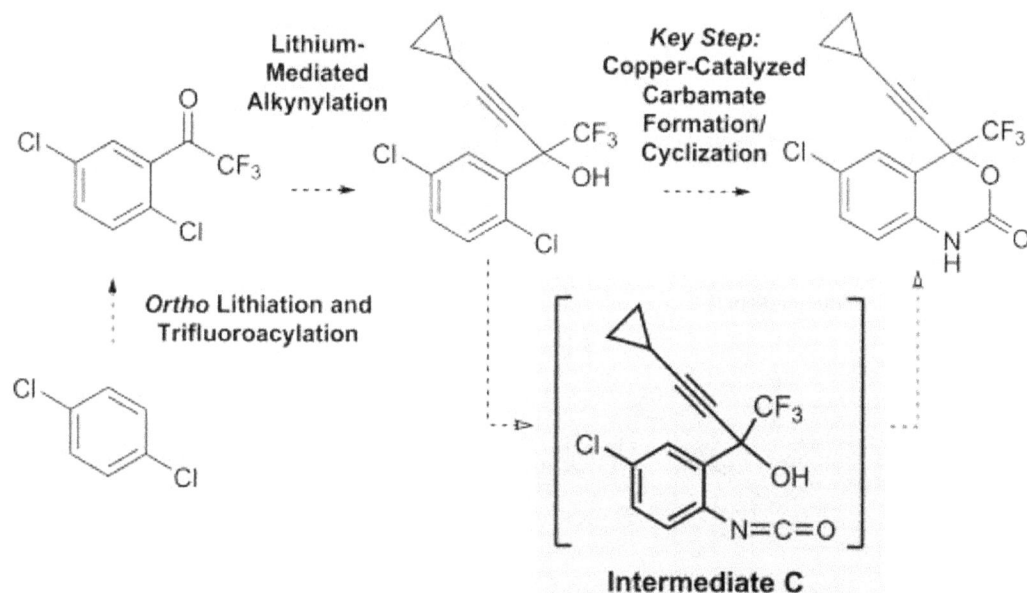

FIGURE 1.77 Flow route towards efavirenz featuring a one-step carbamate formation/cyclization. (Reprinted with permission from Angewandte Chemie – International Edition, "A Concise Flow Synthesis of Efavirenz", Correia, C.A. et al, 2015. Copyright 2015 WILEY-VCH Verlag GmbH & Co. KGaA, Weinheim.)

The initial stage of the Efavirenz synthesis features the ortho-lithiation of 1,2-dichlorobenzene, forming the unstable intermediate 2,5-dichlorophenyllithium. Despite the superior heat transfer and increased reaction rates already offered by flow reaction systems, further attention to detail in maintaining precise consistent temperature over the course of this 3-stage reaction sequence was required to attenuate potential decomposition and clogging. A partitioned cold bath with a submerged passage in the T-junction between the formation of this intermediate and its introduction to the third loop provided the best results for maintaining optimal conversion and flow rate (Figure 1.78).

Telescoping these reaction conditions through the following trifluoroacylation and lithium-mediated alkynylation was carried out. Judicious selection of reagents and solid-support scavengers was made to account for potential byproduct formation that may impede downstream reactions. The final

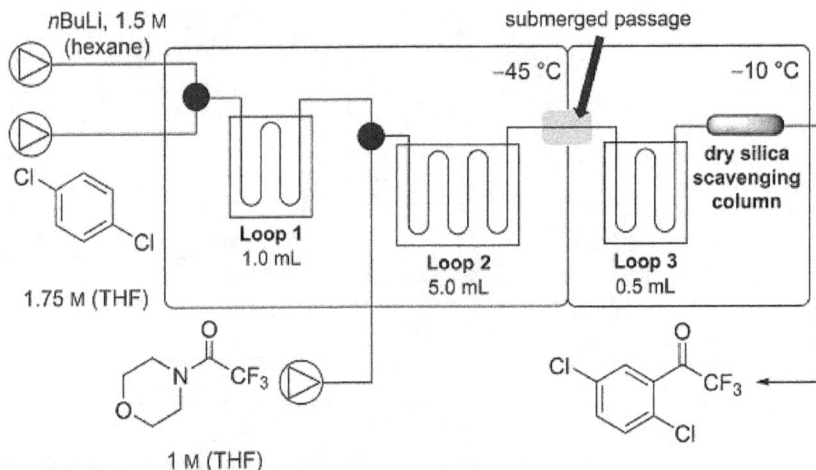

FIGURE 1.78   Continuous flow reactor scheme for the preparation of the trifluoromethyl ketone en route towards efavirenz. (Reprinted with permission from Angewandte Chemie – International Edition, "A Concise Flow Synthesis of Efavirenz", Correia, C.A. et al, 2015. Copyright 2015 WILEY-VCH Verlag GmbH & Co. KGaA, Weinheim.)

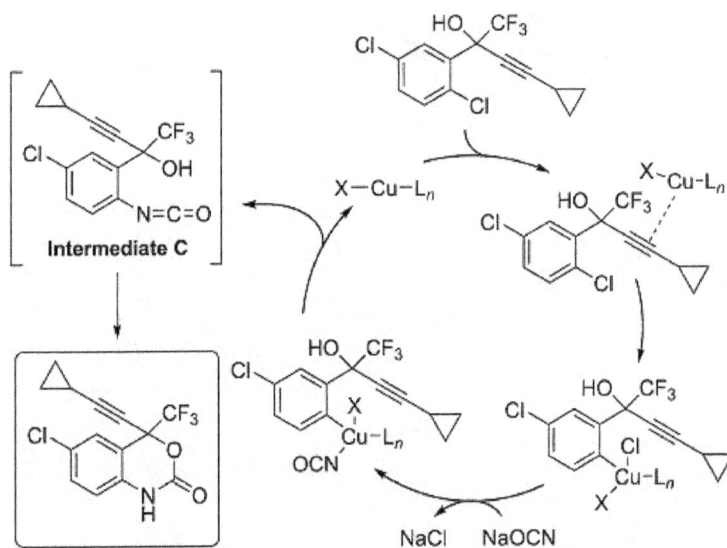

FIGURE 1.79   Proposed mechanism for copper-catalyzed cyclization that proceeds through an isocyanate intermediate C. (Reprinted with permission from Angewandte Chemie – International Edition, "A Concise Flow Synthesis of Efavirenz", Correia, C.A. et al, 2015. Copyright 2015 WILEY-VCH Verlag GmbH & Co. KGaA, Weinheim.)

copper-catalyzed carbamation and tandem cyclization reaction served as the final innovation of this novel continuous sequence, where numerous copper catalysts and ligand combinations were screened for reactivity and solubility purposes. Introduction of sodium cyanate to form an *in-situ* reactive isocyanate is the key feature of the proposed mechanism behind this process (Figure 1.79).

The copper-catalyzed carbamation conditions were developed with additional insights provided from the analogous palladium-catalyzed reaction first reported by Buchwald's group (Vinogradova et al. 2013). The intermediary isocyanate allows for the cyclization to occur under thermodynamic conditions post-reductive elimination, yielding the *rac*-Efavirenz in 62% isolated yield for an overall yield of 45% through three semi-continuous steps. This optimized semi-continuous flow process featuring a heterogeneous catalyst in a PBR provides a significant reduction in processing time, catalyst loading, and PMI in comparison with reported batch manufacturing processes.

1.4.3.5 Hydroxychloroquine

Hydroxychloroquine is a high-volume essential medicine with prohibitively high manufacturing costs in the existing batch process, limiting global access to the API. These costs arise from lengthy processing time, bulky expensive reactors, and expensive advanced starting materials (Yu et al. 2018). Yu et al. at Medicines for All sought to develop a novel, cost-effective continuous flow process starting from cheaper, more abundant commodity chemicals. Key modifications to the batch manufacturing route include avoidance of the ketone protecting group strategy and more expedient reaction conditions to cut down on plant operating time. As the chemistry employed in this strategy is all known, the challenge presented itself in developing reactors and engineering solutions to adapting these research laboratory techniques to an industry-friendly format.

It was believed that swapping chloro-pentanone coupling partner from the commercial route with an iodo-pentanone analogue would boost yield for the desired S_N2 displacement as shown in Figure 1.80. Potential cost concerns were addressed by preparing the material *in situ* from a cheap furan derivative and HI in the absence of solvent.

Implementation of a Zaiput membrane-based separator allowed for in-line purification and removal of excess acid to permit telescoping of the formed material in the following base-mediated amination step, forming ketoxime 16 in 78% isolated yield. The ideal envisaged reductive amination of 16 would proceed through catalytic hydrogenation with commercially available Raney-nickel through adaptation of prior mentioned innovations on continuous catalytic hydrogenations (Yu et al. 2020). By connecting an HPLC pump to a CSTR pressurized under hydrogen gas, the material could be formed in the tank reactor and removed via a dip tube outfitted with a metal filter. In this way the amine product could be isolated while retaining the Raney-nickel in the CSTR, allowing for efficient flow throughput with optimal material consumption and minimized mass loss (Figure 1.81).

The final step in the commercial preparation of hydroxychloroquine is carried out neat in high yields but requires high temperatures and 48 hours reaction time. Therefore, this step was considered ideal for translation into a continuous flow motif to drastically reduce reaction time. Addition of a 1:1 ratio of K_2CO_3/Et_3N was found to speed up reaction time considerably, while the high viscosity of the reaction mixture naturally lent itself towards implementation in a second CSTR for continuous processing purposes. This base-promoted C-N coupling provided hydroxychloroquine in 78% yield in 6 hours at 125°C. Overall, Yu et al. demonstrated that hydroxychloroquine could be prepared semi-continuously in 41% yield with total retention and processing time of 10.5 hours, a drastic reduction in operation time. This

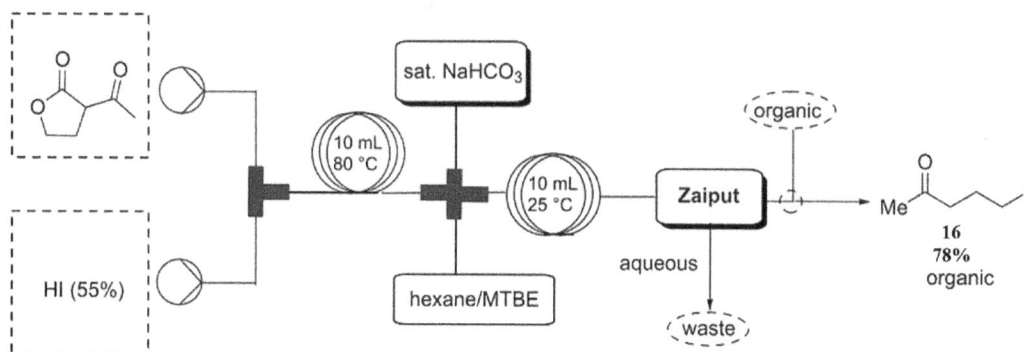

FIGURE 1.80 Flow diagram for the preparation of the iodo-pentanone 16. (Reprinted from https://www.beilstein-journals. org/bjoc/articles/14/45. All further use and permissions should be directed to the license and the Beilstein Journal of Organic Chemistry terms and conditions: (https://www.beilstein-journals.org/bjoc). Copyright 2018.)

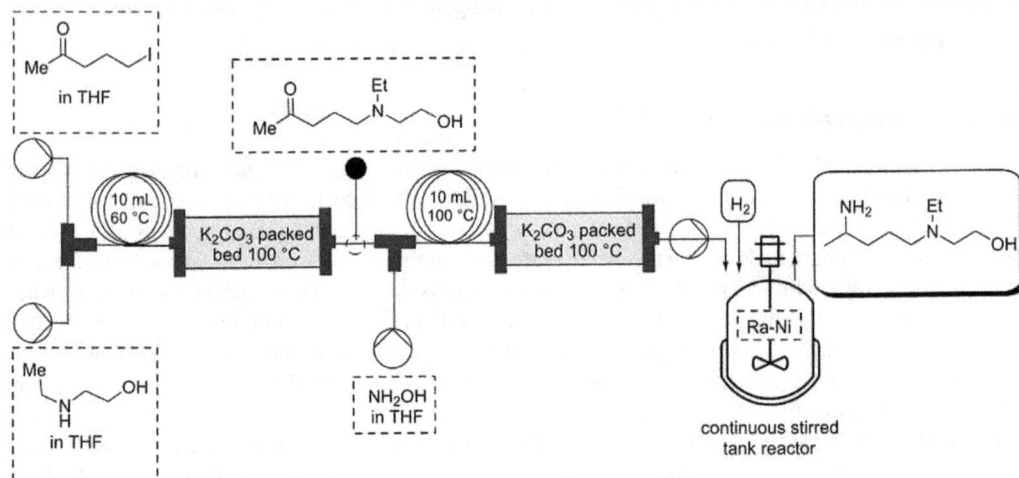

FIGURE 1.81 Optimization of the reductive amination of the iodo-pentanone. (Reprinted from https://www.beilstein-journals.org/bjoc/articles/14/45. All further use and permissions should be directed to the license and the Beilstein Journal of Organic Chemistry terms and conditions: (https://www.beilstein-journals.org/bjoc). Copyright 2018.)

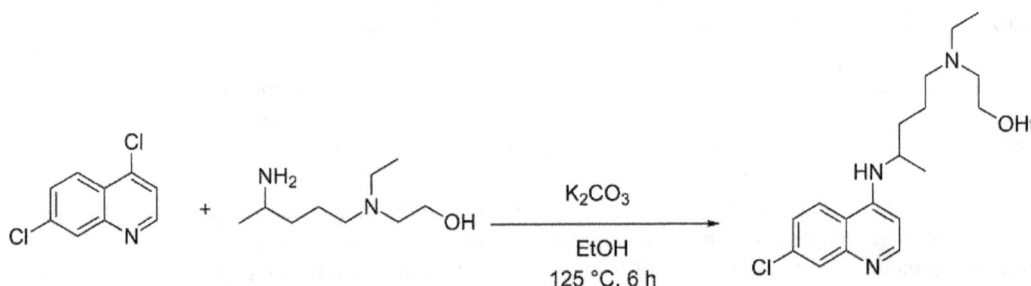

FIGURE 1.82 Optimized conditions for the preparation of hydroxychloroquine. (Reprinted from https://www.beilstein-journals.org/bjoc/articles/14/45. All further use and permissions should be directed to the license and the Beilstein Journal of Organic Chemistry terms and conditions: (https://www.beilstein-journals.org/bjoc). Copyright 2018.)

route offers improvements in raw material cost and availability of starting materials and demonstrates the versatility of reactor platforms that are able to be implemented in series successfully (Figure 1.82).

1.4.3.6 Drug-Like Pyrrolidines Library

Baumann et al. developed a flow synthesis of nitro-pyrrolidines from a [3 + 2] cycloaddition with attenuation of the delayed exotherms attributed to these types of reactions (Baumann et al. 2011). As the pyrrolidine motif is an important pharmacophore in API development, an effort was made towards developing a continuous protocol for the synthesis of drug-like pyrrolidine molecules for the purposes of building a corporate compound drug library (PharmaBlock, n.d.; Yamazaki et al. 2021; Paymode et al. 2020). The bulk of the innovation present came from developing reactors that cut down time as much as possible while making as few modifications to existing synthetic routes as possible, so that the library could be kept as broad as the existing literature precedent allows. To this aim, an emphasis on catalytic reactions and manipulation of timing and thermal regulation was demonstrated in the development of the flow reactor systems (Figure 1.83).

Baumann et al. utilized a Vapourtec R2+/R4 flow system fitted with a back-pressure regulator to allow for superheating of the initial nitroalkene flow stream to make them more reactive. Further modification

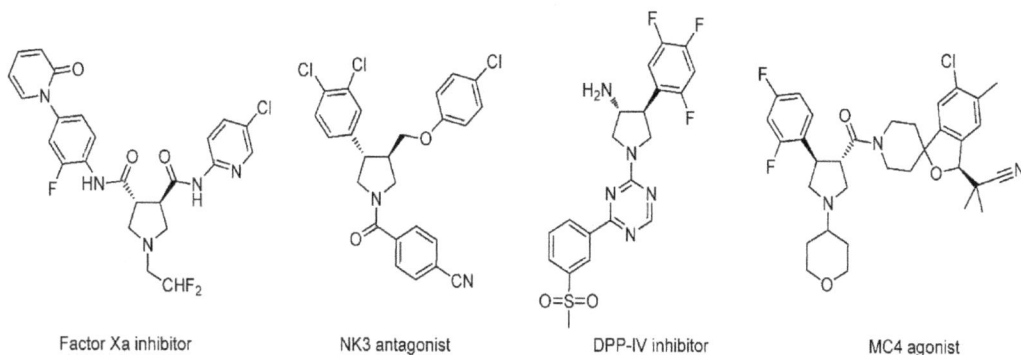

FIGURE 1.83 Advanced pharmaceutical compounds containing pyrrolidine motif. (Reprinted with permission from ACS Combinatorial Science, "Synthesis of a Drug-Like Focused Library of Trisubstituted Pyrrolidines Using Integrated Flow Chemistry and Batch Methods", Baumann, M. et al, 2011. Copyright 2011 American Chemical Society.)

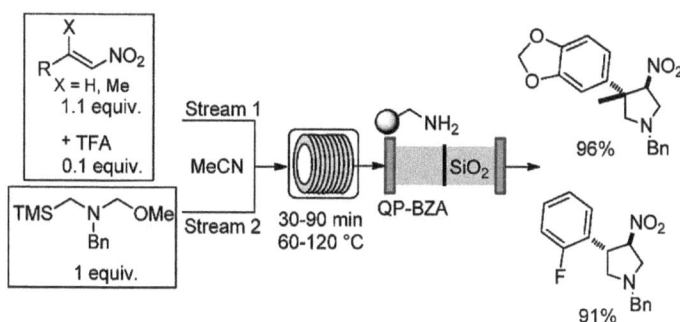

FIGURE 1.84 Flow synthesis of pyrrolidines using in-line purification via QP-BZA column. (Reprinted with permission from ACS Combinatorial Science, "Synthesis of a Drug-Like Focused Library of Trisubstituted Pyrrolidines Using Integrated Flow Chemistry and Batch Methods", Baumann, M. et al, 2011. Copyright 2011 American Chemical Society.)

to the original process was the use of catalytic amounts of TFA in place of a fluoride ion-exchange resin PBR so as to cut down on reaction time and increase overall throughput for large-scale production purposes.

To further reduce unit operations the process adopted in-line purification through a series of solid-support scavengers connected at the end of the reactor, as depicted above in Figure 1.84. The crude material was passed through a packed bed of QuadraPure polymer supported benzylamine (QP-BZA) and silicon dioxide to remove excess nitroalkene, TFA, and other impurities. This permitted telescoping of the nitro compounds through various amination protocols (Figure 1.85).

Two methods for telescoped amination, depicted above, were explored: catalytic hydrogenation under Raney Ni in an H-Cube reactor and comparatively mild excess stannous chloride (SnCl$_2$) at reflux to provide chemoselective reductive amination. The resultant amines were converted to amido-pyrrolidines through addition of triethylamine and varied acid chlorides, then deprotected through catalytic hydrogenation. Acid byproducts were removed from the system in the same manner as the previous step by end-stage addition of a QP-BZA packed column. Repeating this reaction sequence with sulfonyl chloride in lieu of acid chloride afforded the sulfonamide products in yields greater than 90% after normal evaporation of solvent. These three-step protocols featuring in-line purification of intermediates and products provide efficient access to a wide array of trisubstituted pyrrolidines, providing an early framework for API manufacturers looking to develop a cost-effective route to any drug-relevant target from this broad library (Figure 1.86).

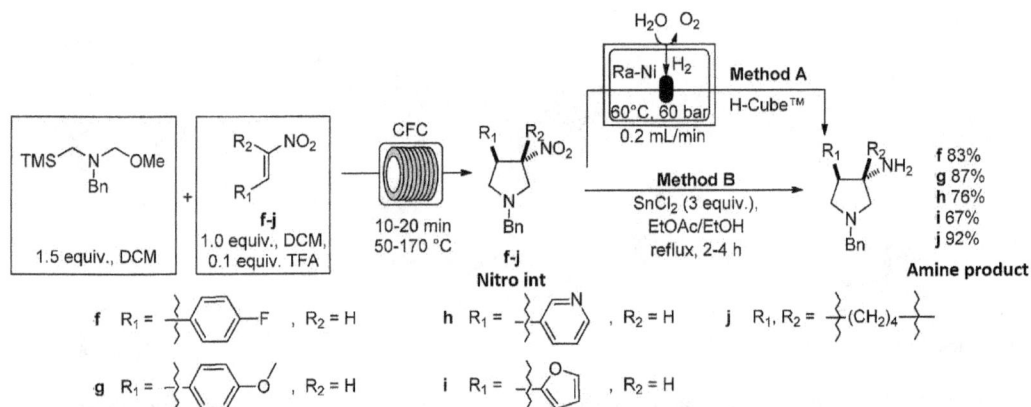

FIGURE 1.85 Flow [3 + 2] cycloaddition of nitro olefins and their subsequent reduction under two different continuous flow conditions to afford amino-pyrrolidines f-j. (Reprinted with permission from ACS Combinatorial Science, "Synthesis of a Drug-Like Focused Library of Trisubstituted Pyrrolidines Using Integrated Flow Chemistry and Batch Methods", Baumann, M. et al, 2011. Copyright 2011 American Chemical Society.)

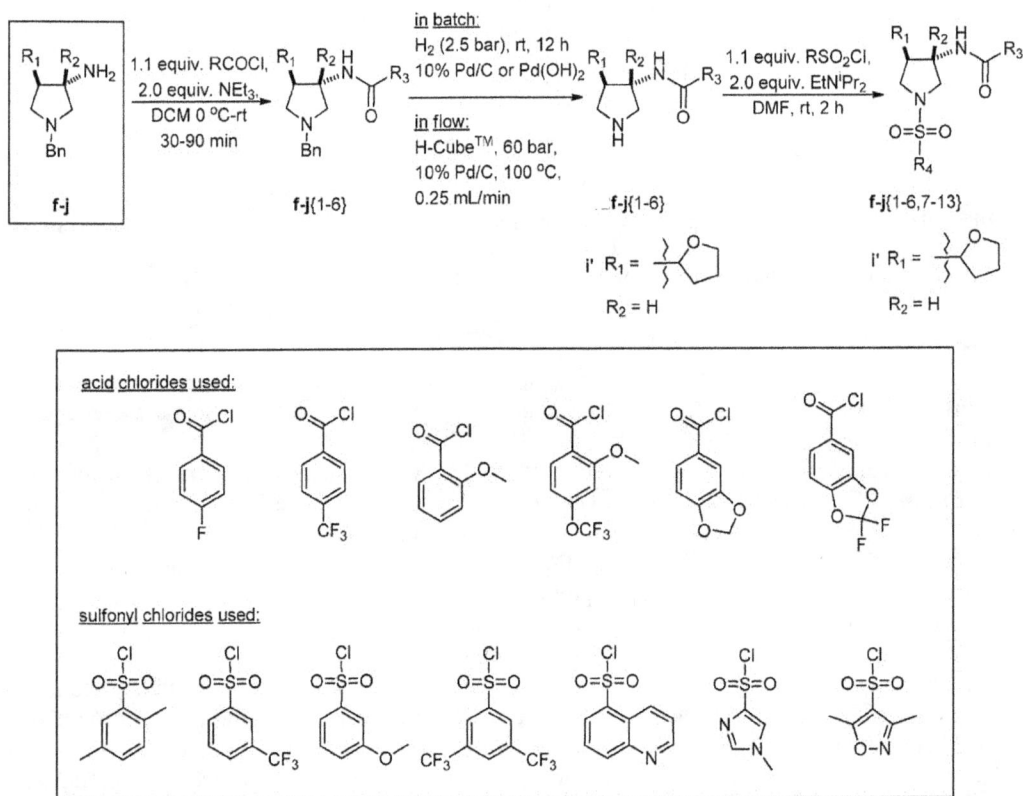

FIGURE 1.86 Amidation of the pyrrolidine intermediates, deprotection, and addition of sulfonyl functional groups to afford target sulfonamides. (Reprinted with permission from ACS Combinatorial Science, "Synthesis of a Drug-Like Focused Library of Trisubstituted Pyrrolidines Using Integrated Flow Chemistry and Batch Methods", Baumann, M. et al, 2011. Copyright 2011 American Chemical Society.)

1.4.3.7 Endoperoxide OZ439

Resistance to antibiotics is a growing concern in the global health industry, in particular for drugs prescribed for the treatment of widespread infections such as malaria (Hastings et al. 2002). For this reason, a number of novel drug candidates with improved pharmacokinetic and pharmacodynamic properties have been developed (Kopetzki et al. 2013; Lévesque and Seeberger 2012; Yu et al. 2018; Flannery et al. 2013). Many of these drug candidates feature 1,2,4-trioxolane cores similar to common malarial treatment drug artemisinin and its derivatives (Flannery et al. 2013). One such endoperoxide, OZ439, has passed Phase 1 clinical trials by the NIH in 2018 and has been identified as having promise for a single-dose treatment for malaria (Vennerstrom et al. 2004; Lau et al. 2015). There is a significant need for a cost-effective route towards this and other trioxolane-core drug candidates to secure a supply of this drug for the economically disadvantaged who are most susceptible to infection by malaria. Towards this aim, Lau et al. in a collaborative effort between the University of Cambridge, Departamento de Química, and GSK developed a continuous flow process for the preparation of OZ439 that features machine-assisted technology and significant improvements in cost and safety (Lau et al. 2015) (Figure 1.87).

The collaborative effort utilized cheaper, more abundant biphenol 7 for selective reduction to afford the cyclohexan-1-one starting material. This material was then telescoped through ozonolysis with the O-methyl oxime moiety 5 from the manufacturing route. Concurrent amidation through simple S_N2 to form the ethyl morpholine precursor 17 and subsequent reduction allowed convenient access *to* OZ439 in four linear steps (Figure 1.88).

Prior art from Ley's group on selective reduction under trickle bed heterogeneous catalysis in an HEL FlowCAT was utilized to convert biphenol to 18 in 58% yield upon crystallization, with a throughput of 400 mg/hr (Ouchi et al. 2014); 18 could then be carried forward upon isolation to the next flow reactor for acetylation in near quantitative yield (Figures 1.89 and 1.90).

The acetyl cyclohexane-1-one was able to be telescoped into the third stage reaction without purification, though this reaction presented challenges of potential blockage as solvent was prone to evaporating under the biphasic reaction conditions. Some clever reaction engineering was implemented to fine-tune the Griesbaum Co-ozonolysis, focused on diluting the concentration of the gas input to increase solvent ratios while still allowing for ideal liquid-gas plug flow (Figure 1.91).

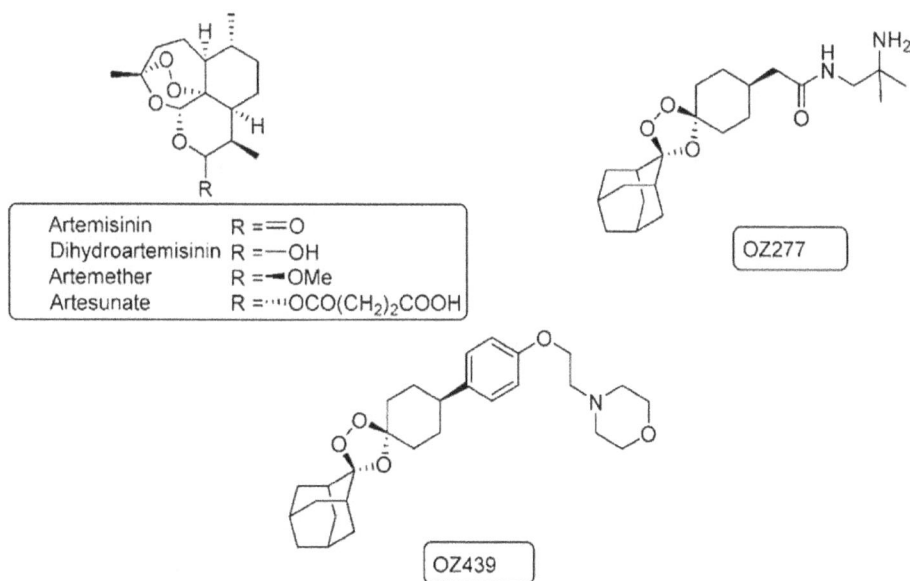

Artemisinin	R ==O
Dihydroartemisinin	R =—OH
Artemether	R =—OMe
Artesunate	R =···OCO(CH₂)₂COOH

FIGURE 1.87 Depiction of artemisinin, its derivatives, OZ277 and OZ439. (Reprinted from https://pubs.acs.org/doi/abs/10.1021/acs.orglett.5b01307. All further use and permissions should be directed to ACS.)

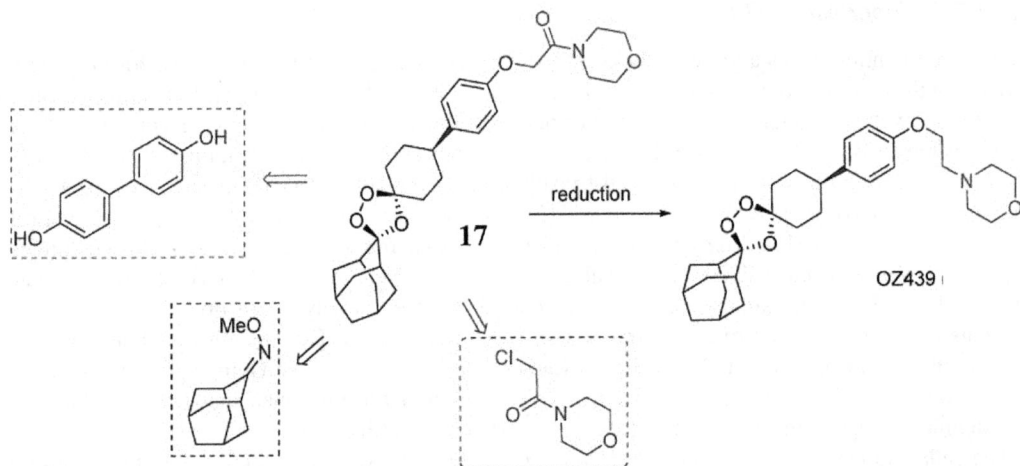

FIGURE 1.88 Retrosynthetic analysis of OZ439 proceeding through 17 prepared from 3 commercially available starting materials. (Reprinted from https://pubs.acs.org/doi/abs/10.1021/acs.orglett.5b01307. All further use and permissions should be directed to ACS.)

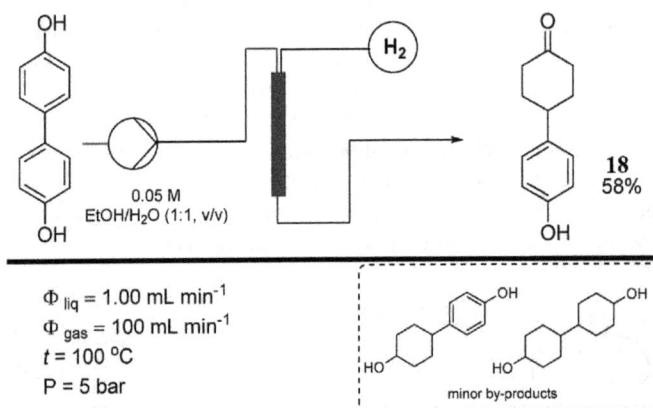

FIGURE 1.89 Selective continuous hydrogenation of 4,4′-Biphenol to 18. (Reprinted from https://pubs.acs.org/doi/abs/10.1021/acs.orglett.5b01307. All further use and permissions should be directed to ACS.)

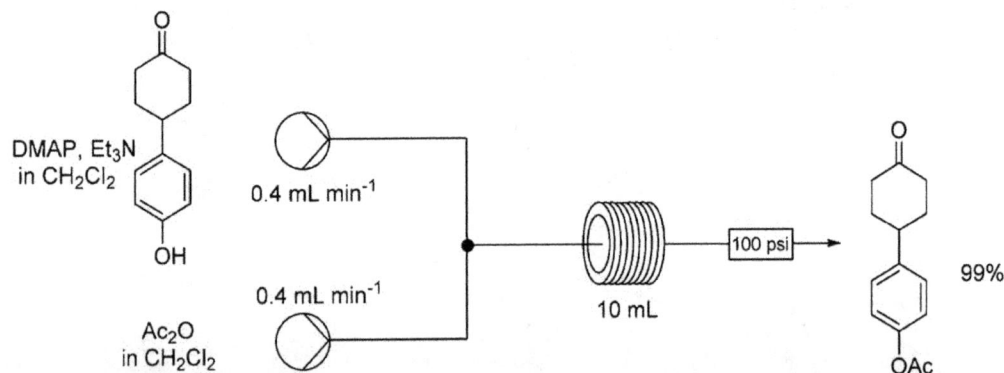

FIGURE 1.90 Flow acetylation of 4-(4-Hydroxyphenyl)cyclohexan-1-one under continuous flow. (Reprinted from https://pubs.acs.org/doi/abs/10.1021/acs.orglett.5b01307. All further use and permissions should be directed to ACS.)

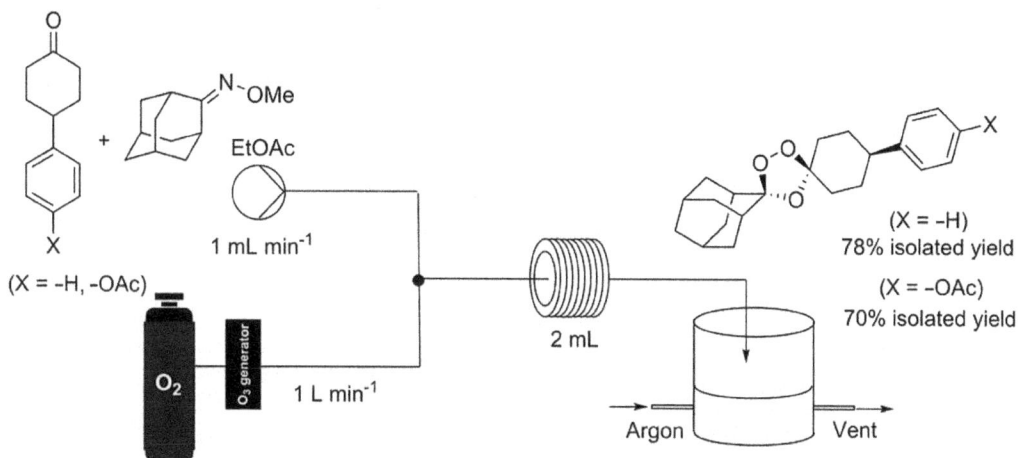

FIGURE 1.91 Flow reactor setup for the Griesbaum co-ozonylsis. (Adapted from https://pubs.acs.org/doi/abs/10.1021/acs. orglett.5b01307. All further use and permissions should be directed to ACS.)

Designing the flow exit stream to pass through an argon-filled chamber allowed for the venting of excess ozone in a safe and efficient manner, overall improving the safety of conducting co-ozonolysis reactions through transfer to this continuous process method. Elimination of the need for genotoxic agent 4-(2-chloroethyl)morpholine by instead focusing on direct amidation and zinc-catalyzed amide-selective reduction in a two-step batch process allowed for production of OZ439 in 86% isolated yield over two steps with an overall yield of 39% across four linear steps. This new flow route demonstrates cost reduction through the use of cheaper, more abundant feedstock, atom economical transformations conducted under continuous flow to boost yield, throughput and scalability, and the elimination of a genotoxic reagent to realize a more accessible route towards OZ439 (Figure 1.92).

1.4.3.8 KRAIC: Continuous Crystallization

While biphasic continuous flow processes are not uncommon, a longstanding setback in the implementation of continuous technology in pharmaceutical development has been the incompatibility of tubing-based flow chemistry and standard crystallization techniques. CSTRs provide a stopgap between this barrier but do not address the inferior scalability offered by these reactors compared to small internal diameter (ID) tubing reactors. For this reason, Robertson et al. developed a plug flow crystallization using a tri-segmented tubular system dubbed the "kinetically regulated automated input crystallizer" (KRAIC) that provided true end-to-end continuous flow synthesis and product crystallization (Robertson et al. 2016). The tri-segmented crystallizer works by segmenting the reaction mixture with air and a selected immiscible solvent to generate plug flow and provide separation of solution droplets (Figures 1.93 and 1.94).

Scott et al. then demonstrated the utility of this continuous crystallizer in the flow synthesis of the tuberculosis API building block pyrazinamide, demonstrating polymorph form selectivity as proof of concept for the utility this process holds for API process design (Daniel Scott et al. 2018) (Figures 1.95 and 1.96).

Controlled nucleation through a swap of organic and supersaturated aqueous solvent offered access to γ and α-pyrazinamide respectively through continuous KRAIC crystallization. This design was also easily attached to the catalytic hydration reactor that prepared the pyrazinamide from pyrazinecarbonitrile, allowing facile continuous crystallization without modification to the reactor system (Figures 1.97 and 1.98).

1.4.3.9 AI Cloud-Based Server Designed Routes to Three APIs

Perhaps one of the most sought-after technologies of the past decade has been the development of AI-assisted automated technology for manufacturing purposes (Epps et al. 2021; Struble et al. 2020; Grisoni et al. 2021). The pharmaceutical industry is no exception to this desired shift in paradigm. The

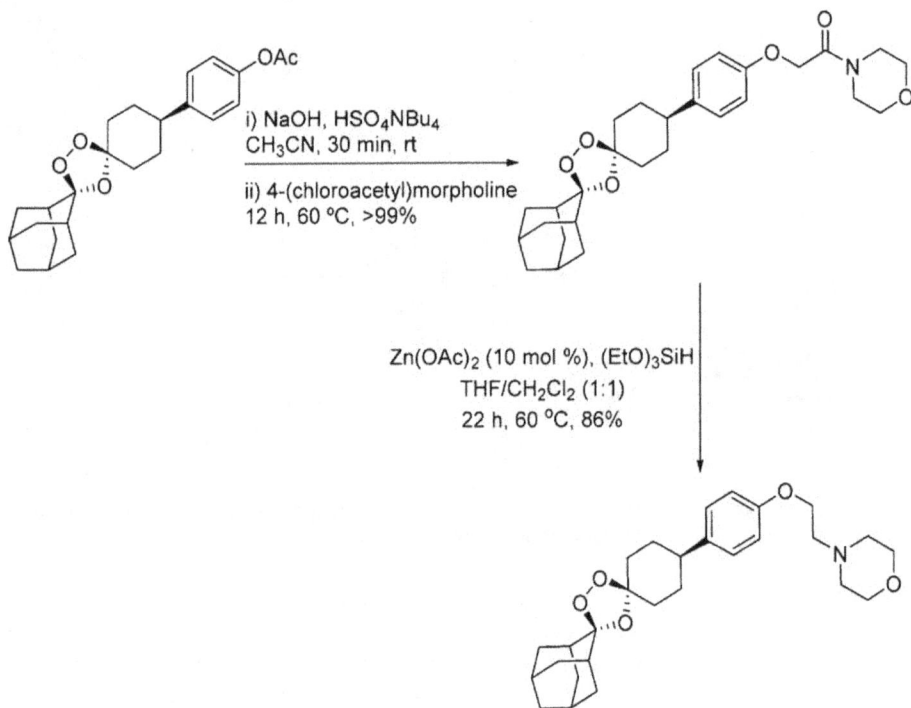

FIGURE 1.92 Final synthesis of OZ439 via amide reduction. (Reprinted from https://pubs.acs.org/doi/abs/10.1021/acs. orglett.5b01307. All further use and permissions should be directed to ACS.)

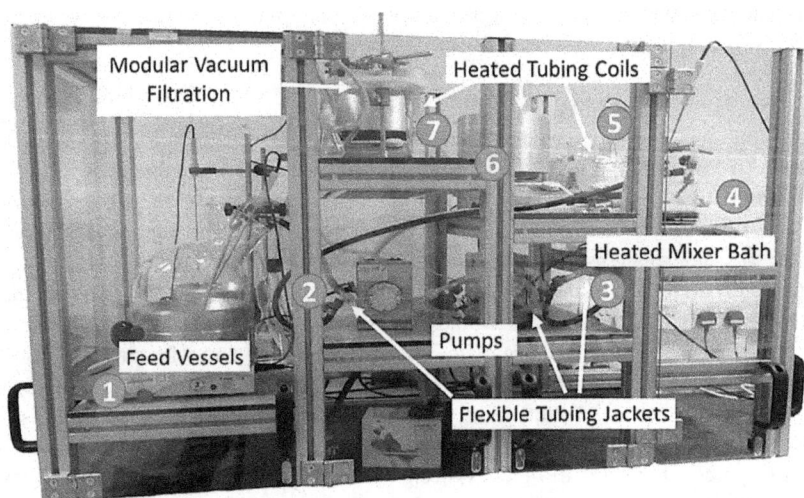

FIGURE 1.93 Depiction of KRAIC (Kinetically-Regulated Automated Input Crystallizer). (Reprinted with permission from Crystal Growth & Design, "Design and Evaluation of a Meso-scale Segmented Flow Reactor (KRAIC)", Roberston, K. et al, 2016. Copyright 2016 American Chemical Society.)

current API manufacturing process involves a planning stage where retrosynthetic viability, cost, efficiency, and sustainability are all taken into consideration and evaluated by process chemists prior to optimization of the predetermined synthetic pathway. Through the use of a cloud-based server, Fitzpatrick et al. demonstrated simultaneous route scouting and optimization of various reaction combinations with automated continuous flow systems for the development of three different APIs: tramadol, lidocaine, and

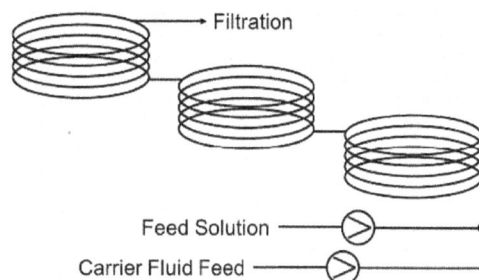

FIGURE 1.94 Schematic of KRAIC with a single-feed setup. (Reprinted with permission from Crystal Growth & Design, "Design and Evaluation of a Meso-scale Segmented Flow Reactor (KRAIC)", Roberston, K. et al, 2016. Copyright 2016 American Chemical Society.)

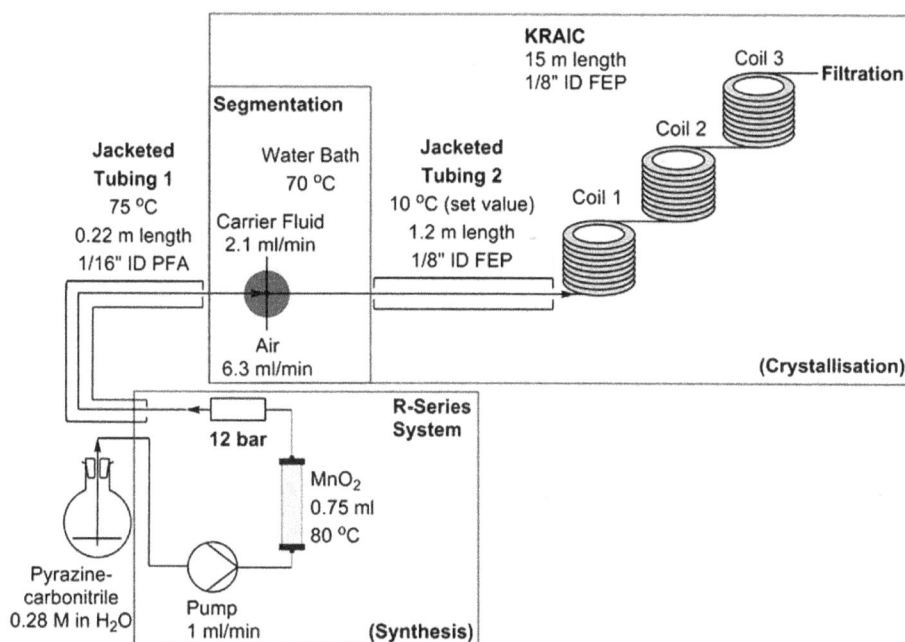

FIGURE 1.95 Diagram of continuous flow synthesis and in-line crystallization for API building block pyrazinamide production featuring controlled nucleation. (Reprinted with permission from C.D. Scott, R. Labes, M. Depardieu, C. Battilocchio, M.G. Davidson, S.V. Ley, C.C. Wilson and K. Robertson, *React. Chem. Eng.*, 2018, **3**, 631 – Published by The Royal Society of Chemistry.)

bupropion (Fitzpatrick et al. 2018). The research team located in Los Angeles was able to access a server in Japan to conduct and supervise the autonomous flow reactors utilized for this study.

A general equipment layout of widely available supply lines, reactor coils, and in-line monitoring equipment such as FlowIR units were acquired so that a single system could be reconfigured to accommodate various reactions of a wide and potentially conflicting nature with minimal oversight. Each API synthesis explored sought to optimize a predetermined number of parameters for each individual reaction step in sequence for successful implementation of the overall process. The below Grignard addition to form tramadol, as depicted in Figure 1.99, was the initial reaction that the team explored using this cloud-based autonomous method, optimizing conversion through automated screens of temperature, residence time, and equivalents of pre-formed Grignard reagent. Autonomous experimentation and evaluation of parameters by the cloud-based server AI determined the ideal reaction conditions within 3 hours and was able to provide 0.172 g/mL per hour of tramadol, far outstripping the previously reported outputs of 0.045 g/mL per hour.

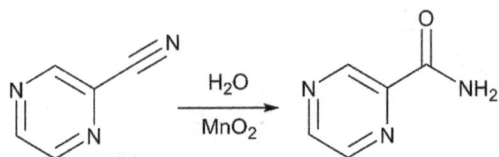

FIGURE 1.96 Catalytic hydration of pyrazinecarbonitrile under continuous flow. (Reprinted with permission from C.D. Scott, R. Labes, M. Depardieu, C. Battilocchio, M.G. Davidson, S.V. Ley, C.C. Wilson and K. Robertson, *React. Chem. Eng.*, 2018, **3**, 631 – Published by The Royal Society of Chemistry.)

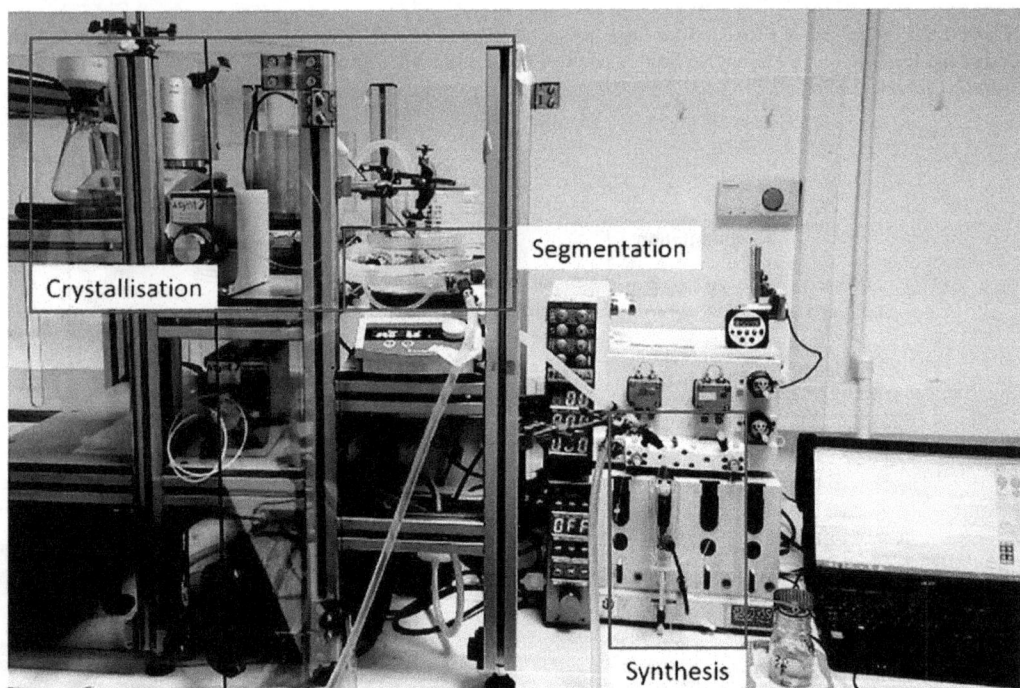

FIGURE 1.97 Connected continuous crystallization and segmentation apparatus. (Reprinted with permission from C.D. Scott, R. Labes, M. Depardieu, C. Battilocchio, M.G. Davidson, S.V. Ley, C.C. Wilson and K. Robertson, *React. Chem. Eng.*, 2018, **3**, 631 – Published by The Royal Society of Chemistry.)

The preparation of lidocaine, which has also been well reported, was further improved upon through the autonomous flow system's AI (Reilly 1999; Karen Goodwin 2009; Britton et al. 2015). Fitzpatrick et al. added the additional consideration of energy usage to the algorithm's evaluation function and then screened the initial acylation reaction outlined below for ideal temperature, residence time, and equivalents of acid chloride similar to the tramadol optimization procedure (Figure 1.100).

The system optimized the reaction and ramped throughput to 39.7 grams of intermediate 19 after just over five hours for reaction optimization the next day. Following optimization of the alkylation step, lidocaine was prepared in 85% isolated yield (15.7 g) after just 8 hours of automated optimization and operation (Figure 1.101).

The final test of this fully automated system was the optimization and implementation of a fully continuous process for a drug that had previously only been reported in batch conditions. Fitzpatrick et al. sought to translate the two-step bromination and N-alkylation steps present in the preparation of the antidepressant Bupropion for this purpose (Figure 1.102).

Given that these reactions had not been telescoped previously, the researchers sought to optimize each reaction independently to maximize conversion prior to the development of the telescoped process. The

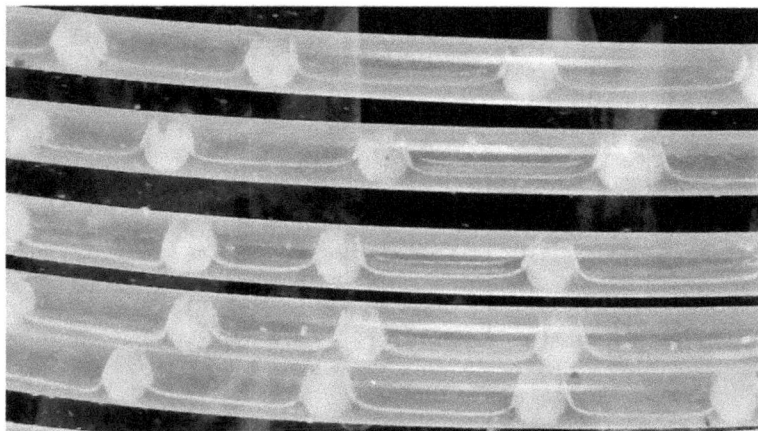

FIGURE 1.98 View of crystals flowing in sluf-flow during a controlled nucleation run. (C.D. Scott, R. Labes, M. Depardieu, C. Battilocchio, M.G. Davidson, S.V. Ley, C.C. Wilson and K. Robertson, *React. Chem. Eng.*, 2018, **3**, 631 – Published by The Royal Society of Chemistry.)

automated system developed an in-line workup procedure by quenching the bromination output stream with aqueous sodium bisulfite and then directing the organic layer output to the second stage reaction after removal of excess solvent via thin-film evaporation (Figure 1.103).

Remarkably, the AI was able to further optimize the reaction post-implementation of the workup stage by treating the full sequence as a single iteration for process intensification. The bromination step was now run in slight excess to reach quantitative yield and eliminate starting material from the output stream, while the concentration of amine coupling partner 20 was increased to provide a more ideal molar ratio of reagents exiting the thin-film evaporator. The AI system was thus able to develop, optimize, and implement a fully continuous process in 4 days with minimal oversight that produced bupropion at a rate of 2.88 g/hr. This ground-breaking autonomous system drastically reduces the need for personnel oversight and enables process scientists to devote their time towards synthetic mapping and other manufacturing concerns (Figure 1.104).

1.4.3.10 Aliskiren: Continuous Preparation from Reagent to Finished Drug Tablet

Heider et al. demonstrated an end-to-end continuous flow process for the preparation of aliskiren that notably features complete production from an advanced starting material to a finished tablet version of the pharmaceutical drug (Heider et al. 2014). Key features of this process include a continuous Boc deprotection with careful management of the salt waste flow stream, continuous liquid-liquid extraction and membrane-based separation, and demonstration of long-term continuous operation over a 240-hour run (Figure 1.105).

Beginning with advanced Boc-protected starting material 21, aminolysis was carried out neat under carboxylic acid catalysis. The reagents were stirred in a CSM and then transferred to a simple tube reactor inside an oven at 100°C where care was taken to evaluate the effects of residence time broadening to select the proper tubing diameter.

The resulting molten product 22 solidified if cooled below 80°C, so a liquid-liquid extraction was carried out using heated water and ethyl acetate. The organic phase was then separated through 12 membrane-based separators as depicted in Figure 1.106. Two backpressure regulators were added to the flow outlets post-separation to accommodate the resultant pressure build due to passing through these 1 μm pore size membranes. The organic outlet was fed into continuous crystallization units to afford 4 in 98.7% purity by HPLC, demonstrating the effectiveness of the membrane separators at purifying the organic flow stream.

a)

0.5 M, dry THF

MeOH

Dry THF

10 mL

BPR

(±)

MgBr

0.5 M, dry THF

Peristaltic

b)

$$F_{eval.} = \frac{1}{\tau} + 3\left(\frac{p}{p+s}\right) + 0.75\left(\frac{1}{x}\right)$$

Throughput   *Conversion*   *Consumption*

c)

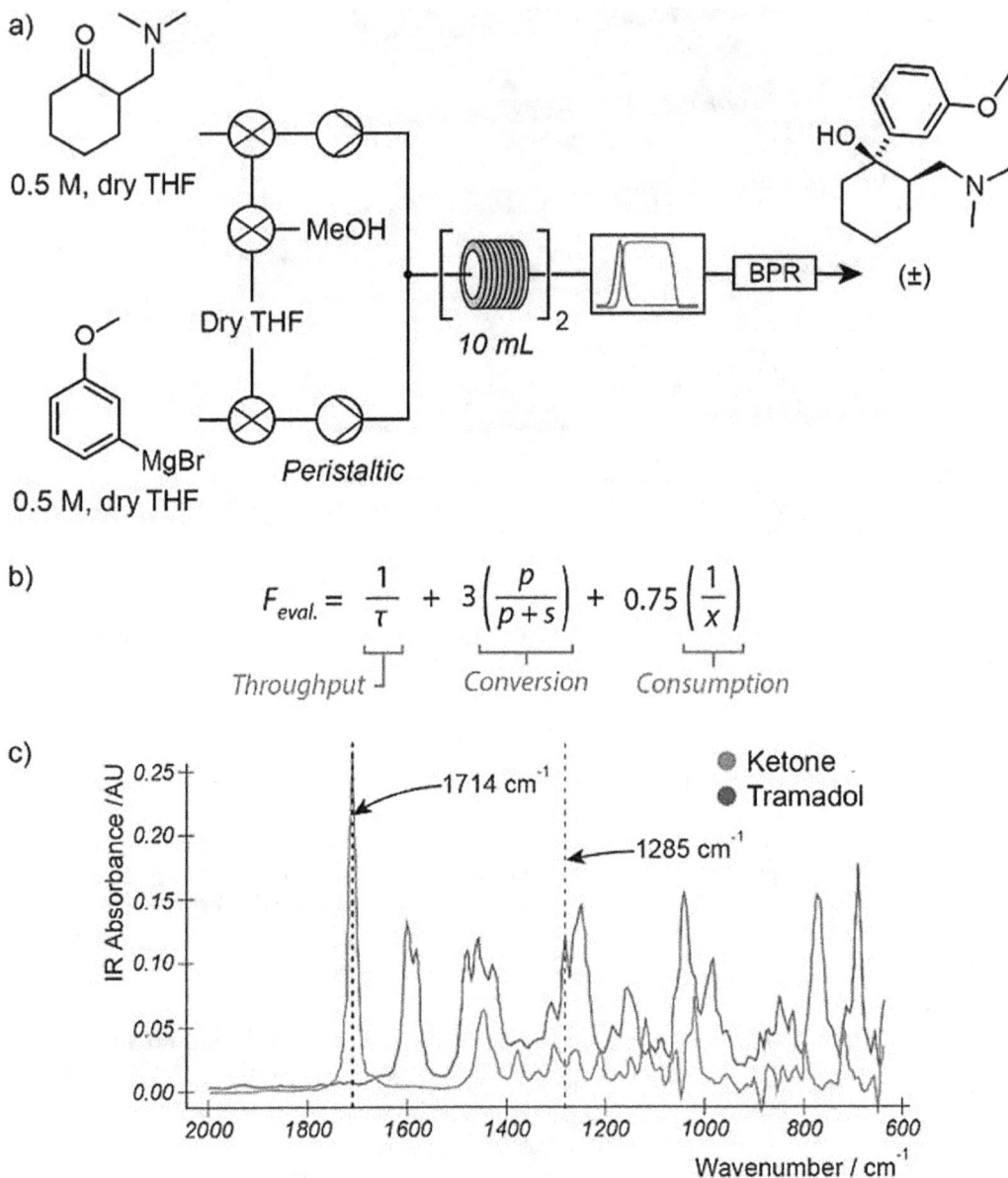

FIGURE 1.99 (a) Diagram of continuous flow synthesis of tramadol (b) calculation for evaluation function used by cloud-based AI in optimization of synthesis where p is Product IR absorbance, s is starting material IR absorbance, and x is equivalents of Grignard reagent (c) overlaid IR spectra of the target tramadol and ketone starting material. (Reprinted with permission from Angewandte Chemie – International Edition, "Across-the-world automated optimization and continuous flow synthesis of pharmaceutical agents operating through a cloud-based server", Fitzpatrick, D.E., 2018. Copyright 2018 The Authors. Published by Wiley-VCH Verlag GmbH & Co. KGaA.)

The ethyl acetate flow stream of 22 was then combined with aqueous HCl to remove the Boc protecting group. As this reaction results in the evolution of CO_2, attenuation of the tubing diameter and flow rate was required to ensure the gas did not disturb the flow rate and cause fouling of the system. It was found that plant scale operation was achievable by feeding the flow reactor with dual-head peristaltic pumps that could flow separate parallel flow lines at the same flow rate, so that the separate HCl and organic

a)

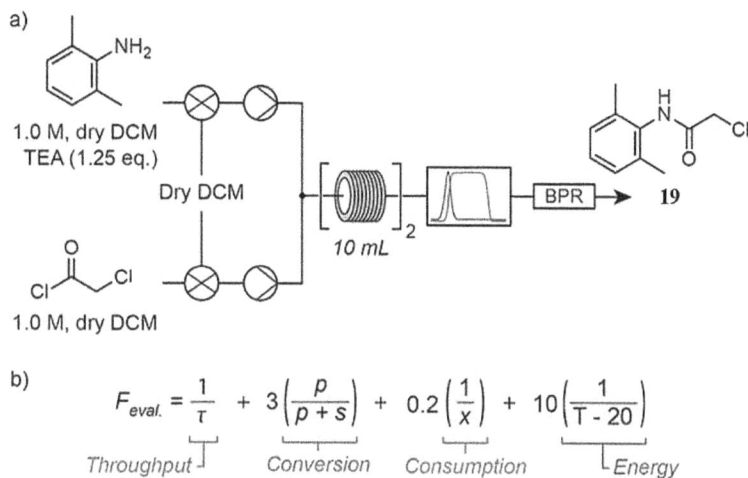

1.0 M, dry DCM
TEA (1.25 eq.)

Dry DCM

10 mL

BPR → **19**

b)

$$F_{eval.} = \frac{1}{\tau} + 3\left(\frac{p}{p+s}\right) + 0.2\left(\frac{1}{x}\right) + 10\left(\frac{1}{T-20}\right)$$

Throughput ⌐ Conversion Consumption ⌐Energy

FIGURE 1.100 (a) Diagram of continuous flow synthesis of 19 en route to lidocaine (b) evaluation function used to optimize the first step of the synthesis where p is Product IR absorbance, s is starting material IR absorbance, and x is equivalents of acid chloride. (Reprinted with permission from Angewandte Chemie – International Edition, "Across-the-world automated optimization and continuous flow synthesis of pharmaceutical agents operating through a cloud-based server", Fitzpatrick, D.E., 2018. Copyright 2018 The Authors. Published by Wiley-VCH Verlag GmbH & Co. KGaA.)

a)

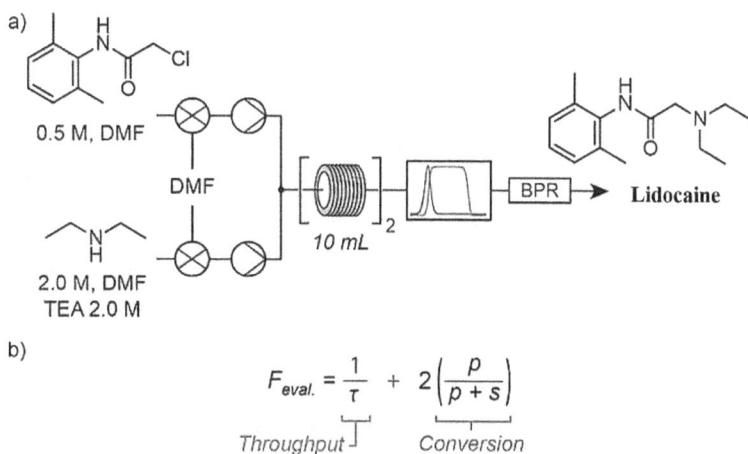

0.5 M, DMF

DMF

10 mL

BPR → **Lidocaine**

2.0 M, DMF
TEA 2.0 M

b)

$$F_{eval.} = \frac{1}{\tau} + 2\left(\frac{p}{p+s}\right)$$

Throughput ⌐ Conversion

FIGURE 1.101 (a) Diagram of continuous flow synthesis of lidocaine (b) the evaluation function of the amine alkylation reaction where p is product IR absorbance and s is starting material IR absorbance. (Reprinted with permission from Angewandte Chemie – International Edition, "Across-the-world automated optimization and continuous flow synthesis of pharmaceutical agents operating through a cloud-based server", Fitzpatrick, D.E., 2018. Copyright 2018 The Authors. Published by Wiley-VCH Verlag GmbH & Co. KGaA.)

mixture of 22 would enter the static mixer at the same rate. This improved the gas-liquid phase distribution through the static mixer, as shown in Figure 1.107.

It was observed that the product degraded quickly in the presence of the excess acid, so an additional line of aqueous NaOH was added to quench the reaction as it exited the flow reactor. Due to issues of clogging when the addition was implemented via tee mixer, a CSM was added to the flow stream so that formed NaCl was distributed more evenly throughout the system and eliminated clogging. Overall yield of aliskiren proceeded between 77–86% of the theoretical yield with an output of 41 g/hr through this continuous flow process (Figure 1.108).

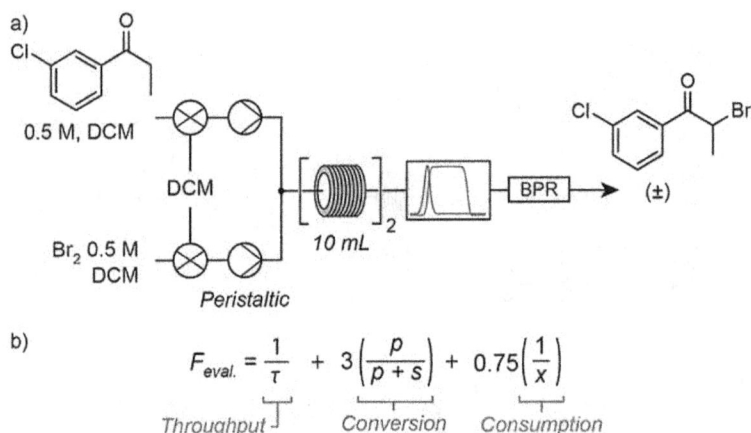

FIGURE 1.102   (a) Diagram of the continuous flow synthesis of the first step to bupropion (b) the evaluation function where p is product IR absorbance, s is starting material IR absorbance and x is equivalents of bromine. (Reprinted with permission from Angewandte Chemie – International Edition, "Across-the-world automated optimization and continuous flow synthesis of pharmaceutical agents operating through a cloud-based server", Fitzpatrick, D.E., 2018. Copyright 2018 The Authors. Published by Wiley-VCH Verlag GmbH & Co. KGaA.)

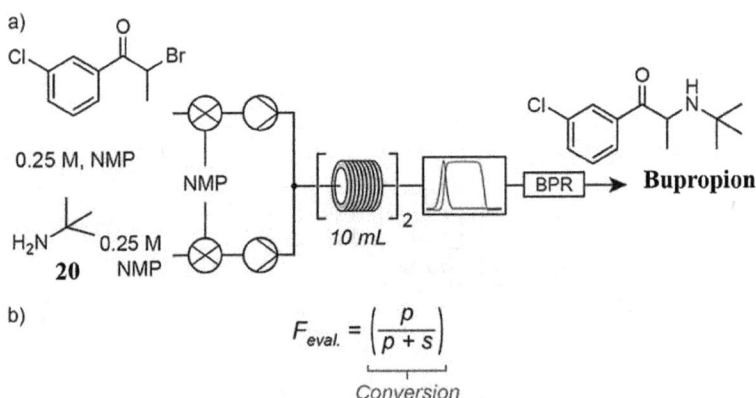

FIGURE 1.103   (a) Diagram of the continuous flow synthesis towards bupropion (b) the evaluation function of the amine alkylation reaction where p is product IR absorbance and s is starting material IR absorbance. (Reprinted with permission from (Angewandte Chemie – International Edition, "Across-the-world automated optimization and continuous flow synthesis of pharmaceutical agents operating through a cloud-based server", Fitzpatrick, D.E., 2018. Copyright 2018 The Authors. Published by Wiley-VCH Verlag GmbH & Co. KGaA.)

1.4.3.11 Real-Time Monitoring of Continuous API Manufacturing with Cutting Edge PAT

Quality control in pharmaceutical manufacturing represents a significant portion of the cost of APIs (Dach et al. 2012; Wiles and Watts 2014). This is due to the strict product quality specification limits as outlined by groups such as the FDA and International Council for Harmonization of Technical Requirements for Pharmaceuticals for Human Use (ICH) which demand demonstration of rigorously tested parametric controls. The ICH further recommends the implementation of continuous processing in the pharmaceutical industry and has developed guidelines outlining both the advantages of continuous manufacturing and procedural guidelines for quality control in these systems (ICH Consensus 2021). The development of real-time monitoring using multivariate tools able to detect a wide range of parameters

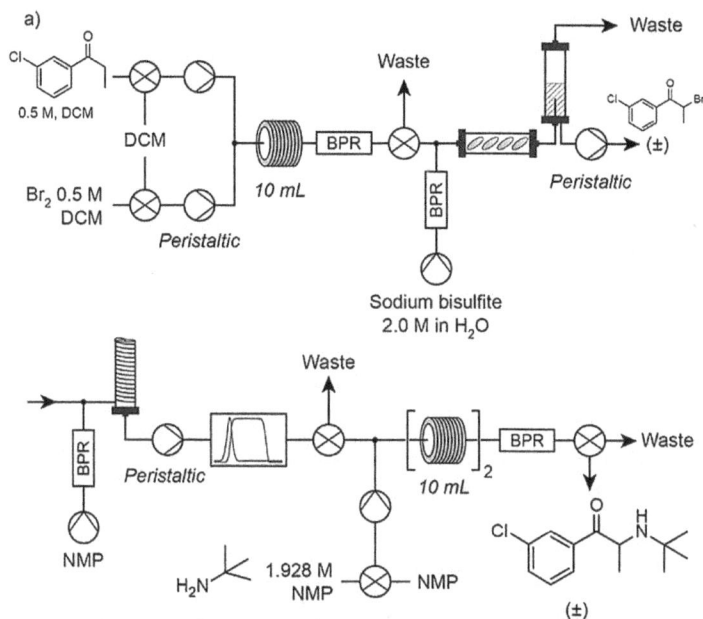

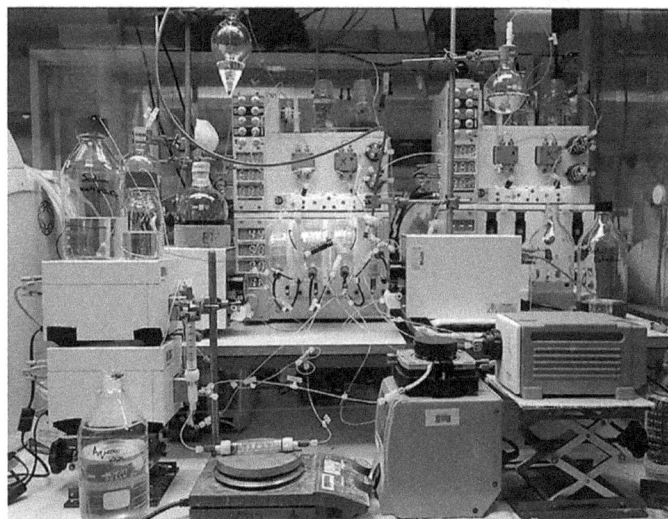

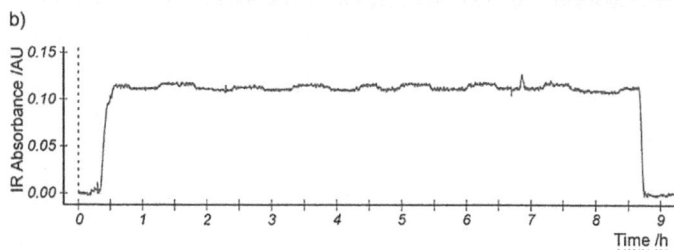

FIGURE 1.104 (a) Diagram of the fully telescoped continuous flow synthesis of bupropion along with an image depicting the actual reactor setup. (b) FlowIR data representing steady state operation indicating process disturbance at 6.9 hours of continuous operation. (Reprinted with permission from Angewandte Chemie – International Edition, "Across-the-world automated optimization and continuous flow synthesis of pharmaceutical agents operating through a cloud-based server", Fitzpatrick, D.E., 2018. Copyright 2018 The Authors. Published by Wiley-VCH Verlag GmbH & Co. KGaA.)

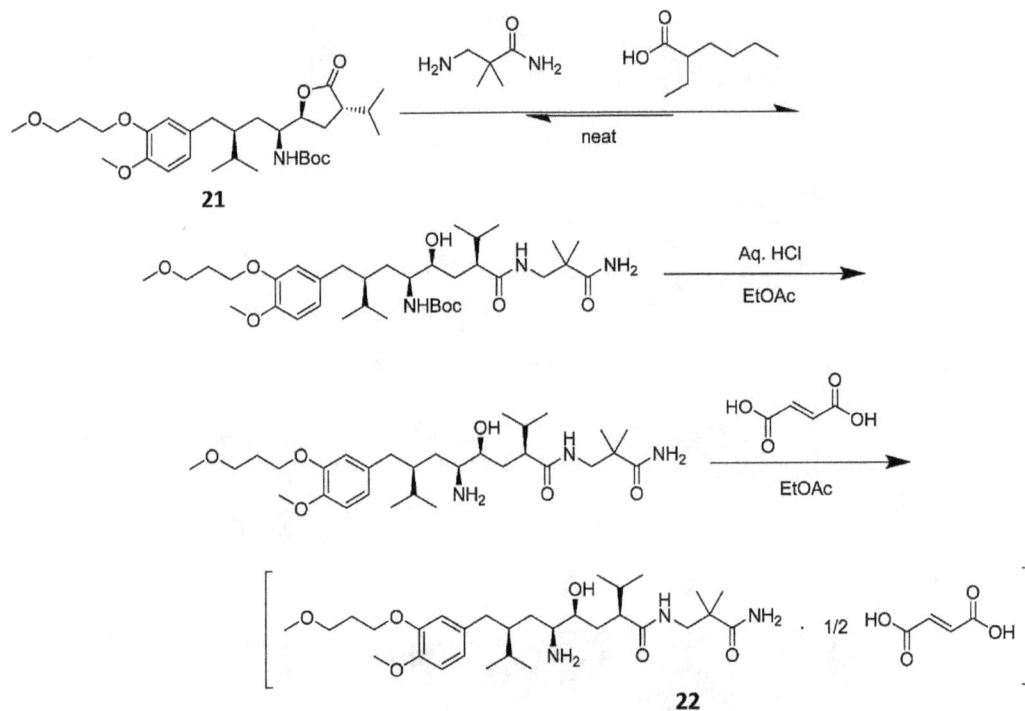

FIGURE 1.105 Reaction diagram for the conversion of 21 to the desired drug salt 22. (Reprinted with permission from Organic Process Research & Development, "Development of a Multi-Step Synthesis and Workup Sequence for an Integrated, Continuous Manufacturing Process of a Pharmaceutical", Heider, P.L. et al, 2014. Copyright 2014 American Chemical Society.)

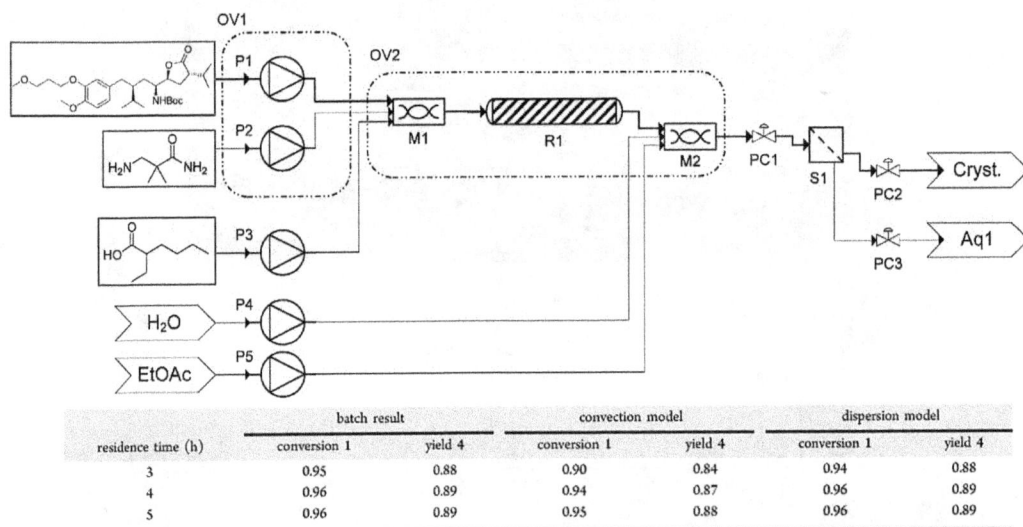

residence time (h)	batch result		convection model		dispersion model	
	conversion 1	yield 4	conversion 1	yield 4	conversion 1	yield 4
3	0.95	0.88	0.90	0.84	0.94	0.88
4	0.96	0.89	0.94	0.87	0.96	0.89
5	0.96	0.89	0.95	0.88	0.96	0.89

FIGURE 1.106 Diagram of continuous flow synthesis and in-line workup and crystallization of aliskiren salt product featuring OV = oven, P = pump, M = mixer, R = reactor, PC = pressure controller, S = liquid-liquid separator, Aq = aqueous waste. (Reprinted with permission from Organic Process Research & Development, "Development of a Multi-Step Synthesis and Workup Sequence for an Integrated, Continuous Manufacturing Process of a Pharmaceutical", Heider, P.L. et al, 2014. Copyright 2014 American Chemical Society.)

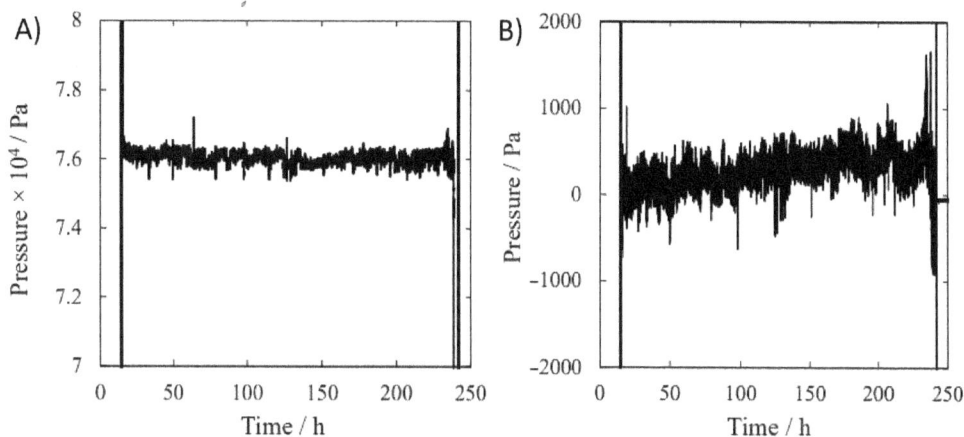

FIGURE 1.107 (A) measure of pressure valves on organic phase exiting the membrane-based liquid-liquid separators (B) measure of the difference in pressure between the aqueous and organic phase outlets of S1. (Reprinted with permission from Organic Process Research & Development, "Development of a Multi-Step Synthesis and Workup Sequence for an Integrated, Continuous Manufacturing Process of a Pharmaceutical", Heider, P.L. et al, 2014. Copyright 2014 American Chemical Society.)

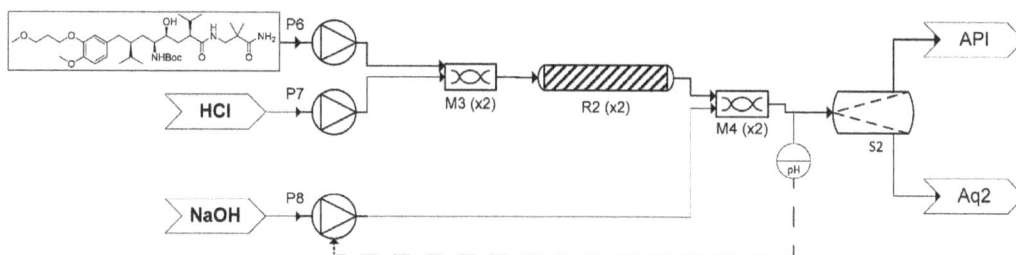

FIGURE 1.108 Diagram for the continuous flow synthesis of aliskiren from 22 where P = pump, M = mixer, R = reactor, pH = pH probe, S = liquid-liquid separator, Aq= aqueous waste, and API = aliskiren final product isolation. (Reprinted with permission from Organic Process Research & Development, "Development of a Multi-Step Synthesis and Workup Sequence for an Integrated, Continuous Manufacturing Process of a Pharmaceutical", Heider, P.L. et al, 2014. Copyright 2014 American Chemical Society.)

would greatly accelerate the root cause analysis timeframe for these quality control testing periods. For this reason, Dumarey et al. from GSK developed and implemented a multivariate statistical process monitoring (MSPM) technique for the continuous production of an API (Dumarey et al. 2019). This model system was demonstrated in the early development stages through the commercial manufacturing stage to demonstrate the effectiveness of this technique through a full API development life cycle.

The principles of MSPM in the context of continuous manufacturing involve "summarizing the variability of multiple process parameters and/or attributes in a few trends based on the collinear features of the investigated process data" (Dumarey et al. 2019). Data is collected through simple process sensors such as measured temperature or flow rate and PAT such as in-line HPLC or IR spectroscopy. In pharmaceutical production where product quality is scrutinized more severely than in other manufacturing processes, it is more common for parameter testing to be conducted by highly trained staff. This is due in part to the increased complexity in drug manufacturing and to the lack of data typically available for transfer from the development stage in the process. Implementing an MSPM process earlier in the development process could provide the necessary stopgap for streamlining the time spent between initial process development and commercial implementation. Gathering data earlier on also allows for a more robust system to be modelled due to the increased amount of data available during the process refinement stage. By using

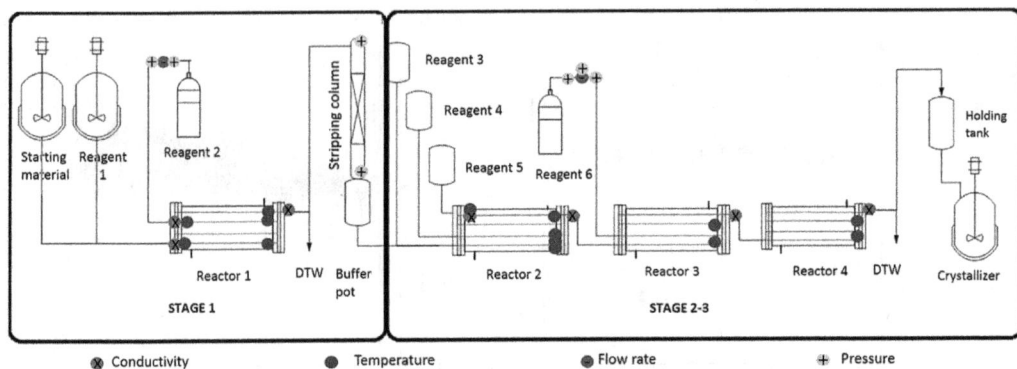

FIGURE 1.109 Depiction of the 5 step, 4-reactor setup with marked sensors and feedback loops used in MSPM approach by GSK. (Reprinted by permission from Springer Science Business Media, LLC: Springer Nature, Journal of Pharmaceutical Innovation. Melanie Dumarey et al., Copyright © 2018.)

MSPM in early-stage development the team at GSK sought to not only improve quality assurance testing but further increase their holistic understanding of the process performance.

A 5-step, 4-reactor API synthesis depicted in Figure 1.109 was studied with this MSPM approach. Sixty-nine process sensors detecting temperature, flow rate, pump speed, pressure, and conductivity were placed intermittently between the three reactors in order to detect variance in these parameters at various stages of the process. Measurement of the product output at each stage combined with the data gathered from these sensors allowed for optimal parameters to be developed and process longevity to be tested with a state-of-control analysis using defined acceptance limits.

Development of a model for the MSPM data analysis consisted of assigning weighted values to the contributions of each process sensor. When a measurement outside the set control limit was observed, real-time analysis quantified which sensors were registering the feedback and to what degree the disturbance could be assigned to each sensor. This greatly accelerated root cause analysis in determining where the system was fouling and permits relatively untrained personnel to expediently identify issues in a manufacturing process by simple data analysis. In this manner, process failures and process inefficiencies could both be addressed in real-time and during early-stage optimization as well as implementation of the commercialized process.

The team was also able to optimize waste collection by determining the precise moment when material began to degrade beyond acceptable limits and building in waste diversion processes. The state-of-control analysis also allowed for the addition of feedback loops that could attenuate process disturbances in real-time by altering parameters such as flow rate, temperature, etc. as an automated system. Addition of PAT such as HPLC provided quantifiable measures of efficiency in terms of yield and elimination of purities from downstream. The use of this advanced MSPM system provided real-time analysis of the entire reaction in an easy-to-comprehend format, expediting the development of a commercial process from early stages of development. The increased output of data also allowed for a more data-driven approach to process optimization, eliminating process disruptions early and redundancies in parameter probing made between plant operators, chemists, and engineers. Demonstrating the value of this methodology for continuous flow production of an API showcases another insight into how continuous technologies can facilitate the production of higher quality pharmaceutical ingredients at a reduced cost.

1.5 Conclusion

Continuous processing is an evolving element of pharmaceutical synthesis that offers significant opportunities to streamline all aspects of process chemistry from drug discovery to commercial operations. This approach also provides a key component to the synthetic toolbox by accessing important pharmacophores via "kinetic pathways" that are currently inaccessible through traditional batch methods. By incorporating this approach across all facets of API process chemistry, synthetic methods can be more effectively translated into scalable processes that have the capability to embrace the principles of process intensification and sustainability.

REFERENCES

Beeler, Aaron B. 2016. "Introduction: Photochemistry in Organic Synthesis." *Chemical Reviews*, 9629–30. https://doi.org/10.1021/acs.chemrev.6b00378.

Afanasyev, Oleg I., Ekaterina Kuchuk, Dmitry L. Usanov, and Denis Chusov. 2019. "Reductive Amination in the Synthesis of Pharmaceuticals." *Chemical Reviews*. https://doi.org/10.1021/acs.chemrev.9b00383.

Afewerki, Samson, Ana Franco, Alina M. Balu, Cheuk-wai Tai, and Rafael Luque. 2020. "Sustainable and Recyclable Heterogenous Palladium Catalysts from Rice Husk-Derived Biosilicates for Suzuki-Miyaura Cross- Couplings, Aerobic Oxidations and Stereoselective Cascade Carbocyclizations." *Scientific Reports*, 1–9. https://doi.org/10.1038/s41598-020-63083-8.

Aken, Koen Van, Lucjan Strekowski, and Luc Patiny. 2006. "EcoScale, a Semi-Quantitative Tool to Select an Organic Preparation Based on Economical and Ecological Parameters." *Beilstein Journal of Organic Chemistry 2*: 1–7. https://doi.org/10.1186/1860-5397-2-3.

Alcázar, Jesús. 2017. "Sustainable Flow Chemistry in Drug Discovery." In *Sustainable Flow Chemistry: Methods and Applications*, 135–64. https://doi.org/10.1002/9783527689118.ch6.

Amara, Zacharias, Martyn Poliakoff, Rubén Duque, Daniel Geier, Giancarlo Franciò, Charles M. Gordon, Rebecca E. Meadows, Robert Woodward, and Walter Leitner. 2016. "Enabling the Scale-Up of a Key Asymmetric Hydrogenation Step in the Synthesis of an API Using Continuous Flow Solid-Supported Catalysis." *Organic Process Research and Development 20* (7): 1321–27. https://doi.org/10.1021/acs.oprd.6b00143.

Archibald, Thomas G., James C. Barnard, and Harlan F. Reese. 2020. "United States Patent : 5861366 United States Patent: 5861366." *New York 2* (19): 1–29. https://patentimages.storage.googleapis.com/30/f4/62/e9b75605352fb0/US10679987.pdf.

Atobe, Mahito, Hiroyuki Tateno, and Yoshimasa Matsumura. 2018. "Applications of Flow Microreactors in Electrosynthetic Processes." *Chemical Reviews 118*: 4541–72. https://doi.org/10.1021/acs.chemrev.7b00353.

Augustine, Robert, Setrak Tanielyan, Stephen Anderson, and Hong Yang. 1999. "A New Technique for Anchoring Homogeneous Catalysts." *Chemical Communications 13*: 1257–58. https://doi.org/10.1039/a903205c.

Baumann, Marcus, Ian R. Baxendale, Christoph Kuratli, Steven V. Ley, Rainer E. Martin, and Josef Schneider. 2011. "Synthesis of a Drug-like Focused Library of Trisubstituted Pyrrolidines Using Integrated Flow Chemistry and Batch Methods." *ACS Combinatorial Science 13* (4): 405–13. https://doi.org/10.1021/co2000357.

Baumann, Marcus, Ian R. Baxendale, Steven V. Ley, Christoper D. Smith, and Geoffrey K. Tranmer. 2006. "Fully Automated Continuous Flow Synthesis of 4,5-Disubstituted Oxazoles." *Organic Letters 8* (23): 5231–34. https://doi.org/10.1021/ol061975c.

Baumann, Marcus, Thomas S. Moody, Megan Smyth, and Scott Wharry. 2020. "A Perspective on Continuous Flow Chemistry in the Pharmaceutical Industry." *Organic Process Research and Development 24* (10): 1802–13. https://doi.org/10.1021/acs.oprd.9b00524.

Beller, Matthias, and Timothy Noe. 2011. "Cross Coupling Reactions in Organic Synthesis Themed Issue." *Chemical Society Reviews 40*: 5010–29. https://doi.org/10.1039/c1cs15075h.

Berton, Mateo, Lena Huck, and Jesús Alcázar. 2018. "On-Demand Synthesis of Organozinc Halides under Continuous Flow Conditions." *Nature Protocols 13* (1): 324–34. https://doi.org/10.1038/nprot.2017.141.

Bleie, Olav, Michael F. Roberto, Thomas I. Dearing, Charles W. Branham, Olav M. Kvalheim, and Brian J. Marquardt. 2015. "Moffat-Swern Oxidation of Alcohols: Translating a Batch Reaction to a Continuous-Flow Reaction." *Journal of Flow Chemistry 5* (3): 183–89. https://doi.org/10.1556/1846.2015.00025.

Bloemendal, Victor R.L.J., Mathilde A.C.H. Janssen, Jan C.M. Van Hest, and Floris P.J.T. Rutjes. 2020. "Continuous One-Flow Multi-Step Synthesis of Active Pharmaceutical Ingredients." *Reaction Chemistry and Engineering 5* (7): 1186–97. https://doi.org/10.1039/d0re00087f.

Bogdan, Andrew R., Sarah L. Poe, Daniel C. Kubis, Steven J. Broadwater, and D. Tyler McQuade. 2009. "The Continuous-Flow Synthesis of Ibuprofen." *Angewandte Chemie – International Edition 48* (45): 8547–50. https://doi.org/10.1002/anie.200903055.

Booker-Milburn, Kevin I, Paul Hirst, Jonathan P.H. Charmant, and Luke H.J. Taylor. 2003. "A Rapid Stereocontrolled Entry to the ABCD Tetracyclic Core of Neotuberostemonine." *Angewandte Chemie – International Edition 42*: 1642–44. https://doi.org/10.1002/anie.50507.

Brinkley, Kendra W., Michael Burkholder, Ali R. Siamaki, Katherine Belecki, and B. Frank Gupton. 2015. "The Continuous Synthesis and Application of Graphene Supported Palladium Nanoparticles: A Highly Effective Catalyst for Suzuki-Miyaura Cross-Coupling Reactions." *Green Processing and Synthesis 4* (3): 241–46. https://doi.org/10.1515/gps-2015-0021.

Britton, Joshua, Justin M. Chalker, and Colin L. Raston. 2015. "Rapid Vortex Fluidics: Continuous Flow Synthesis of Amides and Local Anesthetic Lidocaine." *Chemistry – A European Journal 21* (30): 10660–65. https://doi.org/10.1002/chem.201501785.

Brzozowski, Martin, Matthew O'Brien, Steven V. Ley, and Anastasios Polyzos. 2015. "Flow Chemistry: Intelligent Processing of Gas-Liquid Transformations Using a Tube-in-Tube Reactor." *Accounts of Chemical Research 48* (2): 349–62. https://doi.org/10.1021/ar500359m.

Cantillo, David, Bernd Wolf, Roland Goetz, and C. Oliver Kappe. 2017. "Continuous Flow Synthesis of a Key 1,4-Benzoxazinone Intermediate via a Nitration/Hydrogenation/Cyclization Sequence." *Organic Process Research and Development 21* (1): 125–32. https://doi.org/10.1021/acs.oprd.6b00409.

Cao, Yiran, Gabriele Laudadio, and Timothy Noe. 2019. "The Fundamentals Behind the Use of Flow Reactors in Electrochemistry." *Accounts of Chemical Research 52*: 2858–69. https://doi.org/10.1021/acs.accounts.9b00412.

Carey, John S., David Laffan, Colin Thomson, and Mike T. Williams. 2006. "Analysis of the Reactions Used for the Preparation of Drug Candidate Molecules." *Organic and Biomolecular Chemistry 4* (12): 2337–47. https://doi.org/10.1039/b602413k.

Carneiro, Paula F., Bernhard Gutmann, Rodrigo O.M.A. De Souza, and C. Oliver Kappe. 2015. "Process Intensified Flow Synthesis of 1H-4-Substituted Imidazoles: Toward the Continuous Production of Daclatasvir." *ACS Sustainable Chemistry and Engineering 3* (12): 3445–53. https://doi.org/10.1021/acssuschemeng.5b01191.

Ceylan, Sascha, Ludovic Coutable, Jens Wegner, and Andreas Kirschning. 2011. "Inductive Heating with Magnetic Materials inside Flow Reactors." *Chemistry – A European Journal 17*: 1884–93. https://doi.org/10.1002/chem.201002291.

Changi, Shujauddin M., and Sze Wing Wong. 2016. "Kinetics Model for Designing Grignard Reactions in Batch or Flow Operations." *Organic Process Research and Development 20* (2): 525–39. https://doi.org/10.1021/acs.oprd.5b00281.

Cintas, Pedro, Alessandro Barge, Silvia Tagliapietra, Luisa Boffa, and Giancarlo Cravotto. 2010. "Alkyne-Azide Click Reaction Catalyzed by Metallic Copper under Ultrasound." *Nature Protocols 5* (3): 607–16. https://doi.org/10.1038/nprot.2010.1.

Clarke, Coby J, Wei-Chien Tu, Oliver Levers, Andreas Bro, and Jason P Hallett. 2018. "Green and Sustainable Solvents in Chemical Processes." *Chemical Reviews.* https://doi.org/10.1021/acs.chemrev.7b00571.

Colacot, Thomas, and Johnson Matthey, and Chiral Technologies. 2016. "New Trends in Cross-Coupling : Theory and Applications." *Johnson Matthey Technology Review 60* (2): 99–105.

Correia, Camille A., Kerry Gilmore, D. Tyler McQuade, and Peter H. Seeberger. 2015. "A Concise Flow Synthesis of Efavirenz." *Angewandte Chemie – International Edition 54* (16): 4945–48. https://doi.org/10.1002/anie.201411728.

Coutable, L, A Kirschning, Jan Hartwig, Sascha Ceylan, Lukas Kupracz, Ludovic Coutable, and Andreas Kirschning. 2013. "Heating under High-Frequency Inductive Conditions : Application to the Continuous Synthesis of the Neurolepticum Olanzapine (Zyprexa)." *Angewandte Chemie – International Edition 52*: 1–6. https://doi.org/10.1002/anie.201302239.

Dach, Rolf, Jinhua J. Song, Frank Roschangar, Wendelin Samstag, and Chris H. Senanayake. 2012. "The Eight Criteria Defining a Good Chemical Manufacturing Process." *Organic Process Research and Development 16* (11): 1697–1706. https://doi.org/10.1021/op300144g.

Daniel Scott, C., Ricardo Labes, Martin Depardieu, Claudio Battilocchio, Matthew G. Davidson, Steven V. Ley, Chick C. Wilson, and Karen Robertson. 2018. "Integrated Plug Flow Synthesis and Crystallisation of Pyrazinamide." *Reaction Chemistry and Engineering 3* (5): 631–34. https://doi.org/10.1039/c8re00087e.

Delville, Mariëlle M.E., Pieter J. Nieuwland, Paul Janssen, Kaspar Koch, Jan C.M. van Hest, and Floris P.J.T. Rutjes. 2011. "Continuous Flow Azide Formation: Optimization and Scale-Up." *Chemical Engineering Journal 167* (2–3): 556–59. https://doi.org/10.1016/j.cej.2010.08.087.

Dicks, Andrew P., and Andrei Hent. 2015. "The E Factor and Process Mass Intensity." In *Green Chemistry Metrics*, 45–67. SpringerBriefs in Greem Chemistry for Sustainability. https://doi.org/10.1007/978-3-319-10500-0_3.

Doyle, Michael P., M. Anthony McKervey, and Tao Ye. 1998. *Modern Catalytic Methods for Organic Synthesis with Diazo Compounds: From Cyclopropanes to Ylides.*

Ducry, Laurent, and Dominique M. Roberge. 2005. "Controlled Autocatalytic Nitration of Phenol in a Microreactor." *Angewandte Chemie – International Edition 44* (48): 7972–75. https://doi.org/10.1002/anie.200502387.

Dumarey, Melanie, Martin Hermanto, Christian Airiau, Peter Shapland, Hannah Robinson, Peter Hamilton, and Malcolm Berry. 2019. "Advances in Continuous Active Pharmaceutical Ingredient (API) Manufacturing: Real-Time Monitoring Using Multivariate Tools." *Journal of Pharmaceutical Innovation 14* (4): 359–72. https://doi.org/10.1007/s12247-018-9348-7.

Elliott, Luke D., Malcolm Berry, Bashir Harji, David Klauber, John Leonard, and Kevin I. Booker-Milburn. 2016. "A Small-Footprint, High-Capacity Flow Reactor for UV Photochemical Synthesis on the Kilogram Scale." *Organic Process Research and Development 20* (10): 1806–11. https://doi.org/10.1021/acs.oprd.6b00277.

Endoma-Arias, Mary Ann A., D. Phillip Cox, and Tomas Hudlicky. 2013. "General Method of Synthesis for Naloxone, Naltrexone, Nalbuphone, and Nalbuphine by the Reaction of Grignard Reagents with an Oxazolidine Derived from Oxymorphone." *Advanced Synthesis and Catalysis*, 1–6. https://doi.org/10.1002/adsc.201300284.

Epps, Robert W., Amanda A. Volk, Kristofer G. Reyes, and Milad Abolhasani. 2021. "Accelerated AI Development for Autonomous Materials Synthesis in Flow." *Chemical Science 12* (17): 6025–36. https://doi.org/10.1039/d0sc06463g.

Fanelli, Flavio, Giovanna Parisi, Leonardo Degennaro, and Renzo Luisi. 2017. "Contribution of Microreactor Technology and Flow Chemistry to the Development of Green and Sustainable Synthesis." *Beilstein Journal of Organic Chemistry 13*: 520–42. https://doi.org/10.3762/bjoc.13.51.

Fantoni, Tommaso, Sara Bernardoni, Alexia Mattellone, Giulia Martelli, Lucia Ferrazzano, Paolo Cantelmi, Dario Corbisiero, et al. 2021. "Palladium Catalyst Recycling for Heck-Cassar-Sonogashira Cross-Coupling Reactions in Green Solvent / Base Blend." *ChemSusChem*, 2591–2600. https://doi.org/10.1002/cssc.202100623.

Fitzpatrick, Daniel E., Timothé Maujean, Amanda C. Evans, and Steven V. Ley. 2018. "Across-the-World Automated Optimization and Continuous-Flow Synthesis of Pharmaceutical Agents Operating Through a Cloud-Based Server." *Angewandte Chemie – International Edition 57* (46): 15128–32. https://doi.org/10.1002/anie.201809080.

Flannery, Erika L., Arnab K. Chatterjee, and Elizabeth A. Winzeler. 2013. "Antimalarial Drug Discovery-Approaches and Progress towards New Medicines." *Nature Reviews Microbiology 11* (12): 849–62. https://doi.org/10.1038/nrmicro3138.

Gage, James R., Xiaowen Guo, Jian Tao, and Changsheng Zheng. 2012. "High Output Continuous Nitration." *Organic Process Research and Development 16* (5): 930–33. https://doi.org/10.1021/op2003425.

Gardiner, James, Xuan Nguyen, Charlotte Genet, Mike D. Horne, Christian H. Hornung, and John Tsanaktsidis. 2018. "Catalytic Static Mixers for the Continuous Flow Hydrogenation of a Key Intermediate of Linezolid (Zyvox)." *Organic Process Research and Development 22* (10): 1448–52. https://doi.org/10.1021/acs.oprd.8b00153.

Garrett, Christine E., and Kapa Prasad. 2004. "The Art of Meeting Palladium Specifications in Active Pharmaceutical Ingredients Produced by Pd-Catalyzed Reactions." *Advanced Synthesis and Catalysis 346* (8): 889–900. https://doi.org/10.1002/adsc.200404071.

Goddard-Borger, Ethan D., and Robert V. Stick. 2007. "An Efficient, Inexpensive, and Shelf-Stable Diazotransfer Reagent: Imidazole-1-Sulfonyl Azide Hydrochloride." *Organic Letters 9* (19): 3797–3800.

Goddard-Borger, Ethan D., and Robert V. Stick. 2011. "Additions and Corrections." *Biology of Reproduction 84* (4): 837. https://doi.org/10.1095/biolreprod.111.091843.

Grew, Edward Leon, and Alastair Agnew Roberston. 1974. Reduction of Thebaine. *United States Patent Office*, issued 1974. https://doi.org/10.2307/1190003.

Grisoni, Francesca, Berend J.H. Huisman, Alexander L. Button, Michael Moret, Kenneth Atz, Daniel Merk, and Gisbert Schneider. 2021. "Combining Generative Artificial Intelligence and On-Chip Synthesis for de Novo Drug Design." *Science Advances 7* (24): 1–10. https://doi.org/10.1126/sciadv.abg3338.

Gutmann, Bernhard, Ulrich Weigl, D. Phillip Cox, and C. Oliver Kappe. 2016. "Batch- and Continuous-Flow Aerobic Oxidation of 14-Hydroxy Opioids to 1,3-Oxazolidines—A Concise Synthesis of Noroxymorphone." *Chemistry – A European Journal* 22 (30): 10393–98. https://doi.org/10.1002/chem.201601902.

Hakke, Vikas, Shirish Sonawane, Sambandam Anandan, and Shriram Sonawane. 2021. "Process Intensification Approach Using Microreactors for Synthesizing Nanomaterials – A Critical Review." *Nanomaterials 98.*

Hartwig, Jan, and Andreas Kirschning. 2016. "Flow Synthesis in Hot Water: Synthesis of the Atypical Antipsychotic Iloperidone." *Chemistry – A European Journal* 22 (9): 3044–52. https://doi.org/10.1002/chem.201504409.

Hastings, Ian M., William M. Watkins, and Nicholas J. White. 2002. "The Evolution of Drug-Resistant Malaria: The Role of Drug Elimination Half-Life." *Philosophical Transactions of the Royal Society B: Biological Sciences 357* (1420): 505–19. https://doi.org/10.1098/rstb.2001.1036.

Hatano, Manabu, Tokihiko Matsumura, and Kazuaki Ishihara. 2005. "Highly Alkyl-Selective Addition to Ketones with Magnesium Ate Complexes Derived from Gignard Reagents." *Organic Letters 7* (4): 573–76. https://doi.org/10.1021/ol047685i.

Heck, Richard F. 1982. "Palladium-Catalyzed Vinylation of Organic Halides." In *Organic Reactions.*

Heider, Patrick L., Stephen C. Born, Soubir Basak, Brahim Benyahia, Richard Lakerveld, Haitao Zhang, Rachael Hogan, et al. 2014. "Development of a Multi-Step Synthesis and Workup Sequence for an Integrated, Continuous Manufacturing Process of a Pharmaceutical." *Organic Process Research and Development 18* (3): 402–9. https://doi.org/10.1021/op400294z.

Hein, Christopher D., Xin Ming Liu, and Dong Wang. 2008. "Click Chemistry, a Powerful Tool for Pharmaceutical Sciences." *Pharmaceutical Research 25* (10): 2216–30. https://doi.org/10.1007/s11095-008-9616-1.

Heinz, Benjamin, Dimitrije Djukanovic, Maximilian A. Ganiek, Benjamin Martin, Berthold Schenkel, and Paul Knochel. 2020. "Selective Acylation of Aryl-and Heteroarylmagnesium Reagents with Esters in Continuous Flow." *Organic Letters 22* (2): 493–96. https://doi.org/10.1021/acs.orglett.9b04254.

Heravi, Majid M., Vahideh Zadsirjan, Parvin Hajiabbasi, and Hoda Hamidi. 2019. *Advances in Kumada – Tamao – Corriu Cross – Coupling Reaction: An Update. Monatshefte Für Chemie – Chemical Monthly.* Springer Vienna. https://doi.org/10.1007/s00706-019-2364-6.

Hoffmann, Norbert. 2008. "Photochemical Reactions as Key Steps in Organic Synthesis." *Chemical Reviews 108*: 1052–1103.

Hook, Benjamin D.A., Wolfgang Dohle, Paul R. Hirst, Mark Pickworth, Malcolm B. Berry, and Kevin I. Booker-Milburn. 2005. "A Practical Flow Reactor for Continuous Organic Photochemistry." *Journal of Organic Chemistry 70* (19): 7558–64. https://doi.org/10.1021/jo050705p.

Huck, Lena, Antonio De La Hoz, Angel Díaz-Ortiz, and Jesus Alcázar. 2017. "Grignard Reagents on a Tab: Direct Magnesium Insertion under Flow Conditions." *Organic Letters 19* (14): 3747–50. https://doi.org/10.1021/acs.orglett.7b01590.

ICH Consensus. 2021. *Continuous Manufacturing of Drug Substances and Drug Products Q13.*

Ioannidis, Stephanos, Michelle L. Lamb, Tao Wang, Lynsie Almeida, Michael H. Block, Audrey M. Davies, Bo Peng, et al. 2011. "Discovery of 5-Chloro- N 2-[(1 S)-1-(5-Fluoropyrimidin-2-Yl) Ethyl]- N 4-(5-Methyl-1 H -Pyrazol-3-Yl)Pyrimidine-2,4-Diamine (AZD1480) as a Novel Inhibitor of the Jak/Stat Pathway." *Journal of Medicinal Chemistry 54* (1): 262–76. https://doi.org/10.1021/jm1011319.

Ishitani, Haruro, Yuki Saito, Benjamin Laroche, Xiaofeng Rao, and Shū Kobayashi. 2020. *Chapter 1: Recent Perspectives in Catalysis under Continuous Flow. RSC Green Chemistry.* Vol. 2020-Janua. https://doi.org/10.1039/9781788016094-00001.

Jacks, Thomas E., Daniel T. Belmont, Christopher A. Briggs, Nicole M. Horne, Gerald D. Kanter, Greg L. Karrick, James J. Krikke, et al. 2004. "Development of a Scalable Process for CI-1034, an Endothelin Antagonist." *Organic Process Research and Development 8* (2): 201–12. https://doi.org/10.1021/op034104g.

Jas, Gerhard, and Andreas Kirschning. 2003. "Continuous Flow Techniques in Organic Synthesis." *Chemistry – A European Journal 9* (23): 5708–23. https://doi.org/10.1002/chem.200305212.

Jimenez-Gonzalez, Concepcion, Celia S. Ponder, Quirinus B. Broxterman, and Julie B. Manley. 2011. "Using the Right Green Yardstick: Why Process Mass Intensity Is Used in the Pharmaceutical Industry to Drive More Sustainable Processes." *Organic Process Research and Development 15* (4): 912–17. https://doi.org/10.1021/op200097d.

Karen Goodwin. 2009. *Development of a Greener Synthesis of Lidocaine.* California State University, Sacramento, CA.

King, Anthony O., and Nobuyoshi Yasuda. 2004. "Palladium-Catalyzed Cross-Coupling Reactions in the Synthesis of Pharmaceuticals." In *Topics in Organometallic Chemistry*, 205–45. Springer-Verlag. https://doi.org/10.1007/b94551.

Kinzel, Tom, Yong Zhang, and Stephen L. Buchwald. 2010. "A New Palladium Precatalyst Allows for the Fast Suzuki – Miyaura Coupling Reactions of Unstable Polyfluorophenyl and 2-Heteroaryl Boronic Acids." *Journal of the American Chemical Society*, 14073–75.

Kiso, Yoshihisa, Kohei Tamao, and Makoto Kumada. 1973. "Effects of the Nature of Halides on the Alkyl Group Isomerization in the Nickel-Catalyzed Cross-Coupling of Secondary Alkyl Grignard Reagents with Organic Halides." *Journal of Organometallic Chemistry 50* (1): 4374–76. https://doi.org/10.1016/S0022-328X(00)95063-0.

Knochel, Paul, and Robert D. Singer. 1993. "Preparation and Reactions of Polyfunctional Organozinc Reagents in Organic Synthesis." *Chemical Reviews 93* (6): 2117–88. https://doi.org/10.1021/cr00022a008.

Kong, Caleb J., Daniel Fisher, Bimbisar K. Desai, Yuan Yang, Saeed Ahmad, Katherine Belecki, and B. Frank Gupton. 2017. "High Throughput Photo-Oxidations in a Packed Bed Reactor System." *Bioorganic and Medicinal Chemistry 25* (23): 6203–8. https://doi.org/10.1016/j.bmc.2017.07.004.

Kopach, Michael E., Perry C. Heath, Roger B. Scherer, Mark A. Pietz, Bret A. Astleford, Mary Kay McCauley, Utpal K. Singh, et al. 2015. "Practical Asymmetric Synthesis of an Edivoxetine·HCl Intermediate via an Efficient Diazotization Process." *Organic Process Research and Development 19* (4): 543–50. https://doi.org/10.1021/acs.oprd.5b00014.

Kopetzki, Daniel, Francois Levesque, and Peter H. Seeberger. 2013. "A Continuous-Flow Process for the Synthesis of Artemisinin." *Chemistry – A European Journal*, 5450–56. https://doi.org/10.1002/chem.201204558.

Korwar, Sudha, Somi Amir, Perrer N. Tosso, Bimbisar K. Desai, Caleb J. Kong, Swara Fadnis, Nakul S. Telang, Saeed Ahmad, Thomas D. Roper, and B. Frank Gupton. 2017. "The Application of a Continuous Grignard Reaction in the Preparation of Fluconazole." *European Journal of Organic Chemistry 2017* (44): 6495–98. https://doi.org/10.1002/ejoc.201701002.

Kulkarni, Amol A. 2014. "Continuous Flow Nitration in Miniaturized Devices." *Beilstein Journal of Organic Chemistry 10*: 405–24. https://doi.org/10.3762/bjoc.10.38.

Kunz, Ulrich, Hagen Schönfeld, Wladimir Solodenko, Gerhard Jas, and Andreas Kirschning. 2005. "Manufacturing and Construction of PASSflow Flow Reactors and Their Utilization in Suzuki-Miyaura Cross-Coupling Reactions." *Industrial and Engineering Chemistry Research 44* (23): 8458–67. https://doi.org/10.1021/ie048891x.

Kwon, Tae Hui, Kie Yong Cho, Kyung Youl Baek, Ho Gyu Yoon, and B. Moon Kim. 2017. "Recyclable Palladium-Graphene Nanocomposite Catalysts Containing Ionic Polymers: Efficient Suzuki Coupling Reactions." *RSC Advances 7* (19): 11684–90. https://doi.org/10.1039/c6ra26998b.

Lau, Shing Hing, Alicia Galván, Rohan R. Merchant, Claudio Battilocchio, José A. Souto, Malcolm B. Berry, and Steven V. Ley. 2015. "Machines vs Malaria: A Flow-Based Preparation of the Drug Candidate OZ439." *Organic Letters 17* (13): 3218–21. https://doi.org/10.1021/acs.orglett.5b01307.

Lévesque, François, and Peter H. Seeberger. 2012. "Continuous-Flow Synthesis of the Anti-Malaria Drug Artemisinin." *Angewandte Chemie – International Edition 51* (7): 1706–9. https://doi.org/10.1002/anie.201107446.

Lévesque, Francois, and Peter H. Seeberger. 2011. "Highly Efficient Continuous Flow Reactions Using Singlet Oxygen as a 'Green' Reagent." *Organic Letters 13* (19): 5008–11.

Levin, Daniel. 2014. "Managing Hazards for Scale up of Chemical Manufacturing Processes." *ACS Symposium Series 1181*: 3–71. https://doi.org/10.1021/bk-2014-1181.ch001.

Lin, Hongkun, Chunhai Dai, Timothy F. Jamison, and Klavs F. Jensen. 2017. "A Rapid Total Synthesis of Ciproflaxin Hydrochloride in Continuous Flow." *Angewandte Chemie – International Edition*, 10–15. https://doi.org/10.1002/anie.201703812.

Longstreet, Ashley R., Brian S. Campbell, B. Frank Gupton, and D. Tyler McQuade. 2013. "Improved Synthesis of Mono- and Disubstituted 2-Halonicotinonitriles from Alkylidene Malononitriles." *Organic Letters 15* (20): 5298–5301. https://doi.org/10.1021/ol4025265.

López, Enol, María Lourdes Linares, and Jesús Alcázar. 2020. "Flow Chemistry as a Tool to Access Novel Chemical Space for Drug Discovery." *Future Medicinal Chemistry 12* (17): 1547–63. https://doi.org/10.4155/fmc-2020-0075.

Maeda, Sadao, Mamoru Suzuki, Tameo Iwasaski, Kazuo Matsumoto, and Yoshio Iwasawa. 1984. "Syntheses of 2-Mercapto-4-Substituted Imidazole Derivatives with Antiinflammatory Properties." *Chemical Pharmaceutical Bulletin 32* (7): 2536–43.

Malik, Aslam, Francis Hempenstall, Nicholas Duda, and Ali Suleman. 2016. Methods for Preparing D-Threo-methylphenidate Using Diazomethane, and Compositions Thereof. *US 9,233,924 B2*, issued 2016.

Mandoli, Alessandro. 2019. "Catalyst Recycling in Continuous Flow Reactors." In *Catalyst Immobilization: Methods and Applications*, 257–306. https://doi.org/10.1002/9783527817290.ch8.

Martin, Laetitia J., Andreas L. Marzinzik, Steven V. Ley, and R. Baxendale. 2011. "Safe and Reliable Synthesis of Diazoketones and Quinoxalines in a Continuous Flow Reactor." *Organic Letters 13* (2): 320–23.

Mastronardi, Federica, Bernhard Gutmann, and C. Oliver Kappe. 2013. "Continuous Flow Generation and Reactions of Anhydrous Diazomethane Using a Teflon AF-2400 Tube-in-Tube Reactor." *Organic Letters 15* (21): 5590–93. https://doi.org/10.1021/ol4027914.

Mata, Alejandro, Ulrich Weigl, Oliver Flögel, Pius Baur, Christopher A. Hone, and C. Oliver Kappe. 2020. "Acyl Azide Generation and Amide Bond Formation in Continuous-Flow for the Synthesis of Peptides." *Reaction Chemistry and Engineering 5* (4): 645–50. https://doi.org/10.1039/d0re00034e.

May, Scott A., Martin D. Johnson, Timothy M. Braden, Joel R. Calvin, Brian D. Haeberle, Amy R. Jines, Richard D. Miller, et al. 2012. "Rapid Development and Scale-Up of a 1H-4-Substituted Imidazole Intermediate Enabled by Chemistry in Continuous Plug Flow Reactors." *Organic Process Research & Development 16*: 982–1002.

McQuade, D. Tyler, and Peter H. Seeberger. 2013. "Applying Flow Chemistry: Methods, Materials, and Multi-step Synthesis." *Journal of Organic Chemistry 78*: 6384–89.

Mead, Walter Russell, and Douglas Brinkley. 2003. "Wheels for the World: Henry Ford, His Company, and a Century of Progress, 1903–2003." *Foreign Affairs 82* (5): 176. https://doi.org/10.2307/20033711.

Miyaura, Norio, Kinji Yamada, and Akira Suzuki. 1979. "Our Continuous Discovered." *Tetrahedron Letters 20* (36): 3437–40. http://linkinghub.elsevier.com/retrieve/pii/S0040403901954292.

Moir, Michael, Jonathon J. Danon, Tristan A Reekie, Michael Kassiou, Michael Moir, Jonathon J. Danon, Tristan A. Reekie, and Michael Kassiou. 2019. "Expert Opinion on Drug Discovery An Overview of Late-Stage Functionalization in Today' s Drug Discovery." *Expert Opinion on Drug Discovery*, 1–13. https://doi.org/10.1080/17460441.2019.1653850.

Molnár, Árpád. 2011. "Efficient, Selective, and Recyclable Palladium Catalysts in Carbon-Carbon Coupling Reactions." *Chemical Reviews 111* (3): 2251–2320. https://doi.org/10.1021/cr100355b.

Moore, Jason S., Klavs F. Jensen A. Microfluidic, Wiley Blackwell, Pengfei Li, Jason S. Moore, and Klavs F. Jensen. 2013. "Recycling of Unmodified Homogeneous Palladium A Microfluidic System for Continuous Recycling of Unmodified Homogeneous Palladium Catalysts via Liquid-Liquid Phase Separation." *ChemCatChem*. https://dspace.mit.edu/handle/1721.1/92778.

Murai, T., and F. Asai. 2007. "Three-Component Coupling Reactions of Thioformamides with Organolithium and Grignard Reagents." *Synfacts 2007* (4): 0415–0415. https://doi.org/10.1055/s-2007-968321.

Murrey, Heather E., Joshua C. Judkins, Christopher W. Am Ende, T. Eric Ballard, Yinzhi Fang, Keith Ricca-rdi, Li Di, et al. 2015. "Systematic Evaluation of Bioorthogonal Reactions in Live Cells with Clickable HaloTag Ligands: Implications for Intracellular Imaging." *Journal of the American Chemical Society 137* (35): 11461–75. https://doi.org/10.1021/jacs.5b06847.

Negishi, Ei-ichi, Qian Hu, Zhihong Huang, Mingxing Qian, and Guangwei Wong. 2005. "Palladium-Catalyzed Alkenylation by the Negishi Coupling." *Aldrichimica Acta 38* (3): 71–87.

Noël, Timothy, and Andrew J. Musacchio. 2011. "Suzuki À Miyaura Cross-Coupling of Heteroaryl Halides and Arylboronic Acids in Continuous Flow." *Organic Letters 6*: 14073–75. https://doi.org/10.1039/c1cs15075h.10.1021/ol202052q.

NRC. 2007. "1 @ www.Nap.Edu." http://www.nap.edu/read/11761/chapter/1.

Nunes, Cláudio M., Igor Reva, and Rui Fausto. 2013. "Capture of an Elusive Nitrile Ylide as an Intermediate in Isoxazole-Oxazole Photoisomerization." *Journal of Organic Chemistry 78* (21): 10657–65. https://doi.org/10.1021/jo4015672.

O'Brien, M., I. Baxendale, and S. Ley. 2010. "Flow Ozonolysis Using a Semipermeable Teflon AF-2400 Membrane." *Synfacts 2010* (10): 1199–1199. https://doi.org/10.1055/s-0030-1258661.

Ohba, Masashi, Hiroyuki Kubo, Shigeki Seto, Tozo Fujii, and Hiroyuki Ishibashi. 1998. "A Straightforward Preparation of Chiral 5-(Aminomethyl)Oxazole Derivatives from a-Amino Esters and a-Lithiated Isocyanides." *Chemical Pharmaceutical Bulletin 46* (5): 860–62.

Ötvös, Sándor B., and Ferenc Fülöp. 2015. "Flow Chemistry as a Versatile Tool for the Synthesis of Triazoles." *Catalysis Science and Technology* 5 (11): 4926–41. https://doi.org/10.1039/c5cy00523j.

Ouchi, Takashi, Claudio Battilocchio, Joel M. Hawkins, and Steven V. Ley. 2014. "Process Intensification for the Continuous Flow Hydrogenation of Ethyl Nicotinate." *Organic Process Research and Development* 18 (11): 1560–66. https://doi.org/10.1021/op500208j.

Pastre, Julio C., Philip R.D. Murray, Duncan L. Browne, Guilherme A. Brancaglion, Renan S. Galaverna, Ronaldo A. Pilli, and Steven V. Ley. 2020. "Integrated Batch and Continuous Flow Process for the Synthesis of Goniothalamin." *ACS Omega* 5 (29): 18472–83. https://doi.org/10.1021/acsomega.0c02390.

Paymode, Dinesh J., Flavio S.P. Cardoso, Toolika Agrawal, John W. Tomlin, Daniel W. Cook, Justina M. Burns, Rodger W. Stringham, Joshua D. Sieber, B. Frank Gupton, and David R. Snead. 2020. "Expanding Access to Remdesivir via an Improved Pyrrolotriazine Synthesis: Supply Centered Synthesis." *Organic Letters* 22 (19): 7656–61. https://doi.org/10.1021/acs.orglett.0c02848.

Peltzer, Raphael Mathias, Jürgen Gauss, Odile Eisenstein, and Michele Cascella. 2020. "The Grignard Reaction-Unraveling a Chemical Puzzle." *Journal of the American Chemical Society* 142 (6): 2984–94. https://doi.org/10.1021/jacs.9b11829.

PharmaBlock. n.d. "Pyrrolidine Derivatives in Drug Discovery." https://www.pharmablock.com/cn/web/upload/2020/02/28/1582889792152tj0i7.pdf.

Pieber, Bartholomäus, D. Phillip Cox, and C. Oliver Kappe. 2016. "Selective Olefin Reduction in Thebaine Using Hydrazine Hydrate and O2 under Intensified Continuous Flow Conditions." *Organic Process Research and Development* 20 (2): 376–85. https://doi.org/10.1021/acs.oprd.5b00370.

Pieber, Bartholomäus, Toma Glasnov, and C. Oliver Kappe. 2015. "Continuous Flow Reduction of Artemisinic Acid Utilizing Multi-Injection Strategies – Closing the Gap towards a Fully Continuous Synthesis of Antimalarial Drugs." *Chemistry – A European Journal* 21 (11): 4368–76. https://doi.org/10.1002/chem.201406439.

Pieber, Bartholomäus, Sabrina Teixeira Martinez, David Cantillo, and C. Oliver Kappe. 2013. "In Situ Generation of Diimide from Hydrazine and Oxygen: Continuous-Flow Transfer Hydrogenation of Olefins." *Angewandte Chemie – International Edition* 52 (39): 10241–44. https://doi.org/10.1002/anie.201303528.

Pinho, Vagner D., Bernhard Gutmann, Leandro S.M. Miranda, Rodrigo O.M.A. De Souza, and C. Oliver Kappe. 2014. "Continuous Flow Synthesis of α-Halo Ketones: Essential Building Blocks of Antiretroviral Agents." *Journal of Organic Chemistry* 79 (4): 1555–62. https://doi.org/10.1021/jo402849z.

Plutschack, Matthew B., Bartholomäus Pieber, Kerry Gilmore, and Peter H. Seeberger. 2017. "The Hitchhiker's Guide to Flow Chemistry." *Chemical Reviews* 117 (18): 11796–893. https://doi.org/10.1021/acs.chemrev.7b00183.

Poechlauer, Peter, Juan Colberg, Elizabeth Fisher, Michael Jansen, Martin D. Johnson, Stefan G. Koenig, Michael Lawler, et al. 2013. "Pharmaceutical Roundtable Study Demonstrates the Value of Continuous Manufacturing in the Design of Greener Processes." *Organic Process Research & Development* 17: 1472–78.

Poechlauer, Peter, Julie Manley, Rinus Broxterman, and Mats Ridemark. 2012. "Continuous Processing in the Manufacture of Active Pharmaceutical Ingredients and Finished Dosage Forms: An Industry Perspective." *Organic Process Research & Development* 16: 1586–90.

Porta, Riccardo, Maurizio Benaglia, and Alessandra Puglisi. 2016. "Flow Chemistry: Recent Developments in the Synthesis of Pharmaceutical Products." *Organic Process Research and Development* 20 (1): 2–25. https://doi.org/10.1021/acs.oprd.5b00325.

Proctor, Lee, and John Antony Warr. 2001. Process for the Preparation of Diazonmethane. *WO 01/47869 A1*, issued 2001.

Rehm, Thomas. 2020. "Flow Photochemistry as a Tool in Organic Synthesis." *Chemistry – A European Journal.* https://doi.org/10.1002/chem.202000381.

Reilly, Thomas J. 1999. "The Preparation of Lidocaine." *Journal of Chemical Education* 76 (11): 1557. https://doi.org/10.1021/ed076p1557.

Robertson, Karen, Pierre Baptiste Flandrin, Anneke R. Klapwijk, and Chick C. Wilson. 2016. "Design and Evaluation of a Mesoscale Segmented Flow Reactor (KRAIC)." *Crystal Growth and Design* 16 (8): 4759–64. https://doi.org/10.1021/acs.cgd.6b00885.

Ruiz-Castillo, Paula, and Stephen L Buchwald. 2016. "Applications of Palladium-Catalyzed C – N Cross-Coupling Reactions." *Chemical Reviews.* https://doi.org/10.1021/acs.chemrev.6b00512.

Sagandira, Cloudius R., and Paul Watts. 2019. "Safe and Highly Efficient Adaptation of Potentially Explosive Azide Chemistry Involved in the Synthesis of Tamiflu Using Continuous-Flow Technology." *Beilstein Journal of Organic Chemistry* 15: 2577–89. https://doi.org/10.3762/bjoc.15.251.

Sandberg, Rune V. 1989. Optically Pure Compound and a Process for its Preparation. *4,870,086*, issued 1989.

Shankaraiah, Nagula, Ronaldo Aloise Pilli, and Leonardo S. Santos. 2008. "Enantioselective Total Syntheses of Ropivacaine and Its Analogues." *Tetrahedron Letters 49* (34): 5098–5100. https://doi.org/10.1016/j.tetlet.2008.06.028.

Smith, Christopher D., Ian R. Baxendale, Steve Lanners, John J. Hayward, Stephen C. Smith, and Steven V. Ley. 2007. "[3+27] Cycloaddition of Acetylenes with Azides to Give 1,4-Disubstituted 1,2,3-Triazoles in a Modular Flow Reactor." *Organic and Biomolecular Chemistry 5* (10): 1559–61. https://doi.org/10.1039/b702995k.

Snead, David R., and Timothy F. Jamison. 2013. "End-to-End Continuous Flow Synthesis and Purification of Diphenhydramine Hydrochloride Featuring Atom Economy, in-Line Separation, and Flow of Molten Ammonium Salts." *Chemical Science 4* (7): 2822–27. https://doi.org/10.1039/c3sc50859e.

Sonavane, Sachin, Ravindra Pagire, Dayaghan Patil, Uttam Pujari, Rohan Nikam, and Nitin Pradhan. 2017. "Improved, Solvent Free, Atom Efficient Commercial Process for the Synthesis of Diphenhydramine Hydrochloride." *Current Green Chemistry 4* (3): 161–65. https://doi.org/10.2174/2213346105666171227152717.

Struble, Thomas J., Juan C. Alvarez, Scott P. Brown, Milan Chytil, Justin Cisar, Renee L. Desjarlais, Ola Engkvist, et al. 2020. "Current and Future Roles of Artificial Intelligence in Medicinal Chemistry Synthesis." *Journal of Medicinal Chemistry 63* (16): 8667–82. https://doi.org/10.1021/acs.jmedchem.9b02120.

Suveges, Nícolas S., Rodrigo O.M.A. de Souza, Bernhard Gutmann, and C. Oliver Kappe. 2017. "Synthesis of Mepivacaine and Its Analogues by a Continuous-Flow Tandem Hydrogenation/Reductive Amination Strategy." *European Journal of Organic Chemistry 2017* (44): 6511–17. https://doi.org/10.1002/ejoc.201700824.

Tamura, Hiroshi, and K. Kodama. 2014. "Recent Advances in Organozinc Reagents." In *Comprehensive Organic Synthesis*, edited by Paul Knochel and Gary Molander, 2nd ed., 204–66.

Teoh, Soo Khean, Qiao Yan Toh, Mohammad Salih Noorulameen, and Paul N. Sharratt. 2017. "Sustainability Improvements through Catalyst Recycling in a Liquid-Liquid Batch and Continuous Phase Transfer Catalyzed Process." *Organic Process Research and Development 21* (4): 520–30. https://doi.org/10.1021/acs.oprd.6b00337.

Terao, Jun, and Nobuaki Kambe. 2008. "Cross-Coupling Reaction of Alkyl Halides with Grignard Reagents Catalyzed by Ni, Pd, or Cu Complexes with π-Carbon Ligand(S)." *Accounts of Chemical Research 41* (11): 1545–54. https://doi.org/10.1021/ar800138a.

Tosso, N. Perrer, Bimbisar K. Desai, Eliseu De Oliveira, Juekun Wen, John Tomlin, and B. Frank Gupton. 2019. "A Consolidated and Continuous Synthesis of Ciprofloxacin from a Vinylogous Cyclopropyl Amide." *Journal of Organic Chemistry 84* (6): 3370–76. https://doi.org/10.1021/acs.joc.8b03222.

Tsubogo, Tetsu, Hidekazu Oyamada, and Shu Kobayashi. 2015. "Multistep Continuous-Flow Synthesis of (R)- and (S)-Rolipram Using Heterogeneous Catalysts." *Nature 520* (7547): 329–32. https://doi.org/10.1038/nature14343.

Tullar, B.F., and C.H. Bolen. 1969. Process For The Preparation of 1-n-Butyl-2',6'- pipecoloxylidide. *GB1166802A*, issued 1969. https://www.google.com/patents/US20090286991%5Cnhttp://www.google.com/patents?hl=en&lr=&vid=USPAT3663619&id=APwwAAAAEBAJ&oi=fnd&dq=bromine+water+disinfect+OR+sanitize+OR+purify&printsec=abstract.

Vennerstrom, Jonathan L., Sarah Arbe-Barnes, Reto Brun, Susan A. Charman, Francis C.K. Chiu, Jacques Chollet, Yuxiang Dong, et al. 2004. "Identification of an Antimalarial Synthetic Trioxolane Drug Development Candidate." *Nature 430* (7002): 900–904. https://doi.org/10.1038/nature02779.

Verghese, Jenson, Caleb J. Kong, Daniel Rivalti, Eric C. Yu, Rudy Krack, Jesus Alcázar, Julie B. Manley, et al. 2017. "Increasing Global Access to the High-Volume HIV Drug Nevirapine through Process Intensification." *Green Chemistry 19* (13): 2986–91. https://doi.org/10.1039/c7gc00937b.

Vinogradova, Ekaterina V., Nathaniel H. Park, Brett P. Fors, and Stephen L. Buchwald. 2013. "Palladium-Catalyzed Synthesis of N-Aryl Carbamates." *Organic Letters 15* (6): 1394–97. https://doi.org/10.1021/ol400369n.

Volk, Amanda A, Robert W. Epps, Daniel Yonemoto, and Felix N. Castellano. 2021. "Continuous Biphasic Chemical Processes in a Four-Phase Segmented Flow Reactor." *Reaction Chemistry and Engineering*. https://doi.org/10.1039/d1re00247c.

Wang, Xiao Jun, Li Zhang, Xiufeng Sun, Yibo Xu, Dhileepkumar Krishnamurthy, and Chris H. Senanayake. 2005. "Addition of Grignard Reagents to Aryl Acid Chlorides: An Efficient Synthesis of Aryl Ketones." *Organic Letters 7* (25): 5593–95. https://doi.org/10.1021/ol052150q.

Weeranoppanant, Nopphon. 2019. "Enabling Tools for Continuous-Flow Biphasic Liquid-Liquid Reaction." *Reaction Chemistry and Engineering 4*: 235–43. https://doi.org/10.1039/c8re00230d.

Wei, Xiao Jing, Irini Abdiaj, Carlo Sambiagio, Chenfei Li, Eli Zysman-Colman, Jesús Alcázar, and Timothy Noël. 2019. "Visible-Light-Promoted Iron-Catalyzed C(Sp2)–C(Sp3) Kumada Cross-Coupling in Flow." *Angewandte Chemie – International Edition 58* (37): 13030–34. https://doi.org/10.1002/anie.201906462.

Wiles, Charlotte, and Paul Watts. 2014. "Continuous Process Technology: A Tool for Sustainable Production." *Green Chemistry 16* (1): 55–62. https://doi.org/10.1039/c3gc41797b.

Wu, Bo, Jun Wen, Ji Zhang, Jing Li, Yong Zhe Xiang, and Xiao Qi Yu. 2009. "One-Pot Van Leusen Synthesis of 4,5-Disubstituted Oxazoles in Ionic Liquids." *Synlett 3*: 500–504. https://doi.org/10.1055/s-0028-1087547.

Yamazaki, Ken, Pablo Gabriel, Graziano Di Carmine, Julia Pedroni, Mirxan Farizyan, Trevor A. Hamlin, and Darren J. Dixon. 2021. "General Pyrrolidine Synthesis via Iridium-Catalyzed Reductive Azomethine Ylide Generation from Tertiary Amides and Lactams." *ACS Catalysis 11* (12): 7489–97. https://doi.org/10.1021/acscatal.1c01589.

Yang, Cuixian, Andrew R. Teixeira, Yanxiang Shi, Stephen C. Born, Hongkun Lin, Yunfei Li Song, Benjamin Martin, Berthold Schenkel, Maryam Peer Lachegurabi, and Klavs F. Jensen. 2018. "Catalytic Hydrogenation of: N -4-Nitrophenyl Nicotinamide in a Micro-Packed Bed Reactor." *Green Chemistry 20* (4): 886–93. https://doi.org/10.1039/c7gc03469e.

Yu, Eric, Hari P.R. Mangunuru, Nakul S. Telang, Caleb J. Kong, Jenson Verghese, Stanley E. Gilliland, Saeed Ahmad, Raymond N. Dominey, and B. Frank Gupton. 2018. "High-Yielding Continuous-Flow Synthesis of Antimalarial Drug Hydroxychloroquine." *Beilstein Journal of Organic Chemistry 14*: 583–92. https://doi.org/10.3762/bjoc.14.45.

Yu, Tao, Jiao Jiao, Peidong Song, Wenzheng Nie, Chunhai Yi, Qian Zhang, and Pengfei Li. 2020. "Recent Progress in Continuous-Flow Hydrogenation." *ChemSusChem 13* (11): 2876–93. https://doi.org/10.1002/cssc.202000778.

Zeng, Minfeng, Yijun Du, Chenze Qi, Shufeng Zuo, Xiudong Li, Linjun Shao, and Xian-Man Zhang. 2011. "An Efficient and Recyclable Heterogeneous Palladium Catalyst Utilizing Naturally Abundant Pearl Shell Waste." *Green Chemistry 13* (2): 350–56. https://doi.org/10.1039/c0gc00780c.

Ziegler, Robert E., Bimbisar K. Desai, Jo Ann Jee, B. Frank Gupton, Thomas D. Roper, and Timothy F. Jamison. 2018. "7-Step Flow Synthesis of the HIV Integrase Inhibitor Dolutegravir." *Angewandte Chemie - International Edition 57* (24): 7181–85. https://doi.org/10.1002/anie.201802256.

2

Development of Continuous Pharmaceutical Crystallization[1]

Songgu Wu, Yiming Ma, and Junbo Gong
Tianjin University, Tianjin, People's Republic of China

CONTENTS

2.1 Introduction: Background and Driving Forces

Crystallization is a typical solid–liquid separation unit operation to purify a great diversity of active pharmaceutical ingredients (APIs). It is reported that over 70% of APIs demand the application of crystallization technology to obtain intermediates or final products [1–3]. At present, most crystallization processes in the pharmaceutical industry are performed in batches. Although batch crystallization is well-investigated and widely applied, the problems of batch-to-batch variability and processing inefficiency are still present [5, 6]. Hence, continuous crystallization of inorganic salts and organic compounds, especially in the field of pharmaceutical crystallization [6, 7], has gained increasing interest in recent years.

Continuous crystallization has been implemented for many decades in other manufacturing sectors, typically for large volume commodity chemicals, and shows potential advantages relative to batch crystallization [8–10]. The continuous crystallization also exhibits application prospects in pharmaceutical crystallizations [6]. Firstly, continuous crystallization technology provides considerable flexibility in crystallization control, allowing physical separation by control over each stage of the entire separation process, which is easy to achieve accurate control of the product performance, such as purity, particle size and size distribution, crystal form, and morphology. Secondly, the continuous operation

DOI: 10.1201/9781003149835-3

of the crystallization unit under a constant state of control would reduce batch-to-batch variations, contributing to the robustness of the pharmaceutical production. Additionally, less processing footprints for continuous crystallization equipment could reduce the expenditures and are beneficial for the establishment of a flexible unit to better meet the demand. More importantly, the U.S. Food and Drug Administration (FDA) has come out with relevant regulations to support continuous pharmaceutical manufacturing for better process quality and control [11–14]. Due to these benefits and rationality, continuous pharmaceutical crystallization seems to be an inevitable trend in the development of pharmaceutical production.

In this chapter, we give a general overview of continuous crystallization for pharmaceutical applications, including basic kinetics and thermodynamic principles in crystallization, detailed development, and the application cases of continuous crystallization. In particular, monitoring and control strategies using process analytical technology were also described to provide guides about ensuring the robustness of continuous crystallization.

2.2 Basic Kinetics and Thermodynamic Principles in Crystallization

2.2.1 Solubility and Supersaturation

This section provides a general description of the fundamental principles in crystallization to give a theoretical basis for the design of continuous pharmaceutical crystallization. There are various crystallization methods that could be implemented to purify the solid from solutions, such as slurry, cooling crystallization, evaporation, antisolvent (or drown-out) crystallization, and reactive crystallization. Whichever crystallization approach was used, the yield of crystallization process depends on the equilibrium of solid and liquid phase.

The equilibrium of the solid and liquid phase could be expressed as solubility. Generally, the solubility of organic molecules is associated with the property of the solute, solvent, and temperature. The solubility variations with solvent and temperature are useful for the choice of crystallization method and solvent. In principle, the cooling crystallization would be the best choice when the solubility changes rapidly with temperature. If there are obvious solubility differences in different solvents, antisolvent crystallization could be used to achieve a high yield. The choice of suitable good solvent and antisolvent is based on the solubility in different solvents.

When the solution comes to the solid–liquid equilibrium state, the solid could not crystallize from the solution. Excess solutes beyond the saturation solution are needed to drive crystallization. The area between the solubility curve and supersolubility curve is the metastable zone where solute cannot nucleate spontaneously. The driving force of crystallization is called supersaturation. Supersaturation can be described by the difference between the chemical potential of the solute and the value of the chemical potential at equilibrium:

$$\Delta\mu = \mu - \mu^* \tag{2.1}$$

where μ is the chemical potential of the solute being crystallized and μ^* is the chemical potential of the solute at equilibrium at the same temperature and pressure. When $\mu > \mu^*$, the solution is supersaturated. Then a reduction in the chemical potential through crystallization of the solute can return the system to equilibrium, $\Delta\mu = 0$. Assuming ideal conditions, the supersaturation, S, can be described in terms of the concentrations of the solute by the equation:

$$\ln S = \ln c/c^* = \Delta\mu/RT \tag{2.2}$$

where R is the gas constant (8.314 J mol^{-1} K^{-1}), T is the temperature (K), c is the solute concentration, and c* is the equilibrium solubility. In practical application, it is often expressed as the supersaturation ratio, S [Equation (2.3)] or as the relative supersaturation, σ [Equation (5.4)]:

$$S = c/c^*$$ (2.3)

$$\sigma = (c - c^*)/c^*$$ (2.4)

As the driving force of crystallization, supersaturation should be designed and controlled to ensure the quality of the product, including crystal form and particle size distribution. In principle, a strategy needs to be applied to manage the available growth surface either by primary nucleation or, more commonly by seeding, and subsequently following a trajectory within the MSZW close to the solubility limit, thereby avoiding uncontrolled formation of new particles through nucleation.

2.2.2 Nucleation and Growth

Crystallization from solution can be considered a two-step process. The first step is the phase separation or "birth" of new crystals, which is called nucleation. The second step is the growth of these crystals to larger sizes. Analysis of industrial crystallization processes and design of continuous crystallization require knowledge of both nucleation and crystal growth.

As the first step of crystallization, nucleation plays an important role in product quality, such as polymorph outcomes, crystal size, and size distribution. Herein we give the general concept and classification of nucleation in industrial production. Nucleation can broadly be classified into two categories: primary nucleation and second nucleation. Primary nucleation describes the nucleation occurred when no crystalline matter is present in the system, including homogeneous and heterogeneous. Specifically, primary nucleation expresses the initial formation of crystals in a supersaturated solution. In comparison, secondary nucleation describes the formation of new crystals induced by the existing solids of crystallizing solute, such as seeding and attrition. As mentioned before, primary nucleation can also be classified into two types: homogeneous nucleation and heterogeneous nucleation. Heterogeneous nucleation relies on the presence of a foreign interface for the formation of new crystals. Although it seems like secondary nucleation, it's different in the existing solid in solution before nucleation. Heterogeneous nucleation is initialized by a foreign compound while secondary crystallization relies on the solid of the same solute. Conversely, homogeneous nucleation is therefore the spontaneous formation of new crystals without the assistance of other solids, either foreign interface or solute itself. However, primary nucleation is limited in practical applications since it's very rare in industrial production. But it's still of great significance to investigate this phenomenon, which paves the way for understanding other types of nucleation. Heterogeneous nucleation is therefore the dominant process in pharmaceutical production.

A stable production requires a suitable nucleation rate to ensure the size of the final product. It's thus important to understand the nucleation rate and the effect of operation conditions on the nucleation rate. Nucleation rate, J, is defined as the number of nuclei formed per unit volume per time and is largely dependent on supersaturation. Many efforts have been devoted to modelling and predicting the nucleation rate. Table 2.1 summarizes the empirical equations to describe the nucleation kinetics.

TABLE 2.1

Empirical Nucleation Rate Equations for Different Nucleation Types

Nucleation Type	Expression	Reference
Primary	$J = k_b S^b$	[15]
Homogeneous	$J = A \exp\left[\dfrac{-16\pi\gamma^3 v^2}{3k^3 T^3 (\ln S)^2}\right] J = A \exp\left(-\dfrac{B}{\ln^2 S}\right)$	[16]
Heterogeneous	$J = k_{bhet} \exp\left[\dfrac{-16\pi\gamma^3 v^2 f(\varphi)}{3k^3 T^3 [\ln(\delta + 1)]^2}\right] J = A \exp\left(-\dfrac{B}{\ln^2 S}\right)$	[17]
Secondary	$J = k_b S^b \mu_2$	[18]

After nucleation has occurred, the newly formed nuclei can continue to grow to a larger size. This process is called crystal growth, the second step of nucleation. The crystal growth is highly affected by bulk diffusion and surface integration. The growth kinetics is thus dependent on varieties of factors. The most important factor is supersaturation, which gives the driving force for crystal growth. The existence and properties of impurity can also influence the growth rate. Most of the impurity can inhibit growth, while some can also promote growth. We can also add foreign substances, which we called additives, to modulate the crystal growth. The local mixing, agitation, and solvent properties also have important effects on the growth rate. Besides the crystal growth through molecular attachment, particle breakage, and agglomeration should also be taken into consideration in industrial production. Agglomeration brings a huge challenge in measuring growth kinetics through an online instrument, such as focused beam reflectance measurement (FBRM). The accurate growth rate, which is determined as dL/dt, can also be measured through single crystal growth experiment using optical microscopy. However, it may not always replicate the actual process in industrial production since the hydrodynamic environments are usually different between the static growth cell and crystallizer with agitation. Considering the influence factors, the kinetic growth rate can also be expressed as:

$$G = A \exp(-E_G/RT) \Delta C^g \qquad (2.5)$$

Where G is growth rate (m s^{-1}), A is constant, E_G represents the activation energy (J mol^{-1}), and g is the order of crystal growth. There are a number of variations of this equation for different types of crystal growth and the equations were summarized in Table 2.2.

2.2.3 Mass and Population Balance Equation

Particle size distribution (PSD) is associated with nucleation rate, growth rate, and residence time, which is affected by almost all the operation conditions, including temperature, supersaturation, agitation rate, aggregation, and so on. It's thus very complex to understand the relationship between PSD and various conditions. The application of the population balance equations (PBEs) to industrial crystallization is a milestone in the development of industrial crystallization. The PBE model is a common model formula proposed by Randolph and Larson [19] that is based on the continuity of the mass during a crystallization process and typically has the following forms:

$$\partial n/\partial t + \partial(nG)/\partial L + (n - n0)/\tau = B_{Ag} - D_{Ag} + B_{Br} - D_{Br} + J \qquad (2.6)$$

where n is the joint probability density function, t is time, L is crystal size, τ is the residence time, B_{Ag} and D_{Ag} represent birth and death terms for agglomeration, and B_{Br} and D_{Br} represent birth and dead terms for breakage. Population balance modelling (PBM) can significantly reduce the number of experiments required to develop a crystallization process. At present, there are two main objectives for the research of PBEs: (i) Combined with the measured PSD, we can obtain information about crystallization kinetics, which is very useful for the design of a crystallizer and (ii) the PBEs can provide guides for the operating conditions of crystallizer to achieve the desired particle size and size distribution.

TABLE 2.2

Empirical Crystal Growth Rate Equations for Different Growth Types

Growth Mechanism	Equations	Reference
Size-independent growth	$G = k_g S^g$	[19]
Size-dependent growth	$G = k_g S^g (1 + \gamma L)^p$	[20]
Power law growth	$G = k_g S^g L^p$	[21]

Since the 1980s, the PBE model has been widely investigated in the modelling of solution crystallization in batch and continuous processes [22]. Because of the steady-state condition of the continuous process, the PBE model can be mathematically simplified to some extent. A systematic study developed by PBEs in batch and continuous crystallization that introduces the conceptual design of the crystallization processes was carried out by Vetter et al [23]. It constructed a connection among the variable range of product characteristics, the diversified crystallizer devices, and the independent variables describing them. Actually, quite a lot of researchers tend to focus more on the performance of the model itself. Su et al [24]. presented first-principles dynamic and kinetic models for nucleation and growth of paracetamol crystallizing in a multisegment multiaddition plug flow crystallizer. They figured out that the startup duration could be obviously compressed by the implementation of open-loop optimization techniques determined by the simulation. They also optimized the antisolvent addition position to get the desired particle size distribution. In the same year, they progressively expanded the concentration control strategy from batch crystallization into a continuous MSMPR crystallizer. The PBE was used together with the mass balance equations to provide a rigorous and general mathematical model for the conversion of a conventional batch pharmaceutical crystallization into a continuous mode [25]. However, some PBE models identified by the infinite-dimensional nature hinder their handling in practical controllers. Therefore, precise control of the CSD in a continuous process counting on non-linear reduced-order models with the reduced-order modelling technique (ROM) has been reported [26]. Researchers focused on the expansion of the PBE solution itself, and the study of agglomeration and breakage helped to better simulate the continuous crystallization process.

2.3 Development and Application of Continuous Crystallizers

According to the general classification, there are mainly two continuous crystallization systems: mixed-suspension mixed-product-removal (MSMPR) crystallizers and continuous tubular crystallizers. MSMPR crystallizers have a single stage or multiple stages, while continuous tubular crystallizers can be subdivided into continuous plug flow crystallizers (CPFCs), [27] continuous oscillatory baffled crystallizers (COBCs), [28] and continuous segmented flow crystallizers (CSFCs) [29]. Schematic diagrams of the mentioned crystallizers are shown in Figure 2.1 [30]. Different crystallizer types offer various characteristics relevant to the control of crystallization processes. MSMPR crystallizers feature their well internal

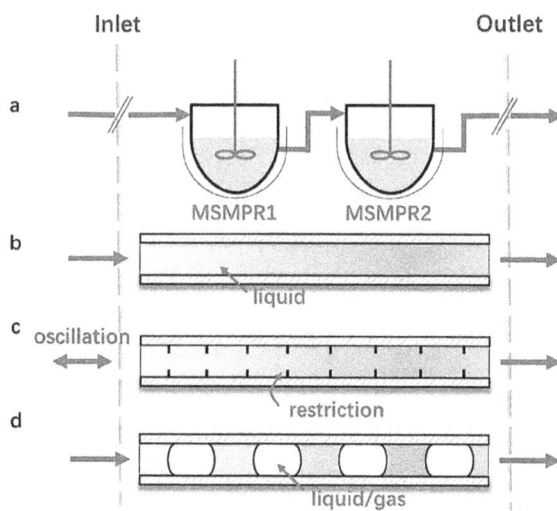

FIGURE 2.1 Schematic diagrams of four types of continuous crystallizer: (a) MSMPR crystallizer cascade; (b) continuous plug flow crystallizer (CPFC); (c) continuous oscillatory baffled crystallizer (COBC); (d) continuous segmented flow crystallizer (CSFC). Reprinted with permission from Ref. [4]. Copyright © 2020 American Chemical Society.

mixing as well as a relatively long residence time. Compared with an MSMPR crystallizer, tubular crystallizers have the advantages of a narrow residence time distribution and a relatively simple scale-up process [31]. However, it suffers from the disadvantages that the continuous tubular crystallizer may not be easy to control [32], and that the system can be easily blocked [33]. In this section, we will focus on the introduction of MSMPR and continuous tubular crystallizers as well as some detailed application examples of them in continuous crystallization processes.

2.3.1 Single Stage and Cascades of Mixed Suspension Mixed Product Removal

Generally, single-stage MSMPR crystallizers are believed to be similar to batch crystallizers and are often commonly used to study nucleation behavior or optimize the particle size distribution in continuous crystallization processes [34, 35]. It provides a degree of familiarity to operators and lowers capital investment. Randolph's work offered a detailed explanation of single-stage MSMPR crystallizers [36]. Multistage MSMPR crystallizers are a cascade of two or more MSMPR crystallizers, in which the former one's outlet line connects directly to the next one as a feed line. In comparison with single-stage MSMPR, MSMPR cascades can enhance production capacity and product quality [37–39]. Plant capacity is a main factor in determining the number of cascading MSMPR crystallizers needed, while total cost minimization should also be considered [40, 41]. Prominent articles are discussed below in relation to some examples of product attribute regulation with single-stage MSMPR and cascades of MSMPR in continuous crystallizations.

Particle Size and Morphology Control. Ferguson et al. [42] compared the antisolvent crystallization of benzoic acid in batch, continuous plug flow, and MSMPR configurations, and found that the continuous modes of operation (plug flow and MSMPR) could obtain crystal size distributions that were both smaller and larger than the equivalent batch crystallizations, in addition to providing huge increases in productivity. Vetter et al. [23] constructed an attainable region of mean particle sizes versus the total residence time for three different pharmaceutical MSMPR cascades. The final results showed that MSMPR crystallizers with a low number of cascades could produce crystals with larger particle sizes. Narducci et al. [43] coupled ultrasound with an adipic acid MSMPR crystallizer and investigated the effect of inlet solute concentration and ultrasound power amplitudes. The crystal size of adipic acid was much smaller (about 60 μm) than with MSMPR alone (about 500 μm) in the presence of ultrasound. Yang et al. [44, 45] demonstrated the crystallization of paracetamol in an MSMPR coupled with a wet milling unit and found that different locations of the wet mill have different impacts on the particle size. Gerard et al. [46] studied the impacts of calcium ion addition on the reaction crystallization of sodium bicarbonate in a single-stage MSMPR crystallizer. The nucleation and growth rates could be determined when the steady state was reached. It was indicated that the calcium-based additives changed the morphology of crystals from elongated needle to almost spheroidal. Tahara et al. [47] used a single-stage MSMPR crystallizer to produce spherical crystals of albuterol sulfate, among which water was used as the solvent and an ethyl acetate/emulsifier mixture was used as the antisolvent. Peña and Nagy [48] divided the continuous spherical crystallization of benzoic acid into two steps. The first step was the nucleation and growth-dominant stage, while the second step was the agglomeration dominant stage. Finally, they continuously obtained spherical crystals with a diameter of about 1 mm with this process.

Yield, Recycle, and Purity. Alvarez et al. [49] used mother liquid recycling to improve the cooling crystallization yield of cyclosporine. It was found that the implementation of a recycle stream increased the yield from 74% to 87%, compared with the yield of a batch process. However, the purity decreased from 95% to 94%. Zhang et al. [50] developed a combined antisolvent and cooling continuous crystallization operation using a two-stage MSMPR process, and generated a model based on the data from the experiments. They found that the stage temperature and the residence time affected the yield, and the increased yield did result in a slight decrease in purity. In later work, Wong et al. [51] simplified the cyclosporine multistage MSMPR crystallizer into a single-stage MSMPR crystallizer by continuously concentrating and recycling the mother liquid, thereby achieving better purity and yield (94.3% and 91.8%, respectively). Figure 2.2 shows the equipment setup with a recycle system and experimental results using the recycle system. In the continuous antisolvent/cooling crystallization of deferasirox [51], the recycled mother liquid was evaporated, mixed with antisolvent, and then re-refluxed into the crystallizer, which

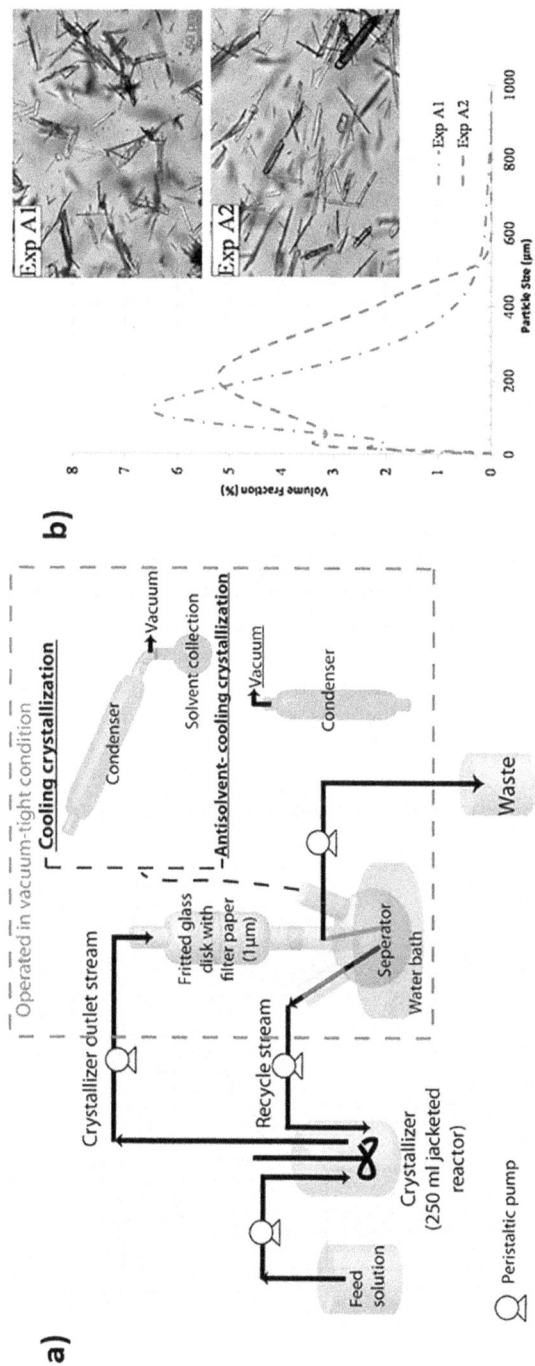

FIGURE 2.2 (a) Schematic diagram of the single-stage MSMPR with recycle (SMR) system; (b) Particle size distribution of two experiments (Exp A2 with higher recycle ratio). Reprinted with permission from Ref. [51]. Copyright © 2012 American Chemical Society.

resulted in a maximum yield of 82.1% and a minimum impurity concentration of 0.2 ppm. Ferguson et al. [52] applied an organic solvent nanofiltration membrane in order to preferentially concentrate the API (deferasirox) from a continuously operated MSMPR and purge the limiting impurity (4-hydrazinobenzoic acid) from the mother liquid recycling stream. Li et al. [53] proposed the incorporation of solids recycling with a two-stage MSMPR system to improve yield so as to overcome the long residence time required for a high yield when the growth kinetics is slow. A 2017 study by Vartak et al. [54] successfully employed solution complexation accompanied by nanofiltration in combination with a recycle line in an MSMPR configuration to control impurity buildup during recycling. The results showed that a 13% improvement in yield was identified relative to MSMPR operation in the absence of recycling, and solution complexation significantly reduced impurity incorporation.

Polymorph, Cocrystal, and Chirality Control. Lai et al. [55] demonstrated that the polymorph of L-glutamic acid crystals could be effectively controlled by varying the residence time and temperature in MSMPR crystallization. They concluded that if the endpoint temperature in a single-stage MSMPR is 25°C, the residence time should be 900 min to obtain a pure stable β polymorph, which is not realistic for the continuous crystallization process. On the basis of kinetic simulations and experimental verification, the authors proved that the seeding could not precisely control the crystal polymorph. Motivated by the abovementioned research, Farmer et al. [56] performed a remarkable work analyzing polymorphism under steady-state conditions and modified the population balance model into a non-dimensional form. Power exponential forms for the descriptions of crystal nucleation and growth kinetics were used, and the two dimensionless parameters characterizing the polymorph results in continuous crystallization at the corresponding temperatures are shown in Figure 2.3. On the basis of the plots, the authors believed that when the homogeneous nucleation process occurred, the crystallization process could be as far as possible from the bifurcation line to control the polymorphism. Lee et al. [57] used continuous co-crystallization to form 1:2 co-crystals of phenazine-vanillin in order to separate vanillin. Powell et al. [58] used a novel periodic MSMPR crystallizer to produce the urea-barbituric acid co-crystal and compared the effect of different operating conditions on the co-crystal form. Their results showed that the pure crystal form I could be obtained using optimal crystallization conditions. Qamar et al. [59] published the first research in transitioning preferential crystallization from batch process to continuous process, among which an MSMPR with continuous seeding and with a fine-dissolving operation was used to continuously produce a preferential enantiomer. Steendam et al. [60] utilized a single-stage MSMPR system to achieve continuous crystallization of enantiopure crystals of sodium bromate from an achiral solution.

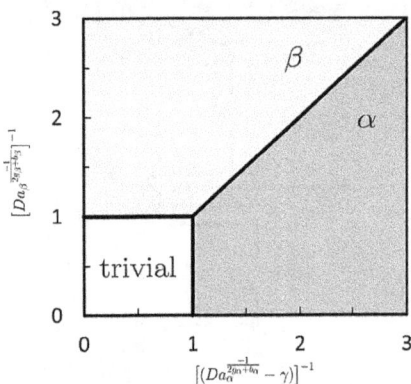

FIGURE 2.3 Three stability regions for polymorphic continuous crystallization. Reprinted with permission from Ref. [56]. Copyright 2016 American Institute of Chemical Engineers.

2.3.2 Continuous Tubular Crystallizers

CPFCs are the most commonly used tubular crystallizers. The supersaturation is rapidly accumulated as a result of antisolvent or reactive solvent addition, and the design of the thin tube largely avoids the occurrence of inefficient mixing [61, 62]. A COBC is a type of continuous tubular crystallizer with periodically spaced baffles that contribute to the combination of the oscillatory motion and net flow in the main tube. This design is beneficial for momentum transfer, mass transfer, and heat transfer [63–65]. In CSFCs, which are also known as continuous slug flow crystallizers, [66, 67] the solution inside the pipeline is divided into microbatch volumes or liquid "bubbles" in a continuous mode by an immiscible fluid. Since the residence time and the physical and chemical environment of each volume unit are consistent, the crystals are precisely produced by the CSFC with uniform mean particle size, morphology, and polymorphism [68].

Eder et al. [69] reported continuous operation on the product. A suspension of acetylsalicylic acid seed mixed with acetylsalicylic acid mother liquid was continuously pumped into a CPFC crystallizer. They investigated the effect of flow rate on the final crystal size distribution and concluded that a high flow rate resulted in a low volume mean diameter, and that blockages in the pipe could be avoided by manipulating the seed flow rate. To control nucleation without seeding, Majumder and Nagy [70] applied a fines dissolution process in plug flow crystallization, and established a population balance model coupled with nucleation and the growth and dissolution kinetics. They systematically studied the key factors that determine fine dissolving. Wong et al. [71] applied a contact nucleation device to generate uniform seeds; the size of the seeds could be controlled by supersaturation and by the residence time of the seeds in the nucleation device. Furuta et al. [72] applied ultrasound in plug flow crystallization and found that the crystal size decreased remarkably (down to 1–7 μm). Ferguson et al. [73] applied a Roughton-type vortex mixer to enhance the mixing efficiency. With this device, the square-weighted chord length was reduced from 152 μm to 52 μm.

Briggs et al. [63] designed and operated a COBC with seeding of L-glutamic acid to optimize control over the crystalline polymorph. The experimental results indicated that when bulk supersaturation remained in the range of 2–3, the polymorphic phase purity of the thermodynamically stable β form was retained within two residence times. Agnew et al. [74] combined COBC and MSMPR systems to produce paracetamol form II with enhanced dissolving ability and compressibility, which showed the system to have better efficiency than individual MSMPR or COBC crystallizers. Zhao et al. [75] applied a COBC to make over 1 kg of α-lipoic acid/nicotinamide cocrystals within 3 h. Besides, the spherical agglomerated product was obtained with good purity and narrow particle size distributions. In the study by Peña et al. [76], a COBC was implemented to strengthen the continuous spherical crystallization operation. The authors attempted to achieve separate control of the nucleation, growth, and agglomeration processes by the use of spatially distributed solutions, solvents, antisolvents, and bridging solutions. They also claimed that the back-mixing effect caused by the excessive residence time and excessive slurry density was the critical factor in the broad agglomerate size distribution.

Neugebauer and Khinast [77] investigated using a CSFC crystallizer to produce protein crystals, and were able to obtain enzyme lysozyme crystals with sizes that ranged between 15 μm and 40 μm within 113.4 min. Jiang et al. [78] used the same type of crystallizer to continuously produce L-asparagine monohydrate. In their research, nucleation and growth were separated in order to enhance the individual control of each phenomenon. By manipulating the gas and liquid flow rates and adjusting the mixing approach of hot and cool fluids that were used for seed generation, Jiang et al. were able to obtain crystals with a maximum size of 588 μm within 5 min. In later work, Jiang et al. [79] used ultrasonic nucleation devices instead of the original nucleation device. Using indirect ultrasonication, Jiang et al. produced crystals with a size of 321 μm within 8.5 min. Rossi et al. [80] used ultrasonication in droplet-based microfluidic crystallization and were able to produce adipic acid crystals with a small mean size (15 μm) at a high production rate and with a narrow distribution. In addition, many researchers use CSFCs to investigate the crystallization mechanism.

2.4 Monitoring and Controlling Continuous Pharmaceutical Crystallization via Process Analytical Technology

2.4.1 Process Monitoring and Analysis

Process Analytical Technology (PAT) was introduced by the FDA in 2004. It was described as a system aiming to design, analyze and control the manufacturing system by measuring the critical parameters and fundamental data of APIs and monitoring the process in real time. During the past two decades, several PAT tools have been focused on the application of the crystallization process control, including focused beam reflectance measurement (FBRM), particle vision and measurement (PVM), attenuated total reflectance Fourier-transform infrared (ATR-FTIR) and ultraviolet-visible (ATR-UV/Vis), and Raman spectroscopy.

ATR-FTIR and ATR-UV/Vis spectroscopy enable monitoring of the API concentration in liquid and solid phase. Several researchers control and monitor the tabletting step during continuous manufacturing of Diclofenac sodium [81], silicified microcrystalline cellulose [82], and mannitol [83] with the near-infrared spectroscopy by the high efficiency and non-destructive characteristics. In situ, ATR-UV/Vis is a comparatively emerging tool which is applied to solutes containing chromophores. Although ATR-UV/Vis is already used in some nanosized crystallizing behavior descriptions [84–87], it still has a long way to go due to its self-limitation.

In situ, FBRM can measure the particle size distribution and particle counts based on the chord length distribution in suspension. FBRM has a wide range of applications in both batch and continuous operation for process monitoring and particle size analysis. Zhang et al. [88] used FBRM to determine the optimal cooling curve for better morphology of crystals in batch seeding cooling crystallization of sodium phosphate tribasic dodecahydrate. They also focused on the nucleation process in the presence of high concentrations of magnesium ions. It was found that the prenucleation clusters gradually converted into more ordered structures by the relative relationship between chord distribution and time. Siddique et al. [89] investigated the combination of FBRM and mid-IR in batch oscillatory baffled crystallizer of alpha lactose monohydrate. The dynamic and thermodynamic parameters determined by the batch crystallization provide the principles of continuous operation. Morris et al. [90] used FBRM to identify the steady-state process in the production of benzoic acid by MSMPR crystallizer, thereby obtaining the nucleation and growth kinetics of cooling crystallization.

Raman spectroscopy is a vibrational spectroscopy technique that enables a non-destructive analysis of chemical composition and microscopic configuration similar to infrared spectroscopy. The change in the molecular polarizability raised by the inelastic scattering of the monochromatic laser light contributes to the distinct response in solid, liquid, and gaseous samples. Due to the absorption, fluorescence and scattering will vary with physical properties, for example, Raman spectra still present differences even with the same samples with different morphology. Thus, repetitive collection of data with long scanning time should be required to achieve stabilized test results [91, 92]. White et al. [93] gave a general introduction to the application of continuous manufacturing in the biological and pharmaceutical industries. Acevedo et al. [94] developed a comprehensive method that could monitor the bulk concentration and quantified the metastable polymorphic form upper the base detection line of carbamazepine in cooling continuous crystallization. Li et al. [95] established a Raman method during batch and continuous manufacturing processes of acetaminophen. It could precisely quantify the content of the API powder during tablet compression.

PVM provides real-time visualization of basic morphological information like crystal shape and size. Besides, it can also identify a series of phenomena in the crystallization process [96], namely, nucleation, growth, polymorphic transformation, agglomeration, breakage, and oiling out. Kacker et al. [97] established an online imaging system to represent the particle size distribution and the crystal shape during the crystallization process in COBC. The outcome of the image analysis probe indicated similar results to the FBRM measurements. Moreover, Jiang et al. [98] described a low-cost system with effective monitoring and controlling ability for continuous crystallization processes. It was composed of a basic stereo microscope and video camera for imaging and characterization of the L-asparagine monohydrate crystals in real time.

In addition to the above widely used crystallization monitoring methods, conductivity measurements, refractive index measurements, turbidity measurements, and acoustic spectroscopy are also available in PAT. The different analysis strategies need to be settled according to the crystallization system and the actual conditions. However, some limitations still cannot be ignored in the application of the PAT tools. Theoretically, the intensity of the illumination source, the sensitivity of the detector, and the light transfer function of the analytical instrument (e.g., monochromator, probe, fiber optics) together with the cross sections constrain the detection limit of many analytes [99]. For example, the at-line near-infrared spectroscopy (NIR) approach showed the limitation of low reliability and high susceptibility to final product moisture content [100]. FBRM is an important PAT tool for detecting the chord length of APIs at the lab level. However, compared to other particle size measurement tools (e.g., single-frequency ultrasound technique, 3D optical reflectance measurement), the measurable concentration of APIs needs to be strictly limited, and the shape of the API will also affect the accuracy of the measurement results. As the slurry becomes denser, easy fouling of the intrusive probe also becomes an important cause of the failure of online monitoring. In addition to fouling, such probes also face challenges like calibration, mixing impact, equipment wear, etc. [101, 102] Once the online determination of the concentration or the particle size distribution is required to achieve or exceed the accuracy of offline measurements (e.g., HPLC, Malvern laser particle size analyzer), the selection should be made for the most suitable PAT tool under the acceptation of the corresponding quantum mechanical and technological limits spectroscopic tools [103].

2.4.2 Advances Crystallization Control Approaches

2.4.2.1 Model-Based Control Strategies

With the gradual maturity and improvement of the numerical solvers and computational hardware, experimental verification has gradually become a crucial supplement while establishing a model. Peng et al. [104] collected the predicted CSD and supersaturation by the combination model of PBE and thermodynamic model platform. The experimentally fitted kinetics parameters were verified with the prediction values, which showed a good agreement in a specific temperature range. A theoretically based control application was completed in Rohani's research group [105], and they successfully obtained metastable crystals with narrow size distribution. Zhao et al. [106] suggested a population balance model that considered the physical constraints to simulate the inseparable shrinkage and breakage of the agglomerated particles during the reactive dissolution by the continuous stir. The coupled equations were solved by high-order moment-conserving method of classes.

The truth is that a large majority of continuous crystallization theoretical models and devices can only realize in the laboratory stage. Therefore, in order to better connect theoretical work with industrial production, application to achieve multiobjective optimization and process synthesis with process control in continuous crystallization are significant development directions in the future. Due to the complex interplay between heat and mass transfer unit operations, multiobjective optimization and process integration require a mathematical modeling approach. A non-dominated set – which was called the "Pareto frontier" – brought possible solutions that allow improving one objective without degrading another [107]. Ridder et al. [108] defined that the vector of objective functions unified the coefficient of variation and weight mean size. The coupled differential equations were solved by either the method of moments or the high-resolution finite volume method to calculate the Pareto frontiers for this integration vector. A neoteric parallel design together with the control approach was provided to realize the best crystallization design that can pursue optimum product properties. Diab and Gerogiorgis [38] treated the lowest total cost and non-significant environmental impact as the optimization objectives in the process configuration. The optimum economical option in attainable crystallization and plantwide yields were determined by performing a steady-state process model and simulation investigation. Similar work is also implemented to assess cost minimization options in MSMPR [40]. Process synthesis refers to an effective combination

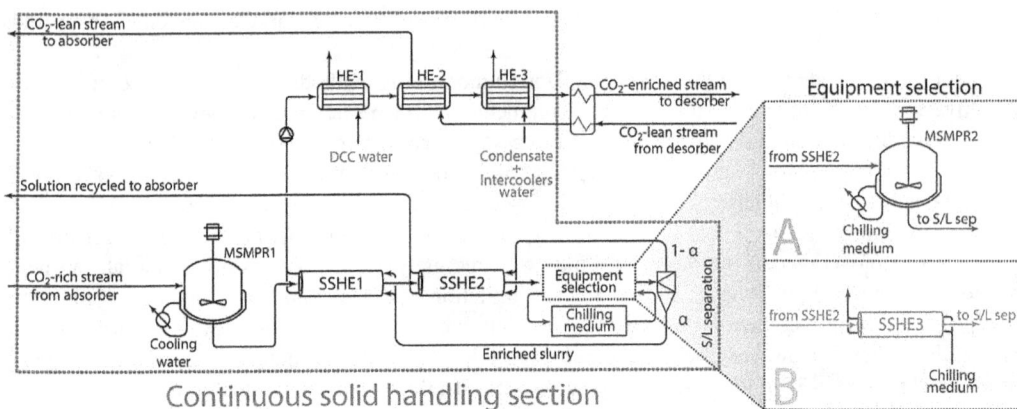

FIGURE 2.4   Flow scheme adopted for the continuous solid handling section produced by Milella et al. The dashed blue box indicates the battery limit of the section. In addition, configurations A (in purple) and B (in green) identify the process alternatives adopted for the continuous cooling crystallization of ammonium bicarbonate. Configuration A exploits an MSMPR for the final crystallization step while configuration B uses scraped surface heat exchangers. Reprinted with permission from Ref. [109]. Copyright © 2018 American Chemical Society.

of independent unit operations, where energy consumption and productivity are as important as product quality requirements. A systematic method presented by Milella et al. [109] was established to capture post-combustion CO_2 in multistage continuous operation with a novelty design of a heat exchanger named scraped surface heat exchanger (Figure 2.4). They developed a rate-based model for describing particle behavior during crystallization and dissolution. Furthermore, the optimization framework emphasized the trade-off between the key performance indicators and the interdependency among individual operating variables. Sen et al. [110] coupled filtration, drying, and mixing of the API with an excipient as an integrated flowsheet by simulation. The main objective was to optimize the integrated flowsheet model such that there was an overall improvement in process operation, and a narrower CSD has been given as well. A milestone work of continuous operation was successfully published in 2016 [111]. They reported the continuous-flow synthesis and formulation of APIs in a compact, reconfigurable manufacturing platform. Continuous end-to-end synthesis in the 1 m^3 system produced sufficient quantities per day, and the productions met U.S. Pharmacopeia standards as well. Yazdanpanah et al. [112] developed a continuous heterogeneous crystallization process in place of the need for complex downstream processing steps. The production was directly compressed into tablet form, and the maximum drug loading of the excipient with API could reach 47%. The continuous crystallization is very demanding on the steady-state, and it is easier to achieve uniform concentration at the lab scale, that is, to achieve the state of the theoretical simulation presetting especially in MSMPR. Factors trigger the deviation in scale-up including the potential for an unstable residence time distribution in crystallizers, which may result in broad PSD, the shrinking of heat transfer areas, and intricate transfer mechanisms at low flow rates. Model-based control approaches require kinetics functions of crystal nucleation and growth to be expressed in a simpler and more accurate form so that it is possible to jointly obtain a numerical solution in conjunction with the mass balance. At present, researchers are more inclined to innovate in advanced theoretical models, but that is hard to be verified experimentally. Compared to the increasing number of new APIs being synthesized, the number of APIs that have established kinetic models is extremely diminutive, which also severely restricts the application of advanced control models to industrialization. Besides, due to the occurrence of back-mixing or dead zone during continuous manufacturing, these unexpected phenomena will lead to theoretical predictions that are far removed from the real results. Experimental work was performed in a non-ideal crystallizer [113]. The authors qualitatively analyzed the effects of the initial supersaturation, loading amount, and CSD of the seed on the product quality in a 75 L draft tube crystallizer. In tubular continuous crystallization, staged heating or cooling is one of the most effective ways to regulate crystal products. However, this can lead to scale formation on the wall of the tube crystallizer. Majumder and Nagy [62] established dynamic fouling behavior on PFC considering the rate of solute transport and shear stress induced by fluid turbulence. Coupling the kinetic model with the PBE can predict the concentration distribution inside the plug and the CSD. To sum up, the currently scalable simulation work and experimentally verifications should have the following characteristics: (a) approximately perfect mixing; (b) no classification at withdrawal; (c) breakage assumed negligible; and (d) uniform shape factor. Steady-state operation requires that the feed rate, composition, and temperature remain constant, and the crystallizer volume and temperature also remain constant.

2.4.2.2 Classical Feedback Loop Control Strategies

In the proposal for renovations in physical separation and manufacturing of crystalline pharmaceutical products, the quality-by-control (QbC) concept was developed from the quality-by-design (QbD) proposed by FDA. By the implementation of closed-loop (feedback) control approaches, the influence of disturbances in the crystallization process and product vibration can be reduced under "design via control" strategy under the optimum operating trajectories. Yang et al. [114] developed a continuous crystallization system with an automated feedback two-stage (MSMPR) crystallization platform. A centralized automation program coded in LabVIEW was organized to achieve feedback/feedforward control on the continuous crystallization of carbamazepine. Besenhard et al. [115] described a crystal size tuning strategy in a continuous tubular crystallizer based on a simple model-free control approach. A feedback controller that precisely controlled the mean crystal size was developed by using a CSD analyzer and empirical studies.

In a general sense, model-free closed-loop control approaches, which are generated on the basis of the QbC concept and application of PAT tools, are classified into direct nucleation control (DNC) and supersaturation (concentration feedback) control (SSC/CFC). These robust control approaches allow a controlled crystallization of the boundaries of the metastable zone and impel the entire process operating in the presupposed crystallization region.

DNC is a closed-loop control strategy to avoid the formation of fine particles. The rapid switching between heating and cooling or adding solvent or antisolvent strategies was implemented diffusely to reach the purpose of the direct control of nucleation and fines removal by the in-situ number of FBRM counts. The superiority of the DNC approach has been proved for the preparation of crystalline products with the desired mean size [84, 116] or polymorphic form, [117] the improved crystal surface properties [118], and the minimizing of the solvent inclusion [102]. The coupling of DNC with PAT is also worthy of attention. Kacker et al. [119] adopted microwave heating to eliminate the limitations of traditional heat exchange methods, which resulted in a very rapid response during DNC applications. The batch time was significantly reduced while achieving the same narrow particle size distribution. A developed direct nucleation control based on image analysis was presented by Borsos et al. [120, 121] The application of image feedback control could perform better data processing on some complicated complexities like crystal sticking and agglomerates disintegration in contrast with the FBRM-based DNC. For continuous crystallization processes, how to quickly reach steady-state operations has always been the key to the startup process, a fact that used to be commonly ignored [90, 122]. When Yang et al. [123] identified this gap, they proposed a feedback control approach to lessening startup duration which conceded to changing the controlled set-point with a rapid response disturbances rejection mechanism. Based on the direct nucleation control of batch crystallization, they proposed a feedback control method based on FBRM and achieved the required particle size control for the continuous crystallization of acetaminophen in single-stage and two-stage continuous MSMPR crystallizers. In their later work, Yang et al. [44] adopted wet-milling in the DNC approach in single-stage paracetamol cooling continuous crystallization. It was found that the choice of wet milling addition in the upstream or the downstream could affect the primary nucleation or secondary nucleation. However, the main framework of the continuous crystallization DNC approach is established by batch operation. Thus, it is necessary to further investigate the well-studied feedback control strategy to achieve continuous operation. Acevedo et al. [124] used developed mathematical models that contrasted five DNC approaches, which included simple DNC, bounds DNC, predictive DNC, reverse DNC, and basic DNC, on a single-stage MSMPR system (Figure 2.5).

Supersaturation drives the nucleation and growth process of crystalline products, so concentration feedback control is a product quality control strategy that relies on an online concentration measurement

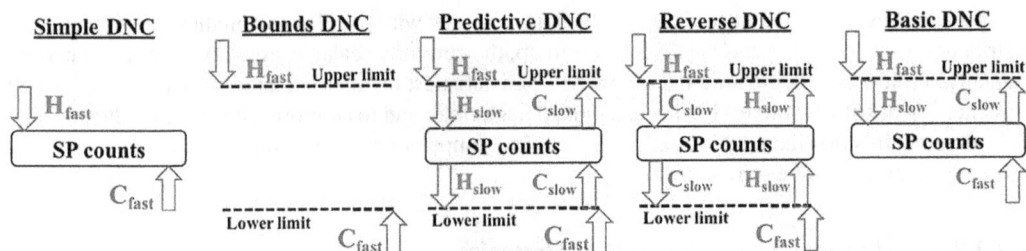

FIGURE 2.5 Algorithm for multiple DNC strategies implemented in a continuous cooling crystallization process by Acevedo et al. Reprinted with permission from Ref. [124]. Copyright © 2017 American Chemical Society.

method. In the last 20 years, ATR-FTIR spectroscopy [125] and ATR-UV/Vis [126] have been applied to monitor the supersaturation level. The SSC needs to meet the following requirements: (i) A calibration model should be established that correlates the collected spectra with solution concentration and temperature; (ii) the operation region relying on the equilibrium solubility and metastable boundary must be determined by offline experiments; and (iii) a programmed controller is the core of the whole process, which calculates the optimum temperature under the current condition [127]. The application of SSC to achieve improved product quality in batch operation has been widely reported in the previous literature [128–132]. Whether it is CFC or SSC, it directly measures the concentration of solute in the solution and converts it into relative supersaturation or absolute supersaturation, and limits the specific operating area in the phase diagram. During the crystallization process, the controller adjusts the feed flow rate or the manufacturing temperature gradient by monitoring the solute concentration and the system temperature in real time. The crystallization process is performed under the optimal target supersaturation according to the offline measurement. Since the solubility curve is a function of temperature and solvent type, the method can be extended to antisolvent crystallization by determining the operating curve for different systems.

In the DNC of a continuous process, FBRM or other CSD analysis equipment detects the chord length distribution of the crystal and then the nucleation, crystal form transformation, aggregation, and breakage behaviors of the target compound are speculated. This is undoubtedly advantageous for obtaining crystals of narrow particle size distribution and better morphology. Although, if the API is polymorphic, solvate, or hydrate, supersaturation control is considered to be more applicable, which is based on the investigation of empirical experiments with the specific set point. Supersaturation drives the entire crystallization process, so controlling the supersaturation of the bulk solution is the most effective way to prepare crystalline products. The precise capturing signals by the detector and timely response to the variation of the concentration are the precondition in judging whether an SSC approach could work out or not, which is easily realized for most APIs. However, since the establishment of an SSC requires offline-assisted experiments and precise calibration models of concentration detection equipment, which is complex and subject to low nucleation or growth rate constants, the supersaturation in the solution is often inconsistent with the product of the batch process. Thus, the actual control strategy of the process needs to be selected and the characteristics of the system should be taken into account. From the results of Nagy's continuous research, if the self-defect of the online CSD detection instrument can be ignored or avoided, [102] the DNC approach is the easiest operating and most efficient control strategy compared to any other open-loop or closed-loop model-based/model-free control strategy [133, 134]. In the future, the prospect of development based on model control lies in the simplification of the solution of higher-order partial differential equations and the deep understanding of the crystallization mechanism of complex systems. The development of a model-free control relies on a smarter detection method (sensor) and a more timely and sensitive feedback algorithm (e.g., first-order approximation) [135].

Whether it is the model-based or the model-free control strategy, the relationship between crystal growth rate and particle density varying with time in the system is always closely related to the process and product quality. For some systems with simple nucleation or growth models, the model-based control approach has the ability to fully describe the crystallization process and provides a safety guarantee of process operation, which is the optimal choice. However, for APIs that are prone to aggregation and breakage behaviors, or have special phenomena (such as oiling-out), the experiment-based model-free control approach has higher accuracy and provides higher margins. It is often more suitable for lab-scale or industrial-scale scaling up. As crystallization belongs to the semi-empirical and semi-theoretical discipline, it can be sure that the combination of model-based or model-free control strategies have stronger development potential.

2.4.3 Obstacles in the Scale-Up to Industrial Scale

The challenges in association with scaling up of continuous crystallization center on the issues of fouling, encrustation, and blockages. Such circumstances are mainly caused by heterogeneous nucleation due to insufficient heat transfer or equipment material differences. In the process of slurry transfer, due to the supersaturated state, the APIs are more likely to encounter undesirable nucleation and growth in comparison with batch operation. Compared to the scaling up of MSMPR, the crystallization in CPFCs is dependent on the temperature gradient or solvent addition to generate the setting supersaturation, which will aggravate the heterogeneous nucleation phenomenon of the inner wall of crystallizers. In addition, since APIs suitable for tubular crystallizers tend to have relatively large nucleation and growth rates, this also provides greater possibilities for the occurrence of fouling and blockages in transfer lines [136, 137]. The main methods of avoidance are: (i) Adding extra additive or solvent [62, 138]; (ii) increasing conveying intensity [139, 140]; and (iii) applying new internals to enhance mixing [73, 141]. In addition, the optimization of operation temperature and residence time can also overcome or improve the fouling situation. But in real situations, due to the minimization of cost requirements and product quality requirements, the implementation of specific continuous crystallization strategies should always be treated as multifactor optimization issues [38, 41].

As on the lab scale, the supersaturation is almost uniformly distributed and solid crystals can suspend well. In this case, data from the PAT sensor can represent the whole crystallization. However, on a larger-scale or industrial-scale, problems can appear due to scale up. For example, mixing such as particle suspension, particle attrition etc. [3] should be considered in cooling crystallizers. Even more remarkable, mixing problems could make scale-up more difficult for reaction crystallization and antisolvent crystallization which are commonly fast. In this case, antisolvent adding mode, adding velocity, adding a position, and configuration of the crystallizer can significantly affect the properties of the final crystals including size, shape, and CSD. Compared to separation operations that rely on thermodynamic equilibrium (such as rectification), product quality is often more sensitive to factors such as heat exchange and residence time. When the quality of crystalline products fluctuates, we are more dependent on empirical judgments currently due to the inability to accurately determine the internal conditions of continuous processes. At present, only a few drugs have achieved industrial-scale continuous crystallization, but most industrial-scale continuous crystallization still stays in the production of inorganic salts (such as sodium chloride and lithium carbonate), which is due to the huge demand for the production of these products. On the other hand, inorganic salt products often require high purity and yield of product. For the continuous crystallization of drugs, in addition to purity and yield, CSD and shape will affect the efficiency of downstream filtration, dry mixing, granulation, tabling, etc. which also puts forward higher requirements for continuous crystallization operation.

2.5 Conclusion

Continuous crystallization has been reviewed with respect to its uptake for pharmaceutical applications. Two types of crystallization configurations have been successfully demonstrated for continuous pharmaceutical crystallization: mixed suspension, mixed-product removal (MSMPR) systems, and tubular crystallizers. MSMPR systems have received the most attention to date, most likely because of historic experience with stirred tank reactors in the pharmaceutical sector. Although U.S. regulators have emphasized for years that the crystallization industry should adopt continuous manufacturing and some famous pharmaceutical companies such as Novartis [142] have proposed a continuous process, they still need to break down the obstacle of the "business as usual" approach [143] by further investigating the mechanism of continuous crystallization and the proof of industrial-scale continuous operation examples. In order to exploit the potential economic advantages of continuous crystallization, more contributions are needed in future research, including (i) more adaptable online detection means, (ii) better hardware design to alleviate fouling and encrustation, (iii) conjunction with other process intensification approaches (e.g., ultrasound, microwave), and (iv) development of a more systematic integrated feedback model.

NOTE

1 http://www.iecp-group.com/

REFERENCES

1. S.K. Teoh, C. Rathi, P. Sharratt, Practical Assessment Methodology for Converting Fine Chemicals Processes from Batch to Continuous, *Organic Process Research & Development 20* (2) (2016) 414–431. https://doi.org/10.1021/acs.oprd.5b00001.
2. M.D. Johnson, S.A. May, J.R. Calvin, J. Remacle, J.R. Stout, W.D. Diseroad, N. Zaborenko, B.D. Haeberle, W.M. Sun, M.T. Miller, J. Brennan, Development and Scale-Up of a Continuous, High-Pressure, Asymmetric Hydrogenation Reaction, Workup, and Isolation, *Organic Process Research & Development 16* (5) (2012) 1017–1038. https://doi.org/10.1021/op200362h.
3. B. Wood, K.P. Girard, C.S. Polster, D.M. Croker, Progress to Date in the Design and Operation of Continuous Crystallization Processes for Pharmaceutical Applications, *Organic Process Research & Development 23* (2) (2019) 122–144. https://doi.org/10.1021/acs.oprd.8b00319.
4. Y.M. Ma, S.G. Wu, E.G.J. Macaringue, T. Zhang, J.B. Gong, J.K. Wang, Recent Progress in Continuous Crystallization of Pharmaceutical Products: Precise Preparation and Control, *Organic Process Research & Development 24* (10) (2020) 1785–1801. https://doi.org/10.1021/acs.oprd.9b00362.
5. D.J. Zhang, S.J. Xu, S.C. Du, J.K. Wang, J.B. Gong, Progress of Pharmaceutical Continuous Crystallization, *Engineering 3* (3) (2017) 354–364. https://doi.org/10.1016/j.Eng.2017.03.023.
6. J. Norman, R.D. Madurawe, C.M.V. Moore, M.A. Khan, A. Khairuzzaman, A New Chapter in Pharmaceutical Manufacturing: 3D-Printed Drug Products, *Advanced Drug Delivery Reviews 108* (2017) 39–50. https://doi.org/10.1016/j.addr.2016.03.001.
7. H. Leuenberger, New Trends in the Production of Pharmaceutical Granules: Batch versus Continuous Processing, *European Journal of Pharmaceutics and Biopharmaceutics 52* (3) (2001) 289–296. https://doi.org/10.1016/s0939-6411(01)00199-0.
8. D. Han, T. Karmakar, Z. Bjelobrk, J. Gong, M. Parrinello, Solvent-Mediated Morphology Selection of the Active Pharmaceutical Ingredient Isoniazid: Experimental and Simulation Studies, *Chemical Engineering Science 204* (2019) 320–328. https://doi.org/10.1016/j.ces.2018.10.022.
9. P. Shi, S.J. Xu, S.C. Du, S. Rohani, S.Y. Liu, W.W. Tang, L.N. Jia, J.K. Wang, J.B. Gong, Insight into Solvent-Dependent Conformational Polymorph Selectivity: The Case of Undecanedioic Acid, *Crystal Growth & Design 18* (10) (2018) 5947–5956. https://doi.org/10.1021/acs.cgd.8b00738.
10. M.Y. Chen, S.G. Wu, S.J. Xu, B. Yu, M. Shilbayeh, Y. Liu, X.W. Zhu, J.K. Wang, J.B. Gong, Caking of crystals: Characterization, mechanisms and prevention, *Powder Technology 337* (2018) 51–67. https://doi.org/10.1016/j.powtec.2017.04.052.
11. S.L. Lee, T.F. O'Connor, X.C. Yang, C.N. Cruz, S. Chatterjee, R.D. Madurawe, C.M.V. Moore, L.X. Yu, J. Woodcock, Modernizing Pharmaceutical Manufacturing: from Batch to Continuous Production, *Journal of Pharmaceutical Innovation 10* (3) (2015) 191–199. https://doi.org/10.1007/s12247-015-9215-8.
12. S. Chatterjee, FDA Perspective on Continuous Manufacturing, *Presented at the IFPAC Annual Meeting*, Baltimore, MD, Jan 22–25 (2012).
13. X.C. Yang, D. Acevedo, A. Mohammad, N. Pavurala, H.Q. Wu, A.L. Brayton, R.A. Shaw, M.J. Goldman, F. He, S.L. Li, R.J. Fisher, T.F. O'Connor, C.N. Cruz, Risk Considerations on Developing a Continuous Crystallization System for Carbamazepine, *Organic Process Research & Development 21* (7) (2017) 1021–1033. https://doi.org/10.1021/acs.oprd.7b00130.

14. B.E. Huff, Continuous Processing in the Pharmaceutical Industry, *Abstracts of Papers of the American Chemical Society 246* (2013).

15. K. Sangwal, Some Features of Metastable Zone Width of Various Systems Determined by Polythermal Method, *CrystEngComm 13* (2) (2011) 489–501. https://doi.org/10.1039/c0ce00065e.

16. D. Kashchiev, A. Borissova, R.B. Hammond, K.J. Roberts, Effect of Cooling Rate on the Critical Undercooling for Crystallization, *Journal of Crystal Growth 312* (5) (2010) 698–704. https://doi.org/10.1016/j.jcrysgro.2009.12.031.

17. G.J. Söhnel, O. Precipitation: *Basic Principles and Industrial Applications*, Butterworth-Heinemann, Oxford (1992).

18. J. Garside, R.J. Davey, Secondary Contact Nucleation-Kinetics, Growth and Scale-Up, *Chemical Engineering Communications 4* (4–5) (1980) 393–424. https://doi.org/10.1080/00986448008935918.

19. J.R. Beckman, A.D. Randolph, Crystal Size Distribution Dynamics in a Classified Crystallizer. 2. Simulated Control of Crystal Size Distribution, *AIChE Journal 23* (4) (1977) 510–520. https://doi.org/10.1002/aic.690230416.

20. J. Garside, S.J. Jancic, Prediction and Measurement of Crystal Size Distribution for Size-Dependent Growth, *Chemical Engineering Science 33* (12) (1978) 1623–1630. https://doi.org/10.1016/0009-2509(78)85138-0.

21. J. Garside, Industrial Crystallization from Solution, *Chemical Engineering Science 40* (1) (1985) 3–26. https://doi.org/10.1016/0009-2509(85)85043-0.

22. Z.K. Nagy, Model Based Robust Control Approach for Batch Crystallization Product Design, *Computers & Chemical Engineering 33* (10) (2009) 1685–1691. https://doi.org/10.1016/j.compchemeng.2009.04.012.

23. T. Vetter, C.L. Burcham, M.F. Doherty, Regions of Attainable Particle Sizes in Continuous and Batch Crystallization Processes, *Chemical Engineering Science 106* (2014) 167–180.

24. Q.L. Su, B. Benyahia, Z.K. Nagy, C.D. Rielly, Mathematical Modeling, Design, and Optimization of a Multisegment Multiaddition Plug-Flow Crystallizer for Antisolvent Crystallizations, *Organic Process Research & Development 19* (12) (2015) 1859–1870. https://doi.org/10.1021/acs.oprd.5b00110.

25. Q.L. Su, Z.K. Nagy, C.D. Rielly, Pharmaceutical Crystallisation Processes from Batch to Continuous Operation Using MSMPR Stages: Modelling, Design, and Control, *Chemical Engineering and Processing Process Intensification 89* (2015) 41–53. https://doi.org/10.1016/j.cep.2015.01.001.

26. T. Chiu, P.D. Christofides, Nonlinear Control of Particulate Processes, *AIChE Journal 45* (6) (1999) 1279–1297. https://doi.org/10.1002/aic.690450613.

27. B. Winter, H. Georgi, An Extended Crystallizer Model for the Sizing and Optimization of Crystallizer Cascades, *International Chemical Engineering 25* (61) (1985) 1.

28. M. Mackley, Process Innovation Using Oscillatory Flow within Baffled Tubes, *Chemical Engineering Research and Design 69* (A3) (1991) 197–199.

29. R. Vacassy, J. Lemaitre, H. Hofmann, J. Gerlings, Calcium Carbonate Precipitation Using New Segmented Flow Tubular Reactor, *AIChE Journal 46* (6) (2000) 1241–1252. https://doi.org/10.1002/aic.690460616

30. Y. Ma, S. Wu, E.G.J. Macaringue, T. Zhang, J. Gong, J. Wang, Recent Progress in Continuous Crystallization of Pharmaceutical Products: Precise Preparation and Control, *Organic Process Research & Development 24* (10) (2020) 1785–1801. https://doi.org/10.1021/acs.oprd.9b00362

31. M. Furuta, K. Mukai, D. Cork, K. Mae, Continuous Crystallization Using a Sonicated Tubular System for Controlling Particle Size in an API Manufacturing Process, *Chemical Engineering and Processing: Process Intensification 102* (2016) 210–218. https://doi.org/10.1016/j.cep.2016.02.002.

32. J. Chen, B. Sarma, J.M. Evans, A.S. Myerson, Pharmaceutical Crystallization, *Crystal Growth & Design 11* (4) (2011) 887–895. https://doi.org/10.1021/cg101556s

33. M. Jiang, Z. Zhu, E. Jimenez, C.D. Papageorgiou, J. Waetzig, A. Hardy, M. Langston, R.D. Braatz, Continuous-Flow Tubular Crystallization in Slugs Spontaneously Induced by Hydrodynamics, *Crystal Growth & Design 14* (2) (2014) 851–860. https://doi.org/10.1021/cg401715e

34. X. Sun, Y. Sun, J. Yu, Cooling Crystallization of Aluminum Sulfate in Pure Water, *Journal of Crystal Growth 419* (2015) 94–101. https://doi.org/10.1016/j.jcrysgro.2015.03.005

35. A.M. Kolbach-Mandel, J.G. Kleinman, J.A. Wesson, Exploring Calcium Oxalate Crystallization: A Constant Composition Approach, *Urolithiasis 43* (5) (2015) 397–409. Doi: https://doi.org/10.1007/s00240-015-0781-5

36. A. Randolph, *Theory of Particulate Processes*, 2nd ed, Academic Press, San Diego (1988).

37. M.-C. Lührmann, J. Timmermann, G. Schembecker, K. Wohlgemuth, Enhanced Product Quality Control through Separation of Crystallization Phenomena in a Four-Stage MSMPR Cascade, *Crystal Growth & Design 18* (12) (2018) 7323–7334. https://doi.org/10.1021/acs.cgd.8b00941

38. S. Diab, D.I. Gerogiorgis, Technoeconomic Evaluation of Multiple Mixed Suspension-Mixed Product Removal (MSMPR) Crystallizer Configurations for Continuous Cyclosporine Crystallization, *Organic Process Research & Development 21* (10) (2017) 1571–1587. https://doi.org/10.1021/acs.oprd.7b00225.

39. J. Li, B.L. Trout, A.S. Myerson, Multistage Continuous Mixed-Suspension, Mixed-Product Removal (MSMPR) Crystallization with Solids Recycle, *Organic Process Research & Development 20* (2) (2016) 510–516. https://doi.org/10.1021/acs.oprd.5b00306

40. S. Diab, D.I. Gerogiorgis, Technoeconomic Optimization of Continuous Crystallization for Three Active Pharmaceutical Ingredients: Cyclosporine, *Paracetamol, and Aliskiren, Industrial & Engineering Chemistry Research 57* (29) (2018) 9489–9499. https://doi.org/10.1021/acs.iecr.8b00679.

41. J. Li, T.-T. C. Lai, B.L. Trout, A.S. Myerson, Continuous Crystallization of Cyclosporine: Effect of Operating Conditions on Yield and Purity, *Crystal Growth & Design 17* (3) (2017) 1000–1007. https://doi.org/10.1021/acs.cgd.6b01212.

42. S. Ferguson, G. Morris, H. Hao, M. Barrett, B. Glennon, Characterization of the Anti-Solvent Batch, Plug Flow and MSMPR Crystallization of Benzoic Acid, *Chemical Engineering Science 104* (2013) 44–54. https://doi.org/10.1016/j.ces.2013.09.006.

43. O. Narducci, A.G. Jones, E. Kougoulos, Continuous Crystallization of Adipic Acid with Ultrasound, *Chemical Engineering Science 66* (6) (2011) 1069–1076. https://doi.org/10.1016/j.ces.2010.12.008.

44. Y. Yang, L. Song, Y. Zhang, Z.K. Nagy, Application of Wet Milling-Based Automated Direct Nucleation Control in Continuous Cooling Crystallization Processes, *Industrial & Engineering Chemistry Research 55* (17) (2016) 4987–4996. https://doi.org/10.1021/acs.iecr.5b04956.

45. Y. Yang, L. Song, T. Gao, Z.K. Nagy, Integrated Upstream and Downstream Application of Wet Milling with Continuous Mixed Suspension Mixed Product Removal Crystallization, *Crystal Growth & Design 15* (12) (2015) 5879–5885. https://doi.org/10.1021/acs.cgd.5b01290.

46. E. Plasari, H. Muhr, A. Gerard, Effect of Calcium Based Additives on the Sodium Bicarbonate Crystallization in a MSMPR Reactor, *Powder Technology An International Journal on the Science & Technology of Wet & Dry Particulate Systems* (2014).

47. K. Tahara, M. O'Mahony, A.S. Myerson, Continuous Spherical Crystallization of Albuterol Sulfate with Solvent Recycle System, *Crystal Growth & Design* 2015, *15*, 10, 5149–5156 https://doi.org/10.1021/acs.cgd.5b01159

48. R. Pena, Z.K. Nagy, Process Intensification through Continuous Spherical Crystallization Using a Two-Stage Mixed Suspension Mixed Product Removal (MSMPR) System, *Crystal Growth & Design* (2015) 4225–4236. https://doi.org/10.1021/acs.cgd.5b00479

49. A.J. Alvarez, A. Singh, A.S. Myerson, Crystallization of Cyclosporine in a Multistage Continuous MSMPR Crystallizer, *Crystal Growth & Design 11* (10) (2011) 4392–4400. https://doi.org/10.1021/cg200546g

50. H. Zhang, J. Quon, A.J. Alvarez, J. Evans, A.S. Myerson, B. Trout, Development of Continuous Anti-Solvent/Cooling Crystallization Process using Cascaded Mixed Suspension, Mixed Product Removal Crystallizers, *Organic Process Research & Development 16* (5) (2012) 915–924. https://doi.org/10.1021/op2002886.

51. S.Y. Wong, A.P. Tatusko, B.L. Trout, A.S. Myerson, Development of Continuous Crystallization Processes Using a Single-Stage Mixed-Suspension, Mixed-Product Removal Crystallizer with Recycle, *Crystal Growth & Design 12* (11) (2012) 5701–5707. https://doi.org/10.1021/cg301221q.

52. S. Ferguson, F. Ortner, J. Quon, L. Peeva, A. Livingston, B.L. Trout, A.S. Myerson, Use of Continuous MSMPR Crystallization with Integrated Nanofiltration Membrane Recycle for Enhanced Yield and Purity in API Crystallization, *Crystal Growth & Design 14* (2) (2014) 617–627. https://doi.org/10.1021/cg401491y.

53. J. Li, B.L. Trout, A.S. Myerson, Multistage Continuous Mixed-Suspension, Mixed-Product Removal (MSMPR) Crystallization with Solids Recycle, *Organic Process Research and Development* 2016, *20*, 2, 510–516. https://doi.org/10.1021/acs.oprd.5b00306.

54. S. Vartak, A.S. Myerson, Continuous Crystallization with Impurity Complexation and Nanofiltration Recycle, *Organic Process Research & Development 21* (2) (2017) 253–261. https://doi.org/10.1021/acs.oprd.6b00438.

55. T. Lai, S. Ferguson, L. Palmer, B.L. Trout, A.S. Myerson, Continuous Crystallization and Polymorph Dynamics in the l-Glutamic Acid System, *Organic Process Research & Development 18* (11) (2014) 1382–1390. https://doi.org/10.1021/op500171n.

56. T.C. Farmer, C.L. Carpenter, M.F. Doherty, Polymorph Selection by Continuous Crystallization, *AIChE Journal 62* (9) (2016) 3505–3514. https://doi.org/10.1002/aic.15343.

57. T. Lee, H.R. Chen, H.Y. Lin, H.L. Lee, Continuous Co-Crystallization As a Separation Technology: The Study of 1:2 Co-Crystals of Phenazine-Vanillin, *Crystal Growth & Design 12* (12) (2012) 5897–5907. https://doi.org/10.1021/cg300763t.

58. K.A. Powell, G. Bartolini, K.E. Wittering, A.N. Saleemi, C.C. Wilson, C.D. Rielly, Z.K. Nagy, Toward Continuous Crystallization of Urea-Barbituric Acid: A Polymorphic Co-Crystal System, *Crystal Growth & Design 15* (10) (2015) 4821–4836. https://doi.org/10.1021/acs.cgd.5b00599.

59. S. Qamar, M.P. Elsner, I. Hussain, A. Seidel-Morgenstern, Seeding Strategies and Residence Time Characteristics of Continuous Preferential Crystallization, *Chemical Engineering Science 71* (2012) 5–17. https://doi.org/10.1016/j.ces.2011.12.030.

60. R.R.E. Steendam, J.H. ter Horst, Continuous Total Spontaneous Resolution, *Crystal Growth & Design 17* (8) (2017) 4428–4436. https://doi.org/10.1021/acs.cgd.7b00761.

61. Y. Zhao, V.K. Kamaraju, G. Hou, G. Power, P. Donnellan, B. Glennon, Kinetic Identification and Experimental Validation of Continuous Plug Flow Crystallisation, *Chemical Engineering Science 133* (2015) 106–115. https://doi.org/10.1016/j.ces.2015.02.019.

62. A. Majumder, Z.K. Nagy, Dynamic Modeling of Encrust Formation and Mitigation Strategy in a Continuous Plug Flow Crystallizer, *Crystal Growth & Design 15* (3) (2015) 1129–1140. https://doi.org/10.1021/cg501431c.

63. A.J. Florence, N. Briggs, U. Schacht, V. Raval, T. McGlone, J. Sefcik, Seeded Crystallization of β-l-Glutamic Acid in a Continuous Oscillatory Baffled Crystallizer, *Organic Process Research and Development 2015, 19*, 12, 1903–1911. https://doi.org/10.1021/acs.oprd.5b00206.

64. S. Lawton, G. Steele, P. Shering, L. Zhao, I. Laird, X.W. Ni, Continuous Crystallization of Pharmaceuticals Using a Continuous Oscillatory Baffled Crystallizer, *Organic Process Research & Development 13* (6) (2009) 1357–1363. https://doi.org/10.1021/op900237x.

65. H.G. Jolliffe, D.I. Gerogiorgis, Process Modelling, Design and Technoeconomic Evaluation for Continuous Paracetamol Crystallisation, *Computer Aided Chemical Engineering 43* (2018) 1637–1642. https://doi.org/10.1016/j.compchemeng.2018.03.020.

66. M. Jiang, R.D. Braatz, Designs of Continuous-Flow Pharmaceutical Crystallizers: Developments and Practice, *CrystEngComm 21* (23) (2019) 3534–3551. DOI: https://doi.org/10.1039/C8CE00042E

67. M. Jiang, C.D. Papageorgiou, J. Waetzig, A. Hardy, M. Langston, R.D. Braatz, Indirect Ultrasonication in Continuous Slug-Flow Crystallization, *Crystal Growth & Design 15* (5) (2015) 2486–2492. https://doi.org/10.1021/acs.cgd.5b00263.

68. N. Jongen, M. Donnet, P. Bowen, J. Lemaitre, H. Hofmann, R. Schenk, C. Hofmann, M. Aoun-Habbache, S. Guillemet-Fritsch, J. Sarrias, A. Rousset, M. Viviani, M.T. Buscaglia, V. Buscaglia, P. Nanni, A. Testino, J.R. Herguijuela, Development of a Continuous Segmented Flow Tubular Reactor and the 'Scale-Out' Concept – In Search of Perfect Powders, *Chemical Engineering & Technology 26* (3) (2003) 303–305. https://doi.org/10.1002/ceat.200390046.

69. R.J.P. Eder, S. Radl, E. Schmitt, S. Innerhofer, M. Maier, H. Gruber-Woelfler, J.G. Khinast, Continuously Seeded, Continuously Operated Tubular Crystallizer for the Production of Active Pharmaceutical Ingredients, *Crystal Growth & Design 10* (5) (2010) 2247–2257. https://doi.org/10.1021/cg9015788.

70. A. Majumder, Z.K. Nagy, Fines Removal in a Continuous Plug Flow Crystallizer by Optimal Spatial Temperature Profiles with Controlled Dissolution, *AIChE Journal 59* (12) (2013) 4582–4594. https://doi.org/10.1002/aic.14196.

71. S.Y. Wong, Y. Cui, A.S. Myerson, Contact Secondary Nucleation as a Means of Creating Seeds for Continuous Tubular Crystallizers, *Crystal Growth & Design 13* (6) (2013) 2514–2521. https://doi.org/10.1021/cg4002303.

72. M. Furuta, K. Mukai, D. Cork, K. Mae, Continuous Crystallization Using a Sonicated Tubular System for Controlling Particle Size in an API Manufacturing Process, *Chemical Engineering and Processing Process Intensification 102* (2016) 210–218. https://doi.org/10.1016/j.cep.2016.02.002.

73. S. Ferguson, G. Morris, H. Hao, M. Barrett, B. Glennon, In-Situ Monitoring and Characterization of Plug Flow Crystallizers, *Chemical Engineering Science 77* (2012) 105–111. https://doi.org/10.1016/j.ces.2012.02.013.

74. L.R. Agnew, T. McGlone, H.P. Heatcroft, A. Robertson, A.R. Parsons, C.C. Wilson, Continuous Crystallization of Paracetamol (Acetaminophen) Form II: Selective Access to a Metastable Solid Form, *Crystal Growth & Design* (2017). https://doi.org/10.1021/acs.cgd.6b01831

75. L. Zhao, V. Raval, N.E. Briggs, R.M. Bhardwaj, T. McGlone, I.D. Oswald, A.J. Florence, From Discovery to Scale-Up: α-Lipoic Acid: Nicotinamide Co-Crystals in a Continuous Oscillatory Baffled Crystalliser, *CrystEngComm* (2014). https://doi.org/10.1039/C4CE00154K

76. R. Peña, J.A. Oliva, C.L. Burcham, D.J. Jarmer, Z.K. Nagy, Process Intensification through Continuous Spherical Crystallization Using an Oscillatory Flow Baffled Crystallizer, *Crystal Growth & Design 17* (9) (2017) 4776–4784.

77. P. Neugebauer, J.G. Khinast, Continuous Crystallization of Proteins in a Tubular Plug-Flow Crystallizer, *Crystal Growth & Design 15* (3) (2015) 1089–1095.

78. J. Mo, Z. Zhu, E. Jimenez, C.D. Papageorgiou, R.D. Braatz, Continuous-Flow Tubular Crystallization in Slugs Spontaneously Induced by Hydrodynamics, *Crystal Growth & Design 14* (2) (2014) 851–860.

79. M. Jiang, C.D. Papageorgiou, J. Waetzig, A. Hardy, M. Langston, R.D. Braatz, Indirect Ultrasonication in Continuous Slug-Flow Crystallization, *Crystal Growth & Design 15* (5) (2015) 2486–2492. https://doi.org/10.1021/acs.cgd.5b00263.

80. D. Rossi, R. Jamshidi, N. Saffari, S. Kuhn, A. Gavriilidis, L. Mazzei, Continuous-Flow Sonocrystallization in Droplet-Based Microfluidics, *Crystal Growth & Design 15* (11) (2015) 5519–5529. https://doi.org/10.1021/acs.cgd.5b01153.

81. V. Pauli, Y. Roggo, L. Pellegatti, N.Q. Nguyen Trung, F. Elbaz, S. Ensslin, P. Kleinebudde, M. Krumme, Process Analytical Technology for Continuous Manufacturing Tableting Processing: A Case Study, *Journal of Pharmaceutical and Biomedical Analysis 162* (2019) 101–111. https://doi.org/10.1016/j.jpba.2018.09.016.

82. J.M. Vargas, S. Nielsen, V. Cárdenas, A. Gonzalez, E.Y. Aymat, E. Almodovar, G. Classe, Y. Colón, E. Sanchez, R.J. Romañach, Process Analytical Technology in Continuous Manufacturing of a Commercial Pharmaceutical Product, *International Journal of Pharmaceutics 538* (1–2) (2018) 167–178. https://doi.org/10.1016/j.ijpharm.2018.01.003.

83. D. Brouckaert, L. De Meyer, B. Vanbillemont, P.J. Van Bockstal, J. Lammens, S. Mortier, J. Corver, C. Vervaet, I. Nopens, T. De Beer, Potential of Near-Infrared Chemical Imaging as Process Analytical Technology Tool for Continuous Freeze-Drying, *Analytical Chemistry 90* (7) (2018) 4354–4362. https://doi.org/10.1021/acs.analchem.7b03647.

84. A. Saleemi, C. Rielly, Z.K. Nagy, Automated Direct Nucleation Control for in situ Dynamic Fines Removal in Batch Cooling Crystallization, *CrystEngComm 14* (6) (2012) 2196. https://doi.org/10.1039/c2ce06288g.

85. E. Simone, A.N. Saleemi, Z.K. Nagy, In Situ Monitoring of Polymorphic Transformations Using a Composite Sensor Array of Raman, NIR, and ATR-UV/vis Spectroscopy, FBRM, and PVM for an Intelligent Decision Support System, *Organic Process Research & Development 19* (1) (2014) 167–177. https://doi.org/10.1021/op5000122.

86. E. Simone, A.N. Saleemi, Z.K. Nagy, Application of Quantitative Raman Spectroscopy for the Monitoring of Polymorphic Transformation in Crystallization Processes Using a Good Calibration Practice Procedure, *Chemical Engineering Research and Design 92* (4) (2014) 594–611. https://doi.org/10.1016/j.cherd.2013.11.004.

87. K.A. Ramisetty, Å.C. Rasmuson, Controlling the Product Crystal Size Distribution by Strategic Application of Ultrasonication, *Crystal Growth & Design 18* (3) (2018) 1697–1709. https://doi.org/10.1021/acs.cgd.7b01619.

88. D. Zhang, L. Liu, S. Xu, S. Du, W. Dong, J. Gong, Optimization of Cooling Strategy and Seeding by FBRM Analysis of Batch Crystallization, *Journal of Crystal Growth 486* (2018) 1–9. https://doi.org/10.1016/j.jcrysgro.2017.12.046.

89. H. Siddique, C.J. Brown, I. Houson, A.J. Florence, Establishment of a Continuous Sonocrystallization Process for Lactose in an Oscillatory Baffled Crystallizer, *Organic Process Research & Development 19* (12) (2015) 1871–1881. https://doi.org/10.1021/acs.oprd.5b00127.

90. G. Morris, G. Power, S. Ferguson, M. Barrett, G. Hou, B. Glennon, Estimation of Nucleation and Growth Kinetics of Benzoic Acid by Population Balance Modeling of a Continuous Cooling Mixed Suspension, Mixed Product Removal Crystallizer, *Organic Process Research & Development 19* (12) (2015) 1891–1902. https://doi.org/10.1021/acs.oprd.5b00139.

91. J. Li, R. Li, B. Zhao, H. Guo, S. Zhang, J. Cheng, X. Wu, Quantitative Measurement of Carbon Isotopic Composition in CO_2 Gas Reservoir by Micro-Laser Raman Spectroscopy, *Spectrochimica Acta Part A, Molecular and Biomolecular Spectroscopy 195* (2018) 191–198. https://doi.org/10.1016/j.saa.2018.01.082.

92. C.J. Smith, J. Dinh, P.D. Schmitt, P.A. Stroud, J. Hinds, M.J. Johnson, G.J. Simpson, Calibration-Free Second Harmonic Generation (SHG) Image Analysis for Quantification of Trace Crystallinity Within Final Dosage Forms of Amorphous Solid Dispersions, *Applied Spectroscopy 72* (11) (2018) 1594–1605. https://doi.org/10.1177/0003702818786506.

93. K.A. Esmonde-White, M. Cuellar, C. Uerpmann, B. Lenain, I.R. Lewis, Raman Spectroscopy as a Process Analytical Technology for Pharmaceutical Manufacturing and Bioprocessing, *Analytical and Bioanalytical Chemistry 409* (3) (2017) 637–649. https://doi.org/10.1007/s00216-016-9824-1.

94. D. Acevedo, X. Yang, A. Mohammad, N. Pavurala, W.-L. Wu, T.F. O'Connor, Z.K. Nagy, C.N. Cruz, Raman Spectroscopy for Monitoring the Continuous Crystallization of Carbamazepine, *Organic Process Research & Development 22* (2) (2018) 156–165. https://doi.org/10.1021/acs.oprd.7b00322.

95. Y. Li, C.A. Anderson, J.K. Drennen, 3rd, C. Airiau, B. Igne, Method Development and Validation of an Inline Process Analytical Technology Method for Blend Monitoring in the Tablet Feed Frame Using Raman Spectroscopy, *Analytical Chemistry 90* (14) (2018) 8436–8444. https://doi.org/10.1021/acs.analchem.8b01009.

96. Y. Wu, N.R. Mirza, G. Hu, K.H. Smith, G.W. Stevens, K.A. Mumford, Precipitating Characteristics of Potassium Bicarbonate Using Concentrated Potassium Carbonate Solvent for Carbon Dioxide Capture. Part 1. Nucleation, *Industrial & Engineering Chemistry Research 56* (23) (2017) 6764–6774. https://doi.org/10.1021/acs.iecr.7b00699.

97. R. Kacker, S. Maaß, J. Emmerich, H. Kramer, Application of Inline Imaging for Monitoring Crystallization Process in a Continuous Oscillatory Baffled Crystallizer, *AIChE Journal 64* (7) (2018) 2450–2461. https://doi.org/10.1002/aic.16145.

98. M. Jiang, R.D. Braatz, Low-Cost Noninvasive Real-Time Imaging for Tubular Continuous-Flow Crystallization, *Chemical Engineering & Technology 41* (1) (2018) 143–148. https://doi.org/10.1002/ceat.201600276.

99. R.W. Kessler, W. Kessler, E. Zikulnig-Rusch, A Critical Summary of Spectroscopic Techniques and their Robustness in Industrial PAT Applications, *Chemie Ingenieur Technik 88* (6) (2016) 710–721. https://doi.org/10.1002/cite.201500147.

100. K. Korasa, G. Hudovornik, F. Vrecer, Applicability of near-infrared spectroscopy in the monitoring of film coating and curing process of the prolonged release coated pellets, *European Journal of Pharmaceutical Sciences: Official Journal of the European Federation for Pharmaceutical Sciences 93* (2016) 484–92. https://doi.org/10.1016/j.ejps.2016.08.038.

101. M. Mostafavi, S. Petersen, J. Ulrich, Effect of Particle Shape on Inline Particle Size Measurement Techniques, *Chemical Engineering & Technology 37* (10) (2014) 1721–1728. https://doi.org/10.1002/ceat.201400212.

102. E. Simone, W. Zhang, Z.K. Nagy, Application of Process Analytical Technology-Based Feedback Control Strategies To Improve Purity and Size Distribution in Biopharmaceutical Crystallization, *Crystal Growth & Design 15* (6) (2015) 2908–2919. https://doi.org/10.1021/acs.cgd.5b00337.

103. Z. Chen, D. Lovett, J. Morris, Process Analytical Technologies and Real Time Process Control a Review of Some Spectroscopic Issues and Challenges, *Journal of Process Control 21* (10) (2011) 1467–1482. https://doi.org/10.1016/j.jprocont.2011.06.024.

104. Y. Peng, Z. Zhu, R.D. Braatz, A.S. Myerson, Gypsum Crystallization during Phosphoric Acid Production: Modeling and Experiments Using the Mixed-Solvent-Electrolyte Thermodynamic Model, *Industrial & Engineering Chemistry Research 54* (32) (2015) 7914–7924. https://doi.org/10.1021/acs.iecr.5b01763.

105. Z. Gao, Y. Wu, J. Gong, J. Wang, S. Rohani, Continuous Crystallization of α-Form L-Glutamic Acid in an MSMPR-Tubular Crystallizer System, *Journal of Crystal Growth 507* (2019) 344–351. https://doi.org/10.1016/j.jcrysgro.2018.07.007.

106. W. Zhao, M.A. Jama, A. Buffo, V. Alopaeus, Population Balance Model and Experimental Validation for Reactive Dissolution of Particle Agglomerates, *Computers & Chemical Engineering 108* (2018) 240–249. https://doi.org/10.1016/j.compchemeng.2017.09.019.

107. M. Trifkovic, M. Sheikhzadeh, and S. Rohani, Kinetics Estimation and Single and Multi-Objective Optimization of a Seeded, Anti-Solvent, Isothermal Batch Crystallizer, *Industrial & Engineering Chemistry Research* 2008, *47*, 1586–1595.

108. B.J. Ridder, A. Majumder, Z.K. Nagy, Population Balance Model-Based Multiobjective Optimization of a Multisegment Multiaddition (MSMA) Continuous Plug-Flow Antisolvent Crystallizer, *Industrial & Engineering Chemistry Research 53* (11) (2014) 4387–4397. https://doi.org/10.1021/ie402806n.

109. F. Milella, M. Gazzani, D. Sutter, M. Mazzotti, Process Synthesis, Modeling and Optimization of Continuous Cooling Crystallization with Heat Integration—Application to the Chilled Ammonia CO2 Capture Process, *Industrial & Engineering Chemistry Research 57* (34) (2018) 11712–11727. https://doi.org/10.1021/acs.iecr.8b01993.

110. M. Sen, A. Rogers, R. Singh, A. Chaudhury, J. John, M.G. Ierapetritou, R. Ramachandran, Flowsheet Optimization of an Integrated Continuous Purification-Processing Pharmaceutical Manufacturing Operation, *Chemical Engineering Science 102* (2013) 56–66. https://doi.org/10.1016/j.ces.2013.07.035.

111. A. Adamo, R. L. Beingessner, M. Behnam, J. Chen, T.F. Jamison, K.F. Jensen, J.C.M. Monbaliu, A.S. Myerson, E.M. Revalor, D.R. Snead, T. Stelzer, Ondemand-Continuous Flow Production of Pharmaceuticals in a Compact Reconfigurable System. *Science.* https://doi.org/10.1126/science.aaf1337

112. N. Yazdanpanah, C.J. Testa, S.R.K. Perala, K.D. Jensen, R.D. Braatz, A.S. Myerson, B.L. Trout, Continuous Heterogeneous Crystallization on Excipient Surfaces, *Crystal Growth & Design 17* (6) (2017) 3321–3330. https://doi.org/10.1021/acs.cgd.7b00297.

113. A.N. Kalbasenka, L.C.P. Spierings, A.E.M. Huesman, H.J.M. Kramer, Application of Seeding as a Process Actuator in a Model Predictive Control Framework for Fed-Batch Crystallization of Ammonium Sulphate, *Particle & Particle Systems Characterization 24* (1) (2007) 40–48. https://doi.org/10.1002/ppsc.200601053.

114. X. Yang, D. Acevedo, A. Mohammad, N. Pavurala, H. Wu, A.L. Brayton, R.A. Shaw, M.J. Goldman, F. He, S. Li, R.J. Fisher, T.F. O'Connor, C.N. Cruz, Risk Considerations on Developing a Continuous Crystallization System for Carbamazepine, *Organic Process Research & Development 21* (7) (2017) 1021–1033. https://doi.org/10.1021/acs.oprd.7b00130.

115. M.O. Besenhard, P. Neugebauer, C.-D. Ho, J.G. Khinast, Crystal Size Control in a Continuous Tubular Crystallizer, *Crystal Growth & Design 15* (4) (2015) 1683–1691. https://doi.org/10.1021/cg501637m.

116. M.R. Abu Bakar, Z.K. Nagy, A.N. Saleemi, C.D. Rielly, The Impact of Direct Nucleation Control on Crystal Size Distribution in Pharmaceutical Crystallization Processes. *Crystal Growth & Design 9* (3) (2009) 1378–1384. https://doi.org/10.1021/cg800595v.

117. M. R. Abu, Z. K. Bakar, C. D. Nagy, Rielly Seeded Batch Cooling Crystallization with Temperature Cycling for the Control of Size Uniformity and Polymorphic Purity of Sulfathiazole Crystals. *Organic Process Research & Development 13* (2009) 1343–1356. https://doi.org/10.1021/op900174b.

118. M.R. Abu Bakar, Z.K. Nagy, C.D. Rielly, Investigation of the Effect of Temperature Cycling on Surface Features of Sulfathiazole Crystals during Seeded Batch Cooling Crystallization, *Crystal Growth & Design 10* (9) (2010) 3892–3900. https://doi.org/10.1021/cg1002379.

119. R. Kacker, P.M. Salvador, G.S.J. Sturm, G.D. Stefanidis, R. Lakerveld, Z.K. Nagy, H.J.M. Kramer, Microwave Assisted Direct Nucleation Control for Batch Crystallization: Crystal Size Control with Reduced Batch Time, *Crystal Growth & Design 16* (1) (2015) 440–446. https://doi.org/10.1021/acs.cgd.5b01444.

120. Á. Borsos, B. Szilágyi, P.Ş. Agachi, Z.K. Nagy, Real-Time Image Processing Based Online Feedback Control System for Cooling Batch Crystallization, *Organic Process Research & Development 21* (4) (2017) 511–519. https://doi.org/10.1021/acs.oprd.6b00242.

121. A. Borsos, A. Majumder, Z.K. Nagy, Multi-Impurity Adsorption Model for Modeling Crystal Purity and Shape Evolution during Crystallization Processes in Impure Media, *Crystal Growth & Design 16* (2) (2015) 555–568. https://doi.org/10.1021/acs.cgd.5b00320.

122. Q. Su, B. Benyahia, Z.K. Nagy, C.D. Rielly, Mathematical Modeling, Design, and Optimization of a Multisegment Multiaddition Plug-Flow Crystallizer for Antisolvent Crystallizations, *Organic Process Research & Development 19* (12) (2015) 1859–1870. https://doi.org/10.1021/acs.oprd.5b00110.

123. Y. Yang, L. Song, Z.K. Nagy, Automated Direct Nucleation Control in Continuous Mixed Suspension Mixed Product Removal Cooling Crystallization, *Crystal Growth & Design 15* (12) (2015) 5839–5848. https://doi.org/10.1021/acs.cgd.5b01219.

124. D. Acevedo, Y. Yang, D.J. Warnke, Z.K. Nagy, Model-Based Evaluation of Direct Nucleation Control Approaches for the Continuous Cooling Crystallization of Paracetamol in a Mixed Suspension Mixed Product Removal System, *Crystal Growth & Design 17* (10) (2017) 5377–5383. https://doi.org/10.1021/acs.cgd.7b00860.

125. D. D. Dunuwila, L. B. Carroll, K. A. Berglund, An Investigation of the Applicability of Attenuated Total Reflection Infrared Spectroscopy for Measurement of Solubility and Supersaturation of Aqueous Citric Acid Solutions. *Journal of Crystal Growth 137* (1994) 561–568. https://doi.org/10.1016/0022-0248(94)90999-7

126. A.N. Saleemi, G. Steele, N.I. Pedge, A. Freeman, Z.K. Nagy, Enhancing Crystalline Properties of a Cardiovascular Active Pharmaceutical Ingredient Using a Process Analytical Technology Based Crystallization Feedback Control Strategy, *International Journal of Pharmaceutics 430* (1–2) (2012) 56–64. https://doi.org/10.1016/j.ijpharm.2012.03.029.

127. L.L. Simon, E. Simone, K.A. Oucherif, Crystallization Process Monitoring and Control Using Process Analytical Technology, *Computer Aided Chemical Engineering 41* (2018) 215–242. https://doi.org/10.1016/b978-0-444-63963-9.00009-9.

128. M. Jiang, M.H. Wong, Z. Zhu, J. Zhang, L. Zhou, K. Wang, A.N. Ford Versypt, T. Si, L.M. Hasenberg, Y.-E. Li, R.D. Braatz, Towards Achieving a Flattop Crystal Size Distribution by Continuous Seeding and Controlled Growth, *Chemical Engineering Science 77* (2012) 2–9. https://doi.org/10.1016/j.ces.2011.12.033.

129. D. Duffy, M. Barrett, B. Glennon, Novel, Calibration-Free Strategies for Supersaturation Control in Antisolvent Crystallization Processes, *Crystal Growth & Design 13* (8) (2013) 3321–3332. https://doi.org/10.1021/cg301673g.

130. N. C. S. Kee, R. B. H. Tan, R. D. Braatz, Selective Crystallization of the Metastable α-Form of l-Glutamic Acid using Concentration Feedback Control. *Crystal Growth & Design 9* (7) (2009) 3044–3051. https://doi.org/10.1021/cg800546u.

131. N. Nonoyama, K. Hanaki, Y. Yabuki, Constant Supersaturation Control of Antisolvent-Addition Batch Crystallization. *Organic Process Research and Development 10* (4) (2006) 727–732. https://doi.org/10.1021/op0600052.

132. E. Simone, A.N. Saleemi, N. Tonnon, Z.K. Nagy, Active Polymorphic Feedback Control of Crystallization Processes Using a Combined Raman and ATR-UV/Vis Spectroscopy Approach, *Crystal Growth & Design 14* (4) (2014) 1839–1850. https://doi.org/10.1021/cg500017a.

133. Y. Yang, Z.K. Nagy, Advanced Control Approaches for Combined Cooling/Antisolvent Crystallization in Continuous Mixed Suspension Mixed Product Removal Cascade Crystallizers, *Chemical Engineering Science 127* (2015) 362–373. https://doi.org/10.1016/j.ces.2015.01.060.

134. A.N. Saleemi, C.D. Rielly, Z.K. Nagy, Comparative Investigation of Supersaturation and Automated Direct Nucleation Control of Crystal Size Distributions using ATR-UV/vis Spectroscopy and FBRM, *Crystal Growth & Design 12* (4) (2012) 1792–1807. https://doi.org/10.1021/cg201269c.

135. F. Holtorf, A. Mitsos, L.T. Biegler, Multistage NMPC with On-Line Generated Scenario Trees: Application to a Semi-Batch Polymerization Process, *Journal of Process Control 80* (2019) 167–179. https://doi.org/10.1016/j.jprocont.2019.05.007.

136. C. Darmali, S. Mansouri, N. Yazdanpanah, M.W. Woo, Mechanisms and Control of Impurities in Continuous Crystallization: A Review, *Industrial & Engineering Chemistry Research 58* (4) (2018) 1463–1479. https://doi.org/10.1021/acs.iecr.8b04560.

137. Y. Ma, Z. Li, P. Shi, J. Lin, Z. Gao, M. Yao, M. Chen, J. Wang, S. Wu, J. Gong, Enhancing Continuous Reactive Crystallization of Lithium Carbonate in Multistage Mixed Suspension Mixed Product Removal Crystallizers with Pulsed Ultrasound, *Ultrasonics Sonochemistry 77* (2021) 105698. https://doi.org/10.1016/j.ultsonch.2021.105698.

138. K.A. Powell, A.N. Saleemi, C.D. Rielly, Z.K. Nagy, Monitoring Continuous Crystallization of Paracetamol in the Presence of an Additive Using an Integrated PAT Array and Multivariate Methods, *Organic Process Research & Development 20* (3) (2016) 626–636. https://doi.org/10.1021/acs.oprd.5b00373.

139. J.L. Quon, H. Zhang, A. Alvarez, J. Evans, A.S. Myerson, B.L. Trout, Continuous Crystallization of Aliskiren Hemifumarate, *Crystal Growth & Design 12* (6) (2012) 3036–3044. https://doi.org/10.1021/cg300253a.

140. Y. Cui, M. O'Mahony, J.J. Jaramillo, T. Stelzer, A.S. Myerson, Custom-Built Miniature Continuous Crystallization System with Pressure-Driven Suspension Transfer, *Organic Process Research & Development 20* (7) (2016) 1276–1282. https://doi.org/10.1021/acs.oprd.6b00113.
141. A.J. Alvarez, A.S. Myerson, Continuous Plug Flow Crystallization of Pharmaceutical Compounds, *Crystal Growth & Design 10* (5) (2010) 2219–2228.
142. N. Variankaval, A.S. Cote, M.F. Doherty, From form to Function: Crystallization of Active Pharmaceutical Ingredients, *AIChE Journal 54* (7) (2008) 1682–1688. https://doi.org/10.1002/aic.11555.
143. S. Byrn, M. Futran, H. Thomas, E. Jayjock, N. Maron, R.F. Meyer, A.S. Myerson, M.P. Thien, B.L. Trout, Achieving Continuous Manufacturing for Final Dosage Formation: Challenges and How to Meet Them May 20–21 2014 Continuous Manufacturing Symposium, *Journal of Pharmaceutical Sciences 104* (3) (2015) 792–802. https://doi.org/10.1002/jps.24247.

3

Residence Time Distribution in Continuous Manufacturing

Sonia M. Razavi
Rutgers, the State University of New Jersey

Atul Dubey
Pharmaceutical Continuous Manufacturing, US Pharmacopeial Convention, Rockville, MD

Fernando J. Muzzio
Chemical and Biochemical Engineering

CONTENTS

3.1 Importance of RTD in CM

Although continuous manufacturing (CM) adoption in the pharmaceutical industry is behind other industries, its recent popularity is driven by several benefits, such as enhanced product quality, reduced manufacturing costs, improved efficiency, and increased flexibility for scale-up [3–9]. However, the transition from batch to continuous manufacturing is not trivial. The major obstacle involves the technical and regulatory requirement of implementing advanced control concepts, in some cases requiring novel sensing methods. Because continuous powder flow through the integrated production system must be maintained over a long period of time, the control strategy should ensure the consistent quality of the product despite any variability in the process, raw materials, or environmental conditions [8]. As a result, real-time release (RTR) strategies typically involve a diversion system to direct any out-of-specification (OOS) product to scrap [10]. Thus, a comprehensive study of the process dynamics is essential, enabling an understanding of how a disturbance in the mass flow rate of an ingredient, often starting from a feeder, would propagate through the system and affect the finished products. Material traceability along the manufacturing line is required to divert any non-conforming product [11]. In simple words, the control system must know precisely and at all times "what" material is "where" and "when" in the integrated line [12].

RTD is a commonly used approach to characterize process dynamics [13]. Knowing the degree of back-mixing in the integrated line is very important. This is possible through the characterization of the RTD in the line. A low degree of back-mixing is sometimes preferable to reduce yield losses in CM as the system responds more nimbly to control actions. However, a certain amount of back-mixing is desirable to smoothen fluctuations [14] due to, for example, feeder refills, which can cause sudden increases in the mass flow rate of a given ingredient [15]. The rate of back-mixing, quantified by the breadth of an RTD profile, is affected by material properties [16, 17] and operating conditions [18–20]. Thus, thorough knowledge of the RTD of the material throughout the continuous manufacturing process is required to understand the system dynamics as the basis for material traceability and advanced process controls.

With the implementation and growing interest in continuous oral solid dose manufacturing in the pharmaceutical industry [5, 21, 22], RTDs are increasingly used to characterize powder-based continuous processes. As a result, in recent years, the RTD has been studied extensively to characterize powder flow and mixing behaviour inside individual unit operations such as in feeders [17, 23, 24], continuous mixers [16, 25–28], granulators [29–31], extruders [32–35], fluidized beds [36], feed frames [19, 37–40], and roller compactors [41, 42]. More recently, the RTD of fully integrated continuous processes, including direct compression lines [43, 44], dry granulation lines [41–43, 45], and wet granulation lines [30, 43, 46], were investigated and determined. In the remaining parts of this chapter, we will discuss the fundamentals of RTD and how it can be determined in a given system.

3.2 Determination of the RTD

Determining the RTD within a system involves the introduction of an input signal, measuring the output signal, and comparing them to characterize the delay time and mixing behaviour. RTD was first theorized in 1935 by MacMullin and Weber [47], followed by a seminal paper on RTD in 1953 published by Danckwerts [1], specifically analyzing ideal and non-ideal fluid flow within a reactor system. Later, numerical solutions of RTD for different systems and boundary conditions were examined [48–50].

In utilizing RTD methods, there are some underlying assumptions [1, 51–53] that need to be considered:

1. The system is continuous, and there is a constant or periodic *unidirectional* flow of the material in the system
2. The system has reached steady flow rates, and flow properties must remain constant as a function of time
3. For repeated RTD experiments, the system is assumed to maintain similar experimental conditions while accounting for intrinsic process fluctuations.

Following these assumptions, it is crucial to establish a clear and reliable methodology for evaluating and performing RTD experiments.

There are two commonly used methods to introduce a perturbation into a continuous powder flow system: a tracer pulse and a step change in an ingredient mass flow rate [48, 54]. Pulse input involves the quick and sudden introduction of a tracer material into the flowing stream [48], whereas, in the step change method, the concentration of the ingredient (or the tracer) is changed instantaneously, evenly, and continuously over the whole time window. In both methods, the outlet concentration is measured over time [48, 54]. Proper tracking of the tracer material with acceptable measurement frequency is required to perform an accurate RTD experiment. Process analytical technology (PAT) monitoring techniques such as near-infrared (NIR) [55] and Raman [56, 57] spectroscopic methods allow for a robust RTD characterization, as they have proven to have high accuracy with adequate sampling frequency. Other detection methods can also be employed to measure the tracer concentration as it exits the system, including colourimetric measurements or UV/Vis spectroscopy using a camera [18, 41, 58, 59], light-induced fluorescence (LIF) spectroscopy [59], and positron emission particle tracking (PEPT) [46]. Among the listed techniques, PEPT uses a different RTD measurement technique, which is tracking the trajectory of single particles. Particle tracking is also the basis of RTD simulations using computational methods such as discrete element method (DEM), computational fluid dynamics (CFD), and population-balance models (PBM) [23, 40, 60–66], where the motion of thousands to millions of particles is tracked to obtain an RTD profile. However, such methods require extensive computational power and ultimately need to be validated using experiments.

Once the outlet concentration of the tracer as a function of time t, $c(t)$, is acquired, the RTD probability distribution function, $E(t)$, for the pulse input experiment can be determined directly using Equation (3.1).

$$E(t) = \frac{c(t)}{\int_0^\infty c(t)\, dt} \tag{3.1}$$

The RTD can also be described by a cumulative distribution function, $F(t)$, which can be determined directly from a step change input, defined as follows:

$$F(t) = \frac{c(t) - c_i}{c_f} \tag{3.2}$$

where c_i and c_f are the initial and final tracer concentrations, respectively. By differentiating $F(t)$, the $E(t)$ profile can be obtained.

The choice of the introduction method (pulse vs. step change) is dependent on various factors. A comparison between the two methods is provided in-depth by Escotet-Espinoza et al. [53]. Here, some main differences are discussed.

In the pulse experiments, generally an external tracer is chosen, and thus careful selection of the tracer is necessary to ensure minimal disturbances in the bulk powder flow. Thus, not only the external material should be selected wisely, but also the amount being inserted needs to be controlled and kept as small as possible. For situations where an expensive tracer needs to be used with no possible alternatives, a pulse input is preferred to minimize the cost. The RTD profile, $E(t)$, showing the pulse response data, provides detailed information on the system compared to the cumulative RTD profile, $F(t)$, resulting from the step response data, as the integration effect of F(t) can potentially smoothen critical aspects of the RTD data [2].

On the other hand, for the step change method, typically, the material within the formulation (e.g., API) is selected to be the tracer by varying the rate of feeding material in the feeder. Thus, the step change method is attractive as it does not require opening the process to insert the tracer. Moreover, the models already built for PAT instruments for inline monitoring are able to detect the "step" easily. However, keeping the constant tracer concentration in the feed is experimentally challenging. Moreover, the step change method requires consistent and continued addition or depletion of tracer material, which could lead to possible changes in the bulk powder flow properties, and thus the size of the step must be small but within the detection limit of the PAT instrument [67]. Even more critically, the introduction of a large step in the mass flow rate of an ingredient, and the resulting large change in blend composition, can cause the blend properties to change during the experiment, introducing an additional source of error in the results.

To characterize an RTD profile and compare RTDs for different processing conditions, the mean residence time, variance, and skewness are traditionally used [13, 16, 39]. These RTD metrics are defined below.

The mean residence time (τ), which is the most used metric to characterize RTD, is the first moment of $E(t)$, which represents the average time that the tracer particles spend in the system, is given by:

$$\tau = \int_0^\infty t * E(t)\, dt \tag{3.3}$$

The mean-centred variance of the RTD curve, σ_τ^2, is calculated using the second mean-centred moment of the curve, which describes the breadth of the curve:

$$\sigma_\tau^2 = \int_0^\infty \frac{(t - \tau)^2 * E(t)}{\tau^2}\, dt \tag{3.4}$$

The third mean-centred moment of the RTD curve, ψ_τ, is called the mean-centred skewness of the RTD describing the asymmetry of the RTD curve and is calculated using the following equation:

$$\psi_\tau = \int_0^\infty \frac{(t-\tau)^3 * E(t)}{\tau^3}\, dt \tag{3.5}$$

Using these metrics to describe the RTD of a system, while extremely popular, relies on the assumption that the shape of the profiles is known. As discussed in the following section, mixing models can also be used to characterize an RTD curve. RTD modelling plays a key role in developing continuous technologies [68].

3.3 RTD Modelling

The RTD curve obtained experimentally or by simulation is then used to characterize the flow and mixing behaviour within the system. The two ideal mixing behaviours are the continuous stirred tank (CST) and the plug flow (PF) pipe. In a CST, perfect instantaneous mixing occurs inside the tank, whereas in the plug flow, perfect mixing occurs across the pipe, but no mixing is assumed to take place in the axial direction [54]. Combining these basic models allows for describing the behaviour of many real unit operations with non-ideal mixing behaviour. A review by Rodrigues [69] presents different compartment models describing scenarios, including effects such as dead zones, recycling, back-mixing, and bypassing that can be modelled using a combination of ideal and non-ideal flow systems.

The two widely used models for RTD in powder systems are the tank-in-series (TiS) model and the axial dispersion (AD) equation (also known as the Fokker-Planck equation, the convection-dispersion model or, incorrectly, the convection-diffusion model) [16, 48, 52, 70]. The TiS model describes the non-ideal flow system as a discrete series of identically sized CSTs. The AD model assumes perfect mixing in the radial direction and simulates mixing in a pipe as a combination of plug flow and dispersive transport of materials along the axial length of the system. In other words, the AD model describes the system as a continuous path where a diffusion-like process is superimposed on the ideal PF unit [54]. In the case where axial convection is dominant, this model reduces to the PF model, while in the limit of infinitely fast axial dispersion, the model reduces to a CST. Intermediate conditions are captured by a finite ratio of convection rate to dispersion rate.

The RTD of the whole continuous line is typically obtained by characterizing the RTD for each unit operation and connecting them together using convolution integrals [13]. This helps develop flowsheet models, which are approximate mathematical representations of the manufacturing line dynamics [71]. Developing a flowsheet model enables in-silico process design and optimization, control strategy assessment and optimization, and an accurate risk assessment tool. Convolution integrals can also be employed to predict the effects of the RTD of multiple unit operations on perturbations and to investigate the damping behaviour of a unit operation on a disturbance, for example, feeder fluctuations. Funnel plots are generally used to visualize the maximum concentration upset due to all possible rectangular disturbances in terms of duration and strength (i.e., excess or defect of the target API concentration) [11, 14, 16]. A funnel plot is generated by convoluting the disturbances by the RTD of the system. It is divided into two regions, one indicating the conditions where the response will be within specifications and the other indicating the parametric region where the OOS product is produced. The OOS window can then be used to design control strategies to divert material.

3.4 Importance of Tracer Selection in RTD Experimental Approach

In RTD characterization, the goal is to describe the residence time of a material in the system, often using a tracer. Implicitly, the tracer is assumed to follow the underlying flow "honestly" [54]. Given the tendency of powders to segregate as a function of their particle size and density, it is self-evident that the accuracy of the experimentally determined RTD relies on proper tracer selection. In selecting an "external" tracer, three main conditions listed below should be met [1, 13, 53]:

1. The tracer should be detectable from other materials in the system
2. The presence of the tracer should not affect the flow properties of the underlying blend
3. The tracer should have the same intrinsic RTD as the material that is being traced (i.e., the API)

To be able to find a material with these specifications, a large material property data library consisting of extensive information about the material flow properties of both active ingredients and excipients is required. Characterizing powders during process development, especially in continuous manufacturing, is essential, and the information can be stored in a material property database [72–77]. Using multivariate analysis tools [78], powders with similar properties can be identified. Among the multivariate analysis tools, principal component analysis (PCA) is the oldest and best-known technique to interpret large datasets by reducing the dimensionality of the dataset while preserving as much variability as possible [79, 80]. Principal components (PCs) are new independent variables constructed as linear combinations of the original variables. Most of the information in the original dataset is squeezed into the first few components. The dataset X can be decomposed, based on the equation below, into a set of scores (T) and loadings (P), while the remaining variability is modelled as a random error (ε):

$$X = TP^T + \varepsilon \qquad (3.6)$$

Scores are the positions of each observation in the new coordinate system of PCs, and loadings describe how much each variable contributes to a particular PC. A loading sign indicates whether a variable and a PC are positively or negatively correlated. There are various software packages that offer PCA. The procedure for selecting a tracer using PCA is described below in detail using a case study.[1]

A material property data library consisting of 162 pharmaceutically relevant powders was used to identify an appropriate tracer for Compap L (Mallinckrodt), which is a directly compressible grade of acetaminophen, to conduct pulse input RTD studies [81]. The material properties were priorly determined using a standard suite of measurements, including particle size distribution, bulk and tapped densities, and flow properties. For more information about the details of the characterization methods, the reader is referred to [81, 82].

PCA was performed on the material property data library to compare Compap L to the remaining 161 powders in the reduced space. Nine principal components (PCs) were selected, which explained more than 90% of the total variability in the material library. Other statistical criteria can also be used for determining how many PCs should be examined and how many to be ignored; in our experience, the different criteria add to the elegance of the method without changing the conclusions.

To find the most similar powders to Compap L in the reduced PC space, the weighted Euclidean distance was calculated, which takes into account the amount of variability explained by each PC, defined as follows:

$$d_{a-b} = \sqrt{\sum_{i=1}^{n} w_i * (a_i - b_i)^2} \quad 0 < w_i < 1 \qquad (3.7)$$

where n is the total number of PCs selected in the model, a_i is the score of Material A (i.e., Compap L) in the ith principal component, b_i is the score of Material B in the ith principal component, and w_i is the statistical weight (the percentage of explained variability) of the ith principal component. A value of "distances" is calculated for each material in the database, which can be ranked from low to high, corresponding to most similar to least similar to Compap L. Based on the richness of the data library in the vicinity of Compap L, there were multiple powders that could be suitable. However, similarity in physical properties is not sufficient in searching for a tracer. One should also keep in mind that the selected powder needs to be detectable, and in the case of using NIR or Raman spectroscopy as a detector, the selected powder tracer needs to have dissimilarities in the chemical properties compared to Compap L and the bulk powder. In general, the stronger the chemical contrast, the better, since this increases the accuracy of the PAT method and also allows the user to minimize the amount of tracer utilized.

In short, the ideal tracer is one that shows the most similarity in physical properties to the API while also having dissimilarities in its chemical properties compared to the bulk blend and the API. For the above example, Mannogem XL (SPI Pharma) was selected as an appropriate tracer for Compap L because of its low Euclidean distance and high level of contrast between its spectral data and the bulk powder, which for this case was Starch 1500 (Colorcon). The following section explains the importance of a proper methodology to compare RTD data. To help understand the method capabilities, we continue our example by validating the tracer selection hypothesis through RTD experiments and comparing RTD profiles of two very different tracers.

3.5 Importance of a Proper Statistical Methodology to Compare RTD Profiles

Typically, the RTD of a unit operation or an integrated system is measured for multiple conditions, for example, different blend compositions, flow rates, and processing conditions. For example, in the case of blending systems, the differences in the mean and distribution of the tracer's RTD profile for various processing conditions can be used and compared to determine the completeness of mixing inside a system [25, 28]. Moreover, for online quality control based on the diversion of RTD-predicted non-compliant products, the RTD profile needs to be validated by comparing it with experimental or simulated data. While some companies are currently engaged in using RTD measurements to characterize the performance of continuous manufacturing lines, there is currently no well-defined statistical method to compare RTD curves from different experiments or corresponding to different conditions. This immediately invites the question – what is the proper mathematical methodology to perform this analysis? Statistical analysis of RTD data is less than trivial for multiple reasons; chief among them is that RTD data points are self-correlated. In simple terms, the multiple measurements that comprise a single RTD curve are not independent of each other. Thus, proper statistical methods are needed to compare RTDs to avoid misallocation of degrees of freedom and miscalculation of statistical significance.

There exist two main comparison approaches for self-correlated distributions: model-dependent and model-independent. Model-independent methods do not make any mechanistic assumptions; they simply apply suitable statistical procedures (such as multivariate analysis of variance [MANOVA] and PCA) designed to address the self-correlation in the data set. A similar approach can be used to ensure that RTD data are analyzed correctly [16, 81]. This approach can be particularly useful for rapid data screening when the data are complex and mechanistic models are unknown or have dubious validity.

Model-dependent methods fit the profile to a specific mechanistic model that is believed to provide a suitable representation of the profile, for example, the Fokker-Planck equation for a blender or CSTs for a feed frame. In this approach, the experimental measurement of the profile is used to obtain optimum estimates of model parameters. Measured profiles corresponding to different experimental sets (e.g., different continuous lines) can be compared based on the estimated values of the parameters using standard methods (such as t-tests for pairwise group comparison or ANOVA for multiple groups) to determine whether the measured difference in profiles is statistically significant or not [16, 81, 83]. This approach is beneficial when the mechanistic models can help elucidate the physical attributes of the system.

The choice between the two approaches mainly relies on comparison purposes. For different applications, different comparison methods are advised. We continue our example from Section 4, where Mannogem XL was selected as an appropriate tracer for Compap L. Pulse input RTD experiments were conducted on a continuous blender to validate the tracer selection methodology, that is, checking whether Mannogem XL has an equivalent RTD as Compap L under similar process settings. The focus of this section is to provide a suitable statistical method to compare RTD profiles. To this end, a tracer with

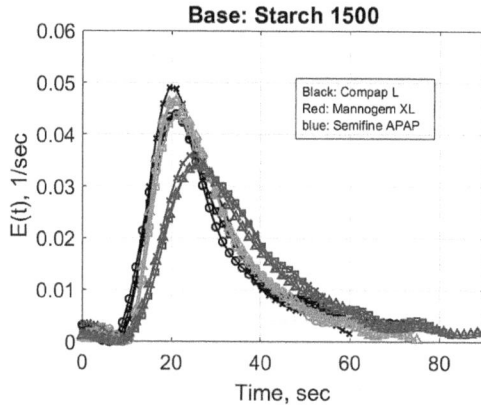

FIGURE 3.1 RTD profiles.

different physical properties was chosen, resulting in a different RTD profile to help understand the method's capabilities.

The experiments were conducted on a Gericke GCM 250 mixer (Gericke USA, Somerset, NJ) fitted with an alternate blade configuration operating at 100 rpm. The blender configuration remained fixed throughout the experimental runs. A K-Tron KT20 feeder (Coperion K-Tron Pitman Inc., Sewell, NJ) fitted with a coarse auger screw configuration and a C-type motor was used to maintain a steady flow of base powder into the mixer. At the exit of the mixer, a vibratory feeder (Eriez Magnetics, Erie, PA) was placed to dispense the powder homogeneously for the PAT. A Bruker Optics (Billerica, MA) Matrix Fourier transform near-infrared (FT-NIR) spectrometer equipped with a Q-412 NIR probe sensor head for non-contact analysis was located on a platform above the vibratory feeder. Capturing an accurate RTD profile depends on a robust NIR method development, which is beyond the scope of this book chapter. However, for full details regarding the NIR model and the experimental procedure, the reader is referred to [81].

Starch 1500 was selected as the bulk flowing powder, and pulses of Compap L and Mannogem XL were injected at the entrance of the blender. Six grams of tracer were chosen, which provided an acceptable tracer concentration profile by the NIR model. Semi-fine APAP was also chosen as the "bad" tracer, which had a large "distance" to Compap L in the PC space. For each tracer, three replicates were performed while the mass flow rate remained constant at 14 kg/h. The E(t) profiles were calculated using Equation (3.1). Figure 3.1 depicts the three replicates of RTD curves as a result of introducing different tracers.

For a quantitative comparison, both model-dependent and model-independent approaches are used to compare these six RTD profiles.

3.6 Model-Dependent Approach

As mentioned earlier, in the model-dependent approach, the RTD profile is fitted to a mechanistic model. This is the foundation of RTD modeling, being able to describe an RTD curve with an equation. Here, we use the fitting parameters acquired from different RTD curves for comparison purposes. In the case of an RTD inside a blender, the axial dispersion model has been shown to describe the RTD profile closely. The degree of back mixing or axial dispersion within a system can be quantified using the Peclet number, which expresses the ratio between the convection and dispersion rates [16, 20, 54]. Large Peclet number values correspond to less dispersive mixing occurring in the system. The delay time (t_{delay}) is associated with the plug flow region in the unit contributing to no mixing. A unit step,

TABLE 3.1

Regression Results for the Axial Dispersion Equation

	Peclet Number					Delay Time (sec)					Dispersion Time (sec)				
	Exp. #					Exp. #					Exp. #				
Tracer	1	2	3	Ave.	St. Dev.	1	2	3	Ave.	St. Dev.	1	2	3	Ave.	St. Dev.
Compap L	6.3	5.0	4.4	5.26	0.97	6.8	6.9	7.0	6.86	0.10	15.6	16.1	15.4	15.69	0.40
Mannogem XL	4.2	4.2	5.0	4.50	0.44	9.2	9.7	8.6	9.16	0.55	14.6	13.6	14.5	14.26	0.54
Semi-fine APAP	6.0	5.9	5.5	5.81	0.25	7.3	7.6	7.1	7.34	0.26	20.8	21.6	21.3	21.26	0.38

representative of the plug flow system, is convoluted with the axial dispersion equation resulting in the following equation:

$$E(t) = \frac{u(t-\tau_{delay})Pe^{0.5}}{(4\pi(t-\tau_{delay})\tau_{dis})^{0.5}} e^{-\left(\frac{Pe\left(1-\frac{(t-\tau_{delay})}{\tau_{dis}}\right)}{\frac{4(t-\tau_{delay})}{\tau_{dis}}}\right)} \tag{3.8}$$

where, τ_{delay} is the delay time, τ_{dis} is dispersion time, and Pe is the Peclet number $Pe = VL/D$ (where V is the powder velocity in the blender, L is the blender length, and D is the dispersion coefficient). The experimental E(t) profiles for each pulse experiment were fitted to Equation (3.7), and the regression results are listed in Table 3.1. A one-way ANOVA with a significance level of $p < 0.05$ was performed to determine whether there were any statistically significant differences between the means of three unrelated groups. The analysis shows statistical dissimilarity for delay time and dispersion time with p-values lower than 0.05 and nearly significant differences for Pe with a p-value of 0.11.

3.7 Model-Independent Approach

Another alternative to compare the RTD profiles is to use a model-independent approach, in particular MANOVA, which is a type of multivariate analysis that allows testing hypotheses regarding the effect of one or more independent variables on two or more dependent variables. To be able to perform this analysis, the RTD profiles were converted to the cumulative distribution functions F(t). Because of the auto-correlated nature of the RTD data, MANOVA repeated measures were employed by selecting all the concentration values as the continuous dependent variables and tracer material as the independent factor. The expression can be written as:

$$y_{hi} = \mu_j + \alpha_h + \varepsilon_{hi}$$
$$h-1,\ldots,s \text{ groups}$$
$$j-1,\ldots,n \text{ repeated measures}$$
$$i=1,\ldots,N_h \text{ samples in group } h \tag{3.9}$$
$$N = \sum N_h \text{ total sample}$$

where y_{hi} is an $n \times 1$ vector of ith sample in the hth group, μ is an $n \times 1$ vector for mean response at jth within-subject tracer, α_h is an $n \times 1$ vector for the between-group effect of the hth group, and ε_{hi} is an $n \times 1$ vector of residuals [84, 85]. To examine differences of between-subjects effects, that is, between tracers, contrast tests were used. Figure 3.2 shows the average F(t) profiles for each tracer and the F-test results corresponding to performing contrast tests between tracers within the MANOVA repeated

(a)

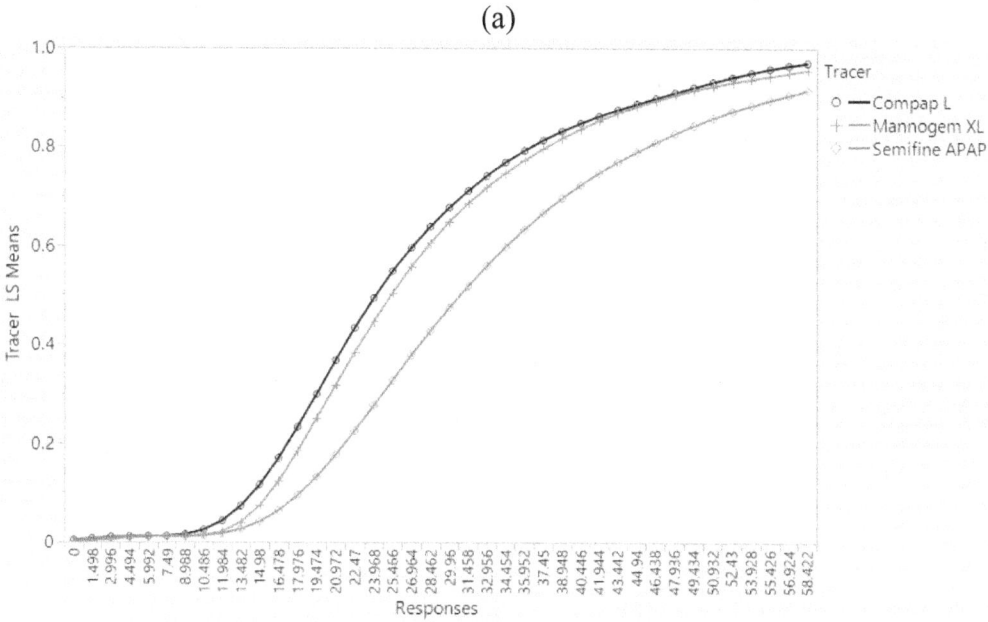

(b)

Material	Compap L	Mannogem XL	Semifine APAP
Compap L		0.2478	0.0020*
Mannogem XL	0.2478		0.0006*
Semifine APAP	0.0020*	0.0006*	

FIGURE 3.2 (a) Average CDF RTD profiles for different tracers (the response refers to the time in seconds) and (b) the comparison of RTD curves using MANOVA repeated measures. *p*-values lower than 5% indicate differences in the RTD curves.

measures test. The results suggested a statistical difference between semi-fine APAP and Mannogem XL (*p*-value = 0.0006), and semi-fine APAP and Compap L (*p*-value = 0.0020). In other words, using MANOVA, it became clear that using semi-fine APAP as a tracer would result in a (statistically) significantly different RTD profile, whereas the RTD profiles of Mannogem XL and Compap L are equivalent.

Based on the example provided, MANOVA repeated measures compare the RTD profiles more scrupulously as it takes into account a majority of the RTD profile, compared to the model-dependent approach. However, the limitation of this approach is that the number of dependent variables (i.e., cumulative tracer concentration measured at each time point) across different RTD profiles should not significantly vary as the number of variables is limited to the profile that recovers the full tracer amount first. Thus, comparison of RTD profiles that are distinctly different from each other is not advised using MANOVA.

3.8 Discussion

Typically, pharmaceutical companies (i) establish the "steady-state" RTD of a continuous manufacturing line by performing tracer experiments across multiple unit operations, (ii) use the obtained results to fit the parameters of models that simulate the response of the combined unit operations to input composition fluctuations (i.e., during feeder refill), and then (iii) use the resulting models to divert to scrap portions of the blend (or tablets compressed within a certain time interval) that might lead to the product being out of compliance.

Except for the described caution required to select a proper tracer, the use of RTD in the characterization, optimization, and control of continuous pharmaceutical manufacturing lines has closely followed the application of RTD for continuous flow fluid systems, which was developed several decades earlier. However, moving forward, we anticipate a substantial degree of specialization in pharmaceutical manufacturing:

1. Pharmaceutical manufacturing systems utilize manufacturing conditions that include intrinsic variability (e.g., the level of powder in the hopper of a feed frame is likely to oscillate, or alternatively, the throughput in the tablet press is dynamically adjusted to keep the hopper level constant. In either case, the RTD of process components [either the feed hopper or the feed frame] can change dynamically as manufacturing proceeds). This is already motivating many researchers, including the authors of this chapter, to create adaptive RTD models capable of responding to such changes in manufacturing conditions.

2. Related to this issue is the ability to predict *de novo* the RTD of a line for a given material. This would require the development of "inner" models enabling the prediction of RTD parameters as a function of ingredient and blend material properties. This is a laborious but feasible undertaking that would advance substantially the ability to design and optimize manufacturing processes.

3. The many difficulties associated with selecting and introducing tracers in cGMP lines are providing a strong impetus for the development of faster and more sensitive instrumentation that would enable the use of the step change method, which can be performed using the blend ingredients instead of an external tracer.

4. As described above, proper statistical procedures are needed to compare RTDs corresponding to different materials or conditions. Moving forward, additional work is needed to complete the development of rigorous procedures:

    a. RTD results are usually noisy, corresponding to both the granular nature of powders and the relatively high level of measurement noise. Many inexperienced users use RTD parameter estimation methods that are significantly affected by this noise. Mathematical methods that characterize and reduce the noise component in the RTD measurement would help avoid making decisions based on faulty estimates.

    b. One particular effect of noise is that the tail of RTD distributions is difficult to characterize. This is typically not an issue for quality control, because the tail of the RTD has minimal, if any, effect on a properly selected exclusion interval. However, the RTD tail plays a major role in any meaningful analysis of materials traceability, in particular, in selecting criteria for "batch" definition. Again, the answer to this question is the development of more sensitive and faster instrumentation, which enables higher accuracy. Instrument suppliers have made very substantial progress in the last few years, and as newer instruments become standard, the ability to address these issues will improve substantially.

Overall, the use of RTD as an essential component of a line design, optimization, and control is expected to expand significantly in the coming years until it becomes a standard component of pharmaceutical manufacturing process development. As RTD methods become essential components of process development and quality control, they are also likely to be carefully examined by regulators. Lack of alignment with regulators regarding the proper implementation of RTD methodologies can become the cause of delays in approvals.

NOTE

1 For readers that are more mathematically inclined, we submit that PCA identifies the eigenvectors/eigenvalues of the covariance matrix, and then rotates the underlying coordinate space so that the eigenvectors (which are liner combinations of the original basis vectors, that is, the material properties) act as a unit vector basis for a new coordinate system where variability of the entire dataset is maximized along each eigenvector.

REFERENCES

1. Danckwerts PV. Continuous flow systems: Distribution of residence times. *Chemical Engineering Science*. 1953;*2*(1):1–13.
2. Levenspiel O. *Tracer technology: Modeling the flow of fluids*: Springer Science & Business Media; 2011.
3. Burcham CL, Florence AJ, Johnson MD. Continuous manufacturing in pharmaceutical process development and manufacturing. *Annual Review of Chemical and Biomolecular Engineering*. 2018;*9*:253–81.
4. Teżyk M, Milanowski B, Ernst A, Lulek J. Recent progress in continuous and semi-continuous processing of solid oral dosage forms: A review. *Drug Development and Industrial Pharmacy*. 2016;*42*(8):1195–214.
5. Schaber SD, Gerogiorgis DI, Ramachandran R, Evans JM, Barton PI, Trout BL. Economic analysis of integrated continuous and batch pharmaceutical manufacturing: A case study. *Industrial & Engineering Chemistry Research*. 2011;*50*(17):10083–92.
6. Karttunen A-P, Wikström H, Tajarobi P, Fransson M, Sparén A, Marucci M, et al. Comparison between integrated continuous direct compression line and batch processing–the effect of raw material properties. *European Journal of Pharmaceutical Sciences*. 2019;*133*:40–53.
7. Byrn S, Futran M, Thomas H, Jayjock E, Maron N, Meyer RF, et al. Achieving continuous manufacturing for final dosage formation: Challenges and how to meet them. May 20–21, 2014 continuous manufacturing symposium. *Journal of Pharmaceutical Sciences*. 2015;*104*(3):792–802.
8. Allison G, Cain YT, Cooney C, Garcia T, Bizjak TG, Holte O, et al. Regulatory and quality considerations for continuous manufacturing. May 20–21, 2014 continuous manufacturing symposium. *Journal of Pharmaceutical Sciences*. 2015;*104*(3):803–12.
9. Vanhoorne V, Vervaet C. Recent progress in continuous manufacturing of oral solid dosage forms. *International Journal of Pharmaceutics*. 2020;*579*:119194.
10. Srai JS, Badman C, Krumme M, Futran M, Johnston C. Future supply chains enabled by continuous processing—Opportunities and challenges. May 20–21, 2014 Continuous Manufacturing Symposium. *Journal of Pharmaceutical Sciences*. 2015;*104*(3):840–9.
11. Tian G, Lee SL, Yang X, Hong MS, Gu Z, Li S, et al. A dimensionless analysis of residence time distributions for continuous powder mixing. *Powder Technology*. 2017;*315*:332–8.
12. Pauli V, Elbaz F, Kleinebudde P, Krumme M. Methodology for a variable rate control strategy development in continuous manufacturing applied to twin-screw wet-granulation and continuous fluid-bed drying. *Journal of Pharmaceutical Innovation*. 2018;*13*(3):247–60.
13. Engisch W, Muzzio F. Using residence time distributions (RTDs) to address the traceability of raw materials in continuous pharmaceutical manufacturing. *Journal of Pharmaceutical Innovation*. 2016;*11*(1):64–81.
14. García-Muñoz S, Butterbaugh A, Leavesley I, Manley LF, Slade D, Bermingham S. A flowsheet model for the development of a continuous process for pharmaceutical tablets: An industrial perspective. *AIChE Journal*. 2018;*64*(2):511–25.
15. Engisch WE, Muzzio FJ. Feedrate deviations caused by hopper refill of loss-in-weight feeders. *Powder Technology*. 2015;*283*:389–400.
16. Escotet-Espinoza MS, Moghtadernejad S, Oka S, Wang Z, Wang Y, Roman-Ospino A, et al. Effect of material properties on the residence time distribution (RTD) characterization of powder blending unit operations. Part II of II: Application of models. *Powder Technology*. 2019;*344*:525–44.
17. Van Snick B, Kumar A, Verstraeten M, Pandelaere K, Dhondt J, Di Pretoro G, et al. Impact of material properties and process variables on the residence time distribution in twin screw feeding equipment. *International Journal of Pharmaceutics*. 2019;*556*:200–16.
18. Dülle M, Özcoban H, Leopold C. Analysis of the powder behavior and the residence time distribution within a production scale rotary tablet press. *European Journal of Pharmaceutical Sciences*. 2018;*125*:205–14.

19. Tanimura S, Singh R, Román-Ospino AD, Ierapetritou M. Residence time distribution modelling and in line monitoring of drug concentration in a tablet press feed frame containing dead zones. *International Journal of Pharmaceutics*. 2021;*592*:120048.

20. Vanarase AU, Osorio JG, Muzzio FJ. Effects of powder flow properties and shear environment on the performance of continuous mixing of pharmaceutical powders. *Powder Technology*. 2013;*246*:63–72.

21. Lee SL, O'Connor TF, Yang X, Cruz CN, Chatterjee S, Madurawe RD, et al. Modernizing pharmaceutical manufacturing: From batch to continuous production. *Journal of Pharmaceutical Innovation*. 2015;*10*(3):191–9.

22. Ierapetritou M, Muzzio F, Reklaitis G. *Perspectives on the continuous manufacturing of powder-based pharmaceutical processes*. Wiley Online Library; 2016. p. 1846–62.

23. Toson P, Khinast JG. Particle-level residence time data in a twin-screw feeder. *Data in Brief*. 2019;*27*:104672.

24. Blackshields CA, Crean AM. Continuous powder feeding for pharmaceutical solid dosage form manufacture: A short review. *Pharmaceutical Development and Technology*. 2018;*23*(6):554–60.

25. Gao Y, Vanarase A, Muzzio F, Ierapetritou M. Characterizing continuous powder mixing using residence time distribution. *Chemical Engineering Science*. 2011;*66*(3):417–25.

26. Sarkar A, Wassgren CR. Simulation of a continuous granular mixer: Effect of operating conditions on flow and mixing. *Chemical Engineering Science*. 2009;*64*(11):2672–82.

27. Marikh K, Berthiaux H, Mizonov V, Barantseva E, Ponomarev D. Flow analysis and Markov chain modelling to quantify the agitation effect in a continuous powder mixer. *Chemical Engineering Research and Design*. 2006;*84*(11):1059–74.

28. Portillo PM, Ierapetritou MG, Muzzio FJ. Characterization of continuous convective powder mixing processes. *Powder Technology*. 2008;*182*(3):368–78.

29. Kumar A, Vercruysse J, Vanhoorne V, Toiviainen M, Panouillot P-E, Juuti M, et al. Conceptual framework for model-based analysis of residence time distribution in twin-screw granulation. *European Journal of Pharmaceutical Sciences*. 2015;*71*:25–34.

30. Kumar A, Alakarjula M, Vanhoorne V, Toiviainen M, De Leersnyder F, Vercruysse J, et al. Linking granulation performance with residence time and granulation liquid distributions in twin-screw granulation: An experimental investigation. *European Journal of Pharmaceutical Sciences*. 2016;*90*:25–37.

31. Ismail HY, Singh M, Darwish S, Kuhs M, Shirazian S, Croker DM, et al. Developing ANN-Kriging hybrid model based on process parameters for prediction of mean residence time distribution in twin-screw wet granulation. *Powder Technology*. 2019;*343*:568–77.

32. Kreimer M, Aigner I, Lepek D, Khinast J. Continuous Drying of Pharmaceutical Powders Using a Twin-Screw Extruder. *Organic Process Research & Development*. 2018;*22*(7):813–23.

33. Wesholowski J, Berghaus A, Thommes M. Inline determination of residence time distribution in hot-melt-extrusion. *Pharmaceutics*. 2018;*10*(2):49.

34. Wesholowski J, Hoppe K, Nickel K, Muehlenfeld C, Thommes M. Scale-Up of pharmaceutical Hot-Melt-Extrusion: Process optimization and transfer. *European Journal of Pharmaceutics and Biopharmaceutics*. 2019;*142*:396–404.

35. Wesholowski J, Podhaisky H, Thommes M. Comparison of residence time models for pharmaceutical twin-screw-extrusion processes. *Powder Technology*. 2019;*341*:85–93.

36. Chen H, Diep E, Langrish TA, Glasser BJ. Continuous fluidized bed drying: Residence time distribution characterization and effluent moisture content prediction. *AIChE Journal*. 2020;*66*(5):e16902.

37. Mateo-Ortiz D, Méndez R. Relationship between residence time distribution and forces applied by paddles on powder attrition during the die filling process. *Powder Technology*. 2015;*278*:111–7.

38. Furukawa R, Singh R, Ierapetritou M. Effect of material properties on the residence time distribution (RTD) of a tablet press feed frame. *International Journal of Pharmaceutics*. 2020;*591*:119961.

39. Dülle M, Özcoban H, Leopold C. The effect of different feed frame components on the powder behavior and the residence time distribution with regard to the continuous manufacturing of tablets. *International Journal of Pharmaceutics*. 2019;*555*:220–7.

40. Puckhaber D, Eichler S, Kwade A, Finke JH. Impact of particle and equipment properties on residence time distribution of pharmaceutical excipients in rotary tablet presses. *Pharmaceutics*. 2020;*12*(3):283.

41. Kruisz J, Rehrl J, Sacher S, Aigner I, Horn M, Khinast JG. RTD modeling of a continuous dry granulation process for process control and materials diversion. *International Journal of Pharmaceutics*. 2017;*528*(1–2):334–44.

42. Mangal H, Kleinebudde P. Experimental determination of residence time distribution in continuous dry granulation. *International Journal of Pharmaceutics*. 2017;*524*(1–2):91–100.

43. Karttunen A-P, Hörmann TR, De Leersnyder F, Ketolainen J, De Beer T, Hsiao W-K, et al. Measurement of residence time distributions and material tracking on three continuous manufacturing lines. *International Journal of Pharmaceutics*. 2019;*563*:184–97.

44. Tian G, Koolivand A, Gu Z, Orella M, Shaw R, O'Connor TF. Development of an RTD-based flow-sheet modeling framework for the assessment of in-process control strategies. *AAPS PharmSciTech*. 2021;*22*(1):1–10.

45. Martinetz M, Karttunen A, Sacher S, Wahl P, Ketolainen J, Khinast J, et al. RTD-based material tracking in a fully-continuous dry granulation tableting line. *International Journal of Pharmaceutics*. 2018;*547*(1–2):469–79.

46. Lee KT, Ingram A, Rowson NA. Twin screw wet granulation: The study of a continuous twin screw granulator using Positron Emission Particle Tracking (PEPT) technique. *European Journal of Pharmaceutics and Biopharmaceutics*. 2012;*81*(3):666–73.

47. Mac Mullin R, Weber M. The theory of short circuiting in continuous-flow mixing vessels in series and the kinetics of chemical reactions in such systems. *Transactions of the American Institute of Chemical Engineers* 1935;*31*(2):409–58.

48. Levenspiel O. *Chemical reaction engineering*: John Wiley & Sons; 1999.

49. Fogler HS, Fogler SH. *Elements of chemical reaction engineering*: Pearson Educación; 1999.

50. Nauman EB. Residence time theory. *Industrial & Engineering Chemistry Research*. 2008;*47*(10):3752–66.

51. Nauman EB. *Residence time distributions*: Wiley; 2003.

52. Bhalode P, Tian H, Gupta S, Razavi SM, Roman-Ospino A, Talebian S, et al. Using residence time distribution in pharmaceutical solid dose manufacturing–a critical review. *International Journal of Pharmaceutics*. 2021:121248.

53. Escotet-Espinoza MS, Moghtadernejad S, Oka S, Wang Y, Roman-Ospino A, Schäfer E, et al. Effect of tracer material properties on the residence time distribution (RTD) of continuous powder blending operations. Part I of II: Experimental evaluation. *Powder Technology* 2019;*342*:744–63.

54. Fogler HS. *Essentials of chemical reaction engineering: Essenti chemica reactio engi*: Pearson Education; 2010.

55. Alam MA, Shi Z, Drennen III JK, Anderson CA. In-line monitoring and optimization of powder flow in a simulated continuous process using transmission near infrared spectroscopy. *International Journal of Pharmaceutics*. 2017;*526*(1–2):199–208.

56. Fonteyne M, Soares S, Vercruysse J, Peeters E, Burggraeve A, Vervaet C, et al. Prediction of quality attributes of continuously produced granules using complementary pat tools. *European Journal of Pharmaceutics and Biopharmaceutics*. 2012;*82*(2):429–36.

57. Nagy B, Farkas A, Gyürkés M, Komaromy-Hiller S, Démuth B, Szabó B, et al. In-line Raman spectroscopic monitoring and feedback control of a continuous twin-screw pharmaceutical powder blending and tableting process. *International Journal of Pharmaceutics*. 2017;*530*(1–2):21–9.

58. Kruisz J, Faulhammer E, Rehrl J, Scheibelhofer O, Witschnigg A, Khinast JG. Residence time distribution of a continuously-operated capsule filling machine: Development of a measurement technique and comparison of three volume-reducing inserts. *International Journal of Pharmaceutics*. 2018;*550*(1–2):180–9.

59. Scheibelhofer O, Kruisz J, Rehrl J, Faulhammer E, Witschnigg A, Khinast JG. LIF or dye: Comparison of different tracing methods for granular solids. *Powder Technology*. 2020;*367*:20–31.

60. Sen M, Singh R, Vanarase A, John J, Ramachandran R. Multi-dimensional population balance modeling and experimental validation of continuous powder mixing processes. *Chemical Engineering Science*. 2012;*80*:349–60.

61. Chen K, Bachmann P, Bück A, Jacob M, Tsotsas E. CFD simulation of particle residence time distribution in industrial scale horizontal fluidized bed. *Powder Technology*. 2019;*345*:129–39.

62. Ismail HY, Singh M, Albadarin AB, Walker GM. Complete two dimensional population balance modelling of wet granulation in twin screw. *International Journal of Pharmaceutics*. 2020;*591*:120018.

63. Zheng C, Zhang L, Govender N, Wu C-Y. DEM analysis of residence time distribution during twin screw granulation. *Powder Technology*. 2021;*377*:924–38.

64. Ketterhagen WR. Simulation of powder flow in a lab-scale tablet press feed frame: Effects of design and operating parameters on measures of tablet quality. *Powder Technology*. 2015;*275*:361–74.

65. Hildebrandt C, Gopireddy SR, Scherließ R, Urbanetz NA. Investigation of powder flow within a pharmaceutical tablet press force feeder–A DEM approach. *Powder Technology*. 2019;*345*:616–32.
66. Siegmann E, Forgber T, Toson P, Martinetz MC, Kureck H, Brinz T, et al. Powder flow and mixing in different tablet press feed frames. *Advanced Powder Technology*. 2020;*31*(2):770–81.
67. Weinekötter R, Gericke H. *Mixing of solids*: Springer Science & Business Media; 2013.
68. ICH. Final Concept Paper ICH Q13: Continuous manufacturing of drug substances and drug products. *International Conference on Harmonisation Q132018*.
69. Rodrigues AE. Residence time distribution (RTD) revisited. *Chemical Engineering Science*. 2020:116188.
70. Gao Y, Muzzio FJ, Ierapetritou MG. A review of the Residence Time Distribution (RTD) applications in solid unit operations. *Powder Technology* 2012;*228*:416–23.
71. Metta N, Ghijs M, Schäfer E, Kumar A, Cappuyns P, Van Assche I, et al. Dynamic flowsheet model development and sensitivity analysis of a continuous pharmaceutical tablet manufacturing process using the wet granulation route. *Processes*. 2019;*7*(4):234.
72. Escotet-Espinoza MS, Moghtadernejad S, Scicolone J, Wang Y, Pereira G, Schäfer E, et al. Using a material property library to find surrogate materials for pharmaceutical process development. *Powder Technology*. 2018;*339*:659–76.
73. Wang Y, O'Connor T, Li T, Ashraf M, Cruz CN. Development and applications of a material library for pharmaceutical continuous manufacturing of solid dosage forms. *International Journal of Pharmaceutics*. 2019;*569*:118551.
74. Wang T, Alston K, Wassgren C, Mockus L, Catlin A, Fernando S, et al. The creation of an excipient properties database to support quality by design (QbD) formulation development. *American Pharmaceutical Review*. 2013;*16*(4):16–25.
75. Yu J, Xu B, Zhang K, Shi C, Zhang Z, Fu J, et al. Using a material library to understand the impacts of raw material properties on ribbon quality in roll compaction. *Pharmaceutics*. 2019;*11*(12):662.
76. Benedetti A, Khoo J, Sharma S, Facco P, Barolo M, Zomer S. Data analytics on raw material properties to accelerate pharmaceutical drug development. *International Journal of Pharmaceutics*. 2019;*563*:122–34.
77. Hayashi Y, Nakano Y, Marumo Y, Kumada S, Okada K, Onuki Y. Application of machine learning to a material library for modeling of relationships between material properties and tablet properties. *International Journal of Pharmaceutics*. 2021;*609*:121158.
78. Ferreira AP, Tobyn M. Multivariate analysis in the pharmaceutical industry: Enabling process understanding and improvement in the PAT and QbD era. *Pharmaceutical Development and Technology*. 2015;*20*(5):513–27.
79. Jolliffe IT, Cadima J. Principal component analysis: A review and recent developments. *Philosophical Transactions of the Royal Society A: Mathematical, Physical and Engineering Sciences*. 2016;*374* (2065):20150202.
80. Loska K, Wiechuła D. Application of principal component analysis for the estimation of source of heavy metal contamination in surface sediments from the Rybnik Reservoir. *Chemosphere*. 2003;*51*(8):723–33.
81. Razavi SM, Roman A, Bhalode P, Scicolone J, Callegari G, Dubey A, et al. Implementation of a methodology for selection of an appropriate tracer to measure the residence time distribution (RTD) of continuous powder blending operations. *Chemical Engineering Science*. 2022.
82. Moghtadernejad S, Escotet-Espinoza MS, Oka S, Singh R, Liu Z, Román-Ospino AD, et al. A training on: Continuous manufacturing (direct compaction) of solid dose pharmaceutical products. *Journal of Pharmaceutical Innovation*. 2018;*13*(2):155–87.
83. Peterwitz M, Jodwirschat J, Loll R, Schembecker G. Tracking raw material flow through a continuous direct compression line Part I of II: Residence time distribution modeling and sensitivity analysis enabling increased process yield. *International Journal of Pharmaceutics*. 2022:121467.
84. Weinfurt KP. *Repeated measures analysis: ANOVA, MANOVA, and HLM*. 2000.
85. Wang Y, Snee RD, Keyvan G, Muzzio FJ. Statistical comparison of dissolution profiles. *Drug Development and Industrial Pharmacy*. 2016;*42*(5):796–807.

4

Powder Electrostatics in Continuous Pharmaceutical Manufacturing

Michela Beretta
Research Center Pharmaceutical Engineering GmbH, Graz, Austria
Institute of Process and Particle Engineering, Graz University of Technology, Graz, Austria

Joana T. Pinto
Research Center Pharmaceutical Engineering GmbH, Graz, Austria

Amrit Paudel
Research Center Pharmaceutical Engineering GmbH, Graz, Austria
Institute of Process and Particle Engineering, Graz University of Technology, Graz, Austria

CONTENTS

DOI: 10.1201/9781003149835-5

4.1 Introduction

In the course of the ongoing shift from batch to continuous manufacturing (CM) of pharmaceutical products, powder electrostatics have gained attention due to the increased likelihood of electrostatic effects taking place during processing. Here, compared to batch processes, particle–particle and particle–wall contacts occur more continuously or frequently yielding a higher chance of electrostatic charge development (Mukherjee et al. 2021).

When particles collide with each other or with the wall of the processing equipment, charge transfer occurs between the two material surfaces leading to oppositely charged surfaces upon separation. Such phenomenon is known as: (i) contact electrification or contact charging, when the materials come into contact and are then separated, (ii) impact charging, when there is only a short contact time, and (iii) frictional electrification, triboelectrification, triboelectric charging, or tribocharging, when the materials are rubbed against each other (Matsusaka and Masuda 2003). However, since the charge transfer is a non-equilibrium process and it is challenging to distinguish among the types of contact mode involved in its generation (i.e., sliding, rolling, impact, fluidization), the use of terms triboelectric charging or tribocharging is broadly accepted (Matsusaka et al. 2010).

Tribocharging is known since antiquity and has been extensively researched. However, given its complexity, our understanding of many aspects is still limited (Lacks and Shinbrot 2019). The electrostatic effects are unpredictable and often responsible for manufacturing and/or safety concerns. Tribocharging has been reported as the root cause of critical manufacturing problems in different industries, including that of pharmaceutical solid products. Representative problems include: powder agglomeration, segregation (Hao et al. 2013), spontaneous demixing (Mehrotra et al. 2007), reduced/erratic flow properties

(Pingali et al. 2009b), and adhesion (Samiei et al. 2017; Ghori et al. 2014). These effects can trigger the risk of failures in the critical quality and process attributes, thereby potentially resulting in significant economic losses (Nwose et al. 2012). Additionally, powder tribocharging tends to generate sparks and unpleasant electrical shocks for operators. In more severe cases, dust explosions can be the dangerous result of an uncontrolled generation of electrostatic charges (Nifuku and Katoh 2003; Glor 1985; Glor 2003; Glor 2005).

The recent advancement of CM operations in the pharmaceutical industry offers a faster way of production (i.e., high throughput) and relies on equipment with a higher inner surface-to-volume ratio compared to batch manufacturing (Domokos et al. 2020; Schaber et al. 2011). This facilitates different types of contact interactions (i.e., particle–particle and particle–wall) and consequently enhances powder triboelectrification. Depending on their physicochemical properties, powders that are more prone to acquire electrostatic charges can accumulate a higher extent of static charge due to their continuous motion throughout the manufacturing line (i.e., with limited time for charge relaxation) and may be challenging to handle in such continuous processes (Beretta et al. 2020a). Cases of severe powder equipment surface adhesion might be encountered in CM due to the long processing times, resulting in process interruptions. For instance, the adhesion of the material to the processing equipment can induce deviations in mass flow, which may propagate throughout the process line and lead to the variability of the active pharmaceutical ingredient (API) content in the final product. In more severe cases, a complete blockage of the line can occur, requiring shut-down and cleaning. Moreover, the adhered material induced by triboelectrification can impair the reliable signal detection by the process analytical technology (PAT) tools (Allenspach et al. 2021).

Therefore, the measurement, prediction, and control of the powder tribocharging phenomenon become key for the stability and success of the long-term operations in CM processes. In this chapter, we aim at the one hand to describe the current knowledge and state-of-the-art techniques for the experimental quantification and modeling of tribocharging and on the other hand to present perspectives for a safer and more cost-effective production.

4.2 Charging Mechanisms

4.2.1 Material Categorization: Conductors, Semi-Conductors, and Insulators

Depending on their ability to transfer electric charge, materials can be broadly categorized into three main groups: conductors, semi-conductors, and insulators. According to the energy band model of solid-state physics shown in Figure 4.1, conductors are characterized by high conductivity as they do not or possess only a short forbidden energy gap (also known as energy gap or band gap), that is, the distance between the valence band (where electrons are bounded to the nucleus) and conduction band (where free electrons are able to conduct current). In insulators instead, the conductivity is limited by the presence of a large forbidden energy gap, thus requiring a high amount of external energy to move electrons from the valence into the conduction band due to their strong bonding with the nucleus. Semi-conductors have intermediate properties and require a low amount of external energy to reach the conduction state.

Only conductor and insulator materials are typically encountered in pharmaceutical applications. Therefore, in this chapter, we focus on these two material types and their interactions to explain the charge transfer mechanisms at the basis of their powder tribocharging.

4.2.2 Charging Mechanisms in Pharmaceutical Applications

Pharmaceutical powders are typically organic materials with insulator properties, such as high resistivity (above 10^{13} Ωm) and slow charge relaxation times (from minutes to hours) (Bailey 1998). In the pharmaceutical industry, such powders are, in most cases, processed using equipment with a metal conductive surface (typically stainless steel). Likewise, the interaction between pharmaceutical powders and processing surfaces involves: (i) insulator–metal and (ii) insulator–insulator contacts.

In contrast to the charge transfer developing between conductive materials (i.e., metal–metal contacts), which is well-known and properly understood, the mechanisms behind the charge transfer of insulators

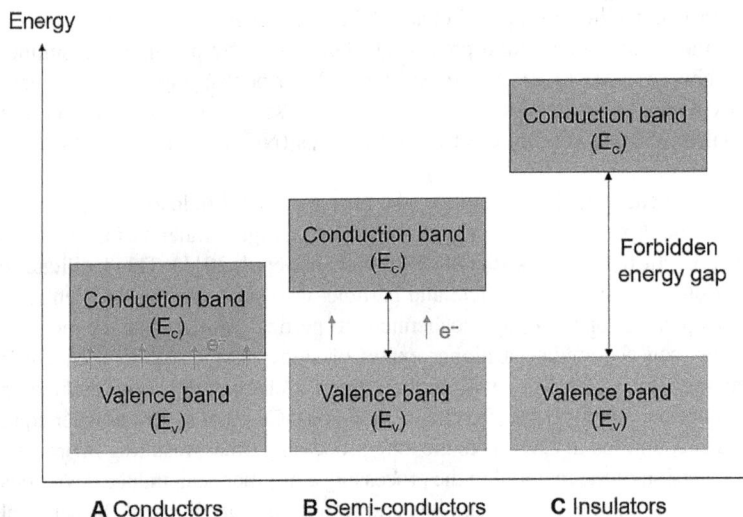

FIGURE 4.1   Energy band model of solid-state physics (conductors, semi-conductors, insulators).

are still unclear. Difficulties in explaining the tribocharging behavior of insulators arise from their complex nature, challenging to properly characterize and for which, the electron band energies are not well defined. Compared to metals, where the charge transfer is known to occur *via* electron tunnelling, for insulators, it is proposed that different species, that is, electron, ion, material fragments, or combinations of them, can transfer.

4.2.2.1 Electron Transfer

The concept of electron transfer is extensively described for metal–metal contacts, and has been extended to insulator contact types. Here, the contact potential difference (CPD), arising from the difference in the work function (WF; for metals) and apparent or effective work function (for insulators) between the two surfaces, is responsible for the electrons transfer from the surface with the lower to the higher WF (equalizing the energy levels of the two materials). Therefore, the magnitude of charge transferred between the two surfaces (Δq) can be expressed as:

$$\Delta q = C_0 \cdot CPD = C_0 \frac{-(WF_1 - WF_2)}{e} \tag{4.1}$$

where C_0 is the effective capacitance (which depends on the characteristics of the surfaces) and e is the elementary charge (Matsusaka et al. 2010). Such a proposed mechanism has been supported by experimental evidence showing a linear relationship between the charge generated and the metal CPD (Davies 1969) and by spectral responses of photoelectric emission experiments performed before and after contact electrification (Murata and Kittaka 1979). Theoretical models have also been proposed for a mechanistic description of such mechanism (Lowell 1979).

The transfer of electrons for insulators may seem counterintuitive as they do not contain free electrons in their conduction bands, however, the surface and the bulk of a solid are energetically different. The presence of surface states is believed to provide intermediate energetic states, which are accessible for electrons and can provide the driving force for the transfer mechanism due to the difference in effective WF (Lowell and Rose-Innes 1980). Such explanation has been recently questioned by the findings of a thermo-luminescence study showing that the presence of electrons in such states would not be sufficient to account for the magnitude of charge observed in the case of same material tribocharging (Waitukaitis et al. 2014). Other theories postulate that the driving force for electron transfer comes from the interactions between the contacting surfaces leading to the delocalization of electrons in inorganic materials

(Xu et al. 2018; Lacks and Gordon 1994) or the formation of electric fields arising from deformations on the crystal lattice (Abdelaziz et al. 2018). Research in the field of electrochemical reduction reactions seems to support the electron transfer mechanism in insulators (Liu and Bard 2008; Liu and Bard 2009a; Liu and Bard 2009b), where it has been hypothesized that the presence of the transferred electrons on negatively charged insulators may promote the chemical reactions (by electron transfer in the reactant solution). It is however not clear whether these electrochemical reductions are indeed promoted by the transferred electrons or by the radicals formed during the mechanochemical process (Baytekin et al. 2012a).

4.2.2.2 Ion Transfer

The concept of ion transfer has been initially proposed by Harper (1967) and since then, the role of ions in the triboelectrification of insulator materials has been the subject of several investigations. This type of transfer mechanism is rather complex and depends on the type, concentration, and mobility of the ions present on the material surface. For molecules that can easily dissociate in ions, experimental evidence has demonstrated the transfer of weakly bound ions from the original surface to a new one (Diaz et al. 1991; McCarty and Whitesides 2008; McCarty et al. 2007a; McCarty et al. 2007b). A lower tribocharging propensity was also observed for molecules containing both anions and cations as mobile ions (Diaz et al. 1991). Ion transfer however could take place also for materials that do not possess mobile ions. In such cases, ions can be supplied from the atmosphere interacting with the surface or by the presence of a water layer on solid surfaces.

Several models have been proposed to describe triboelectrification due to ion transfer, however, no quantitative evaluation of this mechanism has been provided so far. The Harper ion model (Harper 1967), later adapted by McCarty and Whitesides (McCarty and Whitesides 2008), explains the transfer of a single mobile ion during contact and separation of surfaces as a function of its potential energy. The mechanism involved, in the case of a water layer present on particle surfaces, has been described to be highly sensitive to the thickness of the aqueous layer. The thin surface water layer is reported to enhance the charging process, whereas the thick layer is known to mitigate charge. Besides water layer thickness, also the concentration of ions in the adsorbed aqueous layer and the temperature rise during frictional contacts will impact tribocharging (Gu et al. 2013; McCarty and Whitesides 2008; Harris et al. 2019). The hydroxide adsorption model by McCarty and Whitesides explains ion transfer (i.e., OH^- ions) when an adsorbed water layer is present. Later Knorr suggested a bipolar model for the water-layer-mediated transfer of charge involving frictional forces which accounts for the formation of separated and oppositely charged areas (Knorr 2011).

4.2.2.3 Material Transfer

The impact and frictional contacts between surfaces can also lead to the transfer of material fragments, small dust particles, or impurities present on the surfaces. The extent of material transfer depends on the mechanical properties of the materials (Baytekin et al. 2012b; Pandey et al. 2018), surface characteristics (Lowell and Rose-Innes 1980), and mode of contact (Lacks 2012).

Evidence supporting the material transfer from one surface to another is dated back to the late 70s (Salaneck et al. 1976) and has been supported by more recent experiments in the field of mechanochemistry. Kelvin probe microscopy experiments were performed to study charged surfaces and revealed a network of positive and negative charge areas at the microscale (Gonzalez et al. 2017; Burgo et al. 2012; Baytekin et al. 2011; Barnes and Dinsmore 2016) that were attributed to the transfer of material fragments (da Silveira Balestrin et al. 2014). Although so far, no theoretical model exists to describe the material transfer mechanism, recent studies have shown that the extent of material transfer can affect tribocharging in terms of both magnitude (Pandey et al. 2018) and polarity of charge (Baytekin et al. 2012b).

The extent to which each specific transfer mechanism contributes to the overall material triboelectrification is not yet understood (Sakaguchi et al. 2014). However, besides the type of species transferred and mechanisms behind the resulting triboelectrification, there are several other factors which need to be considered and understood.

4.3 Principal Factors Impacting Powder Electrostatics

During pharmaceutical processing, tribocharging can be affected by several factors. These can be generally classified into material- and process-related factors as shown in Table 4.1. More detailed explanations are given below.

4.3.1 Tribocharging Dependence on Material-Related Factors

4.3.1.1 Work Function

As described briefly in Section 4.2, the WF defined for metals or the apparent/effective work function for insulators is considered the driving force for electron transfer. This material-related factor represents, therefore, one of the fundamental properties involved in the charging of pharmaceutical materials (Lowell and Rose-Innes 1980). WF is defined as the minimum energy needed to extract an electron from a solid material surface. And it is more formally expressed as the distance between the Fermi and the vacuum energy level (Kahn 2016). This parameter is frequently used to estimate the direction of charge transfer and a good correlation between the estimated WF and the tribocharging trends has been demonstrated in several studies (Akande and Lowell 1985; Lowell 1976). By ranking the materials according to their WF (from low to high values) as shown in Figure 4.2, triboelectric series have been developed to allow preliminary predictions of the surface charge resulting from the materials' collisions (Zou et al. 2019; Henniker 1962; Gooding and Kaufman 2014; Bailey 1993). However, their applicability has also been frequently questioned since the WF only describes the electronic structure of the material without taking into consideration the additional factors involved in the charging process. For example, Sarkar et al. concluded that the tribocharging of materials during processing cannot be predicted from the WF in vacuum, and suggested that, for more relevant predictions, the latter should be assessed in more 'realistic' environments (Sarkar et al. 2012). The WF is typically determined using techniques such as photoemission spectroscopy (PES) for an absolute determination and Kevin–Zisman method for a relative determination of the probe (Murata and Kittaka 1979; Matsusaka et al. 2010; Itakura et al. 1996). Atomic force microscopy (AFM)-based determination of the WF has also been recently proposed (Herzberg et al. 2021). Alternatively, computational tools such as *ab initio* density functional theory (DFT) or semi-empirical molecular orbital calculations (MOPAC) are also frequently used to compute the WF. More details on the molecular modeling approaches used to predict tribocharging are provided in Section 4.5.1.

As an alternative to the WF, a recent study has shown that the computed ionization potential (IP) can be a better parameter to estimate the charging propensity of materials (Brunsteiner et al. 2019). The IP considers an isolated atom and describes the energy required to remove the outermost electron from its

TABLE 4.1

Overview of Material-Related and Process-Related Factors Influencing Tribocharging

Material-Related Factors	Process-Related Factors
Work function	Unit operation
Surface chemistry	Equipment surface and design
Powder crystallinity	Process parameters
Particle size distribution	Environmental conditions
Particle shape	
Surface roughness	
Mechanical properties	
Hygroscopicity	
Formulation	

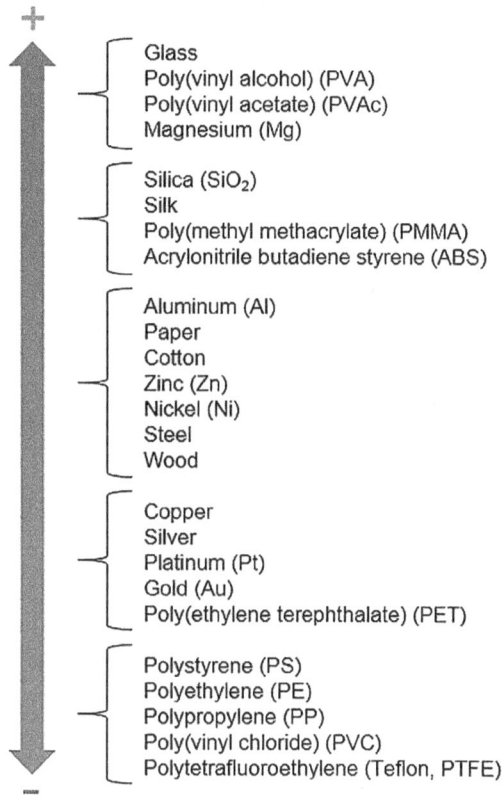

FIGURE 4.2 Tribocharging series. (Adapted from Gooding and Kaufman 2014.)

ground state to infinity (the atom becomes ionized). When calculating the IP, it is important to take into account the structural relaxation of materials, thus computing the IP based on adiabatic energy differences is relevant.

4.3.1.2 Surface Chemistry

Several studies demonstrated the influence of surface chemistry on tribocharging. The changes in the surface chemistry have been obtained by the addition of functionalized comonomers (Kamiyama et al. 1994), dry-coating processes (Jallo and Dave 2015), and silanization reactions (Biegaj et al. 2017; Lee et al. 2018). Kamiyama et al. showed that materials containing easily ionized functional groups on their surfaces possess a higher charging propensity, attributed to a facilitated ion transfer mechanism (Kamiyama et al. 1994). By coating paracetamol particles with titania, hydrophilic, and hydrophobic silica, Jallo and Dave demonstrated that the hydrophilic coatings lead to a lower charge compared to hydrophobic ones (Jallo and Dave 2015). Similar findings were reported by Biegaj et al. using silanization reactions to obtain glass beads with different functional groups (i.e., −OH, −NH$_2$, −CN, −F). Moreover, by studying the charge decay characteristics of the functionalized surfaces, the same authors concluded that hydrophobic surfaces show greater charge retention (Biegaj et al. 2017). Using the same methodology to alter the surface chemistry of materials, Lee et al. found that the contact between hydrophilic and hydrophobic surfaces generates a significant number of positive charges on the hydrophilic surface. Further, it was noted by authors that the latter phenomenon was mitigated when an acidic environment was used and favored when a basic condition was employed (Lee et al. 2018). The substitution groups of methylcellulose (MC) and hydroxypropyl methylcellulose (HPMC) polymers have also been suggested by Ghori et al. as significant contributors to their tribocharging. Generally, materials with a higher hydroxypropyl

(Hpo)/methoxyl (Meo) substitution ratio (in the range of 0 to 0.403) showed lower tribocharging (Ghori et al. 2014).

The functional groups present at the surface will directly influence the surface energetics of materials. Thus, it is not surprising that studies have shown good correlations between the acquired charge and surface energy (Jallo and Dave 2015; Ahfat et al. 2000). A detailed description of the surface energy and measurement techniques is out of scope for this chapter; however, it is important to know that this parameter is composed of a dispersive and polar component. The dispersive component represents the Lifshitz-van der Waals interactions, whereas the polar component refers to the acid–base interactions. More specifically, the acid component indicates the electron-accepting and the base component the electron-donating propensity of the material. Consequently, some literature suggests a correlation between the charge acquired by the material and its acid–base characteristics (Ahfat et al. 2000). However, Jallo and Dave found that the charging trend was influenced not only by the acid-base characteristics of the powders but also by their dispersive component (Jallo and Dave 2015). Likewise, the determination of the surface energy may be a good indicator for material tribocharging.

Tribocharging may occur also between materials with the same chemistry (Henry 1953; Lowell and Truscott 1986; Pähtz et al. 2010a). Thus, in addition to the functional groups, the materials' purity (doped, undoped, clean, contaminated, etc.) can also impact their triboelectrification. The presence of even a small amount of (surface) impurities (e.g., degradation products, atmospheric contaminants, etc. [Zhao et al. 2000; Mukherjee et al. 2016; Modhave et al. 2020]) is believed to induce variations in the effective work function and the vacuum level position (Apodaca et al. 2010). This can alter the electrostatic properties of the material (Kahn 2016). Moreover, surface impurities can also change the mode of particle interactions and/or take part in the charge transfer, affecting triboelectrification (Mukherjee et al. 2016).

4.3.1.3 Powder Crystallinity

Several studies have investigated the effect of crystallinity on tribocharging (Zellnitz et al. 2019a; Wong et al. 2014; Kwok and Chan 2008a; Murtomaa et al. 2002a; Shekunov et al. 2002; Carter et al. 1998; Murtomaa et al. 2004). However, literature is populated with inconsistent results concerning the relationship between crystallinity and tribocharging. For instance, Cartner et al. have investigated the tribocharging of amorphous (spray-dried) and crystalline lactose and observed higher charging for the crystalline material. Conversely, Murtomaa et al. reported an increase in charge density for lactose powders with a higher degree of amorphous contents (up to 1%) (Murtomaa et al. 2002a). Further, the authors also associated the presence of a higher amorphous content (up 95%) with greater variability in the sign and magnitude of charge as well as different particle size distribution (PSD) and morphology of lactose particles (Murtomaa et al. 2004). The higher magnitude and opposite charge polarity found for amorphous forms were confirmed by other studies on micronized and supercritical-fluid conditioned salmeterol xinafoate (Shekunov et al. 2002) and salbutamol sulfate (Zellnitz et al. 2019a; Wong et al. 2014; Kwok and Chan 2008a).

Generally, the aforementioned results reflect the fact that due to crystallinity being highly related to other properties (e.g., hygroscopicity, material hardness, shape, etc.), it is hard to decouple its effect from other physicochemical factors involved in triboelectrification. Likewise, the effect of the crystal structure on tribocharging has been associated with the impact of molecular (dis-) orders on the higher structure of materials, that is, differences in their specific surface area (SSA) (Murtomaa et al. 2004), mechanical properties (Karner and Urbanetz 2011), crystal packing, and moisture content (Wong et al. 2014; Zellnitz et al. 2019a).

4.3.1.4 Particle Size and Particle Size Distribution

The particle size of materials and its distribution has a significant impact on charging and it is one of the most studied material-related factors in this context. Typically, smaller particles are reported to acquire a higher charge than coarse particles due to their larger SSA for charge transfer (Sarkar et al. 2012; Mukherjee et al. 2016). However, in some cases, an opposite trend is observed. The latter has been attributed to the lower inertia upon the impact of small particles (Mountain et al. 2001) and to their lower surface deformation during elastic–plastic collisions (Saleh et al. 2011). For the same material, smaller particles generally tend to charge negatively, whereas the coarser ones positively (Zhao et al. 2000; Zheng et al. 2003; Forward et al. 2009; Zhao et al. 2002; Zhao et al. 2003; Trigwell et al. 2003; Waitukaitis et al. 2014). In some cases, an opposite trend is reported (Sowinski et al. 2010; Mehrani et al. 2005; Sow et al. 2011; Carter and Hartzell 2017). Moreover, materials with a broader PSD have been shown to charge to both a higher magnitude (Zheng et al. 2003) and to a lower magnitude (Wu and Bi 2011, Forward et al. 2009, Bennett et al. 1999), when compared to more monodispersed ones.

For chemically identical materials, the particle size dependence of tribocharging cannot be explained by possible differences in the WF (Gallo and Lama 1976) for particles above 1 μm (Lacks and Sankaran 2011). Thus, other mechanisms are involved in the generation of charge. For instance, Lacks et al. have proposed that asymmetric contacts may be responsible for the bipolar charging of particles of different sizes (Lacks and Sankaran 2016). Asymmetric contacts will result in different contact areas, where small and large areas will charge with an opposite polarity following the transfer of species (i.e., electrons or ions). According to the theory, assuming an equal density of species on the surface of fine and coarse particles, the surface of coarser particles is expected to trap a greater number of high-energy species, leading to the systematic transfer of species from coarse to fine particles during contact. Following the proposed mechanism and assuming that the transferred species are negative (electrons or anions), smaller particles are expected to acquire a negative polarity and larger particles a positive charge. However, this hypothesis has been put into question by thermo-luminescence studies (Waitukaitis et al. 2014).

4.3.1.5 Particle Shape

The role of particle shape on tribocharging has been extensively studied by Ireland using flow along an inclined plane (Ireland 2010a; Ireland 2010b; Ireland 2012). Particle shape was found to influence the mode of contact (sliding, rolling, bouncing), which in turn critically affected the charging process (Ireland 2010a). Irregular particles, characterized by a low roundness ratio, were found to slide with a quasi-fixed orientation, without being able to roll or tumble. For spherical particles (high roundness ratio), rolling was the predominant type of contact which continuously rendered available a fresh surface for the charging process (Ireland 2012). This explained, other sliding-based observations where spherical particles were discovered to gather more charges when compared to irregular-shaped ones (Ireland 2010a; Ireland 2010b; Karner et al. 2014; Sarkar et al. 2012). However, under specific circumstances, irregular particles may undergo violent tumbling and bouncing leading to higher charging compared to the rolling motion of round particles (Ireland 2012). The higher SSA of irregular particles may additionally promote charging as observed, for example, during pneumatic conveying (Saleh et al. 2011).

Extending the effect of shape on triboelectrification to non-granular materials, recent studies have also shown that a change in the shape of flexible materials in the three-dimensional space led to a change in charge. More specifically, the results showed that when the material becomes more compact (from an extended to a bent geometry), the amount of charge decreases. The proposed mechanism behind such observation is that a dynamic charge transfer with the atmosphere occurs, that is, a reversible ionization of air molecules and surface deposition of ions from the air (Pandey et al. 2020). Studies on contact-separation mode of triboelectric nanogenerators (TENG) have also shown that using identical materials with different surface curvatures led to a negative charge polarity for positive curvature surfaces and a positive polarity in the opposite case (Xu et al. 2019).

4.3.1.6 Surface Roughness

The surface roughness of the particles plays an important role in determining the area of contact for tribocharging (Matsusaka et al. 2000) and the frictional properties of the materials (Ivković et al. 2000). A higher tribocharging tendency is often reported by investigators for rough particles compared to smooth ones (Kwek et al. 2013; Karner et al. 2014). For insulator materials, particles of higher roughness are expected to have higher energy states resulting from the accumulation of charges on the peak of the asperities, thus leading to an uneven charge distribution on the surface (Alan et al. 2020). Materials with a higher surface roughness and greater distance among asperities have been also reported to charge more homogenously due to a more uniform distribution of normal force on the points of contact (Neagoe et al. 2017). The higher SSA of rough particles can increase their ability to adsorb moisture and other species, which can affect charge transfer (Kwek et al. 2013; Zhao et al. 2000; Mukherjee et al. 2016; Trigwell et al. 2003).

4.3.1.7 Mechanical Properties

The mechanical properties of materials have also been reported to affect tribocharging. These can directly affect the contact area available for charge transfer (Watanabe et al. 2007a) or influence the extent to which material is transferred from one surface to the other (Pandey et al. 2018; Baytekin et al. 2012b). During contact, materials can deform either elastically or plastically and the respective contact area is inversely related to the elastic modulus (stiffer materials have a higher elastic modulus) and hardness of the materials (Pinto et al. 2020). It is expected that hard materials have a small contact area as they do not deform (or deform to a lower extent) upon contact, and thus, charge to a lower extent. However, if such materials are brittle, they may tend to break more easily and the charge transfer *via* material fragments may take place (Tanoue et al. 1999). Harder materials are expected to enhance the fragmentation of the softer ones in contact, contributing to the charging process (Baytekin et al. 2012b). On the other hand, the higher adhesive forces observed for soft materials upon contact may promote the cleavage of bonds, thus facilitating triboelectrification *via* material transfer (Pandey et al. 2018).

4.3.1.8 Hygroscopicity

Depending on their hygroscopicity, materials can sorb a different amount of water molecules when exposed to a humid atmosphere. The moisture adsorbed on the material surface as well as the one absorbed into its bulk (even if to a lower extent) can affect its charging propensity (Jallo and Dave 2015). It is generally believed that the presence of water molecules reduces electrostatic effects due to an enhanced conductivity (Biegaj et al. 2017; Rowley and Mackin 2003). However, it has been demonstrated that, in certain cases, water may have an opposite effect and facilitate the charge transfer mechanism (Beretta et al. 2020b; Wiles et al. 2004) or have a negligible effect on tribocharging (Beretta et al. 2020b; Rowley and Mackin 2003). It seems, that the overall effect of water on tribocharging is dependent on the amount and location. Different surface-water interactions have been proposed to explain the aforementioned contradicting observations: (i) water could act as a 'source and sink' of ions (Knorr 2011; de Burgo et al. 2011), (ii) water can enhance the material conductivity (Grosvenor and Staniforth 1996; Kwok and Chan 2008b), and (iii) water can act as a lubricant reducing inter-particulate friction (Beretta et al. 2020b). The dominating mechanism(s) at work seem to be material-dependent and may be influenced by changes in the environmental conditions, which can critically affect the thickness of the water layer adsorbed (Schella et al. 2017). Overall, this can also result in different charge relaxation kinetics.

4.3.1.9 Formulation

When considering multicomponent systems, such as powder blends, their composition plays a significant role in the overall tribocharging process. Typically, APIs show a higher charging propensity compared to excipients (Šupuk et al. 2012). Contrary to the hydroxyl groups present in most of the hydrophilic excipients' surfaces, APIs can comprise a wider variety of elements (e.g., halogens and other hetero-atoms) and normally present smaller particle sizes which make them more prone to tribocharging (Biegaj et al. 2017). The prediction of the blend charge is not an easy task, given the numerous types of interaction that might be involved in their processing (i.e., contacts among different materials and equipment). This task is further complicated by the tendency of materials to adhere to the equipment surface and/or other materials. For this reason, also for this material-related factor, careful interpretations are required, depending on the unique combination of factors at play. Based on the assumption that APIs show a higher charging propensity, it would be expected to observe an overall higher charging for formulations comprising APIs in higher concentrations. However, even if some evidence is in line with the previously expected effect (Rescaglio et al. 2019; Engers et al. 2006; Ghori et al. 2014), others show opposite findings (Rowley 2001; Zellnitz et al. 2019b; Soppela et al. 2010). For instance, the studies from Rowley et al. and Zellnitz et al. have shown a decrease in charge when increasing the salbutamol sulfate concentration in one case from 0.5 wt% to 5 wt% in binary blends with α-lactose monohydrate (Rowley 2001) and from 2 wt% to 5 wt% in mannitol-based binary blends (Zellnitz et al. 2019b). Similarly, Soppela et al. observed a decrease in charge density when increasing the concentration of paracetamol from 0 wt% to 25 wt% in binary blends comprising different grades of microcrystalline cellulose (Soppela et al. 2010). By extending the range of API concentration from 0 wt% to 100 wt%, Rescaglio et al. showed different charge evolutions as a function of the API concentration, which, depending on the combination of API and excipient considered in the blend, may show a monotonic or non-monotonic evolution with changes to the charge polarity (Rescaglio et al. 2019).

4.3.2 Impact of Process-Related Factors on Tribocharging

4.3.2.1 Unit Operation

Tribocharging can essentially occur in every unit operation involving granular materials; however, its magnitude can vary depending on the type of process employed in the manufacturing line. Pharmaceutical manufacturing is composed of two major stages: drug substance manufacturing (also known as primary manufacturing) and drug product manufacturing (also known as secondary manufacturing). The first deals with the synthesis, isolation, purification, and finishing of the API(s), whereas the second focuses on the production of the final dosage form by combining the API(s) with other ingredients. Both involve several processing steps and can be operated in a continuous manner. However, most of the unit operations of primary manufacturing involves the presence of a liquid phase, which makes them less sensitive to tribocharging. The tribocharging propensity of the final API crystals in the bulk powder could still be affected by the types of solvent employed during crystallization, washing, and filtration steps. In addition, the presence of residual impurities could also contribute to the change in the tribocharging propensity of the solid-state API. In the final continuous drying step of the API manufacturing process (used to remove the residual liquid obtaining the API in a powder form), the nuisance of tribocharging can lead to agglomeration or adhesion effects altering the particle properties carefully designed during crystallization (Zettl et al. 2021; Aigner et al. 2022). Other mechanically intensive processes such as dry milling and sieving of API, often used as an intermediate step between primary and secondary manufacturing, can lead to the generation of disordered solid surface as well as facilitate the charge transfer (Beretta et al. 2022). Tribocharging can be considered more critical for secondary manufacturing, where every unit operation involves the handling and processing of powder-based materials to produce the final dosage form. Different continuous process routes are available for the production of drug products, with the most popular being continuous direct compression (CDC), continuous dry granulation (CDG), and continuous wet granulation (CWG) (Ierapetritou et al. 2017). A detailed description of these manufacturing routes is out of scope for this chapter, however, a brief overview of the principal unit operations involved is provided below to highlight relevant processing steps for charge generation. Inherent to all manufacturing routes, continuous powder feeding is the initial and most crucial processing step due to its potential implications on the overall process stability and final product quality (Hsiao et al. 2020). Here, API and excipients (e.g., fillers, binders, disintegrants, lubricants, etc.) are typically fed from loss-in-weight (LIW) feeders to gravimetrically control their mass flow according to the desired formulation. The fed mass from the different feeders is either directly conveyed in the blender by means of a hopper funnel or may pass through a mill for de-lumping purposes. Following blending, the powder blend is introduced (i) directly into the tablet press (in CDC we have compression as a final step to produce tablets) in case of CDC lines, (ii) to a dry granulation unit (i.e., roller compactor) in CDG lines, or (iii) to wet granulation unit (i.e., high-shear, twin-screw, or fluid bled) with a subsequent drying step in CWG lines. After granulation, the granules are typically milled to tailor their PSD prior to tableting or capsule

TABLE 4.2

Extent of Electrostatic Charging as Function of
the Processing Operation

Operation	Charge Density (μc/kg)
Sieving	$10^{-5} - 10^{-3}$
Pouring	$10^{-3} - 10^{-1}$
Scroll feed transfer	$10^{-2} - 1$
Milling	$10^{-1} - 1$
Pneumatic conveying	$1 - 10^{2}$

Source: Adapted from Gibson 1997.

filling. To convey the powder through the different unit operations, pneumatic conveying or transfer by gravity are commonly employed.

For several of the operations present in CM lines, the range of charge densities that may develop has been indicated by Gibson, as shown in Table 4.2 (Gibson 1997). Generally, higher charging is observed for operations where a high amount of energy and/or a high frequency of particulate contacts are involved. For this reason, lower charge densities are found in simple sieving or pouring operations but the acquired charge can be significantly higher in milling and pneumatic conveying. In pneumatic conveying, the presence of particles in a more dispersed phase enhances even further their triboelectrification due to the facilitated particle contact interactions (Norouzi et al. 2020).

Tribocharging has been suggested to be the potential source of problems in powder feeding (Muehlenfeld and Thommes 2014; Gold and Palermo 1965; Engisch and Muzzio 2014) and therefore, investigated as a critical parameter affecting performance (Bostijn et al. 2019; Stauffer et al. 2019; Bekaert et al. 2021). In the specific context of CM, a couple of recent studies have focused on the evaluation of feeding-induced charge for commonly used pharmaceutical powders in CM (Beretta et al. 2020a) and on the impact of tribocharging on the performance of the gravimetric feeding operation including hopper refilling (Allenspach et al. 2021). Both studies showed that materials undergoing higher tribocharging tend to adhere more to feeder surfaces (i.e., powder stagnation in the hopper, adhesion to the screws, bearding effects at the outlet, and alteration to the powder trajectory during free-fall). Powder stagnation in the feeder hopper or a reduction in the screw-free volume caused by material build-up can result in poor accuracy and consistency of the dosed mass, and, if refill systems are used, their operation may be detrimentally affected requiring manual intervention. When the material build-up is located at the screw outlet (i.e., bearding), the material accumulation may increase over time and suddenly be dislodged leading to mass flow deviations. This may become even more critical when such material build-up occurs at the outlet of the hopper funnel, typically used to collect the dosed materials from the different feeders in the line, thus becoming undetected by the feeder control algorithm (Allenspach et al. 2021). Beretta et al. showed that the magnitude and polarity of charge acquired following the feeding process are material-dependent, and therefore it may be possible to mitigate such effects if the powder blend to be processed is rationally designed (Beretta et al. 2020a). To the best of the authors' knowledge, no tribocharging study has been performed on a continuous blender, however, the knowledge gained in batch-blending processes is expected to be applicable also in a continuous environment. It is well-known, that blending may be affected by the presence of charged materials, with materials of the same polarity repelling each other and materials of opposite polarity attracting each other. Therefore, the rational control of the respective component sizes (Naik et al. 2016b) and polarity (Pu et al. 2009) has been demonstrated to enhance blend homogeneity and its stability against segregation.

Tribocharging can also impact the tableting operation, although the extent of electrostatic charging developing during this operation is unknown. For instance, it has been shown that tribocharging may alter the die-filling step (Nwose et al. 2012) and/or may induce material sticking to the punches (Samiei et al. 2017). The study by Samiei et al. clearly showed that punch sticking is dominated by the charge decay kinetics of the API (even for a formulation comprising only 10 wt% of API). Based on a similar filling principle, the smooth operation of capsule filling machines may be likewise affected by the generation of electrostatic charges.

4.3.2.2 Equipment Surface and Design

The design of the equipment, including the material of construction, equipment's internal surface area as well as its geometry, can impact the material tribocharging. It is known that powders of the same product processed using equipment made of distinct materials will charge to a different extent depending on the WF difference (Carter et al. 1992; Eilbeck et al. 1999; Engers et al. 2006; Rowley and Mackin 2003; Watanabe et al. 2007a). This effect could be, however, altered by the adhesion of particulate material on the surface of the processing equipment, as suggested by Elajnaf et al. (2006) and Eilbeck et al. (2000). The lower particle–wall interactions obtained after coating stainless-steel containers with excipients or APIs by Elajnaf et al. led to a reduction of their tribocharging during the mixing process (Elajnaf et al. 2006). Similarly, replicated experiments performed in a non-cleaned cyclone showed a progressive adhesion of particles and a decrease in charge (Eilbeck et al. 2000). Following the same rationale, it has been shown that the internal area of the processing equipment will also play a role in the triboelectrification, as it can influence the number of particle–wall contacts in relation to particle–particle ones (Zhu et al. 2007; Mukherjee et al. 2019). Other geometry factors such as hopper angles (Mukherjee et al. 2021), auxiliary devices, for example, impellers, secondary conveyors, piping, etc. (Schwindt et al. 2017), may also affect the contact mechanisms, and in turn, impact tribocharging. For instance, Zhu et al. found that a horizontal oscillating mixer would lead to a higher material charging compared to a tumble mixer (turbula). These findings were proposed to be a result of the larger contact area produced by the sliding motion of the oscillating mixer compared to the impacts that the material undergoes in the turbula device (Zhu et al. 2007).

4.3.2.3 Process Parameters

4.3.2.3.1 Number, Time, and Energy of Contact

The selection of process parameters such as feed rate, blending speed and time, as well as others will determine the number, length, and energy of contacts that the material experiences during processing and will, therefore, affect tribocharging. A recent study conducted by Allenspach et al. has investigated the feeding performance of a standard and direct compression (DC) grade of HPMC. The poorer performance of the standard HPMC grade, that is, higher mass flow deviations and failed hopper refills, were correlated to its higher charging propensity leading to greater material adhesion. The accumulation of material on the feeder barrel was found to correlate to the set feed rate, that is, higher when increasing the feed rate from 1 kg/h to 15 kg/h (Allenspach et al. 2021). Similarly, Zhu et al. reported a higher level of charge and material adhesion during blending when increasing the blender speed from 34 rpm to 72 rpm (Zhu et al. 2007). At higher processing speeds, the occurrence of tribocharging effects is believed to be facilitated by the high number and frequency of particle–wall contacts as well as lowering of the possibility of charge relaxation (i.e., short interval time between repeated collisions). Moreover, the charging kinetics are highly dependent on the processing time and typically follow a monotonic trend until the charge saturation level is reached (Zhu et al. 2007). In contrast, a mathematical model developed by Shinbrot et al. to predict the charging of insulators during repeated contacts surprisingly revealed the reduction of charge at higher contact frequency. The model predictions were validated experimentally using a vibrated bed of glass beads (Shinbrot et al. 2018).

4.3.2.3.2 Shear and Normal Forces

In many cases, the dense state of a powder bulk requires a certain amount of shear to produce a flow or for this to be mixed properly with other materials. The application of such shear can, however, induce tribocharging, as demonstrated by Šupuk et al. In their study, a modified annular shear cell was used to apply shear strain to α-lactose monohydrate particles and to simultaneously record the development of electrostatic charge (measuring the current flowing through the powder bed). It was found that when a normal load (20 kPa) and shear rates (from 0.0021 s^{-1} up to 0.0057 s^{-1}) were applied on the powder bed, the magnitude of the current and charge generated increased due to enhanced particle–particle and particle–wall collisions. Moreover, a significantly higher charge was observed when increasing the compaction of the powder bed (shear strain up to 6.84) (Šupuk et al. 2007). Similar results were obtained by Pingali et al. who showed that the electrostatic properties of various pharmaceutical blends were significantly impacted by the shear rate and, even to a higher extent, by the strain (i.e., total energy) experienced by the powders. The impact of shear on the acquired charge density seems to be however formulation-dependent. The charge density and the impedance (i.e., measure of conductivity) were generally found to increase when increasing the shear strain (from 40 to 640 rev), however when a lubricant, that is, magnesium stearate, was added to the blend, an opposite trend was observed. Such opposite results may be possibly driven by an enhanced delamination and coating propensity of the non-conductive and shear-sensitive magnesium stearate (Pingali et al. 2010).

Besides the effect of shear, normal forces might also have an impact on the tribocharging propensity of the materials as indicated by the investigations conducted by Ireland et al. In their study, an increase in tribocharging was found for thicker beds of particulate materials flowing down through an inclined chute, suggesting that the formation of a larger contact area (less bouncing and rolling effects) and a higher normal force acting on the particle layer in contact with the surface of the processing material led to higher charging (Ireland 2010b; Ireland 2010a). Likewise, the same mechanism has been hypothesized to explain the higher charging observed at lower chute inclination angles where normal forces are expected to dominate (Naik et al. 2015; Yao et al. 2016).

4.3.2.3.3 Environmental Conditions

The environmental conditions to which the materials are exposed during processing are well-known to critically affect tribocharging. Temperature, external electric fields, relative humidity (RH) as well as their combinations will contribute to the generation of tribocharging effects. Generally, higher temperatures tend to reduce the charge generation, most likely due to a lower electric resistance helping toward charge dissipation (Greason 2000; Xu et al. 2018). The presence of external electric fields has been instead proposed as a pre-requisite for the same material tribocharging of insulators upon collision (Pähtz et al. 2010b) and its contribution to the separation of water ions responsible for charging under a humid atmosphere (Zhang et al. 2015b).

With regard to RH, this is the environmental factor mostly studied in the literature. In combination with the material properties (i.e., hygroscopicity and SSA) of the powder, the RH in the environment will impact the kinetics of water adsorption impacting triboelectrification. Another mechanism by which RH could affect tribocharging is due to the alteration of the air conductivity. The presence of water vapor in the humid air is expected to enhance the conductivity of the air promoting charge dissipation (Karner and Urbanetz 2011). This mechanism is, however, believed to be less dominant compared to the effect of water molecules on the material surfaces (Schella et al. 2017). Typically, a higher RH is associated with lower tribocharging levels (Nifuku and Katoh 2003; Elajnaf et al. 2006; Zhu et al. 2007); however, as discussed in Section 4.3.1.8, this assumption cannot be generalized as materials with different physicochemical properties may show different tribocharging trends when increasing RH such as: (i) decrease in charge density; (ii) initial increase in charge density, followed by a decrease after a certain RH threshold; (iii) a progressive increase in charge density; and (iv) an independent relation between RH and tribocharging (Beretta et al. 2020b). Some researchers have also proposed that different RH levels will lead to distinct types of charge transfer mechanisms, with electron transfer taking place at low RH and an ion transfer at a higher RH (Németh et al. 2003). Electrons may tunnel easier when increasing the RH in a relatively low range due to the initial increase of surface conductivity, however, electron tunnelling is significantly reduced after reaching a critical RH value (Zheng et al. 2014).

4.4 Principles and Techniques for Charge Measurement

Relying on distinct physical principles (e.g., friction, impaction, collision, fluidization, shear, etc.), different measurement techniques have been developed for the quantification of electrostatic charge (Karner and Urbanetz 2011; Matsusaka et al. 2010; Wong et al. 2013, 2015a; Kwok and Chan 2009; Peart 2001; Hoe et al. 2011). In general, the techniques used for charge measurement can be divided into two categories:

TABLE 4.3

Overview of the Available Methods for the Quantification of Electrostatic Charge that may be Relevant in Continuous Manufacturing with Related Advantages and Disadvantages

	Device	Advantage	Disadvantage
Static measurement methods	Faraday cup	Simple, reliable Widely applicable	Measures only the net charge unless a tailored design is developed (e.g., vertical array)
	Induction/grid probes	In-situ charge measurement Widely applicable Charge measured as function of time	Measures only the net charge Accuracy may be affected by the adhesion of the material to the probe
Dynamic measurement methods	Ring-shaped induction sensor	Simple, reliable Measures the magnitude and polarity of single particles	Measures particles during free-fall motion from a vibrating feeder Requires signal processing
	High-speed videography combined with acoustic levitation	Precision techniques for particle contacts	Not widely applicable Relevant only for particle–particle interactions
	Electrical single particle aerodynamic relaxation time (E-SPART)	Measurement of bipolar charge	Complex set-up design Determination of particle charge is based on count (not on mass) Cannot operate at high flow rates
	Phase doppler particle analyzer (PDPA)	Measurement of bipolar charge Simultaneous determination of charge and particle size	Accuracy dependent on velocity and particle size measurements The presence of highly agglomerated and highly charged particles may introduce errors Limited to low flow rates
	Charge spectrometer	Measurement of bipolar charge Measurement of the charge to diameter ratio	Consists of two separate devices Large and heavy set-up
Others	Atomic force microscopy (AFM)	Precise control of the contact process Simultaneous information on several particle properties	Requires sample preparation Measure single particle interactions Gives qualitative information

Adapted from (Wong et al. 2013).

(i) static methods, where the measured value is based on the charge transferred or induced by the material to the measuring device, and (ii) dynamic methods, where the charge is measured based on its mobility in a given electric field (Wong et al. 2013; Kwok and Chan 2009; Hoe et al. 2011). The selection of the most suitable method depends on the application of interest. For instance, static methods are considered more appropriate for powder mixing, pouring, or filling operations, but have the limitation of measuring only the net charge (i.e., net charge resulting from the sum of electrostatic charges of different polarity). Dynamic methods are instead, more suitable for powder fluidization or aerosolization (Hoe et al. 2011). An overview of the type of devices available for each category of measurement method is provided in Table 4.3 and described in detail in Sections 4.4.1, 4.4.2 and 4.4.3.

4.4.1 Static Measurement Methods

4.4.1.1 Faraday Cup

The Faraday cup is the most frequently used instrument for measuring the net charge of materials, due to its simplicity and reliability. The construction of the Faraday cup (shown in Figure 4.3) is based on two conducting containers (i.e., protection and measuring cup), separated by an insulator layer (Matsusaka et al. 2010; Karner and Urbanetz 2011; Wong et al. 2013). The outer container (i.e., protection cup) serves to protect the inner one from external influences and it is therefore grounded. The inner container

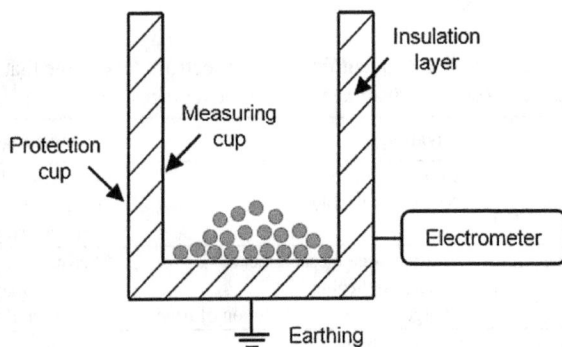

FIGURE 4.3   Schematic of a Faraday cup. (Adapted from Wong et al. 2013.)

(i.e., measuring cup) is used for the measurement and it is therefore connected to an electrometer. When the charged material is introduced inside the Faraday cup, a charge of the same magnitude and opposite polarity is induced on the inner wall and quantified by the electrometer.

Besides the simple operation of manually pouring the charged material into the Faraday cup, different conveying and tribocharging mechanisms exist to assess the propensity of the material to attain electrostatic charge during processing. One of the first Faraday cup-based tribocharging measurement methods was proposed by Murtomaa and Laine, who used a glass pipe inclined by 55° to measure the charge obtained after sliding lactose and glucose mixtures (Murtomaa and Laine 2000). The commercially available GranuCharge™ device (GranuTools, Belgium) is based on a similar method for the determination of the electrostatic charge of materials after flow and impact with specifically designed pipes (Rescaglio et al. 2019). The device is also equipped with RH controlling accessory. Such a device has been used in several studies to evaluate the tribocharging propensity of the powders for CM operations, that is, twin-screw feeding (Bostijn et al. 2019; Stauffer et al. 2019; Bekaert et al. 2021) and its correlation with the feeding-induced charge has also been demonstrated (Beretta et al. 2020a).

The Faraday cup can also be used in an open-end fashion, known as a through-type Faraday cup (Watanabe et al. 2007a, b; Matsusaka et al. 2000; Watanabe et al. 2006), to perform in-situ charge measurements without altering the movement of the charged materials (i.e., the material of interest flows through the cup). On-line Faraday cups have been developed to measure the charge development, for example, in fluidized beds (Mehrani et al. 2005; Song et al. 2016; Sowinski et al. 2010; Sowinski et al. 2012; Sowinski et al. 2009).

Also based on the measurement principle of the Faraday cup, an aerodynamic dispenser system has been integrated to enable the charge characterization of low quantities of powders. This technique, used for the first time by Zarrebini et al., is particularly attractive at the early stage of product development (especially for high-value materials such as APIs) as it requires only a small amount of material (e.g., typically few milligrams) (2013). Here, a commercially available dispersion unit is used to investigate the tribocharging tendency of the powder which is sandwiched between two thin metal foils in the dispersion unit. A pulse of pressurized gas (typically air) is applied to disperse the particles and the net charge transfer after repeated collisions with the internal surfaces of the unit is measured on a conventional Faraday cup, mounted immediately below. Recently, in a similar fashion, Zafar et al. have used the dispersion unit of Morphologi G3® static image analysis system (Malvern Panalytical, UK) to evaluate the tribocharging propensity of a series of powders in contact with materials presenting different WFs (i.e., dispersion units made of different materials) (2018). Van Snick et al. used the same device to characterize the triboelectrification of 55 pharmaceutical powders relevant for CM with a material consumption of only 30 mg (Van Snick et al. 2018).

The main limitation of the Faraday cup is that it is capable of measuring only the net charge, thus providing an indication of the overall charge of the system resulting from the balance of positive and negative charges. However, systems presenting low levels of net charge may still be composed of highly charged particles with opposite polarity (i.e., bipolar charging), whose characterization may be crucial to

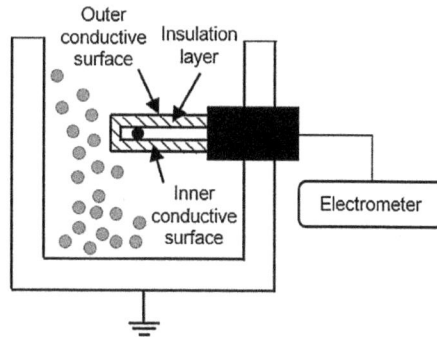

FIGURE 4.4   Schematic of an induction probe. (Adapted from Wong et al. 2013.)

to advance the design and process of formulations with optimal blending characteristics and reduced risk of segregation. To this end, a series of Faraday cups have been used in a vertical array to measure bipolar charging (Zhao et al. 2000; Zhao et al. 2002).

4.4.1.2 Induction Probe

Induction probes (Figure 4.4) are often used for online measurement of charge in fluidized beds, pneumatic conveying, and inhalation systems (Murtomaa et al. 2003a, b; Ciborowski and Wlodarski 1962; Zhou et al. 2013; Kwok et al. 2006; Singh and Hearn 1985). Their mechanism and construction are similar to the Faraday cup, however here outer shielding and insulator layers are used to protect the conducting probe. An opposite charge of the same magnitude is induced on the conducting probe by the material and an electrometer is used to measure the voltage or current generated (Wong et al. 2013). Likewise, the charge density can be measured as a function of time. For fluidized bed systems, coaxial types of probes have been specifically developed for the simultaneous measurement of charge, size, and distance of the solids being processed (Murtomaa and Salonen 2015; Peltonen et al. 2015; Peltonen et al. 2016), whereas in-situ measurements of particle charge and bubble properties could be assessed through dual-tip electrostatic probes (He et al. 2015). Grid-type probes have instead been successfully applied in the field of inhalation to study the charge aerosols emitted from dry powder inhalers (Murtomaa et al. 2003b).

4.4.1.3 Other Static Measurement Techniques

Other static measurement methods exist for more specialized applications, such as the measurement of the charge of inhaled formulations (e.g., electrical next generation impactor (eNGI) (Hoe et al. 2009a, b), electrical low-pressure impactor (ELPI) (Glover and Chan 2004; Young et al. 2007; Kwok et al. 2006) and its modifications (Hickey et al. 2007; Telko et al. 2007; Kwok and Chan 2008b), and modified twin stage impinger (TSI) (Zhu et al. 2008); however these are less relevant for the characterization of CM operations and thus, out of the scope of this chapter.

4.4.2 Dynamic Measurement Methods

4.4.2.1 Ring-Shaped Electrostatic Inductive Sensor

The ring-shaped electrostatic inductive sensor proposed by Hussain et al. offers the possibility to measure both the magnitude and polarity of charge of individual particles (Hussain et al. 2013; Hussain et al. 2016). Here, an inductive sensor is used to detect the magnitude and polarity of the charged particles while being fed from a vibratory feeder into a pipe. When the charged particles pass through the sensing zone, they induce a current that is amplified to detect the direction and amplitude of the peaks in the signal. Signal processing is then applied to evaluate the charge distribution of the particles in terms of both polarity (peak direction) and magnitude (peak amplitude).

4.4.2.2 High-Speed Videography Combined with Acoustic Levitation

The charge transfer arising from the impact of a particle against a target has been largely studied (Lee et al. 2018; Xie et al. 2016; Watanabe et al. 2006; Haeberle et al. 2018). Recently, a new technique combining high-speed videography and acoustic levitation has been proposed by Kline et al. to control the collisions among the particle (through stable levitation positions within the acoustic field) and measure the evolution of their electric charges by applying a frequency-swept AC electrical field (Kline et al. 2020). This method was able to provide complete isolation from the environment and allowed detailed tribocharging investigations into particle–particle contacts having different surface chemistry, size, shape, etc.

4.4.2.3 Electrical Single Particle Aerodynamic Relaxation Time

For the simultaneous measurement of the size and charge of individual particles in the micrometer size range, Mazumder et al. have developed an electrical single-particle aerodynamic relaxation time (E-SPART) analyzer (Mazumder and Ware 1987). This device is suitable for the characterization of aerosols and can supply information about electrical mobility and aerodynamic diameter fast and reliably. The size measurement of individual particles by the E-SPART is based on laser Doppler velocimetry (LDV), where particles in the sample chamber are oscillated by an AC electric field, while in the measurement chamber laser beams are scattered by the device to obtain information about the particle size. Information on the extent and bipolarity of charge can be extracted by their interaction with the applied electric field. The main limitation of E-SPART is that the measurement is limited to low airflow rates (0.5–1l/min), which was proved to be an obstacle when characterizing highly charged, inhomogeneous aerosols. Moreover, the device geometry is rather complex and the determination of the particle charge is based on the count, which could be the source of errors with particles of different mass showing the same charge (Ali et al. 2008). The instrument is however used in several industries, for example for the characterization of toner (Mazumber et al. 1991) and dust particles (Zhang et al. 2007), and it is widely employed in the pharmaceutical industry to determine the charge distribution in inhalation systems (Ali et al. 2008; Philip et al. 1997; Saini et al. 2007), to study the electrostatic effect on the dispersion, transport, and deposition of fine powders (Yurteri et al. 2002; Mountain et al. 2001), or to analyze the electrostatic charge distribution of particles in gas-solid pipe flow (Matsusaka et al. 2002).

4.4.2.4 Phase Doppler Particle Analyzer

A phase doppler particle analyzer (PDPA) able to measure bipolar charging and particle size has been developed by Kulon et al. (2003) and was subsequently modified by Beleca et al. (2010). In this, the measurement chamber is equipped with a pair of laser beams for the determination of the particle size through light scattering and a pair of electrodes with opposite polarity are used for the determination of the charge of the passing particle (i.e., from the deflection of a direct current electric field).

4.4.2.5 Charge Spectrometer

Charge spectrometers allow measuring the charge distribution of particles as a charge-to-diameter ratio (i.e., q/d). The measurement principle of q/d-meters is based on the deflection of a charged particle in an electric field, from which the polarity and magnitude of charge are obtained (Epping and Kuettner 2002). According to their movement pattern, particles are deposited on a glass slide and scanned in a parscan device (equipped with a microscope for image analysis) to calculate the charge-to-diameter ratio of the particles. This measurement technique, mainly used for toners, has been also applied for charge determination during powder delivery in a selective laser sintering (SLS) process (Hesse et al. 2019).

4.4.2.6 Other Dynamic Measurement Techniques

Other dynamic measurement techniques designed for inhalation products include the use of a bipolar Next Generation Impactor (bp-NGI) (Rowland et al. 2019), a multistage precipitator (O'Leary et al. 2008), a bipolar charge measurement system (BCMS) (Balachandran et al. 2003; Kulon and Balachandran 2001), a bipolar charge aerosol classifier (Kulon et al. 2001), a differential mobility analyzer (Knutson and Whitby 1975), laser-based velocimetry (Alois et al. 2017), and a bipolar charge analyzer (BOLAR™) developed by Dekati (Wong et al. 2016; Wong et al. 2015b; Leung et al. 2017, 2016). All those methods are capable of detecting the bipolar charge distribution of particles.

4.4.3 Atomic Force Microscopy Measurement Method

Atomic force microscopy (AFM) has been employed to study contact charging given its inherent ability to measure the force-distance curves during particle-surface separation. Here, single particles have been initially charged by contact with a given surface (Gady et al. 1996; Bunker et al. 2007) *via* the application of electric fields (Mizes et al. 2000; Kwek et al. 2011) and with the beam in a scanning electron microscope (Zhou et al. 2003). The presence of electrostatic forces results in a distinctive curvature in the force–distance profiles (long-range interactions) that clearly separates them from short-range van der Waals forces (Bunker et al. 2007). This technique allows direct control of the contact process and is suitable for the simultaneous characterization of the work of adhesion, surface energy, and electrostatic charge under pre-defined conditions. However, as it can only account for single particle interactions, it may be a more attractive technique for screening purposes at the early stages of development.

4.4.4 Advancement in Process Analytical Technology for Direct and Indirect In-Process Measurement of Powder Charging

Following the concepts of quality by design (QbD), real-time release testing (RTRT), and continuous process verification (CPV), extensive research has focused on the implementation of process analytical technology (PAT) tools in CM lines (Kim et al. 2021). Such PAT tools rely on different measurement methods which can be classified into at-line, online, and in-line. At-line methods are based on the collection and analysis of a sample in close proximity to the actual process, online ones on the measurement of a sample in the process (i.e., the sample is returned to the process after measurement), and in-line methodologies consist on the real-time monitoring during the process flow (i.e., no sampling required). As shown in Sections 4.4.1 and 4.4.2, techniques for at-line and online charge measurements have been widely applied, together with offline ones, to measure charging in lab or pilot scale equipment; however, there are often concerns that such measurement techniques may not be applicable to the industrial scale (Kaialy 2016). It has been suggested that (i) PAT tools may not be able to accurately capture the shear and packing conditions that the material experiences during processing, (ii) sampling may induce further charging, and (iii) it may not be possible to account for the charge relaxation process leading to inaccurate estimation of the in-process charge. However, so far, only a limited number of studies have focused on the in-line measurement of charge, and currently no commercial instrument exists for this purpose. Electrostatic sensors are, so far, the only technology that has been successfully applied for the real-time determination of flow and electrostatic charge in fluidized beds (Shi et al. 2017; Zhang et al. 2018) and pneumatic conveying systems (Gao et al. 2018). Given its simple design, ease of installation, robustness to fouling, and relatively low costs, this technique is considered promising for the development of advanced PAT tools providing a cost-effective method to obtain in-process information such as blend uniformity (Hao et al. 2013). However, so far, only one report could be found on the integration of electrostatic sensors into pharmaceutical manufacturing operations. A dual-electrode, electrostatic powder flow sensor (EPFS) developed by Hill-Izani was used to obtain information on relevant powder flow and tribocharging characteristics under different powder flow conditions (i.e., lean and dense phase) (Hill-Izani 2019).

The EPFS technology consists of an industrial-scale stainless-steel pipe, modified using flanges (Figure 4.5) to accommodate the ring-shaped sensing element and two SubMiniature version A (SMA) bulkheads (each of which is connected to a single electrode). The device was successfully applied at the

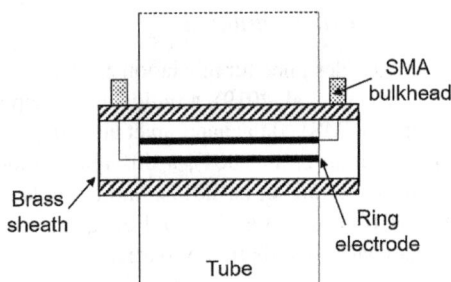

FIGURE 4.5   Schematic of the industrial-scale electrostatic powder flow sensor (EPFS). (Adapted from Hill-Izani 2019.)

outlet of a twin-screw feeder and at the outlet of a tablet press hopper and proved to be suitable for the in-line charge characterization of pharmaceutical powders with a different range of cohesion propensities (Hill-Izani 2019).

The measurement of the powder charging was obtained using the root-mean-square (RMS) of the electrostatic signal normalized against the mass flow rate (expressed as charge per gram per second). Thus, limited information is provided by the technique (no information on the absolute magnitude and polarity of charge could be obtained).

Given the limitation of in-line probes, soft sensors could represent an alternative to the direct determination of powder charge. For example, in a fluidized bed dryer, an arc electrode array was applied to measure the charge of powders at different air velocities and used to indirectly determine moisture content changes in the granules (Zhang et al. 2018). Following an opposite approach, one could imagine that soft sensors relying on models able to link the moisture content of materials to their charging could be used for the indirect determination of the charge density.

4.4.5 Best Measurement Practices

Although pharmaceutical development operates under strict quality requirements and a range of pharmacopeial methods and international conference on harmonization (ICH) guidelines are recommended for their assessment, there is currently a lack of standardized techniques and procedures for measuring the electrostatic charge of materials. Techniques based on different measurement principles can be widely found across the scientific community and measurement devices often present custom-made designs. This makes the reproducibility and comparability of the results found through literature difficult, and thus, limits the applicability of the findings to very specific conditions. Especially for highly sensitive devices such as the Faraday cup, a measurement variability of up to 50% has been reported if standardized procedures are not followed (Peart 2001). It is, therefore, generally recommendable that charge determinations are performed under tightly controlled environmental conditions and with defined quantities of materials. The use of a vibrating chute at a fixed rate is preferred to manual pouring and the materials need to be stored in containers of defined nature (e.g., metal, plastic, glass, etc.) prior to measurement (Peart 2001). Additionally, to improve the reproducibility of the charge results, the operator is advised to be grounded (e.g., with grounding bracelets) to prevent the electrostatic field of the analyst from influencing the measurements (Karner and Urbanetz 2011).

It is important to pay attention to the pre-processing history of the materials (e.g., sieving, homogenization, handling, storage conditions, etc.), which could induce charging prior to analysis and affect the final measurement accuracy and reproducibility. Karner et al. suggested to pre-condition the material prior to the measurement by storing it in a grounded conductive container for a minimum of 48 h at controlled RH (Karner and Urbanetz 2011). Peltonen et al. discharged the samples with an AC neutralizer and placed them in grounded metallic plates to dissipate any possible initial charge prior to the measurements (Peltonen et al. 2018).

The device-cleaning procedure is crucial and so are the materials coming into contact with the device surface (e.g., dry cleaning, use of organic solvent, etc.) (Eilbeck et al. 2000). Eilbeck et al. showed that the cleaning step has an effect on the final charge measured and found to be lower for the acetone-rinsed surface (Eilbeck et al. 2000). Zhou et al. dried the mixing vessels using compressed air and stored them under the same environmental conditions as the material of interest to improve the measurement reproducibility (Zhu et al. 2007). Further, Sarkar et al. employed distilled water and 70% isopropyl alcohol for cleaning and the cleaned surfaces were dried and deionized prior to the next experimental run (Sarkar et al. 2012).

Presently, there is a critical need to identify, compile, and harmonize a set of best measurement practices for the quantification of tribocharging in order to expand the knowledge in the field and minimize the contradictory results found among investigations performed under distinct settings. Figure 4.6 presents a

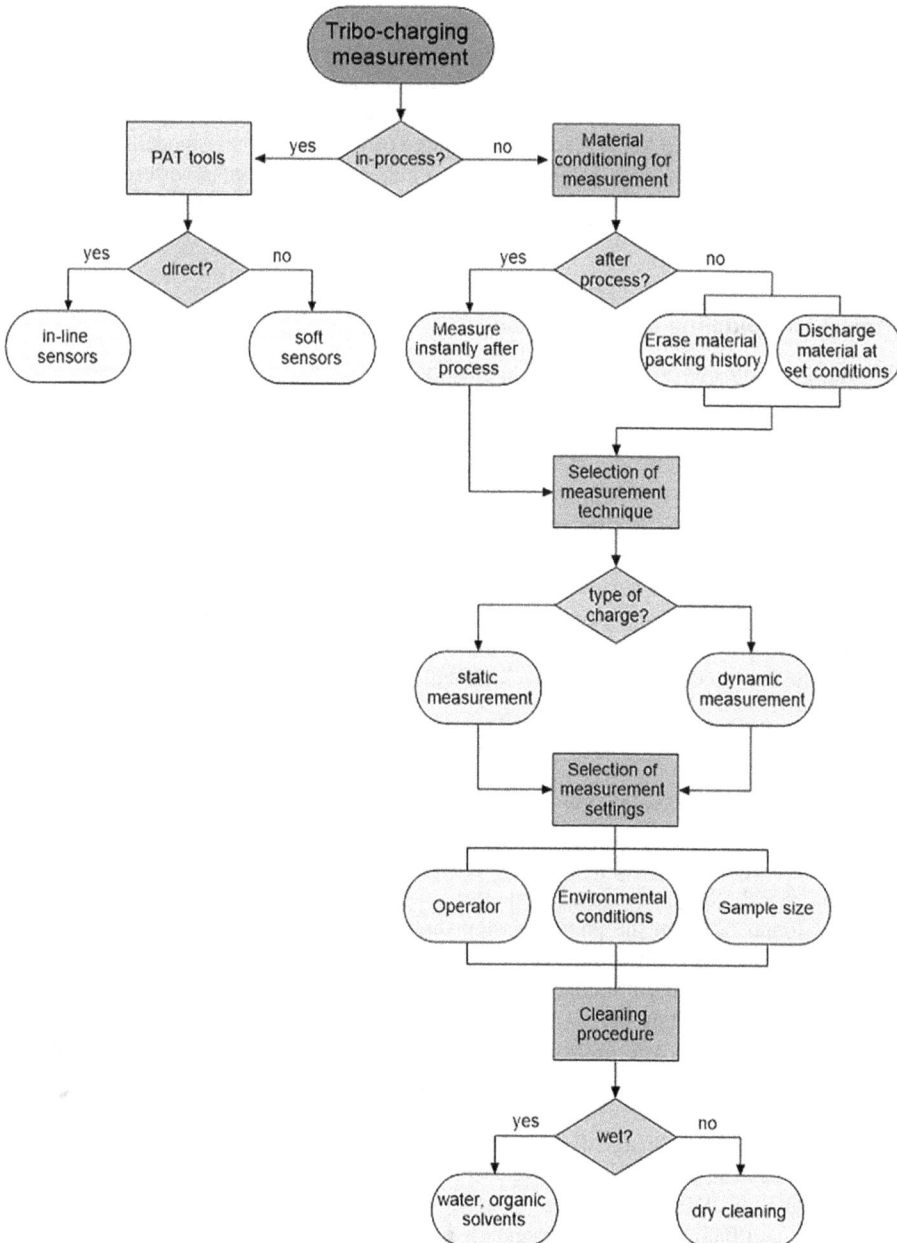

FIGURE 4.6 Generic flowchart of best measurement practices of powder electrostatics.

generic flowchart considering all the critical aspects that, in our practical experience, are considered when performing charge measurements of powder/granular samples.

4.5 Modeling Approaches of Powder Tribocharging

Given the inherent complexity of tribocharging involving hierarchical effects, its accurate prediction and control are a challenge, and so far not completely feasible. As described in Sections 4.2 and 4.3, our understanding of the electrostatic interaction is still limited even at the fundamental level and also challenged by the numerous factors influencing it (material properties, process conditions, and environmental factors). Modeling approaches could help expand the knowledge in this field by applying scientific principles that could support the determination of critical parameters (e.g., contact area, pressure, duration, and contacting frequency between surfaces) difficult to quantify experimentally (Rowley 2001). In this context, different modeling approaches have been demonstrated to be powerful methods for the quantification of effects related to the electrostatic charge of materials. These modeling approaches can, generally, be categorized as follows: (i) molecular modeling and simulation, (ii) discrete element method (DEM), (iii) discrete element method and computational fluid dynamics (DEM-CFD), and (iv) statistical modeling and machine learning (ML).

4.5.1 Molecular Modeling and Simulation

Molecular modeling aims to predict the relative charging trends of materials *in-silico* using first principles. This could provide an efficient tool for the early phase of particle/formulation design, where only a limited amount of material is available (Brunsteiner et al. 2019). In such a modeling approach, theoretical estimations of the polarity and magnitude of charge for a given material are based on the computation of the effective WF. This quantity, which reflects the electronic structure of the material, can be computed using semi-empirical MOPAC or different quantum mechanical methods such as *ab initio* DFT. Due to the simplicity of the method, semi-empirical MOPAC is applied in many studies to determine the electronic states of various materials using the modified neglect of diatomic overlap (MNDO) method. Here, the charging tendency of organic materials can be estimated by determining the energy level of the highest occupied molecular orbitals (HOMO) and the lowest unoccupied molecular orbitals (LUMO), and computing the WF accordingly, as shown in Equation (4.2):

$$WF = IP - 0.5\, E_g \qquad (4.2)$$

where *IP* is the ionization potential, and E_g is the energy band gap, that is, the difference between the HOMO and LUMO levels, which depends on the functional groups present in the chemical structure. The WF values computed applying this method have been shown to correlate with the ones estimated *via* photoemission techniques (Yanagida et al. 1993; Trigwell et al. 2003). More specifically, a direct correlation was found between the photoemission threshold energy and the HOMO level for several polymers, indicating a strong relationship between their WF values and chemical structure. Simulations of the charge transfer using first-principle calculations are instead less reported in literature as they are computationally expensive. However, *ab initio* DFT calculations have been employed in several cases. DFT has been applied for the determination of the WF and charge transfer for metal–insulator contacts (Yoshida et al. 2006) as well as in two-dimensional materials due to flexo-electricity and piezo-electricity (Tan et al. 2021). Further, DFT has been proposed to evaluate the impact of surface defects on charge transfer (Wang et al. 2019; Feshanjerdi and Malekan 2019) and to detect the electron and ion transfer mechanism (Nikitina et al. 2009). The relative charging propensity of pharmaceutical materials has been predicted *in-silico* using DFT (Brunsteiner et al. 2019) and a relationship between their electrostatic spark sensitivities and their electrostatic potentials and energy gaps has been established (Huang et al. 2015). Compared to the semi-empirical MOPAC, DFT is a first principle quantum mechanical method. A recent study comparing these two modeling approaches to calculate the electronic structures of different pharmaceutical materials using distinct approximations and levels of theory showed a better prediction of the tribocharging trends when a higher level of theory was used in the calculations of the electronic structures (Brunsteiner et al. 2019). The authors suggested that even if the improvement is small, it is still advantageous to use the highest level of theory as the calculations can be performed in a few hours with moderate computational resources.

Besides its direct correlation with the material tribocharging propensity, molecular modeling could also be applied to obtain useful information on crucial parameters for tribocharging such as the material hygroscopicity (Ren et al. 2020), wettability (Jarray et al. 2020), surface energy (Saxena et al. 2007), adhesion propensity (Tian et al. 2018), mechanical properties (Chowdhury et al. 2016; Li et al. 2014), etc.

4.5.2 Discrete Element Method Models

DEM is a numerical modeling approach able to simulate charge transfer due to collisional and mechanical factors, among others, and its ability to resolve the physics at the particle level can aid the understanding of the complex physics behind triboelectrification. DEM models can simulate the collisional nature of powder flow (i.e., particle–particle and particle–wall collisions) by dynamically tracking particle trajectories (Mukherjee et al. 2021). Allowing the simulated particles to overlap (a characteristic of soft sphere models), DEM can account for local deformations upon collisions. DEM models are flexible and allow a direct relation between material properties and model parameters for tribocharging modeling (Ketterhagen et al. 2009). DEM is a powerful modeling approach for the quantification of effects related to the electrostatic charge of materials for a variety of processes including pneumatic conveying (Watano 2006), vibrating cylindrical container (Matsuyama et al. 2009), hopper–chute flow (Hogue et al. 2008; Hogue et al. 2009; Mukherjee et al. 2016; Naik et al. 2015), pneumatic flow (Pei et al. 2013), electrostatic separation in a vertically vibrated bed (Laurentie et al. 2013), hopper discharge (Mukherjee et al. 2021), and blending (Naik et al. 2016a, b). The main limitations of the DEM are: (i) difficulty in calibration of the input parameters to mimic the real behavior of the materials to be simulated and their validation with experimental results; (ii) simulations are based on fundamental simplifications (e.g., shape, surface properties of particles, etc.); (iii) current numerical capabilities allow either detailed simulations of small-scale systems, or approximated large-scale models, but not the full-scale simulation of the whole manufacturing devices with arbitrary particle-level precision; (iv) the charge mechanisms are based on the assumption of electron transfer (e.g., WF differences); and (v) charge relaxation processes are usually not considered.

4.5.3 Discrete Element Method and Computational Fluid Dynamics

CFD is a Eulerian method applied to accurately model fluid or particulate systems in a dilute phase. This approach considers the material as a continuum and mass, momentum and energy balances are solved numerically, mainly using either the Eulerian–Eulerian or the Eulerian–Lagrangian approach. In the Eulerian–Eulerian approach, the presence of solids is considered a second continuous phase for which mass, momentum, and energy balances also need to be solved. This simulation technique has been successfully used to predict the charge transfer for more dense phases (higher solid concentration) in fluidized beds (Ray et al. 2019) and in bi-disperse systems (Ray et al. 2020). However, for systems of dense solids, the material is usually assumed to be elastic or elastoplastic, and other modeling approaches, such as the finite element method (FEM), maybe more suitable (Ketterhagen et al. 2009).

In the Eulerian–Lagrangian approach, the solids are modeled in a discrete fashion using DEM and the respective results are coupled with the Eulerian method of CFD. Such a combined DEM-CFD approach has been used to simulate particle–fluid interactions under a wide range of packing and flow conditions. For instance, a CFD-DEM model was built to simulate particle tribocharging during dispersion (Ali and Ghadiri 2017), pneumatic conveying (Korevaar et al. 2014; Norouzi et al. 2020), gas–solid two phases flow (Tanoue et al. 2001), fluidized beds (Hassani et al. 2013; Lim 2013; Kolehmainen et al. 2016), pharmaceutical particle processing (Naik et al. 2015), aerodynamic dispersion (Alfano et al. 2021), powder die filling during tableting operations (Nwose et al. 2012), and to explain the charging mechanism of sands with adsorbed water (Gu et al. 2013).

4.5.4 Statistical Modeling and Machine Learning

As described in Section 4.3, tribocharging is a multifactorial phenomenon, often occurring stochastically (Haeberle et al. 2018). The application of statistical and ML models could therefore be beneficial.

Statistical approaches have been used to effectively design experiments in order to maximize knowledge gained and minimize experimental efforts. For instance, a statistical design of experiments (DOE) has been applied by Karner and Urbanetz (2012, 2013) to investigate the influence of powder properties and blending parameters (i.e., particle size, container size, and concentration of fines) on the tribocharging during mixing. Mukherjee et al. used a statistical formalism to develop a DEM model able to predict the effect of variations in humidity on moisture-dependent cohesion (expressed as a granular Bond number) for multicomponent systems. In this study, an augmented simplex-centroid design (SCD) for tertiary mixtures was applied to efficiently select the most appropriate mixture concentrations (Mukherjee et al. 2019). Additionally, multivariate data analysis (MVDA) approaches such as principal component analysis (PCA) and partial least squares (PLS) models could provide valuable information on the most influencing factors affecting tribocharging. Such models rely on the statistical analysis of the data and have been used in the tribocharging framework for both raw powders and their blends (Soppela et al. 2010; Beretta et al. 2020a). The main disadvantages of these data-driven models are that accurate analyses and predictions require an extensive database and are based solely on linear correlations. Statistical process control (SPC) techniques have also been employed to monitor and improve the performance of electrostatic processes such as frictional sliding (Prawatya et al. 2019) and electrostatic separation (Medles et al. 2009). Artificial neural network (ANN) has also been proposed as a suitable method to model non-linear correlations. This numerical estimation method is able to learn from a given set of inputs and predict the corresponding output by determining the hidden governing rules. This approach has been used to model the electrostatics in a separation process (Lai et al. 2016), and has been suggested as a faster alternative to time-consuming high-level quantum mechanics calculations to generate electrostatic potential (ESP) of surfaces for ligand molecules in interactive drug design (Rathi et al. 2020).

4.6 Strategies for the Control and Mitigation of Powder Tribocharging during (Continuous) Pharmaceutical Operations

The manufacturing problems associated with the occurrence of triboelectrification can lead to significant product losses. Therefore, many studies have focused on the control and mitigation of tribocharging following two main approaches: (i) particle/formulation engineering, where material characteristics are modified and (ii) optimization of the process space, focusing on the manufacturing conditions. As summarized in Table 4.4, given the variety of influencing factors in tribocharging, several strategies could be applied for its mitigation.

4.6.1 Particle/Formulation Engineering

By tailoring particle and/or formulation characteristics, tribocharging can be mitigated in several ways such as *via* surface functionalization, doping, surface coating, modifications of material and particle

TABLE 4.4

Overview of Strategies Available for Charge Mitigation

Particle/Formulation Engineering	Optimization of the Process Space
Surface functionalization	Equipment design and process parameters
Doping	Grounding
Surface coating	Auxiliary equipment for in-process charge mitigation
Modification of material and particle properties	Environmental conditions
Addition of antistatic additives or fines	

properties (e.g., tailoring of crystallinity, size, shape, roughness, hydrophilicity, etc.), and the addition of antistatic additives (i.e., conductive materials or antistatic agents) or fines.

4.6.1.1 Surface Functionalization

Based on the mechanism of ion transfer described in Section 4.2.2.2., material surfaces can be functionalized using weakly bound ions to produce a systematic charge polarity (Lacks and Shinbrot 2019). In the work of Shin et al., a polyethylene terephthalate (PET) surface was successfully functionalized using a series of halogens and amines to tune its triboelectric properties with positive or negative polarity (Shin et al. 2017).

4.6.1.2 Doping

Doping is commonly used in polymeric materials to alter their electrostatic properties. Based on the hypothesis of charge transfer driven by the formation and exchange of ions and radicals upon contact (Sakaguchi et al. 2014; Baytekin et al. 2011), a charge mitigation method has been proposed by doping polymers with free-radical scavengers, such as vitamin E (Baytekin et al. 2013). Charge mitigation is therefore obtained by the chemical removal of radicals formed during contacts. The advantage of such a methodology is that, while giving antistatic properties to the polymers, it preserves the electrical and mechanical properties of the materials. A similar method is reported on the use of radical-scavenging polydopamine (PDA) and tannic acid (TA) in surface coating, which is described in more detail in the surface coating section below (Fang et al. 2017). In addition to the permanent inhibition of tribocharging, an approach for the controlled modification of tribocharging has been proposed by Cezan et al. and relies on the photoexcitation of organic dyes. In their study, common polymers were doped with organic fluorescent dyes to provide a light-controlled discharging process at specific wavelengths (Cezan et al. 2019).

4.6.1.3 Surface Coating

Reduction of the tribocharging properties of materials could be achieved by applying a uniform coating of an antistatic agent around the particulates to be handled. Coating processes, such as magnetically assisted impaction coating (MAIC) or continuous fluid energy mill (FEM), could be used, as shown by Jallo and Dave (2015) and Han et al. (2011), to dry coat pharmaceutical powders with nanoparticles for charge mitigation purposes. Materials like titania, hydrophobic, and hydrophilic silica nanoparticles were used to coat micronized paracetamol and led to an improved flowability and reduced tribocharging tendency at all the different RH levels investigated (Jallo and Dave 2015). The particles were found to charge to the lowest extent when coated with titania, due to their relatively conductive nature, whereas the highest charging propensity was observed for hydrophobic silica coating. The use of hydrophilic silica had instead an intermediate charge mitigation effect and, compared to its hydrophobic counterpart, is expected to attract moisture increasing the overall conductivity. The mitigation properties of hydrophilic nano-silica were also observed after the simultaneous micronization and surface modification of ibuprofen in a FEM device leading to fine surface-modified particles with improved flowability, bulk densities, electrostatic, and dissolution properties (Han et al. 2011).

Alternatively, to the exemplary dry coating processes described so far, wet methods could also be applied in a similar fashion to obtain coated particles with a minimized charging propensity. For example, in their study, Fang et al. dipped polymeric films into a solution containing PDA or TA at room temperature to provide a homogeneous antistatic coating with radical-scavenging property (Fang et al. 2017).

4.6.1.4 Modifications to Material and Particle Properties

Based on the effect of material and particle attributes described in Section 4.3.1, the tribocharging properties of the materials could be mitigated by tailoring their crystallinity, size, shape, roughness, hydrophilicity, mechanical properties, etc. To this end, various particle engineering methods, such as milling, spray-drying, spray freeze-drying, supercritical fluid technology, etc. have been employed as co-processing processes (Shoyele and Cawthorne 2006; Khadka et al. 2014). For instance, Zellnitz et al. and Kwock et al. engineered salbutamol sulfate particles *via* air-jet milling and spray-drying to obtain particles of different physicochemical properties (i.e., shape, solid-state, mechanical properties, and moisture content) (Kwok and Chan 2008a; Zellnitz et al. 2019b). In turn, Wong et al. conditioned the spray-dried salbutamol sulfate with supercritical CO_2 and menthol to obtain particles of similar shape but with different crystallinity and surface roughness (Wong et al. 2014). Sharma et al. treated mannitol particles with argon plasma and observed mitigation of charge, which was attributed to the higher surface roughness of the particles after treatment (Sharma et al. 2008).

4.6.1.5 Addition of Antistatic Additives or Fines

One of the possible strategies to reduce the accumulation of electrostatic charges consists of the addition of antistatic additives, including conductive materials and antistatic agents (Guardiola et al. 1992). Antistatic agents in the pharmaceutical industry comprise cationic ammonium material called Larostat 519 (Wu and Bi 2011; Zhu et al. 2004) or lubricants with antistatic properties such as magnesium stearate (MgSt), stearic acid, and L-ascorbic acid (Sarkar et al. 2012), typically consisting of fine powders. The addition of fine powders to the formulation is in fact believed to (i) coat the surface of the coarse particles having a lubrication effect and (ii) increase the area upon particles contact, thus increasing the conductivity, and consequently, the rate of charge dissipation. Moreover, in case the added particles are able to adsorb moisture (e.g., as for Larostat 519), the water present on the surface can enhance even the overall conductivity (Zhang et al. 2015a). Already in 1983, Wolny and Opaliński demonstrated the charge neutralization effect of adding fines to insulator particles in a fluidized bed and questioned if this effect was related to changes in the electrical conductivity (Wolny and Opaliński 1983). In more recent work, Wu and Bi have used and compared the efficiency of charge reduction in a mechanical shaking device when adding fine particles of carbon nanotubes (CNTs), Larostat 519, aluminum and activated carbon to glass beads, polyethylene resins, and starch powders in a concentration range of 0.3–2.0 wt% (Wu and Bi 2011). Their results evidenced that the addition of fine particles leads to charge dissipation in all cases, however, given their high conductivity and ultrafine particle size, CNTs showed optimal mitigation performance. In contrast, the aluminum powders had poor performance suggesting that their efficiency for charge neutralization could not be explained only by their conductivity, supporting previous findings. Most likely, the mitigation effect is due to the difference in charge polarity obtained during same-material tribocharging for coarse and fine fractions (Zhao et al. 2000; Zheng et al. 2003; Forward et al. 2009; Zhao et al. 2002; Zhao et al. 2003; Trigwell et al. 2003; Waitukaitis et al. 2014; Sowinski et al. 2010; Mehrani et al. 2005; Sow et al. 2011). In fact, when adding a small fraction of finer glass beads (150–170 µm) to coarser counterparts (210–300 µm), Wu and Bi could observe a charge mitigation effect indicating that a broader PSD could be beneficial for engineering materials with a lower tribocharging sensitivity (Wu and Bi 2011). Similar trends have been demonstrated for soda lime glasses and a polyethylene resin (Forward et al. 2009) and both crystalline and spray-dried lactose (Bennett et al. 1999) but opposite results have been reported with wind-blown sand (Zheng et al. 2003).

4.6.2 Optimization of Process Space

The pharmaceutical manufacturing processes and unit operations can be optimized by the engineering of the equipment and refinement of the processing parameters (i.e., equipment-tailored antistatic designs and type of material used in its construction, use of antistatic coatings, in-process charge eliminators, etc.) as well as by the targeted control of the environmental conditions (i.e., temperature and relative humidity) at which the process is carried out.

4.6.2.1 Equipment Design and Process Parameters

The design of the equipment such as material(s) selected for construction and geometry should be opportunely selected to reduce electrostatic build-up. Typically, equipment with conductive surfaces (e.g., stainless steel) should be preferred over ones made out of insulator materials such as plastic (Grossel 2012;

Lachiver et al. 2006). To obtain a low level of tribocharge, Sarkar et al. have shown that the equipment surface material should be selectively chosen depending on the nature of the sample to be processed and the WF difference between the two (Sarkar et al. 2012). Jallo and Dave have suggested that compared to surface modifications on the particulate material, changes in the material of construction of the processing equipment play a lesser role in powder triboelectrification (Jallo and Dave 2015). However, the material of construction and/or the application of antistatic coatings to the equipment surfaces, in combination with tailored particle properties, could still lead to a more effective mitigation of tribocharging. Although the application of antistatic coatings is not a common practice in routine pharmaceutical operations, it could help prevent the development of electrostatic charges. Alternatively, the surface of the equipment could be coated with excipients prior to processing to limit the in-process development of particle–wall contacts, hence reducing the tribocharging effects to particle–particle interactions (Eilbeck et al. 2000; Murtomaa et al. 2002b).

Besides the material of construction and possible coating strategies, other design parameters such as hopper/chute angles and equipment size-to-loaded mass ratio could be adjusted to alter the number and time of particle–wall contacts as well as the normal forces acting on the particles (Mukherjee et al. 2021; Karner and Urbanetz 2012; Mukherjee et al. 2019; Naik et al. 2015; Yao et al. 2016). Typically, steeper chute/hopper angles are associated with lower tribocharging due to the reduced particle–wall contact times (Mukherjee et al. 2021) and normal forces (Naik et al. 2015; Yao et al. 2016), whereas high equipment size-to-loaded mass ratios facilitate tribocharging due to the higher surface wall area available for particle–wall contacts (Karner and Urbanetz 2012; Mukherjee et al. 2019). In addition, the selection of process parameters aimed at the minimization of impact energy, shear, and normal forces experienced by the materials during processing may also contribute to limiting charge accumulation (e.g., lower blending speeds).

4.6.2.2 Grounding

To reduce the risk of electrostatic charge accumulation, the equipment used in pharmaceutical operations is normally grounded. However, as demonstrated in several studies (Engers et al. 2006; Karner and Urbanetz 2012; Pu et al. 2009; LaMarche et al. 2010; LaMarche et al. 2009), this common practice seems to be less efficient than generally thought and may even aggravate the extent of particle adhesion and agglomeration induced by tribocharging (LaMarche et al. 2010). The type of formulation and the hold time after processing were found to be more effective for a faster charge decay compared to grounding practices (Engers et al. 2006). Alternative approaches for in-process charge mitigation could include the use of auxiliary devices implemented within the process.

4.6.2.3 Auxiliary Equipment for In-Process Charge Mitigation

The generation of charge during the process could be mitigated by the use of auxiliary equipment specifically designed for in-process charge mitigation. For instance, static charge eliminators could be applied to this end. Essentially, static eliminators ionize the air to deliver a neutral cloud of ions (i.e., with both positive and negative polarity) to the charged materials, mitigating the charge. These eliminators have been applied to different operations to reduce the charge generated, that is, blending (Pu et al. 2009; Pingali et al. 2009a), pneumatic conveying (Kodama et al. 2002), and in a fluidized bed (Revel et al. 2003) and it was found that their efficacy depends on the accessibility that powder particles have to it. Therefore, the installation of static charge eliminators needs to be strategically planned.

4.6.2.4 Environmental Conditions

It is well-known that environmental conditions play an important role in tribocharging, as such, the temperature and RH levels used in manufacturing sites should be specifically adjusted to optimize powder performance (Murtomaa et al. 2012). However, recent studies have pointed out that the impact of environmental conditions is material/formulation dependent and a one-fits-all approach should be avoided

(Beretta et al. 2020b; Schella et al. 2017). Likewise, it is advised that, in early development phases, a careful assessment of the impact of environmental conditions and material-specific tribocharging should take place.

4.7 Current Gaps and Future Perspectives

The shift of pharmaceutical product manufacturing from a traditional batch approach to a continuous, modular, on-demand (e.g., 3D powder printing), and automated type of process is raising the importance of improving our understanding of material properties in relation to their processability and finished product quality (Arden et al. 2021). This has led the pharmaceutical industry to sharply increase the adoption of scientific tools and techniques that de-risk potential failures throughout the development life cycle. Such measures are first being implemented in the development of solid dosage forms wherein their manufacture heavily involves powder/granular material processing and handling steps. Eventually, this has led to renewed traction in the research of powder electrostatics, a distinguished precursor of diverse manufacturing-related problems. In recent years, prominent contributions to electrostatic charging research were made as collaborative efforts with pharmaceutical companies, equipment, and excipient manufacturers (Pinto et al. 2020; Šupuk et al. 2012; Pingali et al. 2009a; Allenspach et al. 2021).

Despite powder electrostatics being a mature stream in powder technology, pharmaceutical material and manufacturing communities have embraced the available methods and understanding at a relatively slower pace. Several fundamental aspects of tribocharging are yet to be fully elucidated, rendering them highly unpredictable and stochastic in nature. This necessitates harmonized procedures in measuring powder tribocharging using laboratory instrumentations as well as within relevant manufacturing conditions. The adoption of best practices and guidance could help the selection of the right measurement tools, configurations, and parameters as well as data analytics of electrostatics based on analytical capabilities and weaknesses. This could become the foundation for setting the limit of detection/quantification for pharmaceutical materials in relation to their processability and thereby defining specifications and control strategies. Given the stochastic nature of the electrostatic charging, this would facilitate interoperability among analyst, equipment, laboratory, and unit operations/manufacturing sites. For this, the relevant stakeholders among academia, industry, pharmacopeias, and regulators would need to align on the standardized testing principles and procedures for tribocharging measurements. In the case of potential PAT applications, novel in-process sensors for electrostatic for electrostatic measurement demonstrating affordability, retrofitting to unit operation machinery, as well as measurement speeds will become requisites. Overall, it is imperative to holistically consider the analytical procedures for powder electrostatic charge measurements within analytical quality by design (AQbD) and analytical procedure lifecycle (APL) frameworks as endorsed by pharmacopeia and regulatory guidances (Weitzel et al. 2021). This would help the focus on analytical procedures with improved measurement reliability and interoperability through the understanding, reduction, and control of the measured value and polarity of electrostatic charge of pharmaceutical materials. Overall, such an outcome could be achieved be achieved through several well-designed systematic benchmarking studies across a broad range of pharmaceutical materials and the involvement of several stakeholders.

The development of digital twins of manufacturing processes using predictive modeling approaches is a growing paradigm in the pharmaceutical product development and manufacturing sector. In the context of modeling and simulation applicable for powder tribocharging, some encouraging developments have been made over the recent years. While quantum mechanics and DFT methods help derive molecular scale descriptors (e.g., WP and IP) related to materials tribocharging propensities, the extent of their applicability to a large number of solid-state drugs and excipients of different crystallinity, moisture content, and under process simulating conditions is envisioned next. Likewise, it is early for mesoscale computational models of DEM to successfully implement long-range particle surface interactions relevant for the prediction of powder tribocharging. With progressively evolving multiscale physics and computational power, improved *in-silico* tools capable of predicting key aspects of electrostatic charging of pharmaceutical materials are expected to rise in the coming years.

As aforementioned, there are several innovative surface structuring and material designs available in polymer and allied material science for the mitigation of electrostatic charges. A wide variety of antistatic agents is also available. However, their working mechanisms and efficiency for pharmaceutical materials are yet to be tested, and if successful, their safe use in engineering drug substances, excipients, or formulations need to be verified *via* toxicological studies. The innovative equipment design of processes, excipients, and engineered particles for the charge mitigation of pharmaceuticals will need to inherit the knowledge and technologies existing in other disciplines. Adoption of standard antistatic agents from food and fine chemical field to pharmaceuticals will also necessitate meeting the desired quality requirements.

Analytical and computational technologies with improved accuracy are the prerequisite for the rational design of materials and processes with none to minimal electrostatic charge retention. For this, a focused research collaboration involving pharmaceutical drug substance and drug product manufacturers, excipient companies, processing equipment vendors, analytical equipment vendors, computational experts, and software vendors should be encouraged.

ACKNOWLEDGMENTS

The Research Center Pharmaceutical Engineering (RCPE) is funded within the framework of Competence Centers for Excellent Technologies (COMET) by BMK, BMDW, Land Steiermark, and SFG. The COMET program is managed by the FFG. The authors would like to thank Luca Orefice for revising the modeling approaches section of this book chapter.

REFERENCES

Abdelaziz, K.M., Chen, J., Hieber, T.J., and Leseman, Z.C. 2018. "Atomistic Field Theory for Contact Electrification of Dielectrics." *Journal of Electrostatics 96*: 10–15.

Ahfat, N.M., Buckton, G., Burrows, R., and Ticehurst, M.D. 2000. "An Exploration of Inter-Relationships between Contact Angle, Inverse Phase Gas Chromatography and Triboelectric Charging Data." *European Journal of Pharmaceutical Sciences 9*: 271–276.

Aigner, I., Zettl, M., Schroettner, H., van der Wel, P., Khinast, J.G., and Krumme, M. 2022. "Industrial-Scale Continuous Vacuum Drying of Active Pharmaceutical Ingredient Paste: Determination of the Process Window." *Organic Process Research & Development 26*(2): 323–334.

Akande, A.R., and Lowell, J. 1985. "Contact Electrification of Polymers by Metals." *Journal of Electrostatics 16*: 147–156.

Alan, B.O., Barisik, M., and Ozcelik, H.G. 2020. "Roughness Effects on the Surface Charge Properties of Silica Nanoparticles." *Journal of Physical Chemistry C 124* (13): 7274–7286.

Alfano, F.O., Di Renzo, A., Di Maio, F.P., and Ghadiri, M. 2021. "Computational Analysis of Triboelectri Fi Cation Due to Aerodynamic Powder Dispersion." *Powder Technology 382*: 491–504.

Ali, M., and Ghadiri, M. 2017. "Analysis of Triboelectric Charging of Particles Due to Aerodynamic Dispersion by a Pulse of Pressurised Air Jet." *Advanced Powder Technology 28*: 2735–2740.

Ali, M., Reddy, R., and Mazumder, M. 2008. "Simultaneous Characterization of Aerodynamic Size and Electrostatic Charge Distributions of Inhaled Dry Powder Inhaler Aerosols." *Journal of Current Respiratory Medicine Reviews 4* (1): 2–5.

Allenspach, C., Timmins, P., Lumay, G., Holman, J., and Minko, T. 2021. "Loss-in-Weight Feeding, Powder Flow and Electrostatic Evaluation for Direct Compression Hydroxypropyl Methylcellulose (HPMC) to Support Continuous Manufacturing." *International Journal of Pharmaceutics 596*: 120259.

Alois, S., Merrison, J., Iversen, J.J., and Sesterhenn, J. 2017. "Contact Electrification in Aerosolized Monodispersed Silica Microspheres Quantified Using Laser Based Velocimetry." *Journal of Aerosol Science 106*. 1–10.

Apodaca, M.M., Wesson, P.J., Bishop, K.J.M., Ratner, M.A., and Grzybowski, B.A. 2010. "Contact Electrification between Identical Materials." *Angewandte Chemie, International Edition 49*: 946–949.

Arden, N.S., Fisher, A.C., Tyner, K., Yu, L.X., Lee, S.L., and Kopcha, M. 2021. "Industry 4.0 for Pharmaceutical Manufacturing: Preparing for the Smart Factories of the Future." *International Journal of Pharmaceutics 602*: 120554.

Bailey, A.G. 1993. "Charging of Solids and Powders." *Journal of Electrostatics 30*: 167–180.

Bailey, A.G. 1998. "The Science and Technology of Electrostatic Powder Spraying, Transport and Coating." *Journal of Electrostatics 45*: 85–120.

Balachandran, W., Kulon, J., Koolpiruck, D., Dawson, M., and Burnel, P. 2003. "Bipolar Charge Measurement of Pharmaceutical Powders." *Powder Technology 135–136*: 156–163.

Barnes, A.M., and Dinsmore, A.D. 2016. "Heterogeneity of Surface Potential in Contact Electrification under Ambient Conditions: A Comparison of Pre- and Post-Contact States." *Journal of Electrostatics 81*: 76–81.

Baytekin, B., Baytekin, H.T., and Grzybowski, B.A. 2012a. "What Really Drives Chemical Reactions on Contact Charged Surfaces?" *Journal of the American Chemical Society 134*: 7223–7226.

Baytekin, H., Baytekin, B., Hermans, T., Kowalczyk, B., and Grzybowski, B. 2013. "Control of Surface Charges by Radicals as a Principle of Antistatic Polymers Protecting Electronic Circuitry." *Science 341*: 1368–1371.

Baytekin, H.T., Baytekin, B., Incorvati, J.T., and Grzybowski, B.A. 2012b. "Material Transfer and Polarity Reversal in Contact Charging." *Angewandte Chemie, International Edition 51*: 4843–4847.

Baytekin, H.T., Patashinski, A.Z., Branicki, M., Baytekin, B., Soh, S., and Grzybowski, B.A. 2011. "The Mosaic of Surface Charge in Contact Electrification." *Science 333*: 308–312.

Bekaert, B., Penne, L., Grymonpre, W., Van Snick, B., Dhondt, J., Boeckx, J., Vogeleer, J., De Beer, T., Vervaet, C., and Vanhoorne, V. 2021. "Determination of a Quantitative Relationship between Material Properties, Process Settings and Screw Feeding Behavior via Multivariate Data-Analysis." *International Journal of Pharmaceutics 602*: 120603.

Beleca, R., Abbod, M., Balachandran, W., and Miller, P.R. 2010. "Investigation of Electrostatic Properties of Pharmaceutical Powders Using Phase Doppler Anemometry." *IEEE Transactions on Industry Applications 46* (3): 1181–1187.

Bennett, F.S., Carter, P.A., Rowley, G., and Dandiker, Y. 1999. "Modification of Electrostatic Charge on Inhaled Carrier Lactose Particles by Addition of Fine Particles." *Drug Development and Industrial Pharmacy 25* (1): 99–103.

Beretta, M., Hörmann, T.R., Hainz, P., Hsiao, W., and Paudel, A. 2020a. "Investigation into Powder Tribo-Charging of Pharmaceuticals. Part I: Process-Induced Charge via Twin-Screw Feeding." *International Journal of Pharmaceutics 591*: 120014.

Beretta, M., Hörmann, T.R., Hainz, P., Hsiao, W.K., and Paudel, A. 2020b. "Investigation into Powder Tribo-Charging of Pharmaceuticals. Part II: Sensitivity to Relative Humidity." *International Journal of Pharmaceutics 591*: 120015.

Beretta, M., Pinto, J.T., Laggner, P., and Paudel, A. 2022. "Insights into the Impact of Nanostructural Properties on Powder Tribocharging: The Case of Milled Salbutamol Sulfate." *Molecular Pharmaceutics 19* (2): 547–557.

Biegaj, K.W., Rowland, M.G., Lukas, T.M., and Heng, J.Y.Y. 2017. "Surface Chemistry and Humidity in Powder Electrostatics: A Comparative Study between Tribocharging and Corona Discharge." *ACS Omega 2*: 1576–1582.

Bostijn, N., Dhondt, J., Ryckaert, A., Szabó, E., Dhondt, W., Van Snick, B., Vanhoorne, V., Vervaet, C., and De Beer, T. 2019. "A Multivariate Approach to Predict the Volumetric and Gravimetric Feeding Behavior of a Low Feed Rate Feeder Based on Raw Material Properties." *International Journal of Pharmaceutics 557*: 342–353.

Brunsteiner, M., Zellnitz, S., Pinto, J.T., Karrer, J., and Paudel, A. 2019. "Can We Predict Trends in Tribo-Charging of Pharmaceutical Materials from First Principles?" *Powder Technology 356*: 892–898.

Bunker, M.J., Davies, M.C., James, M.B., and Roberts, C.J. 2007. "Direct Observation of Single Particle Electrostatic Charging by Atomic Force Microscopy." *Pharmaceutical Research 24* (6): 1165–1169.

Burgo, T.A.L., Ducati, T.R.D., Francisco, K.R., Clinckspoor, K.J., Galembeck, F., and Galembeck, S.E. 2012. "Triboelectricity: Macroscopic Charge Patterns Formed by Self-Arraying Ions on Polymer Surfaces." *Langmuir 28*: 7407–7416.

Carter, D., and Hartzell, C. 2017. "Extension of Discrete Tribocharging Models to Continuous Size Distributions." *Physical Review E 95*: 012901.

Carter, P.A., Cassidy, O.E., Rowley, G., and Merrifield, R. 1998. "Triboelectrification of Fractionated Crystalline and Spray-Dried Lactose." *Pharmacy and Pharmacology Communications 4*: 111–115.

Carter, P.A., Rowley, G., Fletcher, E.J., and Hill, E.A. 1992. "An Experimental Investigation of Triboelectrification in Cohesive and Non-Cohesive Pharmaceutical Powders." *Drug Development and Industrial Pharmacy 18* (14): 1505–1526.

Cezan, S.D., Nalbant, A.A., Buyuktemiz, M., Dede, Y., Baytekin, H.T., and Baytekin, B. 2019. "Control of Triboelectric Charges on Common Polymers by Photoexcitation of Organic Dyes." *Nature Communications 1* (10): 1–8.

Chowdhury, S.C., Haque, B.Z., and Gillespie, J.W. 2016. "Molecular Dynamics Simulations of the Structure and Mechanical Properties of Silica Glass Using ReaxFF." *Journal of Materials Science 51* (22): 10139–10159.

Ciborowski, J., and Wlodarski, A. 1962. "On Electrostatic Effects in Fluidized Beds." *Chemical Engineering Science 17*: 23–32.

da Silveira Balestrin, L.B., Del Duque, D., da Silva, S., and Galembeck, F. 2014. "Triboelectricity in Insulating Polymers: Evidence for a Mechanochemical Mechanism." *Faraday Discussions 170*: 369–383.

Davies, D.K. 1969. "Charge Generation on Dielectric Surfaces." *Journal of Physics D: Applied Physics 2*: 1533–1537.

de Burgo, T.A., Rezende, C.A., Bertazzo, S., Galembeck, A., and Galembeck, F. 2011. "Electric Potential Decay on Polyethylene: Role of Atmospheric Water on Electric Charge Build-up and Dissipation." *Journal of Electrostatics 69*: 401–409.

Diaz, A.F., Wollmann, D., and Dreblow, D. 1991. "Contact Electrification: Ion Transfer to Metals and Polymers." *Chemistry of Materials 3*: 997–999.

Domokos, A., Nagy, B., Gyürkés, M., Farkas, A., Tacsi, K., Pataki, H., Liu, Y.C., et al. 2020. "End-to-End Continuous Manufacturing of Conventional Compressed Tablets: From Flow Synthesis to Tableting through Integrated Crystallization and Filtration." *International Journal of Pharmaceutics 581*: 119297.

Eilbeck, J., Rowley, G., Carter, P.A., and Fletcher, E.J. 1999. "Effect of Materials of Construction of Pharmaceutical Processing Equipment and Drug Delivery Devices on the Triboelectrification of Size-Fractionated Lactose." *Pharmacy and Pharmacology Communications 5*: 429–433.

Eilbeck, J., Rowley, G., Carter, P.A., and Fletcher, E.J. 2000. "Effect of Contamination of Pharmaceutical Equipment on Powder Triboelectrification." *International Journal of Pharmaceutics 195*: 7–11.

Elajnaf, A., Carter, P., and Rowley, G. 2006. "Electrostatic Characterisation of Inhaled Powders: Effect of Contact Surface and Relative Humidity." *European Journal of Pharmaceutical Sciences 29*: 375–384.

Engers, D.A., Fricke, M.N., Storey, R.P., Newman, A.W., and Morris, K.R. 2006. "Triboelectrification of Pharmaceutically Relevant Powders during Low-Shear Tumble Blending." *Journal of Electrostatics 64*: 826–835.

Engisch, W.E., and Muzzio, F.J. 2014. "Loss-in-Weight Feeding Trials Case Study: Pharmaceutical Formulation." *Journal of Pharmaceutical Innovation 10*: 56–75.

Epping, R.H., and Kuettner, A. 2002. "Free Air Beam in an Electric Field for Determination of the Electrostatic Charge of Powders between 1 and 200 Mm." *Journal of Electrostatics 55* (3–4): 279–288.

Fang, Y., Gonuguntla, S., and Soh, S. 2017. "Universal Nature-Inspired Coatings for Preparing Non-Charging Surfaces." *ACS Applied Materials and Interfaces 9*: 32220–32226.

Feshanjerdi, M., and Malekan, A. 2019. "Contact Electrification between Randomly Rough Surfaces with Identical Materials." *Journal of Applied Physics 125*: 165302.

Forward, K.M., Lacks, D.J., and Sankaran, R.M. 2009. "Charge Segregation Depends on Particle Size in Triboelectrically Charged Granular Materials." *Physical Review Letters 102*: 028001.

Gady, B., Schleef, D., Reifenberger, R., Rimai, D., and DeMejo, L.P. 1996. "Identification of Electrostatic and van Der Waals Interaction Forces between a Micrometer-Size Sphere and a Flat Substrate." *Physical Review B 53* (12): 8065–8070.

Gallo, C.F., and Lama, W.L. 1976. "Some Charge Exchange Phenomena Explained by a Classical Model of the Work Function." *Journal of Electrostatics 2*: 145–150.

Gao, H., Wang, X., Chang, Q., Yan, K., and Liu, J. 2018. "Particle Charging and Conveying Characteristics of Dense-Phase Pneumatic Conveying of Pulverized Coal under High-Pressure by N_2/CO_2." *Powder Technology 328*: 300–308.

Ghori, M.U., Šupuk, E., and Conway, B.R. 2014. "Tribo-Electric Charging and Adhesion of Cellulose Ethers and Their Mixtures with Flurbiprofen." *European Journal of Pharmaceutical Sciences 65*: 1–8.

Gibson, N. 1997. "Static Electricity - An Industrial Hazard under Control?" *Journal of Electrostatics 40–41*: 21–30.

Glor, M. 1985. "Hazards Due to Electrostatic Charging of Powders." *Journal of Electrostatics 16*: 175–191.

Glor, M.. 2003. "Ignition Hazard Due to Static Electricity in Particulate Processes." *Powder Technology 135–136*: 223–233.

Glor, M.. 2005. "Electrostatic Ignition Hazards in the Process Industry." *Journal of Electrostatics 63*: 447–453.

Glover, W., and Chan, H.K. 2004. "Electrostatic Charge Characterization of Pharmaceutical Aerosols Using Electrical Low-Pressure Impaction (ELPI)." *Journal of Aerosol Science 35*: 755–764.

Gold, G., and Palermo, B.T. 1965. "Hopper Flow Electrostatics of Tableting Material I. Instrumentation and Acetaminophen Formulations." *Journal of Pharmaceutical Sciences 54* (2): 310–312.

Gonzalez, J.F., Somoza, A.M., and Palacios-Lidón, E. 2017. "Charge Distribution from SKPM Images." *Physical Chemistry Chemical Physics 19*: 27299–27304.

Gooding, D.M., and Kaufman, G.K. 2014. "Tribocharging and the Triboelectric Series." *Encyclopedia of Inorganic and Bioinorganic Chemistry*, 1–9.

Greason, W.D. 2000. "Investigation of a Test Methodology for Triboelectrification." *Journal of Electrostatics 49*: 245–256.

Grossel, S.S. 2012. "Design and Operating Practices for Safe Conveying of Particulate Solids." *Journal of Loss Prevention in the Process Industries 25*: 848–852.

Grosvenor, M.P., and Staniforth, J.N. 1996. "The Influence of Water on Electrostatic Charge Retention and Dissipation in Pharmaceutical Compacts for Powder Coating." *Pharmaceutical Research 13* (11): 1725–1729.

Gu, Z., Wei, W., Su, J., and Yu, C.W. 2013. "The Role of Water Content in Triboelectric Charging of Wind-Blown Sand." *Scientific Reports 3*: 1–6.

Guardiola, J., Ramos, G., and Romero, A. 1992. "Electrostatic Behaviour in Binary Dielectric/Conductor Fluidized Beds." *Powder Technology 73*: 11–19.

Haeberle, J., Schella, A., Sperl, M., Schröter, M., and Born, P. 2018. "Double Origin of Stochastic Granular Tribocharging." *Soft Matter 14*: 4987–4995.

Han, X., Ghoroi, C., To, D., Chen, Y., and Davé, R. 2011. "Simultaneous Micronization and Surface Modification for Improvement of Flow and Dissolution of Drug Particles." *International Journal of Pharmaceutics 415*: 185–195.

Hao, T., Tukianen, J., Nivorozhkin, A., and Landrau, N. 2013. "Probing Pharmaceutical Powder Blending Uniformity with Electrostatic Charge Measurements." *Powder Technology 245*: 64–69.

Harper, W.R. 1967. *Contact and Frictional Electrification*. Oxford: Clarendon Press.

Harris, I.A., Lim, M.X., and Jaeger, H.M. 2019. "Temperature Dependence of Nylon and PTFE Triboelectrification." *Physical Review Materials 3*: 085603.

Hassani, M.A., Zarghami, R., Norouzi, H.R., and Mostoufi, N. 2013. "Numerical Investigation of Effect of Electrostatic Forces on the Hydrodynamics of Gas-Solid Fluidized Beds." *Powder Technology 246*: 16–25.

He, C., Bi, X.T., and Grace, J.R. 2015. "Simultaneous Measurements of Particle Charge Density and Bubble Properties in Gas-Solid Fluidized Beds by Dual-Tip Electrostatic Probes." *Chemical Engineering Science 123*: 11–21.

Henniker, J. 1962. "Triboelectricity in Polymers." *Nature 196*: 474.

Henry, P.S.H. 1953. "The Role of Asymmetric Rubbing in the Generation of Static Electricity." *British Journal of Applied Physics 4* (2): S31–S36.

Herzberg, M., Zeng, G., Mäkilä, E., Murtomaa, M., Søgaard, S.V., Garnæs, J., Madsen, A., and Rantanen, J. 2021. "Effect of Dehydration Pathway on the Surface Properties of Molecular Crystals." *CrystEngComm 23*: 5788–5794.

Hesse, N., Dechet, M.A., Bonilla, J.S.G., Lübbert, C., Roth, S., Bück, A., Schmidt, J., and Peukert, W. 2019. "Analysis of Tribo-Charging during Powder Spreading in Selective Laser Sintering: Assessment of Polyamide 12 Powder Ageing Effects on Charging Behavior." *Polymers 11*: 609.

Hickey, A.J., Mansour, H.M., Telko, M.J., Xu, Z., Smyth, H.D.C., Mulder, T., McLean, R., Langridge, J., and Papadopoulos, D. 2007. "Physical Characterization of Component Particles Included in Dry Powder Inhalers. II. Dynamic Characteristics." *Journal of Pharmaceutical Sciences 96* (5): 1302–1319.

Hill-Izani, N.Y. 2019. *In-Line Powder Flow Behaviour Measured Using Electrostatic Technology*. United Kingdom: De Montfort University.

Hoe, S., Traini, D., Chan, H.K., and Young, P.M. 2009a. "Measuring Charge and Mass Distributions in Dry Powder Inhalers Using the Electrical Next Generation Impactor (ENGI)." *European Journal of Pharmaceutical Sciences 38*: 88–94.

Hoe, S., Young, P.M., Chan, H.K., and Traini, D. 2009b. "Introduction of the Electrical Next Generation Impactor (ENGI) and Investigation of Its Capabilities for the Study of Pressurized Metered Dose Inhalers." *Pharmaceutical Research 26* (2): 431–437.

Hoe, S., Young, P.M., and Traini, D. 2011. "A Review of Electrostatic Measurement Techniques for Aerosol Drug Delivery to the Lung: Implications in Aerosol Particle Deposition." *Journal of Adhesion Science and Technology 25* (4–5): 385–405.

Hogue, M.D., Calle, C.I., Curry, D.R., and Weitzman, P.S. 2009. "Discrete Element Modeling (DEM) of Tribo-electrically Charged Particles: Revised Experiments." *Journal of Electrostatics 67*: 691–694.

Hogue, M.D., Calle, C.I., Weitzman, P.S., and Curry, D.R. 2008. "Calculating the Trajectories of Triboelectri-cally Charged Particles Using Discrete Element Modeling (DEM)." *Journal of Electrostatics 66*: 32–38.

Hsiao, W.K., Hörmann, T.R., Toson, P., Paudel, A., Ghiotti, P., Stauffer, F., Bauer, F., et al. 2020. "Feeding of Particle-Based Materials in Continuous Solid Dosage Manufacturing: A Material Science Perspective." *Drug Discovery Today 25* (4): 800–806.

Huang, H., Li, Z., Zhang, T., Zhang, G., and Zhang, F. 2015. "Theoretical Study of the Correlation between Electrostatic Hazard and Electronic Structure for Some Typical Primary Explosives." *Journal of Molecular Modeling 21*: 200.

Hussain, T., Deng, T., Bradley, M.S.A., Armour-Chélu, D., Gorman, T., and Kaialy, W. 2016. "Evaluation Studies of a Sensing Technique for Electrostatic Charge Polarity of Pharmaceutical Particulates." *IET Science, Measurement and Technology 10* (5): 442–448.

Hussain, T., Kaialy, W., Deng, T., Bradley, M.S.A., Nokhodchi, A., and Armour-Chélu, D. 2013. "A Novel Sensing Technique for Measurement of Magnitude and Polarity of Electrostatic Charge Distribution across Individual Particles." *International Journal of Pharmaceutics 441*: 781–789.

Ierapetritou, M., Sebastian Escotet-Espinoza, M., and Singh, R. 2017. "Process Simulation and Control for Continuous Pharmaceutical Manufacturing of Solid Drug Products." In Peter Kleinebudde, Johannes Khinast, Jukka Rantanen, eds. *Continuous Manufacturing of Pharmaceuticals*, 33–105. doi:10.1002/9781119001348

Ireland, P.M. 2010a. "Triboelectrification of Particulate Flows on Surfaces: Part I – Experiments." *Powder Technology 198*: 189–198.

Ireland, P.M. 2010b. "Triboelectrification of Particulate Flows on Surfaces: Part II - Mechanisms and Models." *Powder Technology 198* (2): 199–210.

Ireland, P.M. 2012. "Dynamic Particle-Surface Tribocharging: The Role of Shape and Contact Mode." *Journal of Electrostatics 70*: 524–531.

Itakura, T., Masuda, H., Ohtsuka, C., and Matsusaka, S. 1996. "The Contact Potential Difference of Powder and the Tribo-Charge." *Journal of Electrostatics 38* (3): 213–226.

Ivković, B., Djurdjanović, M., and Stamenković, D. 2000. "The Influence of the Contact Surface Roughness on the Static Friction Coefficient." *Tribology in Industry 22* (3–4): 41–44.

Jallo, L.J., and Dave, R.N. 2015. "Explaining Electrostatic Charging and Flow of Surface-Modified Acetamino-phen Powders as a Function of Relative Humidity through Surface Energetics." *Journal of Pharmaceutical Sciences 104* (7): 2225–2232.

Jarray, A., Wijshoff, H., Luiken, J.A., and den Otter, W.K. 2020. "Systematic Approach for Wettability Prediction Using Molecular Dynamics Simulations." *Soft Matter 16* (17): 4299–4310.

Kahn, A. 2016. "Fermi Level, Work Function and Vacuum Level." *Materials Horizons 3* (1): 7–10.

Kaialy, W. 2016. "A Review of Factors Affecting Electrostatic Charging of Pharmaceuticals and Adhesive Mixtures for Inhalation." *International Journal of Pharmaceutics 503*: 262–276.

Kamiyama, M., Maeda, M., Okutani, H., Koyama, K., Matsuda, H., and Sano, Y. 1994. "Effect of Functional Groups on the Triboelectric Charging Property of Polymer Particles." *Journal of Applied Polymer Science 51*: 1667–1671.

Karner, S., Littringer, E.M., and Urbanetz, N.A. 2014. "Triboelectrics: The Influence of Particle Surface Roughness and Shape on Charge Acquisition during Aerosolization and the DPI Performance." *Powder Technology 262*: 22–29.

Karner, S., and Urbanetz, N.A. 2011. "The Impact of Electrostatic Charge in Pharmaceutical Powders with Specific Focus on Inhalation-Powders." *Journal of Aerosol Science 42*: 428–445.

Karner, S., and Urbanetz, N.A. 2012. "Arising of Electrostatic Charge in the Mixing Process and Its Influencing Factors." *Powder Technology 226*: 261–268.

Karner, S., and Urbanetz, N.A. 2013. "Triboelectric Characteristics of Mannitol Based Formulations for the Application in Dry Powder Inhalers." *Powder Technology 235*: 349–358.

Ketterhagen, W.R., Am Ende, M.T., and Hancock, B.C. 2009. "Process Modeling in the Pharmaceutical Industry Using the Discrete Element Method." *Journal of Pharmaceutical Sciences 98* (2): 442–470.

Khadka, P., Ro, J., Kim, H., Kim, I., Kim, J.T., Kim, H., Cho, J.M., Yun, G., and Lee, J. 2014. "Pharmaceutical Particle Technologies: An Approach to Improve Drug Solubility, Dissolution and Bioavailability." *Asian Journal of Pharmaceutical Sciences 9*: 304–316.

Kim, E.J., Kim, J.H., Kim, M.S., Jeong, S.H., and Choi, D.H. 2021. "Process Analytical Technology Tools for Monitoring Pharmaceutical Unit Operations: A Control Strategy for Continuous Process Verification." *Pharmaceutics 13*: 919.

Kline, A.G., Lim, M.X., and Jaeger, H.M. 2020. "Precision Measurement of Tribocharging in Acoustically Levitated Sub-Millimeter Grains." *Review of Scientific Instruments 91* (2): 023908.

Knorr, N. 2011. "Squeezing out Hydrated Protons: Low-Frictional-Energy Triboelectric Insulator Charging on a Microscopic Scale." *AIP Advances 1*: 022119.

Knutson, E.O., and Whitby, K.T. 1975. "Aerosol Classification by Electric Mobility: Apparatus, Theory, and Applications." *Journal of Aerosol Science 6*: 443–451.

Kodama, T., Suzuki, T., Nishimura, K., Yagi, S., and Watano, S. 2002. "Static Charge Elimination on Pellets in a Silo Using a New Nozzle-Type Eliminator." *Journal of Electrostatics 55*: 289–297.

Kolehmainen, J., Ozel, A., Boyce, C.M., and Sundaresan, S. 2016. "A Hybrid Approach to Computing Electrostatic Forces in Fluidized Beds of Charged Particles." *AICHE Journal 62*: 2282–2295.

Korevaar, M.W., Padding, J.T., Van der Hoef, M.A., and Kuipers, J.A.M. 2014. "Integrated DEM-CFD Modeling of the Contact Charging of Pneumatically Conveyed Powders." *Powder Technology 258*: 144–156.

Kulon, J., and Balachandran, W. 2001. "The Measurement of Bipolar Charge on Aerosols." *Journal of Electrostatics 51–52*: 552–557.

Kulon, J., Malyan, B., and Balachandran, W. 2001. "The Bipolar Charge Aerosol Classifier." In *Conference Record IEEE-IAS Annual Meeting*, 2241–2248.

Kulon, Janusz, Malyan, B.E., and Balachandran, W. 2003. "Simultaneous Measurement of Particle Size and Electrostatic Charge Distribution in DC Electric Field Using Phase Doppler Anemometry." *IEEE Transactions on Industry Applications 39* (5): 1522–1528.

Kwek, J.W., Heng, D., Lee, S.H., Ng, W.K., Chan, H.K., Adi, S., Heng, J., and Tan, R.B.H. 2013. "High Speed Imaging with Electrostatic Charge Monitoring to Track Powder Deagglomeration upon Impact." *Journal of Aerosol Science 65*: 77–87.

Kwek, Jin W., Vakarelski, I.U., Ng, W.K., Heng, J.Y.Y., and Tan, R.B.H. 2011. "Novel Parallel Plate Condenser for Single Particle Electrostatic Force Measurements in Atomic Force Microscope." *Colloids and Surfaces A: Physicochemical and Engineering Aspects 385*: 206–212.

Kwok, P., and Chan, H.-K. 2008a. "Solid Forms and Electrostatic Properties of Salbutamol Sulfate." *Respiratory Drug Delivery 3* (January): 919–922.

Kwok, P.C.L., and Chan, H. 2008b. "Effect of Relative Humidity on the Electrostatic Charge Properties of Dry Powder Inhaler Aerosols." *Pharmaceutical Research 25* (2): 277–288.

Kwok, P.C.L., and Chan, H. 2009. "Electrostatics of Pharmaceutical Inhalation Aerosols." *Journal of Pharmacy and Pharmacology 61*: 1587–1599.

Kwok, P.C.L., Collins, R., and Chan, H.-K. 2006. "Effect of Spacers on the Electrostatic Charge Properties of Metered Dose Inhaler Aerosols." *Aerosol Science 37*: 1671–1682.

Lachiver, E.D., Abatzoglou, N., Cartilier, L., and Simard, J.S. 2006. "Insights into the Role of Electrostatic Forces on the Behavior of Dry Pharmaceutical Particulate Systems." *Pharmaceutical Research 23* (5): 997–1007.

Lacks, D.J. 2012. "The Unpredictability of Electrostatic Charging." *Angewandte Chemie, International Edition 51*: 6822–6823.

Lacks, D.J., and Gordon, R.G. 1994. "Tests of Nonlocal Kinetic Energy Functionals." *Journal of Chemical Physics 100*: 4446.

Lacks, D.J., and Sankaran, M.R. 2011. "Contact Electrification of Insulating Materials." *Journal of Physics D: Applied Physics 44*: 453001.

Lacks, D.J., and Sankaran, R.M. 2016. "Triboelectric Charging in Single Component Particle Systems." *Particulate Science and Technology 34*: 55–62.

Lacks, D.J., and Shinbrot, T. 2019. "Long-Standing and Unresolved Issues in Triboelectric Charging." *Nature Reviews Chemistry 3*: 465–476.

Lai, K.C., Lim, S.K., Teh, P.C., and Yeap, K.H. 2016. "Modeling Electrostatic Separation Process Using Artificial Neural Network (ANN)." *Procedia Computer Science 91*: 372–381.

LaMarche, K.R., Liu, X., Shah, S.K., Shinbrot, T., and Glasser, B.J. 2009. "Electrostatic Charging during the Flow of Grains from a Cylinder." *Powder Technology 195*: 158–165.

LaMarche, K.R., Muzzio, F.J., Shinbrot, T., and Glasser, B.J. 2010. "Granular Flow and Dielectrophoresis: The Effect of Electrostatic Forces on Adhesion and Flow of Dielectric Granular Materials." *Powder Technology 199*: 180–188.

Laurentie, J.C., Traoré, P., and Dascalescu, L. 2013. "Discrete Element Modeling of Triboelectric Charging of Insulating Materials in Vibrated Granular Beds." *Journal of Electrostatics 71*: 951–957.

Lee, V., James, N.M., Waitukaitis, S., and Jaeger, H.M. 2018. "Collisional Charging of Individual Sub-Millimeter Particles: Using Ultrasonic Levitation to Initiate and Track Charge Transfer." *Physical Review Materials 2*: 035602.

Leung, S.S.Y., Chiow, A.C.M., Kwok, P.C.L., Ukkonen, A., and Chan, H.K. 2017. "Effect of Spacers on the Bipolar Electrostatic Charge Properties of Metered Dose Inhaler Aerosols—A Case Study With Tilade®." *Journal of Pharmaceutical Sciences 106* (6): 1553–1559.

Leung, S.S.Y., Chiow, A.C.M., Ukkonen, A., and Chan, H.K. 2016. "Applicability of Bipolar Charge Analyzer (BOLAR) in Characterizing the Bipolar Electrostatic Charge Profile of Commercial Metered Dose Inhalers (MDIs)." *Pharmaceutical Research 33*: 283–291.

Li, C., Coons, E., and Strachan, A. 2014. "Material Property Prediction of Thermoset Polymers by Molecular Dynamics Simulations." *Acta Mechanica 225* (4–5): 1187–1196.

Lim, E.W.C. 2013. "Mixing Behaviors of Granular Materials in Gas Fluidized Beds with Electrostatic Effects." *Industrial and Engineering Chemistry Research 52*: 15863–15873.

Liu, C.-Y., and Bard, A.J. 2008. "Electrostatic Electrochemistry at Insulators." *Nature Materials 7*: 505–509.

Liu, C.-Y., and Bard, A.J. 2009a. "Electrons on Dielectrics and Contact Electrification." *Chemical Physics Letters 480*: 145–156.

Liu, C.-Y., and Bard, A.J. 2009b. "Chemical Redox Reactions Induced by Cryptoelectrons on a PMMA Surface." *Journal of the American Chemical Society 131*: 6397–6401.

Lowell, J. 1976. "The Electrification of Polymers by Metals." *Journal of Physics D: Applied Physics 9*: 1571–1585.

Lowell, J. 1979. "Tunnelling between Metals and Insulators and Its Role in Contact Electrification." *Journal of Physics D: Applied Physics 12*: 1541–1554.

Lowell, J., and Rose-Innes, A.C. 1980. "Contact Electrification." *Advances in Physics 29*: 947–1023.

Lowell, J., and Truscott, W.S. 1986. "Triboelectrification of Identical Insulators. II. Theory and Further Experiments." *Journal of Physics D: Applied Physics 19*: 1281–1298.

Matsusaka, S., Ghadiri, M., and Masuda, H. 2000. "Electrification of an Elastic Sphere by Repeated Impacts on a Metal Plate." *Journal of Physics D: Applied Physics 33*: 2311–2319.

Matsusaka, S., Maruyama, H., Matsuyama, T., and Ghadiri, M. 2010. "Triboelectric Charging of Powders: A Review." *Chemical Engineering Science 65*: 5781–5807.

Matsusaka, S., and Masuda, H. 2003. "Electrostatics of Particles." *Advanced Powder Technology 14*: 143–166.

Matsusaka, S., Umemoto, H., Nishitani, M., and Masuda, H. 2002. "Electrostatic Charge Distribution of Particles in Gas-Solids Pipe Flow." *Journal of Electrostatics 55*: 81–96.

Matsuyama, T., Šupuk, E., Ahmadian, H., Hassanpour, A., and Ghadiri, M. 2009. "Analysis of Tribo-Electric Charging of Spherical Beads Using Distinct Element Method." *AIP Conference Proceedings 1145*: 127–130.

Mazumber, M.K., Ware, R.E., Yokoyama, T., Rubin, B.J., and Kamp, D. 1991. "Measurement of Particle Size and Electrostatic Charge Distributions on Toners Using E-SPART Analyzer." *IEEE Transactions on Industry Applications 27* (4): 611–619.

Mazumder, M.K., and Ware, R.E. 1987. "Aerosol Particle Charge and Size Analyzer."

McCarty, L.S., and Whitesides, G.M. 2008. "Electrostatic Charging Due to Separation of Ions at Interfaces: Contact Electrification of Ionic Electrets." *Angewandte Chemie, International Edition 47*: 2188–2207.

McCarty, L.S., Winkleman, A., and Whitesides, G.M. 2007a. "Electrostatic Self-Assembly of Polystyrene Microspheres by Using Chemically Directed Contact Electrification." *Angewandte Chemie, International Edition 46*: 206–209.

McCarty, L.S., Winkleman, A., and Whitesides, G.M. 2007b. "Ionic Electrets: Electrostatic Charging of Surfaces by Transferring Mobile Ions upon Contact." *Journal of the American Chemical Society 129* (13): 4075–4088.

Medles, K., Senouci, K., Tilmatine, A., Bendaoud, A., Mihalcioiu, A., and Dascalescu, L. 2009. "Capability Evaluation and Statistical Control of Electrostatic Separation Processes." *IEEE Transactions on Industry Applications 45* (3): 1086–1094.

Mehrani, P., Bi, H.T., and Grace, J.R. 2005. "Electrostatic Charge Generation in Gas-Solid Fluidized Beds." *Journal of Electrostatics 63*: 165–173.

Mehrotra, A., Muzzio, F.J., and Shinbrot, T. 2007. "Spontaneous Separation of Charged Grains." *Physical Review Letters 99*: 058001.

Mizes, H., Ott, M., Eklund, E., and Hays, D. 2000. "Small Particle Adhesion: Measurement and Control." *Colloids and Surfaces A: Physicochemical and Engineering Aspects 165*: 11–23.

Modhave, D., Saraf, I., Karn, A., and Paudel, A. 2020. "Understanding Concomitant Physical and Chemical Transformations of Simvastatin During Dry Ball Milling." *AAPS PharmSciTech 21*: 152.

Mountain, J.R., Mazumder, M.K., Sims, R.A., Wankum, D.L., Chasser, T., and Pettit, P.H. 2001. "Triboelectric Charging of Polymer Powders in Fluidization and Transport Processes." *IEEE Transactions on Industry Applications 37* (3): 778–784.

Muehlenfeld, C., and Thommes, M. 2014. "Small-Scale Twin-Screw Extrusion - Evaluation of Continuous Split Feeding." *The Journal of Pharmacy and Pharmacology 66*: 1667–1676.

Mukherjee, R., Gupta, V., Naik, S., Sarkar, S., Sharma, V., Peri, P., and Chaudhuri, B. 2016. "Effects of Particle Size on the Triboelectrification Phenomenon in Pharmaceutical Excipients: Experiments and Multi-Scale Modeling." *Asian Journal of Pharmaceutical Sciences 11*: 603–617.

Mukherjee, R., Sansare, S., Nagarajan, V., and Chaudhuri, B. 2021. "Discrete Element Modeling (DEM) Based Investigation of Tribocharging in the Pharmaceutical Powders during Hopper Discharge." *International Journal of Pharmaceutics 596*: 120284.

Mukherjee, R., Sen, K., Fontana, L., Mao, C., and Chaudhuri, B. 2019. "Quantification of Moisture-Induced Cohesion in Pharmaceutical Mixtures." *Journal of Pharmaceutical Sciences 108*: 223–233.

Murata, Y., and Kittaka, S. 1979. "Evidence of Electron Transfer as the Mechanism of Static Charge Generation by Contact of Polymers with Metals." *Japanese Journal of Applied Physics 18*: 421.

Murtomaa, M., Harjunen, P., Mellin, V., Lehto, V.P., and Laine, E. 2002a. "Effect of Amorphicity on the Triboelectrification of Lactose Powder." *Journal of Electrostatics 56*: 103–110.

Murtomaa, M., and Laine, E. 2000. "Electrostatic Measurements on Lactose-Glucose Mixtures." *Journal of Electrostatics 48*: 155–162.

Murtomaa, M., Mäkilä, E., and Salonen, J. 2012. "One-Step Method for Measuring the Effect of Humidity on Powder Resistivity." In *Proceeding 2012 Joint Electrostatics Conference*, 1–9.

Murtomaa, M., Mellin, V., Harjunen, P., Lankinen, T., Laine, E., and Lehto, V. 2004. "Effect of Particle Morphology on the Triboelectrification in Dry Powder Inhalers." *International Journal of Pharmaceutics 282*: 107–114.

Murtomaa, M., Ojanen, K., and Laine, E. 2002b. "Effect of Surface Coverage of a Glass Pipe by Small Particles on the Triboelectrification of Glucose Powder." *Journal of Electrostatics 54*: 311–320.

Murtomaa, M., Räsänen, E., Rantanen, J., Bailey, A., Laine, E., Mannermaa, J.P., and Yliruusi, J. 2003a. "Electrostatic Measurements on a Miniaturized Fluidized Bed." *Journal of Electrostatics 57*: 91–106.

Murtomaa, M., and Salonen, J. 2015. "Simultaneous Measurement of Particle Charge, Distance and Size Using Coaxial Induction Probe." *Journal of Physics: Conference Series 646*: 012038.

Murtomaa, M., Strengell, S., Laine, E., and Bailey, A. 2003b. "Measurement of Electrostatic Charge of an Aerosol Using a Grid-Probe." *Journal of Electrostatics 58*: 197–207.

Naik, S., Hancock, B., Abramov, Y., Yu, W., Rowland, M., Huang, Z., and Chaudhuri, B. 2016a. "Quantification of Tribocharging of Pharmaceutical Powders in V-Blenders: Experiments, Multiscale Modeling, and Simulations." *Journal of Pharmaceutical Sciences 105*: 1467–1477.

Naik, S., Sarkar, S., Gupta, V., Hancock, B.C., Abramov, Y., Yu, W., and Chaudhuri, B. 2015. "A Combined Experimental and Numerical Approach to Explore Tribocharging of Pharmaceutical Excipients in a Hopper Chute Assembly." *International Journal of Pharmaceutics 491*: 58–68.

Naik, S., Sarkar, S., Hancock, B., Rowland, M., Abramov, Y., Yu, W., and Chaudhuri, B. 2016b. "An Experimental and Numerical Modeling Study of Tribocharging in Pharmaceutical Granular Mixtures." *Powder Technology 297*: 211–219.

Neagoe, M.B., Prawatya, Y.E., Zeghloul, T., and Dascalescu, L. 2017. "Influence of Surface Roughness on the Tribo-Electric Process for a Sliding Contact between Polymeric Plate Materials." *IOP Conference Series: Materials Science and Engineering 174*: 012003.

Németh, E., Albrecht, G., Schubert, G., and Simon, F. 2003. "Polymer Tribo-Electric Charging: Dependence on Thermodynamic Surface Properties and Relative Humidity." *Journal of Electrostatics 58*: 3–16.

Nifuku, M., and Katoh, H. 2003. "A Study on the Static Electrification of Powders during Pneumatic Transportation and the Ignition of Dust Cloud." *Powder Technology 135–136*: 234–242.

Nikitina, E., Barthel, H., and Heinemann, M. 2009. "Electron Transfer in Electrical Tribocharging Using a Quantum Chemical Approach." *Journal of Imaging Science and Technology 53* (4): 040503.

Norouzi, Y., Golshan, S., Zarghami, R., and Saleh, K. 2020. "CFD-DEM Simulation of Tribo-Electric Charging of Powders during Pneumatic Conveying." *International Journal of Plasma Environmental Science and Technology 14*: e02002.

Nwose, E.N., Pei, C., and Wu, C.-Y. 2012. "Modelling Die Filling with Charged Particles Using DEM/CFD." *Particuology 10*: 229–235.

O'Leary, M., Balachandran, W., and Chambers, F. 2008. "Nebulised Aerosol Electrostatic Charge Explored Using Bipolar Electrical Mobility Chambers." In *Industry Applications Society Annual Meeting*.

Pähtz, T., Herrmann, H.J., and Shinbrot, T. 2010a. "Why Do Particle Clouds Generate Electric Charges?" *Nature Physics 6*: 364–368.

Pähtz, T., Herrmann, H.J., and Shinbrot, T. 2010b. "Why Do Particle Clouds Generate Electric Charges?" *Nature Physics 6*: 364–368.

Pandey, R.K., Ao, C.K., Lim, W., Sun, Y., Di, X., Nakanishi, H., and Soh, S. 2020. "The Relationship between Static Charge and Shape." *ACS Central Science 6*: 704–714.

Pandey, R.K., Kakehashi, H., Nakanishi, H., and Soh, S. 2018. "Correlating Material Transfer and Charge Transfer in Contact Electrification." *Journal of Physical Chemistry C 122*: 16154–16160.

Peart, J. 2001. "Powder Electrostatics: Theory, Techniques and Applications." *Kona Powder and Particle Journal 19*: 34–45.

Pei, C., Wu, C.Y., England, D., Byard, S., Berchtold, H., and Adams, M. 2013. "Numerical Analysis of Contact Electrification Using DEM-CFD." *Powder Technology 248*: 34–43.

Peltonen, J., Murtomaa, M., Saikkonen, A., and Salonen, J. 2016. "A Coaxial Probe with a Vertically Split Outer Sensor for Charge and Dimensional Measurement of a Passing Object." *Sensors and Actuators, A: Physical 244*: 44–49.

Peltonen, J., Murtomaa, M., and Salonen, J. 2015. "A Coaxial Induction Probe for Measuring the Charge, Size and Distance of a Passing Object." *Journal of Electrostatics 77*: 94–100.

Peltonen, J., Murtomaa, M., and Salonen, J. 2018. "Measuring Electrostatic Charging of Powders On-Line during Surface Adhesion." *Journal of Electrostatics 93*: 53–57.

Philip, V.A., Mehta, R.C., Deluca, P.P., and Mazumder, M.K. 1997. "E-SPART Analysis of Poly (D, L-Lactide-Co-Glycolide) Microspheres Formulated for Dry Powder Aerosols." *Particulate Science and Technology 15* (3–4): 303–316.

Pingali, K.C., Hammond, S.V., Muzzio, F.J., and Shinbrot, T. 2009a. "Use of a Static Eliminator to Improve Powder Flow." *International Journal of Pharmaceutics 369*: 2–4.

Pingali, K.C., Shinbrot, T., Hammond, S.V., and Muzzio, F.J. 2009b. "An Observed Correlation between Flow and Electrical Properties of Pharmaceutical Blends." *Powder Technology 192*: 157–165.

Pingali, K.C., Tomassone, M.S., and Muzzio, F.J. 2010. "Effects of Shear and Electrical Properties on Flow Characteristics of Pharmaceutical Blends." *AICHE Journal 56* (3): 570–583.

Pinget, G., Tan, J., Janac, B., Kaakoush, N.O., Angelatos, A.S., O'Sullivan, J., Koay, Y.C., et al. 2019. "Impact of the Food Additive Titanium Dioxide (E171) on Gut Microbiota-Host Interaction." *Frontiers in Nutrition 6*: 57.

Pinto, J.T., Wutscher, T., Stankovic-Brandl, M., Zellnitz, S., Biserni, S., Mercandelli, A., Kobler, M., et al. 2020. "Evaluation of the Physico-Mechanical Properties and Electrostatic Charging Behavior of Different Capsule Types for Inhalation under Distinct Environmental Conditions." *AAPS PharmSciTech 21*: 128.

Prawatya, Y.E., Senouci, K., Zeghloul, T., Neagoe, M.B., Dascalescu, L., and Medles, K. 2019. "Control Charts for Statistical Process Control of the Tribocharging of Polymer Slabs in Frictional Sliding Contact." *IEEE Transactions on Industry Applications 55* (5): 5253–5260.

Pu, Y.U., Mazumder, M., and Cooney, C. 2009. "Effects of Electrostatic Charging on Pharmaceutical Powder Blending Homogeneity." *Journal of Pharmaceutical Sciences 98*: 2412–2421.

Rathi, P.C., Ludlow, R.F., and Verdonk, M.L. 2020. "Practical High-Quality Electrostatic Potential Surfaces for Drug Discovery Using a Graph-Convolutional Deep Neural Network." *Journal of Medicinal Chemistry 63*: 8778–8790.

Ray, M., Chowdhury, F., Sowinski, A., Mehrani, P., and Passalacqua, A. 2019. "An Euler-Euler Model for Mono-Dispersed Gas-Particle Flows Incorporating Electrostatic Charging Due to Particle-Wall and Particle-Particle Collisions." *Chemical Engineering Science 197*: 327–344.

Ray, M., Chowdhury, F., Sowinski, A., Mehrani, P., and Passalacqua, A. 2020. "Eulerian Modeling of Charge Transport in Bi-Disperse Particulate Flows Due to Triboelectrification." *Physics of Fluids 32* (2): 023302.

Ren, Z., Chen, X., Yu, G., Wang, Y., Chen, B., and Zhou, Z. 2020. "Molecular Simulation Studies on the Design of Energetic Ammonium Dinitramide Co-Crystals for Tuning Hygroscopicity." *CrystEngComm 22* (31): 5237–5244.

Rescaglio, A., De Smet, F., Aerts, L., and Lumay, G. 2019. "Tribo-Electrification of Pharmaceutical Powder Blends." *Particulate Science and Technology*: 1–8.

Revel, J., Gatumel, C., Dodds, J.A., and Taillet, J. 2003. "Generation of Static Electricity during Fluidisation of Polyethylene and Its Elimination by Air Ionisation." *Powder Technology 135–136*: 192–200.

Rowland, M., Cavecchi, A., Thielmann, F., Kulon, J., Shur, J., and Price, R. 2019. "Measuring The Bipolar Charge Distributions of Fine Particle Aerosol Clouds of Commercial PMDI Suspensions Using a Bipolar Next Generation Impactor (Bp-NGI)." *Pharmaceutical Research 36*: 1–14.

Rowley, G. 2001. "Quantifying Electrostatic Interactions in Pharmaceutical Solid Systems." *International Journal of Pharmaceutics 227*: 47–55.

Rowley, G., and Mackin, L.A. 2003. "The Effect of Moisture Sorption on Electrostatic Charging of Selected Pharmaceutical Excipient Powders." *Powder Technology 135–136*: 50–58.

Saini, D., Biris, A.S., Srirama, P.K., and Mazumder, M.K. 2007. "Particle Size and Charge Distribution Analysis of Pharmaceutical Aerosols Generated by Inhalers." *Pharmaceutical Development and Technology 12*: 35–41.

Sakaguchi, M., Makino, M., Ohura, T., and Iwata, T. 2014. "Contact Electrification of Polymers Due to Electron Transfer among Mechano Anions, Mechano Cations and Mechano Radicals." *Journal of Electrostatics 72*: 412–416.

Salaneck, W.R., Paton, A., and Clark, D.T. 1976. "Double Mass Transfer during Polymer-Polymer Contacts." *Journal of Applied Physics 47* (1): 144–147.

Saleh, K., Traore Ndama, A., and Guigon, P. 2011. "Relevant Parameters Involved in Tribocharging of Powders during Dilute Phase Pneumatic Transport." *Chemical Engineering Research and Design 89*: 2582–2597.

Samiei, L., Kelly, K., Taylor, L., Forbes, B., Collins, E., and Rowland, M. 2017. "The Influence of Electrostatic Properties on the Punch Sticking Propensity of Pharmaceutical Blends." *Powder Technology 305*: 509–517.

Sarkar, S., Cho, J., and Chaudhuri, B. 2012. "Mechanisms of Electrostatic Charge Reduction of Granular Media with Additives on Different Surfaces." *Chemical Engineering and Processing 62*: 168–175.

Saxena, A., Kendrick, J., Grimsey, I., and Mackin, L. 2007. "Application of Molecular Modelling to Determine the Surface Energy of Mannitol." *International Journal of Pharmaceutics 343*: 173–180.

Schaber, S.D., Gerogiorgis, D.I., Ramachandran, R., Evans, J.M.B., Barton, P.I., and Trout, B.L. 2011. "Economic Analysis of Integrated Continuous and Batch Pharmaceutical Manufacturing: A Case Study." *Industrial and Engineering Chemistry Research 50* (17): 10083–10092.

Schella, A., Herminghaus, S., and Schröter, M. 2017. "Influence of Humidity on Tribo-Electric Charging and Segregation in Shaken Granular Media." *Soft Matter 13*: 394–401.

Schwindt, N., von Pidoll, U., Markus, D., Klausmeyer, U., Papalexandris, M.V., and Grosshans, H. 2017. "Measurement of Electrostatic Charging during Pneumatic Conveying of Powders." *Journal of Loss Prevention in the Process Industries 49*: 461–471.

Sharma, R., Trigwell, S., and Mazumder, M.K. 2008. "Interfacial Processes and Tribocharging: Effect of Plasma Surface Modification and Physisorption." *Particulate Science and Technology 26*: 587–594.

Shekunov, B.Y., Feeley, J.C., Chow, A.H.L., Tong, H.H.Y., and York, P. 2002. "Physical Properties of Supercritically-Processed and Micronised Powders for Respirator y Drug Delivery." *Kona Powder and Particle Journal 20*: 178–187.

Shi, Q., Zhang, Q., Han, G., Zhang, W., Wang, J., Huang, Z., Yang, Y., Yang, Y., Wu, W., and Yan, Y. 2017. "Simultaneous Measurement of Electrostatic Charge and Its Effect on Particle Motions by Electrostatic Sensors Array in Gas-Solid Fluidized Beds." *Powder Technology 312*: 29–37.

Shin, S.H., Bae, Y.E., Moon, H.K., Kim, J., Choi, S.H., Kim, Y., Yoon, H.J., Lee, M.H., and Nah, J. 2017. "Formation of Triboelectric Series via Atomic-Level Surface Functionalization for Triboelectric Energy Harvesting." *ACS Nano 11*: 6131–6138.

Shinbrot, T., Ferdowsi, B., Sundaresan, S., and Araujo, N.A.M. 2018. "Multiple Timescale Contact Charging." *Physical Review Materials 2*: 125003.

Shoyele, S.A., and Cawthorne, S. 2006. "Particle Engineering Techniques for Inhaled Biopharmaceuticals." *Advanced Drug Delivery Reviews 58*: 1009–1029.

Singh, S., and Hearn, G.L. 1985. "Development and Application of an Electrostatic Microprobe." *Journal of Electrostatics 16*: 353–361.

Song, D., Salama, F., Matta, J., and Mehrani, P. 2016. "Implementation of Faraday Cup Electrostatic Charge Measurement Technique in High-Pressure Gas – Solid Fl Uidized Beds at Pilot-Scale." *Powder Technology 290*: 21–26.

Soppela, I., Airaksinen, S., Murtomaa, M., Tenho, M., Hatara, J., Räikkönen, H., Yliruusi, J., and Sandler, N. 2010. "Investigation of the Powder Flow Behaviour of Binary Mixtures of Microcrystalline Celluloses and Paracetamol." *Journal of Excipients and Food Chemicals 1*: 55–67.

Sow, M., Crase, E., Rajot, J.L., Sankaran, R.M., and Lacks, D.J. 2011. "Electrification of Particles in Dust Storms: Field Measurements during the Monsoon Period in Niger." *Atmospheric Research 102*: 343–350.

Sowinski, A., Mayne, A., and Mehrani, P. 2012. "Effect of Fluidizing Particle Size on Electrostatic Charge Generation and Reactor Wall Fouling in Gas-Solid Fluidized Beds." *Chemical Engineering Science 71*: 552–563.

Sowinski, A., Miller, L., and Mehrani, P. 2010. "Investigation of Electrostatic Charge Distribution in Gas – Solid Fluidized Beds." *Chemical Engineering Science 65*: 2771–2781.

Sowinski, A., Salama, F., and Mehrani, P. 2009. "New Technique for Electrostatic Charge Measurement in Gas-Solid Fluidized Beds." *Journal of Electrostatics 67*: 568–573.

Stauffer, F., Vanhoorne, V., Pilcer, G., Chavez, P.F., Schubert, M.A., Vervaet, C., and De Beer, T. 2019. "Managing Active Pharmaceutical Ingredient Raw Material Variability during Twin-Screw Blend Feeding." *European Journal of Pharmaceutics and Biopharmaceutics 135*: 49–60.

Šupuk, E., Antony, J., Seiler, C., and Ghadiri, M. 2007. "Electrostatic Charge Generation Due to Shear Deformation of Pharmaceutical Powders." http://eprints.hud.ac.uk/12606/.

Šupuk, E., Zarrebini, A., Reddy, J.P., Hughes, H., Leane, M.M., Tobyn, M.J., Timmins, P., and Ghadiri, M. 2012. "Tribo-Electrification of Active Pharmaceutical Ingredients and Excipients." *Powder Technology 217*: 427–434.

Tan, D., Willatzen, M., and Wang, Z.L. 2021. "Electron Transfer in the Contact-Electrification between Corrugated 2D Materials: A First-Principles Study." *Nano Energy 79*: 105386.

Tanoue, K., Ema, A., and Masuda, H. 1999. "Effect of Material Transfer and Work Hardening of Metal Surface on the Current Generated by Impact of Particles." *Journal of Chemical Engineering of Japan 32*: 544–548.

Tanoue, K.I., Tanaka, H., Kitano, H., and Masuda, H. 2001. "Numerical Simulation of Tribo-Electrification of Particles in a Gas-Solids Two-Phase Flow." *Powder Technology 118* (1–2): 121–129.

Telko, M.J., Kujanpää, J., and Hickey, A.J. 2007. "Investigation of Triboelectric Charging in Dry Powder Inhalers Using Electrical Low Pressure Impactor (ELPI™)." *International Journal of Pharmaceutics 336*: 352–360.

Tian, Y., Ina, M., Cao, Z., Sheiko, S.S., and Dobrynin, A.V. 2018. "How to Measure Work of Adhesion and Surface Tension of Soft Polymeric Materials." *Macromolecules 51* (11): 4059–4067.

Trigwell, S., Grable, N., Yurteri, C.U., Sharma, R., and Mazumder, M.K. 2003. "Effects of Surface Properties on the Tribocharging Characteristics of Polymer Powder as Applied to Industrial Processes." *IEEE Transactions on Industry Applications 39* (1): 79–86.

Van Snick, B., Dhondt, J., Pandelaere, K., Bertels, J., Mertens, R., Klingeleers, D., Di Pretoro, G., et al. 2018. "A Multivariate Raw Material Property Database to Facilitate Drug Product Development and Enable In-Silico Design of Pharmaceutical Dry Powder Processes." *International Journal of Pharmaceutics 549*: 415–435.

Waitukaitis, S.R., Lee, V., Pierson, J.M., Forman, S.L., and Jaeger, H.M. 2014. "Size-Dependent Same-Material Tribocharging in Insulating Grains." *Physical Review Letters 112*: 218001.

Wang, L., Tao, J., Ma, T., and Dai, Z. 2019. "The Electronic Behaviors and Charge Transfer Mechanism at the Interface of Metals: A First-Principles Perspective." *Journal of Applied Physics 126*: 205301.

Watanabe, H., Ghadiri, M., Matsuyama, T., Ding, Y.L., Pitt, K.G., Maruyama, H., Matsusaka, S., and Masuda, H. 2007a. "Triboelectrification of Pharmaceutical Powders by Particle Impact." *International Journal of Pharmaceutics 334*: 149–155.

Watanabe, H., Ghadiri, M., Matsuyama, T., Long Ding, Y., and Pitt, K.G. 2007b. "New Instrument for Tribocharge Measurement Due to Single Particle Impacts." *Review of Scientific Instruments 78*: 024706.

Watanabe, H., Samimi, A., Ding, Y.L., Ghadiri, M., Matsuyama, T., and Pitt, K.G. 2006. "Measurement of Charge Transfer Due to Single Particle Impact." *Particle and Particle Systems Characterization 23*: 133–137.

Watano, S. 2006. "Mechanism and Control of Electrification in Pneumatic Conveying of Powders." *Chemical Engineering Science 61*: 2271–2278.

Weitzel, J., Pappa, H., Banik, G.M., Barker, A.R., Bladen, E., Chirmule, N., DeFeo, J., et al. 2021. "Understanding Quality Paradigm Shifts in the Evolving Pharmaceutical Landscape: Perspectives from the USP Quality Advisory Group." *The AAPS Journal 23*: 112.

Wiles, J.A., Fialkowski, M., Radowski, M.R., Whitesides, G.M., and Grzybowski, B.A. 2004. "Effects of Surface Modification and Moisture on the Rates of Charge Transfer between Metals and Organic Materials." *Journal of Physical Chemistry B 108*: 20296–20302.

Wolny, A., and Opaliński, I. 1983. "Electric Charge Neutralization by Addition of Fines to a Fluidized Bed Composed of Coarse Dielectric Particles." *Journal of Electrostatics 14*: 279–289.

Wong, J., Chan, H.-K., and Kwock, P.C.L. 2013. "Electrostatics in Pharmaceutical Aerosols for Inhalation." *Therapeutic Delivery 4* (8): 981–1002.

Wong, J., Kwok, P.C.L., and Chan, H.K. 2015a. "Electrostatics in Pharmaceutical Solids." *Chemical Engineering Science 125*: 225–237.

Wong, J., Kwok, P.C.L., Niemelä, V., Heng, D., Crapper, J., and Chan, H.K. 2016. "Bipolar Electrostatic Charge and Mass Distributions of Powder Aerosols - Effects of Inhaler Design and Inhaler Material." *Journal of Aerosol Science 95*: 104–117.

Wong, J., Kwok, P.C.L., Noakes, T., Fathi, A., Dehghani, F., and Chan, H.K. 2014. "Effect of Crystallinity on Electrostatic Charging in Dry Powder Inhaler Formulations." *Pharmaceutical Research 31*: 1656–1664.

Wong, J., Lin, Y.W., Kwok, P.C.L., Niemelä, V., Crapper, J., and Chan, H.K. 2015b. "Measuring Bipolar Charge and Mass Distributions of Powder Aerosols by a Novel Tool (BOLAR)." *Molecular Pharmaceutics 12*: 3433–3440.

Wu, J., and Bi, H.T. 2011. "Addition of Fines for the Reduction of Powder Charging in Particle Mixers." *Advanced Powder Technology 22*: 332–335.

Xie, L., Bao, N., Jiang, Y., Han, K., and Zhou, J. 2016. "An Instrument for Charge Measurement Due to a Single Collision between Two Spherical Particles." *Review of Scientific Instruments 87*: 014705.

Xu, C., Zhang, B., Wang, A.C., Zou, H., Liu, G., Ding, W., Wu, C., et al. 2019. "Contact-Electrification between Two Identical Materials: Curvature Effect." *ACS Nano 13*: 2034–2041.

Xu, C., Zi, Y., Wang, A.C., Zou, H., Dai, Y., He, X., Wang, P., et al. 2018. "On the Electron-Transfer Mechanism in the Contact-Electrification Effect." *Advanced Materials 30*: 1706790.

Yanagida, K., Okada, O., and Oka, K. 1993. "Low-Energy Electronic States Related to Contact Electrification of Pendant-Group Polymers: Photoemission and Contact Potential Difference Measurement." *Japanese Journal of Applied Physics 32*: 5603–5610.

Yao, J., Ge, S., Zhao, Y., Cong, S., Wang, C.H., and Li, N. 2016. "Investigation of Granule Electrostatic Charge Generation with Normal Stress Effect." *Advanced Powder Technology 27*: 2094–2101.

Yoshida, M., Ii, N., Shimosaka, A., Shirakawa, Y., and Hidaka, J. 2006. "Experimental and Theoretical Approaches to Charging Behavior of Polymer Particles." *Chemical Engineering Science 61* (7): 2239–2248.

Young, P.M., Sung, A., Traini, D., Kwok, P., Chiou, H., and Chan, H.K. 2007. "Influence of Humidity on the Electrostatic Charge and Aerosol Performance of Dry Powder Inhaler Carrier Based Systems." *Pharmaceutical Research 24* (5): 963–970.

Yurteri, C.U., Mazumder, M.K., Grable, N., Ahuja, G., Trigwell, S., Biris, A.S., Sharma, R., and Sims, R.A. 2002. "Electrostatic Effects on Dispersion, Transport, and Deposition of Fine Pharmaceutical Powders: Development of an Experimental Method for Quantitative Analysis." *Particulate Science and Technology 20* (1): 59–79.

Zafar, U., Alfano, F., and Ghadiri, M. 2018. "Evaluation of a New Dispersion Technique for Assessing Triboelectric Charging of Powders." *International Journal of Pharmaceutics 543*: 151–159.

Zarrebini, A., Ghadiri, M., Dyson, M., Kippax, P., and McNeil-Watson, F. 2013. "Tribo-Electrification of Powders Due to Dispersion." *Powder Technology 250*: 75–83.

Zellnitz, S., Pinto, J.T., Brunsteiner, M., Schroettner, H., Khinast, J., and Paudel, A. 2019a. "Tribo-Charging Behaviour of Inhalable Mannitol Blends with Salbutamol Sulphate." *Pharmaceutical Research 36*: 80.

Zhang, J., Srirama, P.K., and Mazumder, M.K. 2007. "E-SPART Analyzer for Mars Mission: A New Approach in Signal Processing and Sampling." *IEEE Transactions on Industry Applications 43* (4): 1084–1090.

Zhang, L., Bi, X., and Grace, J.R. 2015a. "Measurements of Electrostatic Charging of Powder Mixtures in a Free-Fall Test Device." *Procedia Engineering 102*: 295–304.

Zhang, W., Cheng, X., Hu, Y., and Yan, Y. 2018. "Measurement of Moisture Content in a Fluidized Bed Dryer Using an Electrostatic Sensor Array." *Powder Technology 325*: 49–57.

Zhang, Y., Pähtz, T., Liu, Y., Wang, X., Zhang, R., Shen, Y., Ji, R., and Cai, B. 2015b. "Electric Field and Humidity Trigger Contact Electrification." *Physical Review X 5*: 011002.

Zhao, H., Castle, G.S.P., and Inculet, I.I. 2002. "The Measurement of Bipolar Charge in Polydisperse Powders Using a Vertical Array of Faraday Pail Sensors." *Journal of Electrostatics 55*: 261–278.

Zhao, H., Castle, G.S.P., Inculet, I.I., and Bailey, A.G. 2000. "Bipolar Charging in Polydisperse Polymer Powders in Industrial Processes." In *Conference Record - IAS Annual Meeting (IEEE Industry Applications Society) 2*: 835–841.

Zhao, H., Castle, G.S.P., Inculet, I.I., and Bailey, A.G. 2003. "Bipolar Charging of Poly-Disperse Polymer Powders in Fluidized Beds." *IEEE Transactions on Industry Applications 39* (3): 612–618.

Zheng, X., Zhang, R., and Huang, H.J. 2014. "Theoretical Modeling of Relative Humidity on Contact Electrification of Sand Particles." *Scientific Reports 4*.

Zheng, X.J., Huang, N., and Zhou, Y.H. 2003. "Laboratory Measurement of Electrification of Wind-Blown Sands and Simulation of Its Effect on Sand Saltation Movement." *Journal of Geophysical Research-Atmospheres 108* (D10): 4322.

Zhou, H., Götzinger, M., and Peukert, W. 2003. "The Influence of Particle Charge and Roughness on Particle-Substrate Adhesion." *Powder Technology 135–136*: 82–91.

Zhou, Y., Ren, C., Wang, J., Yang, Y., and Dong, K. 2013. "Effect of Hydrodynamic Behavior on Electrostatic Potential Distribution in Gas – Solid Fluidized Bed." *Powder Technology 235*: 9–17.

Zhu, K., Ng, W.K., Shen, S., Tan, R.B.H., and Heng, P.W.S. 2008. "Design of a Device for Simultaneous Particle Size and Electrostatic Charge Measurement of Inhalation Drugs." *Pharmaceutical Research 25* (11): 2488–2496.

Zhu, K., Rao, S.M., Huang, Q.H., Wang, C.H., Matsusaka, S., and Masuda, H. 2004. "On the Electrostatics of Pneumatic Conveying of Granular Materials Using Electrical Capacitance Tomography." *Chemical Engineering Science 59* (15): 3201–3213.

Zhu, K., Tan, R.B.H., Chen, F., Ong, K.H., and Heng, P.W.S. 2007. "Influence of Particle Wall Adhesion on Particle Electrification in Mixers." *International Journal of Pharmaceutics 328*: 22–34.

Zou, H., Zhang, Y., Guo, L., Wang, P., He, X., Dai, G., Zheng, H., et al. 2019. "Quantifying the Triboelectric Series." *Nature Communications 10* (1427): 1–9.

5

Continuous Impregnation Processes

Thamer A. Omar and Fernando J. Muzzio
Rutgers, the State University of New Jersey
Chemical and Biochemical Engineering

CONTENTS

5.1 Introduction

Solid dosage forms such as tablets and capsules are the most common dosage forms among all prescription drugs [1]. Tablets and capsules currently represent more than 70% of the total dosage forms made worldwide [1].

Solid dosage forms consist of a mixture of excipients and active pharmaceutical ingredients (API), which are uniformly distributed throughout the blend. The degree of uniformity in drug content in the product depends on the material properties of the ingredients, the mixing process, and the handling of the blend after mixing. The extent to which the ingredients are homogeneously distributed throughout the blend during the manufacturing process is mostly a function of the particle size distributions, densities, and particle shapes of all the components. Large differences in properties of the APIs and excipients can result in a mixture with poor homogeneity. This invariably influences adversely the drug content uniformity of finished products. Moreover, inhomogeneous distribution of excipients can also affect product quality attributes, including tablet hardness, and, most critical, API release profiles.

Intensive scientific and regulatory efforts have been devoted to ensuring safe products with acceptable content uniformity [2, 3]. In this context, the Food and Drug Administration (FDA) usually requires companies to demonstrate that the relative standard deviation (RSD) of the drug concentration in blend samples is not more than 5% as evidence of acceptable blend homogeneity, and that the RSD of finished product drug content is not more than 6% as evidence of acceptable product content uniformity [4].

Acceptable blend homogeneity and content uniformity are increasingly difficult to achieve as the API content in the blend and the finished product decrease. The amount of API in some dosage forms is lower than 0.1% by weight [5]. In this case, it is very difficult to ensure a uniform distribution of API throughout the excipients by dry blending. The problem is aggravated when drugs are poorly soluble. In such situations, a fairly common approach is to micronize the API, which leads to an increase in particle cohesion and the resulting increase in the tendency to form API agglomerates. Therefore, ensuring high homogeneity for products with low API concentration is a big challenge in pharmaceutical manufacturing, especially for poorly soluble drugs.

More generally, poor homogeneity of the blend and poor content uniformity of the final dosage forms can be attributed to several overlapping factors [5–9]. Segregation caused by differences in both the particle size distributions and densities of the blend's components, insufficient mixing, and inappropriate operation of blending equipment are some of the main factors that can lead to problems in the homogeneity of the blends and uniformity of the final dosage forms.

Controlling the particle size of the drug substance can be a beneficial step in solving problems of content uniformity, inasmuch as it reduces segregation tendencies, but it is necessary to make sure that any change in the particle size will not significantly change the drug release profile. Moreover, the particle sizes of other additives are also important to ensure products with good flowability and high homogeneity. Significant differences in particle size and particle size distribution between the drug and excipients can lead to inhomogeneous products [10].

Intrinsic drug substance solubility and dissolution kinetics of a given grade of the API are also critical properties, which should be thoroughly evaluated before incorporating any drug into the final dosage form. These properties can have a direct influence on drug bioavailability. In 1995, Amidon et al. [11] proposed the Biopharmaceutical Classification System (BCS). In BCS, drugs were classified according to their intestinal permeability and their intrinsic solubility (and more loosely, their dissolution behavior). In this system, the drugs were classified into four classes, where drugs in class II and IV have low intrinsic solubility. It has been estimated that 90% of new chemical entities, 40% of the top 200 marketed drugs in the USA, and 33% of drugs in the USP fall in the low solubility classes [12–14]. Therefore, substantial efforts have been conducted to develop novel formulation approaches to improve the solubility and dissolution behavior of drugs.

The problem of homogeneity of a low-dose product has been addressed through multiple approaches of increasing complexity. Dry processing methods primarily include micronizing the API and then implementing geometric dilution steps, often involving iterative mixing and milling steps. Also, very common has been the implementation of a wet granulation step seeking to enable dispersion of drug aggregates. In cases where these approaches fail, companies have resorted to dissolving or dispersing the drug substance in a liquid carrier, which is then used as a granulation fluid; in this approach, surfactants, complexing agents, electrolytes, and viscosity modifiers are often introduced to promote deagglomeration of the drug particles.

For poorly soluble drugs, the drug particles are either dissolved or dispersed in a liquid medium, and then further dispersed in a polymer carrier; the two most common approaches are spray drying, which employs large amounts of organic solvents, and hot melt extrusion, which requires a complex process and yields an intermediate extrudate that is difficult to process further. All of these methods are complex and expensive to implement, difficult to control, and often utilize large amounts of expensive polymeric excipients.

This situation has motivated a significant level of interest in developing new formulation and manufacturing processes designed to overcome the above-mentioned problems. One such approach developed by the Rutgers Pharmaceutical Engineering group is presented in this chapter.

5.2 Impregnation Onto Porous Carriers

Impregnation is defined as a process of placing chemicals (including drugs) inside the pores of a host particle using a drug solution (or dispersion). This technology has been used for decades by the catalyst manufacturing industry [15], but it has only been used in the pharmaceutical industry in the last decade. The technology mainly includes dissolving the drug in a suitable volatile organic solvent. The solution is sprayed onto the porous carrier, where it is driven into the pores by capillary action, displacing any gas present in the pores. Subsequently, the particles are dried to evaporate the solvent and form the dry drug-impregnated porous carrier. The goal is to create a deposit of the drug substance on the internal surface of the porous carrier. If the carrier pore size is sufficiently small, the drug substance will form a stable amorphous coating of the pore surface, greatly enhancing dissolution. If the amount of solution is carefully selected to correspond to the total internal volume of the pores, the drug solution will completely fill the pores, and, after evaporation of the solvent, will form an extremely uniform distribution of the drug substance across the volume of the carrier.

Loading drugs into porous carriers has many applications and benefits in the development of pharmaceutical dosage forms. Launching a new drug into the market consumes significant resources and research effort and it involves a number of complex steps in drug substance and drug product development. The essential component of drug product development is often the optimization of the physical properties of the drug substance. The effect of a drug's physical properties on pharmaceutical development can be seen from the first step to the final step of the development process. For instance, choosing the preferred solid-state form of the drug can influence the early steps of drug manufacturing such as the drug-substance isolation method, and it can also alter some properties of the final dosage form such as the stability and dissolution behavior of the finished product. A simpler approach to product development is desirable to shorten the required development steps, preferably by excluding some unit operations. Therefore, it is of interest to develop a pharmaceutical manufacturing method that can simplify drug substance and product development and manufacturing. In this chapter, the impregnation of drugs into porous carriers is thoroughly explored as an approach to achieving these aims.

As mentioned early in this chapter, controlling the particle size of drugs and excipients is essential to prevent segregation and produce homogenous blends. Placing the drug inside the pores of porous carriers (instead of forming a monolayer at the surface of the carriers) results in impregnated carriers with a known and predictable particle size distribution of the carrier. Because preformed carriers usually have narrow particle size distribution that is carefully optimized to enable good flow and compaction properties as well as optimal rates of drug release, preservation of these distributions ensures suitable and predictable properties of the impregnated material and the products made from them.

Also, it is very important to reduce dust formation during manufacturing, especially if the product involves potent drugs. Moreover, fines can influence the distribution of drugs within the blend during the mixing or granulation process. Oka et al. (2007) conducted a study to investigate the causes of drug content non-uniformity in granules, which were prepared by wet granulation using a high shear mixer [3]. They pointed out that in their case study the active pharmaceutical ingredient was concentrated in fine granules more than in large granules in a process termed "differential granulation". As a result, fine granules were super potent, which, coupled with size-segregation of the granulated blend, lead to non-homogeneity of drug content in blend samples.

Importantly, agglomeration of particles during the impregnation process can also occur, resulting in segregation of the impregnated intermediate blend. This is a failure mode for the impregnation process. Usually, this type of agglomeration occurs when the drying rate of the solvent is too fast relative to the impregnation rate, or when mixing during spraying is insufficient; both of these situations can lead to conditions where the liquid is in excess on the external surface of particles, leading to the formation of inter-particle bonds. Consequently, the impregnation process must be designed to results in products with a narrow particle size distribution, showing no increase either in fines or in agglomerates [16, 17].

As mentioned, poor drug solubility leads to numerous challenges in drug development, including formulation and storage. Low solubility of a hydrophobic drug, resulting in slow drug release in aqueous media, can be particularly challenging and various strategies to improve solubility and release have been developed. Often low solubility and slow-release rate of a drug can be the rate-limiting step for oral bioavailability, and different approaches have been applied to increase the aqueous solubility and the oral bioavailability of such drugs, such as size reduction, drug amorphization, spray drying [18], complex formation with cyclodextrin [19] and with other materials, and hot-melt extrusion (HME) [20]. All of these approaches rely, in some way, on increasing the surface area between the drug and the dissolution medium. In general, it has been verified that increasing the surface area of poorly soluble drugs is an effective tool to improve the dissolution rate (and therefore the release rate) of a drug [21]. In this context, different approaches have been implemented, which include milling the API into fine particles [22, 23], emulsification [24], and spray drying of the suspension where the API is dispersed at a molecular level into fine particles of the polymer [22].

Drug amorphization is also considered a promising strategy to improve the solubility of the drug substance. The amorphous state has greater free energy, which leads both to greater solubility and to an enhanced kinetic rate of dissolution, than the crystalline state. However, the high surface energy of the amorphous state is often associated with physical and chemical stability problems. Stabilizing the amorphous state usually involves the addition of polymers that are often expensive, can lead to toxicity problems, and reduce the achievable loading of the drug substance in the dosage form. Therefore, techniques that can *simultaneously* increase the surface area of the drug, amorphize it, and stabilize it are highly desirable.

Impregnation can achieve all these goals by loading drug solution into porous carriers and then evaporating the solvent. In particular, loading drugs into mesoporous and nanoporous materials has gained significant attention in the pharmaceutical industry [25]. A silicate mesoporous carrier has recently been used for adjusting drug release rates, targeting drugs, and producing and isolating metastable polymorphs of drugs [26–30]. Silicate mesoporous materials display outstanding properties such as narrow particle size distribution, good flowability, excellent compactability, large surface area, small pores with a narrow size distribution, which is able to create stable drug deposits, and reproducible surface properties. Moreover, both small and large drug molecules have been successfully loaded into the pores using an impregnation technique and the release profile from these products showed diffusion-controlled behavior [31].

Small pores provide good physical stability to the amorphous form by inhibiting or suppressing the crystallization of the drug substance. As such, significant efforts have been applied to invent new porous carriers with new applications. M. Saffari et al. (2016) used porous mannitol to load nifedipine and indomethacin. The results showed that in all the resulting products, the RSD was less than 4% and 80% drug release was obtained within 15 minutes [10]. Similarly, the amenability of using ordered mesoporous silicate SBA-15 to improve the dissolution behavior of poorly soluble drugs was tested. All the loaded products presented improvement in their dissolution behaviors [27]. Grigorov et al. (2013) developed a new method to load drugs into porous carriers, which includes spraying the drug solution into porous carriers using a fluidized bed dryer (FB) [16]. Impregnation and drying occur simultaneously, achieving controlled levels of drug loadings independently of the drug's solubility. This method produced impregnated products with narrow particle size distribution and excellent flow properties [16, 17]. Furthermore, solid products (tablets and capsules) compounded from impregnated carriers showed a significantly improved dissolution profile of tranilast, a poorly soluble drug [31].

As a result, the loading of drugs into porous carriers can be used to create composite materials with tailored physical and chemical properties. These properties can be examined using a variety of characterization techniques. For instance, differential scanning calorimetry (DSC), powder X-ray diffraction (PXD), and Raman spectroscopy can be used to confirm the amorphous state of drug substances inside the pores of porous carriers. Also, particle size distribution and flow properties can be used to demonstrate that the drug substance is inside the pores and not at the surfaces of the porous carriers. Furthermore, dissolution profiles and droplet penetration can be included to characterize the improvement in the solubility and wettability of the composite, as compared to the pure drug substance [32].

5.3 Materials Selection

In impregnation, three main types of materials are used to form a composite particle: the porous carrier, the API, and the solvent. In order to ensure a successful impregnation process, the materials used in this work were carefully selected, as per the description below.

5.3.1 Carrier Properties

The typical porous carriers suitable for impregnation should have a large internal surface area, good flow properties, narrow particle size distribution, be insoluble in the selected organic solvent, and be physically stable under impregnation conditions. The carrier should also be chemically compatible with the drug substance, that is, should be free of undesirable impurities and should not promote chemical decomposition of the API. Because impregnation includes placing chemicals (drugs, and possibly surfactants, pH modifiers, drug release modifiers, etc.) inside the pores of the carrier, the internal surface area and the pore size of porous carriers play crucial roles in the impregnation process. High internal pore volume and surface area provide enough absorption capacity for API solution, which results in a high loading of API into the porous carrier. Moreover, a small pore size ensures a stable amorphization of API inside the pores of the carrier. Impregnation also aims to improve the flow properties of the API particles.

Selecting a carrier with excellent flow properties is necessary to ensure good manufacturability of the resulting impregnated intermediates. Furthermore, the impregnation process by itself requires a carrier with good flow properties because an efficient mixing step is essential to the success of impregnation in general, and to achieving homogeneous distribution of the API in particular. In addition, as mentioned, the particle size distribution of the porous carrier is a critical property in impregnation. The particle size distribution has an impact on blend and content uniformity, which are very important (critical) quality attributes used in making release decisions of the finished product. In order to avoid segregation and poor content uniformity of the finished pharmaceutical product, the particle size distribution of the porous carrier should be narrow. Also, because in impregnation, we need to dissolve the API in volatile organic solvents, the porous carrier should be insoluble in such solvents. If the porous carrier is soluble in the organic solvents used in the process, this will damage or destroy the internal structure of these carriers and also result in carrier granulation. Moreover, the porous carriers should be stable during the impregnation process. If the carrier is soluble in the API solvent, it is possible to use solvents saturated with the carrier material, but this adds a significant level of complexity, including, for example, a need for very accurate temperature control. Porous carriers are also exposed to shear and attrition during the process, and potentially to elevated temperature. Thus, they should be stable under these conditions. For all of these reasons, preserving the original particle size distribution (PSD) of the carrier is essential to the success of the impregnation process.

5.3.2 API Properties and Solvent Selection

The API used in impregnation should possess three main properties: it should be stable under relevant experimental conditions, it should be soluble to a significant extent in the selected solvent, and it should not react with the solvent, the carrier, or any impurities therein. As mentioned previously, the impregnation process includes some potentially harsh conditions such as elevated temperature and process attrition. The API should be physically and chemically stable under these conditions. For instance, if the API is heat labile, and the solvent has low vapor pressure, the high temperature needed to evaporate the solvent may decompose the API; such a condition should be avoided by selecting a different solvent. Also, the API should have a relatively high solubility in the selected organic solvent; the key element (and a factor limiting drug loading) in impregnation is dissolving the required amount of drug in a suitable amount of solvent and then spraying the solution onto a porous carrier. Finally, the API should be inert in the solvent and also when combined with the porous carrier. If there is any possible chemical interaction between the carrier and the API, such a carrier should be excluded from the process.

5.4 Continuous Impregnation

While many industries such as petrochemicals, catalysts, and food manufacturing transitioned large fractions of their production processes to continuous manufacturing (CM) procedures decades ago, the pharmaceutical industry still depends predominantly on conventional batch manufacturing processes, especially in the generic and OTC sectors. The delay in implementing CM processes is partly due to rigid regulatory rules that make it difficult in many countries to modify a process once it has been approved, partly due to the industry's conservative attitude toward new manufacturing technologies, and partly also to the lack of familiarity of many pharmaceutical companies with engineering-intensive processes such as continuous manufacturing. Until about 15 years ago, this led to a decades-long "freeze" of the process development toolbox in pharmaceutical manufacturing [33, 34]. However, batch manufacturing is not an efficient approach for either manufacturing or development of pharmaceuticals. Batch manufacturing methods require many sequential manufacturing steps and necessitate complex, expensive, and risky scale-up studies [35].

In recent years, large efforts have been devoted to finding alternative processes that are feasible, efficient, and robust. Continuous processes can be considered a useful and efficient approach for developing and optimizing pharmaceutical manufacturing and it has recently attracted substantial interest from both industry and regulatory authorities [36–40]. CM has many advantages, including reproducibility, faster development, lower operating cost, robustness, enhanced quality, reduced footprint, and better observability [35]. Accordingly, the USFDA has characterized CM as an emerging technology [40–44]. Recently, six drug manufacturing processes depending on CM methods have been approved in the USA by FDA and many others are expected in the coming years [45]; additional products have also been approved in other jurisdictions. Furthermore, process analytical technologies (PAT) and closed-loop quality control can be more easily implemented for the purposes of in-line process monitoring and real-time quality assurance [46, 47].

A continuous impregnation process refers to the continuous addition of a drug solution into a porous carrier flowing along a continuous "contactor" (e.g., a continuous blender). In this process, the drug solution quickly contacts the porous carrier and uniformly impregnated material is generated.

To get a successful continuous impregnation process, the time window for impregnation should be much shorter than for a batch process. In the batch process, there is a set amount of material and solution that needs to be sprayed over time onto a set amount of carrier. In the continuous process, the powder constantly moves through the system; therefore, the solution addition rate needs to be adjusted to be in a fixed proportion to the carrier mass flow rate to reach the desired fixed ratio of API impregnated in the porous material. That is why in a continuous impregnation process, it is important to adjust the carrier mass flow rate and the corresponding API spraying rate to enable the desired mean residence time in the blender. A residence time that is too long will decrease productivity, while a residence time that is too short will fail to achieve a uniform API-to-carrier mass ratio.

Also, it is important to determine the maximum allowed spray rate that will avoid carrier agglomeration. This step depends highly on the properties of the porous carrier, the throughput of the material, and the process parameters. Therefore, it is essential to choose the porous carriers according to the desired impregnated carrier properties, which were mentioned early in Section 5.3.1 of this chapter. The required devices and process set up to achieve successful continuous impregnation will be discussed below.

5.4.1 Requirements of Continuous Processing and Online Testing Equipment

To enhance the manufacturing of impregnated products, the most important characteristic of the impregnation device is providing good mixing. The resulting API "blend homogeneity", and the consequential "content uniformity", are very important criteria for regulatory agencies. To achieve them, the API should be uniformly distributed within the entire blend and between the final solid dosage forms. In order to get a uniform composition of product units, the "contactor" should provide efficient mixing of the porous carrier and the API solution. In continuous impregnation, four main devices are required to achieve this goal: a weight-in loss feeder for the carrier, an accurate pump for the solution, a contactor that is an efficient mixer, providing enough shear to disperse the solution and any wet lumps that might form in the contactor, and NIR spectroscopy to monitor blend composition. The overall equipment arrangement is used in Figure 5.1. A Case Study is presented next.

5.4.1.1 A Suitable Gravimetric Feeder for the Carrier: The K-Tron KT20

A K-Tron KT20 (Coperion K-Tron Pitman Inc., NJ) loss-in-weight feeder configured with a pair of twin coarse-concave screws was used to dispense material at a controlled mass flow rate. The KT20 loss-in-weight feeder consists of three parts: a volumetric feeder, a weighing platform, and a gravimetric controller. The controller adjusts the screw speed based on the feedback from the load cell, which records weight change over time of the material in the hopper. The first step is to take the feeder and calibrate it with standard weights. Next, the powder is loaded into the hopper and a "feed-factor" (e.g., capacity) calibration is performed according to the K-Tron protocol, to determine the maximum mass flow for the

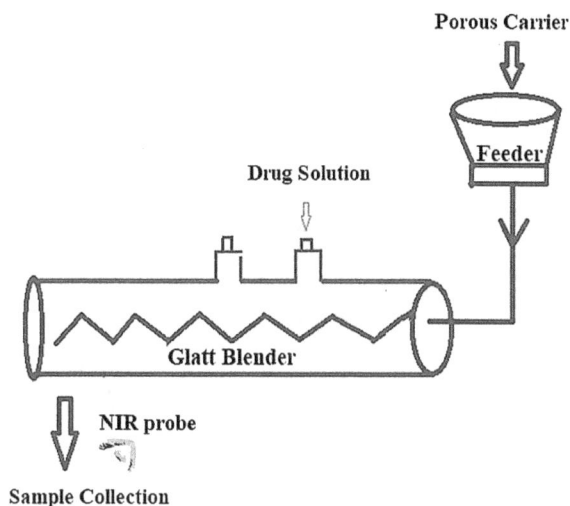

FIGURE 5.1 Continuous Impregnation Set Up displaying the gravimetric feeder, the continuous blender, and the location of the NIR probe.

given material, screw size, and screw configuration. Subsequently, when a mass flow rate set-point is inputted, the feeder determines an initial screw speed based on the ratio between the given set point and the feed factor. The gravimetric controller then adjusts this initial screw speed as necessary to dispense the specified mass flow rate. The accuracy of the instantaneous mass flow rate can be confirmed using a catch scale, and equipment settings can be adjusted if necessary.

5.4.1.2 A Useful Continuous Contactor: The Glatt Continuous Powder Mixer

A modified continuous blender, **the** Glatt GCG-70 **continuous powder mixer,** which is also commonly utilized in continuous dry blending applications, was used to elicit rapid dispersion of the solution onto the carrier particles. This blender is supplied with a nozzle and a peristaltic pump for spraying the API solution so that ingredients are mixed and impregnated simultaneously as they flow along the tubular mixer. The loss-in-weight feeder is used to accurately dispense the host particles, which flowed to the continuous blender. The impregnation step occurs in the continuous blender, after which the powder falls into a transition vibratory feeder where the NIR probe scans the powder bed to monitor API loading.

The continuous blender applies enough shear and achieves excellent mixing performance. Figure 5.2 shows the blender tube. The transparent section allows the view of the impeller. The rightmost port on top of the mixer displays the entry point of the powder ingredient(s), in this case, the porous carrier. The third port from the right displays the pipe dispensing the API solution. The leftmost port shows the discharge of the impregnated carrier onto the subsequent processing step. The discharge port is at an angle to ensure sufficient residence time of the mixture in the blender.

The unit was set up with a 1/3-1/3-1/3 forward-alternating-forward blade configuration originally developed by our group at Rutgers University [35]. The first eight paddles and the last eight paddles all were angled in the forward direction to convey the powder forward through the process. The middle eight blades were angled in an alternating forward and backward direction, creating a back-mixing zone where most of the blender hold-up is located. This blade configuration was fixed throughout all the experiments discussed here. Figure 5.3 illustrates the blending shaft with the blades in the described arrangement.

5.4.1.3 An Efficient ONLINE Monitoring Tool: The Matrix NIR Spectrometer

An FT-NIR (near infrared) Matrix spectrometer (Bruker Optics, Billerica, MA, USA) is a process analyzer often utilized for spectral acquisition in continuous pharmaceutical processes. Keeping the NIR

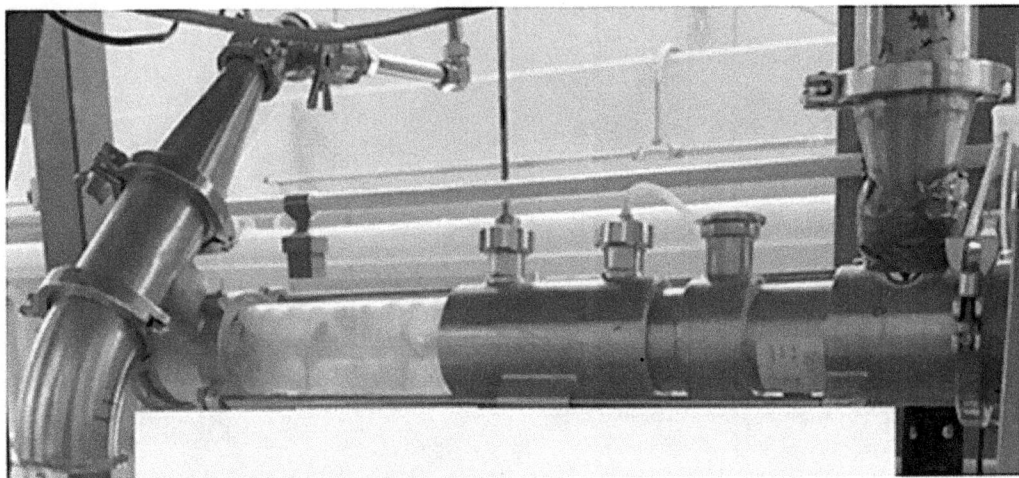

FIGURE 5.2   The continuous blender tube (Glatt GCG-70).

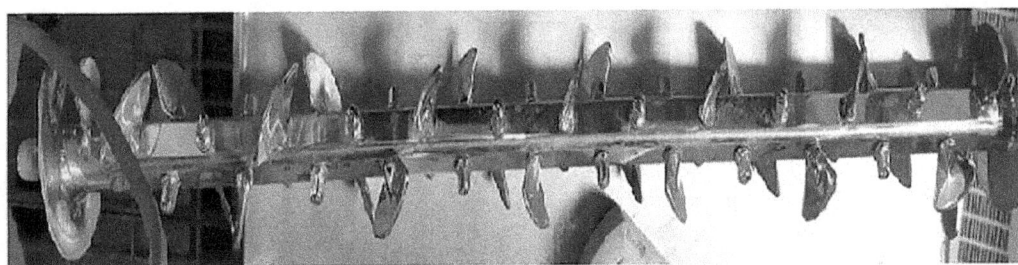

FIGURE 5.3   The blending shaft of the continuous blender.

device at a fixed distance to the flowing powder is crucial to obtaining reproducible data, minimizing sampling errors, and allowing all portions of the flowing powder to have the same probability of being analyzed [48]. In the data discussed below, the OPUS 7.0 software from Bruker is used to control the NIR instrument and construct the calibration models. Figure 5.4 shows an example of the NIR instrument setup, which included a vibratory feeder that transports the impregnated carrier continuously with no interference of the instrument on the material flow.

This near-infrared (NIR) spectroscopy setup can be utilized to measure critical characteristics, including the relative standard deviation (RSD) of the drug content and the residence time distribution (RTD) of the material in the contactor and to monitor. In an RTD study, a tracer pulse of high-contrast material is introduced into the system at the desired point, and it is measured as it leaves the system, enabling the determination of residence time, back-mixing capacity, presence and extent of dead zones, and other important phenomena. The use of online real-time measurements has many advantages. For instance, it can provide accurate and precise data while the experimental runs are occurring. It provides instantaneous and clear knowledge of when the tracer pulse starts exiting the system to when it has fully exited the blender, which allows the experimenter to determine when to conduct the next experiment [49–52]. Since NIRs acquisition is fast and does not require any sample preparation, it is an optimal approach to obtaining inline data acquisition. Furthermore, NIR spectroscopy is flexible enough to detect the concentration of a tracer in the liquid phase.

Another interesting application of inline NIR spectroscopy is evaluating the blend uniformity of the impregnated products. To evaluate the quality of mixing (mixing performance) over time, the relative standard deviation (RSD) of the API content in the impregnated product should be computed. Once the powder flow reached a steady state, the drug solution should constantly pump into the blender and be

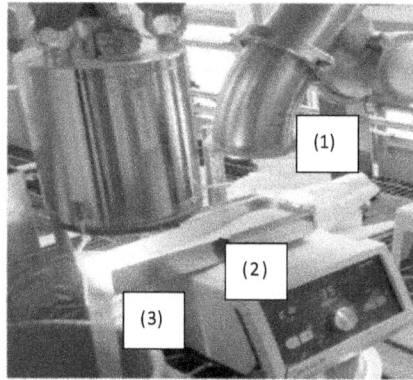

FIGURE 5.4 Bruker NIR instrument set up, displaying the blender discharge (1), the vibratory feeder (2), and the data acquisition zone (3).

allowed to reach the steady state. When the steady state is achieved by observing constant NIR readings, it can be concluded that NIR spectra have been collected over the course of the entire run. The average API concentration should be calculated along with the standard deviation. The RSD can then be calculated as the ratio of the standard deviation over the average of the data set.

In this case study, some impregnation experiments were conducted to monitor content homogeneity of carrier exiting the continuous blender using Neusilin US2 as a host material and Ibuprofen in methanol (IBU solution) as a drug solution. In these experiments, the pumping rate was 25 ml/min, the feeding rate was 50 g/min, and the blender was operated at 150 and 300 rpm. In the beginning, the host material (NEU) was fed until reaching the steady state mass flow rate, which was determined by monitoring the weight vs. time of the material exiting the blender. Then, the IBU solution was pumped and monitored until it reached a steady state. After that, 100 NIR spectra were collected for each experiment. These spectra were analyzed to predict the IBU amount at the steady state (as shown in Figure 5.5 and Table 5.1).

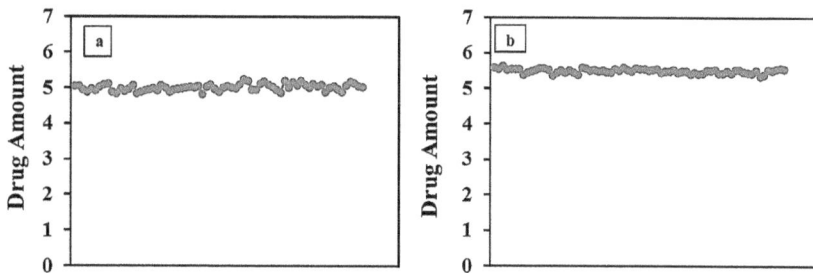

FIGURE 5.5 Measuring %RSD of Ibuprofen impregnated onto a NEU host carrier in a continuous blender (Glatt GCG-70) operated at (a) 150 rpm and (b) 300 rpm.

TABLE 5.1

Drug Loading and RSD Values of Ibuprofen Impregnated Products Using Neusilin US2 as a Host Carrier

Carrier	Blender RPM	Drug Loading*	%RSD
NEU	150	5.01	1.89
	300	5.59	1.11

Note: Other experimental conditions: Feeding rate: 3 Kg/h and 25 gm/ml pumping rate.
*Gram of IBU in 50-gram carrier.

In both cases, the RSD% values were very low (equal to or less than 2.5%), which indicates that the impregnated products showed very good homogeneity. These results demonstrate that impregnation of API in a porous carrier can result in highly homogenous products [16, 17, 53].

Figure 5.5 demonstrates the schematic setup used for continuous impregnation.

5.5 Chapter Summary

Impregnation is the loading of drugs into porous carriers using a suitable solvent as a transporter. In impregnation, some unit operations, which are required for regular manufacturing routes, are excluded. Therefore, impregnation simplifies and shortens the development of pharmaceutical products. Using a continuous blender allows the impregnation process to occur much quicker with more control than using a batch device. Successful continuous impregnation requires a thorough understanding of a diverse array of factors including physical and chemical properties of drugs, solvent properties, porous carriers' properties, blender selection and characterization, and process parameters.

REFERENCES

1. Nickerson B. Sample preparation of pharmaceutical dosage forms: Challenges and strategies for sample preparation and extraction. *Am Assoc Pharm Sci* 2011; 145. doi:10.1007/978-1-4419-9631-2.
2. Oka S, Sahay A, Meng W, Muzzio F. Diminished segregation in continuous powder mixing. *Powder Technol* 2017; *309*:79–88.
3. Oka S, Smrčka D, Kataria A, Emady H, Muzzio F, Štěpánek F, et al. Analysis of the origins of content non-uniformity in high-shear wet granulation. *Int J Pharm* 2017;*528*(1–2):578–85.
4. FDA. *Guidance for Industry: Powder Blends and Finished Dosage Units – Stratified In-Process Dosage Unit Sampling and Assessment*; 2003.
5. Zheng J. *Formulation and Analytical Development for Low-Dose Oral Drug Products*. Hoboken: John Wiley & Sons, Inc.;2009.
6. Cartilier LH, Moës AJ. Effect of drug agglomerates upon the kinetics of mixing of low dosage cohesive powder mixtures. *Drug Dev Ind Pharm* 1989;*15*(12):1911–31.
7. Prescott JK, Garcia TP. A solid dosage and blend content uniformity troubleshooting diagram. *Pharm Technol* 2001;*25*(3):68–88.
8. Sahay N, Ierapetritou M. Nihar SCM. *IFAC Proceeding*;2009;7(PART 1):405–10.
9. Huang CY, Sherry Ku M. Prediction of drug particle size and content uniformity in low-dose solid dosage forms. *Int J Pharm* 2010;*383*(1–2):70–80.
10. Saffari M, Ebrahimi A, Langrish T. A novel formulation for solubility and content uniformity enhancement of poorly water-soluble drugs using highly porous mannitol. *Eur J Pharm Sci* 2016;*83*: 52–61.
11. Amidon GL, Lennernäs H, Shah VP, Crison JR. A theoretical basis for a biopharmaceutic drug classification: The correlation of in vitro drug product dissolution and in vivo bioavailability. *Pharm Res* 1995;*12*(3):413–20.
12. Rodriguez Aller MR, Guillarme D, Veuthey J-L, Gurny R. Strategies for formulating and delivering poorly water-soluble drugs. *J Drug Deliv Sci Technol* 2015;*30*: 342–51.
13. Di L, Kerns EH, Carter GT. Drug-like property concepts in pharmaceutical design. *Curr Pharm Des* 2009;*15*(19):2184–94.
14. Takagi T, Ramachandran C, Bermejo M, Yamashita S, Yu LX, Amidon GL. A provisional biopharmaceutical classification of the top 200 oral drug products in the United States, Great Britain, Spain, and Japan. *Mol Pharm* 2006;*3*(6):631–43.
15. Chester AW, Kowalski JA, Coles ME Muegge EL, Muzzio FJ, Brone D. Mixing dynamics in catalyst impregnation in double-cone blenders. *Powder Technol* 1999;*102*:85–94.
16. Grigorov PI, Glasser BJ, Muzzio FJ. Formulation and manufacture of pharmaceuticals by fluidized-bed impregnation of active pharmaceutical ingredients into porous carriers. *AIChE J* 2013;*59*(12):4538–52.
17. Omar TA, Oka S, Muzzio FJ, Glasser BJ. Manufacturing of pharmaceuticals by impregnation of an active pharmaceutical ingredient into a mesoporous carrier: Impact of solvent and loading. *J Pharm Innov* 2019;*14*:194–205.

18. Jang DJ, Sim T, Oh E. Formulation and optimization of spray-dried amlodipine solid dispersion for enhanced oral absorption. *Drug Dev Ind Pharm* 2013;*39*(7):1133–41.

19. Fei Y, Kostewicz ES, Sheu MT, Dressman JB. Analysis of the enhanced oral bioavailability of fenofibrate lipid formulations in fasted humans using in vitro-in silico-in vivo approach. *Eur J Pharm Biopharm* 2013;*85*(3 PART B):1274–84.

20. Maniruzzaman M, Rana MM, Boateng JS, Mitchell JC, Douroumis D. Dissolution enhancement of poorly water-soluble APIs processed by hot-melt extrusion using hydrophilic polymers. *Drug Dev Ind Pharm* 2013;*39*(2):218–27.

21. Ahern RJ, Hanrahan JP, Tobin JM, Ryan KB, Crean AM. Comparison of fenofibrate-mesoporous silica drug-loading processes for enhanced drug delivery. *Eur J Pharm Sci* 2013;*50*(3–4):400–9.

22. Savjani KT, Gajjar AK, Savjani JK. Drug solubility: Importance and enhancement techniques. *ISRN Pharmaceutics* 2012; 195727. doi:10.5402/2012/195727.

23. Joshi JT. A Review on micronization techniques. *J Pharm Sci Technol* 2011;*3*(7):651–81.

24. Bora Pk. A review on solid dispersion. *Indian Res J Pharm Sci* 2012;*1*(12):1–9.

25. Vallet-Regi M, Rámila A, Del Real RP, Pérez-Pariente J. A new property of MCM-41: *Drug delivery system*. *Chem Mater* 2001;*13*(2):308–11.

26. Mallick S, Pattnaik S, Swain K, De PK, Saha A, Ghoshal G, Mondal A. Formation of physically stable amorphous phase of ibuprofen by solid state milling with kaolin. *Eur J Pharm Biopharm* 2008;*68*:346–51.

27. Van Speybroeck M, Barillaro V, Do Thi T, Mellaerts R, Martens J, Van Humbeeck J, Vermant J, Annaert P, Van Den Mooter G, Augustijns P. Ordered mesoporous silica material SBA-15: A broad-spectrum formulation platform for poorly soluble drugs. *J Pharm Sci* 2009;*98*(8):2648–58.

28. Bahl D, Hudak J, Bogner RH. Comparison of the ability of various pharmaceutical silicates to amorphize and enhance dissolution of indomethacin upon co-grinding. *Pharm Dev Technol* 2008;*13*(3):255–69.

29. Mellaerts R, Mols R, Jammaer JAG, Aerts CA, Annaert P, Van Humbeeck J, et al. Increasing the oral bio-availability of the poorly water-soluble drug itraconazole with ordered mesoporous silica. *Eur J Pharm Biopharm* 2008;*69*(1):223–30.

30. Meer T, Fule R, Khanna D, Amin P. Solubility modulation of bicalutamide using porous silica. *J Pharm Investig* 2013;*43*(4):279–85.

31. Maniruzzaman M, Ross SA, Islam MT, Scoutaris N, Nair A, Douroumis D. Increased dissolution rates of tranilast solid dispersions extruded with inorganic excipients. *Drug Dev Ind Pharm* 2017;*43*(6):947–57.

32. Grigorov PI, Glasser BJ, Muzzio FJ. Improving dissolution kinetics of pharmaceuticals by fluidized bed impregnation of active pharmaceutical ingredients. *AIChE J* 2016;*62*(12):4201–14.

33. Engisch W, Muzzio F. Using residence time distributions (RTDs) to address the traceability of raw materials in continuous pharmaceutical manufacturing *J. Pharm Innov* 2016;*11*(1):64–81.

34. Abboud L, SHSR of TWSJ. New prescription for drug makers: Update the plants. *Wall St J* 2003.

35. Vanarase AU, Muzzio FJ. Effect of operating conditions and design parameters in a continuous powder mixer. *Powder Technol* 2011;*208*(1):26–36.

36. Poechlauer P, Manley J, Broxterman R, Ridemark M. Continuous processing in the manufacture of active pharmaceutical ingredients and finished dosage forms: An industry perspective. *Org Process Res Dev* 2012;*16*:1586–1590.

37. Leuenberger H. New trends in the production of pharmaceutical granules: Batch versus continuous processing. *Eur J Pharm Biopharm* 2001;*52*:279–88.

38. Betz G, Junker-Bürgin P, Leuenberger H. Batch and continuous processing in the production of pharmaceutical granules. *Pharm Dev Technol* 2003;*8*(3):289–97.

39. Warman M. Continuous processing in secondary production. *Chem Eng Pharm Ind RD Manuf* 2011;837–851. doi:10.1002/9780470882221.CH43

40. Chatterjee S. *Perspective on continuous manufacturing*. IFPAC Annual Meeting, Baltimore, MD;2012.

41. Yu LX, Kopcha M. The future of pharmaceutical quality and the path to get there. *Int J Pharm* 2017;*528*(1–2):354–9.

42. Lee SL, Connor TFO, Yang X, Cruz CN, Yu LX, Woodcock J. Modernizing pharmaceutical manufacturing: From batch to continuous production. *J Pharm Innov* 2015;*10*(3):191–9.

43. Allison G, Cain YT, Cooney C, Garcia T, Bizjak TG, Holte O, et al. Regulatory and quality considerations for continuous manufacturing May 20–21, 2014 continuous manufacturing symposium. *J Pharm Sci* 2015;*104*(3):803–12.

44. O'Connor T, Lee S. Chapter37 – Emerging Technology for Modernizing Pharmaceutical Production: Continuous Manufacturing, Qiu Y Chen Y, Zhang GG, Yu L, Mantri RV (eds.). *Developing Solid Oral Dosage Forms*. 2nd ed. Boston, MA: Academic Press;2017:1031–1046.
45. Escotet-Espinoza MS, Moghtadernejad S, Oka S, Wang Y, Roman-Ospino A, Schäfer E, et al. Effect of tracer material properties on the residence time distribution (RTD) of continuous powder blending operations. Part I of II: Experimental evaluation. *Powder Technol* 2019;*342*:744–63.
46. Maniruzzaman M, Nair A, Scoutaris N, Bradley MSA, Snowden MJ, Douroumis D. One-step continuous extrusion process for the manufacturing of solid dispersions. *Int J Pharm* 2015;*496*(1):42–51
47. Tiwari RV, Patil H, Repka MA. Contribution of hot-melt extrusion technology to advance drug delivery in the 21st century. *Expert Opin Drug Deliv* 2016;*13*(3):451–64.
48. Esbensen KH, Paasch-Mortensen P. *Process Sampling: Theory of Sampling – The Missing Link in Process Analytical Technologies (PAT)*. *Process Analytical Technology*. John Wiley & Sons, Ltd.;2010:37–80.
49. Sekulic SS, Ward HW, Brannegan DR, Stanley ED, Evans CL, Sciavolino ST, et al. On-line monitoring of powder blend homogeneity by near-infrared spectroscopy. *Anal Chem* 1996;*68*(3):509–13.
50. Shi Z, Cogdill RP, Short SM, Anderson CA. Process characterization of powder blending by near-infrared spectroscopy: Blend endpoints and beyond. *J Pharm Biomed Anal* 2008;*47*(4–5):738–45.
51. Popo M, Romero-Torres S, Conde C, Romañach RJ. Blend uniformity analysis using stream sampling and near infrared spectroscopy. *AAPS Pharm Sci Tech* 2002;*3*(3):1–11.
52. Rantanen J, Wikström H, Turner R, Taylor LS. Use of in-line near-infrared spectroscopy in combination with chemometrics for improved understanding of pharmaceutical processes. *Anal Chem* 2005;*77*(2):556–63.
53. Muzzio FJ, Glasser BJ, Omar TA. Continuous Processes for Manufacturing Impregnated Porous Carriers and for Manufacturing Pharmaceuticals Containing Impregnated Porous Carriers (WO 2021/126829-A1). World Intellectual Property Organization International Bureau; 2021.

6

Leveraging a Mini-Batchwise Continuous Direct Compression (CDC) Approach to Optimize Efficiency in Process Development, On-Demand Manufacturing, and Continuous Process Verification (CPV)

Martin Warman, Patrick M. Piccione, and Reto Maurer
Pharmaceutical R&D, F. Hoffmann-La Roche AG, Basel, Switzerland
University of Strathclyde, UK

CONTENTS

DOI: 10.1201/9781003149835-7

6.1 Introduction

6.1.1 Definitions

Because of the novel status of mini-batch processing, there is not yet a common source of definitions. The following are provided to give a good basis and context for this chapter.

Continuous unit operation: An operation where the material is introduced at the same rate as the material is being removed. For example, a feeder dosing at a constant flow rate; a horizontal blender where input equals output rate; tablet compression; or spray drying.

Batch feeding: An operation where a desired mass of material is dispensed within a given time window. By using multiple batch feeders, several individual, pre-mixed, or co-processed materials can be added to a batch blender.

Batch blending: An operation where individual components are mixed to achieve the desired uniformity. Typically, the controlled process parameters are fill mass and speed, to deliver uniformity within a time window because the blending process is controlled to ensure the entire mass within the blender has uniform character. This means, typically an individual blend operation produces tablets of a single batch – hence the term batch blending. However, by repeating batch blending, it is possible to feed materials to a continuous unit operation. For example, repeated batch blending can feed a tablet compression operation, provided the refill rate of the press inlet hopper matches that of the input/output rate of the press. In this case, additional controls will need to be applied to ensure each repeating blend operation is uniform, that is, we need uniformity between and as well as within each blend operation.

Mini-batch blender (MBB): A variation on the concept of batch blending, whereby the size of each batch is reduced to minimize the mass of material 'in-process' and therefore reduce the impacts of segregation, caused by variability in physical properties of the in-process materials, large mass transfers, and the impact of the environment (such as vibration) on the materials held in process. Because of the reduced scale, it is possible to have higher accuracy and precision around control of quality attributes such as blend assay, intra-blend uniformity, and inter-blend uniformity. This means that not only one can ensure quality attributes of a single mini-batch, but also between mini-batches, thus ensuring the uniform character of all the mini-batches that go to make up the batch. Because of the pulsing nature of material transfers, typically, the downstream process of the MBB includes a 'surge capacity' (see explanation below). This also means that the DSp (the approved operating range of the process, but also the operating range demonstrated to give a product with acceptable quality attributes), needs to include the impact of changing levels in the surge capacity. Although in CM, one tends to think in terms of scaling out in time, rather than scaling up in terms of size of unit operations, we cannot forget the impact of factors such as changing levels in the system even if the line rate is kept constant.

Surge capacity: The buffer capacity needed to receive the incoming mass, and provide input to feed a continuous operation. As an example, if the mini-batch mass is 1 kg and a dispensing/blending/discharge cycle takes 6 minutes, the surge capacity of a tablet press will fluctuate depending on the transfer time of that 1 kg from the blender. It will typically be at the low level immediately before a new mini-batch arrives, and go to the high level when the mini-batch has been fully transferred (level control). The time taken to process the powder mass through the press equals the rate at which the mini-batch is produced. In the example given, 1 kg/6 min through both the press and MMB – which means the overall line runs at 10 kg/hr.

Continuous manufacturing (CM): An overall manufacturing line consisting of two, or more, unit operations. For example, a batch dispensing feeder/MBB/tablet press is described as a CM process even though it consists of two batch unit operations feeding a continuous operation. The press runs continuously because of the rate of feeding/blending and the surge capacity of the press inlet.

Start-up phase: The period of time taken to reach a point when the process is making a product of conforming quality. Quantitative characterizations of this concept include the residence time (how long it takes materials to reach that location in the process) and the residence time distribution (RTD; leading to the amount of intermixing that has occurred with adjustment materials to reaching that location).

Shut-down phase: The period of time taken to empty the line (therefore sometimes called 'line empty'). This is the time taken for the final unit operation to stop making conforming products after the feeding of materials into the overall process stops.

CM yield: In the case of CM, yield is defined as the total accumulated mass of conforming materials as a percentage of the total mass input. It can be calculated as the difference between the total mass input and the sum of the mass remaining in the equipment at the end of shut-down, and any mass removed as non-conforming, divided by the total mass input.

Intermixing: When running CM, the entirety of the process does not go through the same transformations, at the same time. This means the material 'in process' experiences its own, unique, process history. Intermixing describes what happens at the boundaries of adjacent process material. To give two examples, if two discrete plugs of material have gone through the MBB, those two plugs will be unique, but it is possible for mixing to occur at the boundaries of those plugs when they come in contact. This would cause the material in that 'mixed-zone' to have a mixture of the properties of the individual plugs. Critical in this example is that the two plugs (or the remainder of the mini-batches, which will make up the batch) have fully mixed, the mixing is only at the boundary. The situation is much more complex with continuous processes, as not only is the process history changing constantly, but also many of the process steps rely on the subsequent steps to achieve the final product quality attributes. So, for example, the feeders are attempting to achieve a constant dosing rate, but there is a fluctuation in rate. This means the blender not only tries to achieve perfect mixing of what has been dosed, but also minimizes any fluctuations in dose rate during the period of dosing. This means intermixing, in continuous processes, is not only a consequence of the process, but is actually used to achieve the desired product quality. Because of the complex nature of intermixing in continuous processes, it is typical to take longer to respond to control decisions and require process models (residence time, RTD, and mass flow predictions based on process data) to provide material tracking.

6.1.2 Background and Driving Forces

6.1.2.1 Historical Challenges

The introduction of continuous manufacturing (CM) can be described as the third wave in the application of manufacturing science within the pharmaceutical industry. Prior to the launch of the FDA 21st Century Quality Initiative in Sept 2004, the pharmaceutical industry strived to prevent material with non-confirming specifications from reaching patients (Miggliaccio, 2004) after manufacturing. At that time, pharmaceutical quality systems (PQS) were built on sampling/testing regimes that themselves were laid out in regional pharmacopeia (such as United States Pharmacopeia (USP) and European Pharmacopeia (EP)). These strategies/approaches were focused on demonstrating compliance through testing rather than preventing their manufacture. An important process metric is the process capability index (*Cpk*). *Cpk* is a metric of how centered and variable a process is in relationship to the specification limits. A low

Cpk (under 1.0) shows that either the process variance and/or the process mean is not within the requirements of the specifications. Closer observation of the manufacturing processes at that time, revealed that it was common to have values of less than 1.0, and an average standard deviation of a normal distribution (sigma) level of ~2.8. This translated to an average 20% defect rate.

At the time, many causes were suggested for this poor process performance, with the largest suspect being the limited previous experience of operating at a commercial scale. Often commercial processes had only operated at full scale during process validation (PV). However, PV was deemed successful if able to operate at a commercial scale three times (often called 'three batch validation'), whilst making a product of acceptable quality. The only other previous experience was at a smaller scale, after which so-called scaling factors were applied to claim equivalency to commercial operations. Furthermore, these earlier development activities were not designed or intended to establish the causes of variability in product quality.

Combined, the previous practices around process development and validation led to a lack of understanding of the typical extent and causes of variability. This would only be seen once a product went into commercial manufacturing. It also posed the question, "what is the true product performance?". Quality was being seen by the testing regimes employed – but were the testing regimes not seeing variability because they were simply not looking?

6.1.2.2 *The Emergence of QbD and PAT*

The challenges above led to the FDA Guidance for Industry: PAT – A Framework for Innovative Pharmaceutical Development, Manufacturing, and Quality Assurance, Sept 2004. This guide laid out the concept of using PAT (later defined as a "system for designing, analyzing, and controlling manufacturing through timely measurements of critical quality and performance attributes of raw and in-process materials and processes with the goal of ensuring final product quality" (ICH Q8 (R2), 2014).

The introduction of PAT itself caused a conundrum. When applied to existing (i.e., already approved) products, it could uncover variabilities that had not previously been seen. Therefore, the Guidance specifically added a requirement that the application of PAT to legacy products be managed under the sites' PQS. This requirement included a justification for the implementation, even if used for process development (R&D) purposes. This barrier to adoption for legacy products resulted in PAT use being focused on process development. In particular, there was a focus on the application of PAT during Design of Experiments (DoE), to help establish the correlations between process parameters and product attributes. Those process parameters that need to be controlled in order to ensure product quality were named critical process parameters (CPP), and the attributes that describe the product performance were named critical quality attributes (CQA). Data generated by PAT systems were also used to help set the action and control limits, which act as thresholds for preventing non-conforming material to be manufactured. The application of PAT to legacy products became limited to 'root-cause analysis', often triggered as part of investigations into low process capability, or as part of a deviation investigation. If an existing process was staying within a state of control (i.e., manufacturing a product with acceptable specifications), it was challenging to justify the use of PAT. Why attempt to improve quality, when the quality being achieved was 'good enough'? This is in contrast to other industry sectors where there is a threshold of acceptable quality, but also where further increases in quality have additional value.

To place greater importance on using PAT to establish process understanding, further initiatives such as Quality by Design (QbD) were launched, and backed-up by regulatory guidance. The FDA whitepaper, Pharmaceutical cGMPs For The 21st Century – A Risk-Based Approach) added expectations around process development. In addition, expectations were changed around PV activity, with the publication of FDA's Guidance for Industry: Process Validation: General Principles and Practices.

This new guide included the concept of three stages for PV, and for the first time highlighted the importance of Process Design (PD, stage 1), Process Performance Qualification (PPQ, stage 2), and Process Monitoring (PM, stage 3) (Figure 6.13).

PD builds and captures process knowledge and understanding, and also establishes a control strategy. The process control may consist of both parametric and DSp control, but the control strategy also confirms that the quality attributes stay within acceptable limits. PPQ demonstrates that the process can be operated in a state of control (i.e., a demonstration that the control strategy ensures product quality). PM describes that the programs are in place to maintain process understanding as well as trend process performance going forward as part of a continued process verification (CPV) program. CPV is also known by alternate names, such as "ongoing process verification", in other regions/by other health authorities.

Critically, the QbD initiative introduced a requirement to build/maintain process understanding at a scale that is truly representative of commercial production. Furthermore, this process understanding needs to be captured across the process space in which we would like to operate (and seek to get approval for in the filing). This approved process space, now better known as Design Space (DSp), needs to be confirmed by running experiments at a commercially representative scale, and across the intended operating range. This introduces the requirement to run DoE campaigns at a commercial scale. These campaigns, often called Design Space Confirmation (DSC) or Control Strategy Confirmation (CSC) runs, are executed at a point in the product lifecycle when large amounts of API are not typically available. At this point, the API will still be a development molecule, and still be extremely expensive.

To illustrate this impact, the following theoretical example will be used: *formulation*: a direct compression (DC) formulation, with an API concentration of 20%, and 80% excipients (of which 1% is the lubricant); *intended commercial batch size*: 1000 kg. In order to execute a DSC for a batch commercial process (assuming a 1000 kg batch size), an API- sparing DSC design would require 6 data points + center point. These seven conditions lead to an API consumption of $7 \times 1000 \times 20\% = 1400$ kg. In phase III development, a typical small molecule API costs approximately \$10,000/kg. This means the API costs alone would be around \$14M to execute the DSC above. In addition, it is not typical to have 1400 kg of API available until the drug substance (DS) process is finalized so that the API is in commercial production. This challenge led to a similar barrier to implementation seen with PAT. Everyone accepted QbD as an excellent concept but in many cases, the approach was not viable, because of the cost or availability of API.

The conundrum was worsened by the requirement that the registration stability batches be executed during the commercial process. Often the commercial process is only confirmed after the DSC runs. Samples from those runs are put up on stability testing, meaning confirmation of the pivotal stability batches may not come until 12 months after DSC. This means that although QbD approaches may result in much-improved process understanding and higher process robustness/*Cpk* than for batch processes, they take much longer to achieve approval. Therefore, neither the use of PAT nor QbD could be mandated, only encouraged by the health authorities.

6.1.2.3 CM as a Third Wave of the FDA 21st-Century Quality Initiative

Once CM (concepts) started to be demonstrated around 2004, innovator companies readily engaged in pilot programs. These programs investigated linking together several continuous unit operations (feeding, blending, granulation, and compression) in order to transform starting materials into medicines. Interestingly, even at this early time, it was recognized that small-scale batch unit operations could be run in a repeating batchwise mode. Many early CM examples were wet granulations using segmented/small batch fluidized bed drying, in which small discrete masses of wet granulate are dried. By loading a mass into the cell of the dryer, and then advancing through multiple drying phases before discharging, a significant drying time could be generated for each individual cell and the cells had overlapping drying profiles. Each of these dried masses was then passed to repeating small-scale batch (often now called mini-batch) blending operations. This allows the drying and blending step to have the same line rate as the downstream continuous unit operations, that is, tablet compression.

The introduction of CM is seen as a third wave of quality innovation (following PAT and then QbD), but why is it seen as being a game-changer? Simply because the process (including process dynamics) and equipment can be the same as later commercial manufacturing. Because with CM one can scale out in time (run for longer) not scale up (mass of material being processed), one finds equivalent process setpoints (DSp), the same quality attributes, and equivalent material transfers. As a direct consequence, the mid-development program (phase IIb) can be truly representative of the commercial process. Once the initial start-up phase (identical to the commercial process) has passed, the material being manufactured conforms to specifications and is the same as the material made by the commercial process. Furthermore, if the early unit operations (feeding and blending) operate in discrete plug flow (and so no intermixing with adjacent material occurs), the operation of standalone units is representative of the integrated unit operation. This means the final composition, manufacturing process, and control strategy can be developed on standalone unit operations whilst being identical to the integrated CM process, provided they also take into account the impact of material transfers.

Using the previous formulation/process example, a CM DSC can be carried out using only enough material for the process to reach a state of control (pass through the start-up phase), and then run at a commercially representative line rate long enough to demonstrate the commercial process. At this point, one can switch to the next DoE conditions or empty the line. Although previously demonstrated using a theoretical example, Thomas et al. presented savings for 1817 kg API requirement down to 418 kg by the application of CM in their presentation at IFPAC Cortona 2012 (Thomas, 2012). This is not only a cost saving of ~$14M, but furthermore, this reduced mass of API is more in line with the quantity that would be available during phase IIb of development.

The challenge is "how long do you need to run the process, at the commercial line rate, to be commercially representative"?

6.1.2.4 Recent Filings

Continuous manufacturing is receiving a lot of attention recently, with four companies and seven filings listed (Vanhoorne & Vervaet, 2020). A perspective on what incentives are required to help establish CM as a more standard DP alternative is also available (Badman et al., 2019).

6.1.2.5 Benefits Analysis at Roche

Roche conducted a formal business case analysis prior to the procurement of its development Mini-Batch line. The learnings from the development line at the date of writing have led to the articulation of benefits along three main axes, as shown in Table 6.1. These fundamentally derive from four differentiating aspects of Roche's Mini-Batch technology: the lack of scale-up required, the simplicity of DC (discussed further below), the enhanced process control, and the flexibility in batch size (Table 6.2).

The quality aspect has been highlighted by several industrial participants (Gordon, 2018). Indeed, the production of 15 million tablets under a continuous state of control has been co-published by Merck and GEA as "A very boring 120 hours" (Holman, Tantuccio, Palmer, van Doninck, & Meyer, 2021).

6.1.3 Direct Compression

Historically, direct compression (DC) has been applied only when the powder blend has very good flowability/low cohesivity whilst having acceptable compressibility. If these material properties cannot be achieved/maintained for the mass in-flight of the batch and at the line rates used for batch production, a wet or dry granulation pre-step is typically added. The introduction of CM, however, has given rise to new opportunities, with slower line rates/less material in-flight resulting in an extension of the previous batch DC materials properties regime map. This extension makes DC more amenable to materials with poorer

TABLE 6.1

Main Benefits for Roche Mini-Batch Line

Fast to patients	Shorter development timelines
	Enabler of fast market introduction
Efficient operations	Lower production costs
	On-demand production
	Less product write-offs
Robust processes	Throughout and reliable process control
	Increased yield
	Less non-conforming material

TABLE 6.2

Fundamental Levers for Roche Mini-Batch Line Benefits

Like-to-like transfer to commercial	No scale-up required (less API)
	Minimal transfer efforts
	Commercial scale locked in earlier
Simple process	Established DC technology
	Fewer operators
	Lower production costs
Flexible batch size	On-demand manufacturing
	Commercial supply agility
	Less waste, increased yield
Enhanced process control	Enabling real-time monitoring
	Increased process data available
	Enhanced process control
	Meets Health Authority expectations
	Extendable to Real-Time Release Testing

flowability/higher cohesivity and worse compression characteristics. Industry estimates show the percentage of future formulations using DC increasing from ~15% or current products to between 50–70% of future products.

The unit operations for continuous DC (CDC) are very similar to batch, and consist of feeders to add materials to the blender, followed by a single or sometimes multistage blend process when additional components can be added before the final powder blend is transferred to the tablet press for compression. Typically, all material transfers (feeder to blender, then blender to press) happen under gravity, with the drop height minimized to prevent possible segregation.

In order to minimize the impact of settling/compaction and segregation under vibration during CDC, the mass retained in any/each hopper is kept to a minimum. For example, the retained mass in the feeder hoppers is typically equivalent to less than 1 hour of process run time. Regular top-ups and transfers in the process line are therefore necessary, and the impact thereof (both in terms of mixing and segregation) needs to be well-understood and characterized (Engisch, 2012).

6.1.4 Description of the Different Scales of Production

Before diving into discussions around continuous vs. mini-batch (or small repeating batchwise) processes, we have to consider the overall line rate of the system. Even within simple CM processes such as CDC, matching the scale of production to the required capacity is critical. For comparison of scale, we will assume a common duty-cycle/use rate of 20 h/day, and an 85% annual equipment utilization rate. These are typical maximal operating conditions for Real-time Release control strategies, and where operational activities such as cleaning/change-over and a seven-day shift pattern are included. For the materials, we assume a blend bulk density of 0.5 kg/l.

6.1.4.1 Mass CDC

The largest scale that is typically used by innovator companies, even for high-volume products, is 50–250 kg/h line rate (Figure 6.1, courtesy of GEA Group); 50 kg/h results in 100 kg/day or 220,000 kg/year (Holman, Tantuccio, Palmer, van Doninck, & Meyer, 2021). This scale is known as "mass CDC" and is typically delivered by using continuous feeding/blending. Assuming the same example as used previously of 20% API composition, it means the API feeder needs to deliver at 10 kg/h for API (and so the feeder hopper is typically sized at or near 20 L). In addition, near 40 kg/h needs to be delivered for functional and filler excipients, yet only around 500 g/h for the lubricant component. Even if the excipient feeds are added individually, rather than as a pre-mix, it means the feeders need to be exchangeable and an appropriate configuration selected for the mass required.

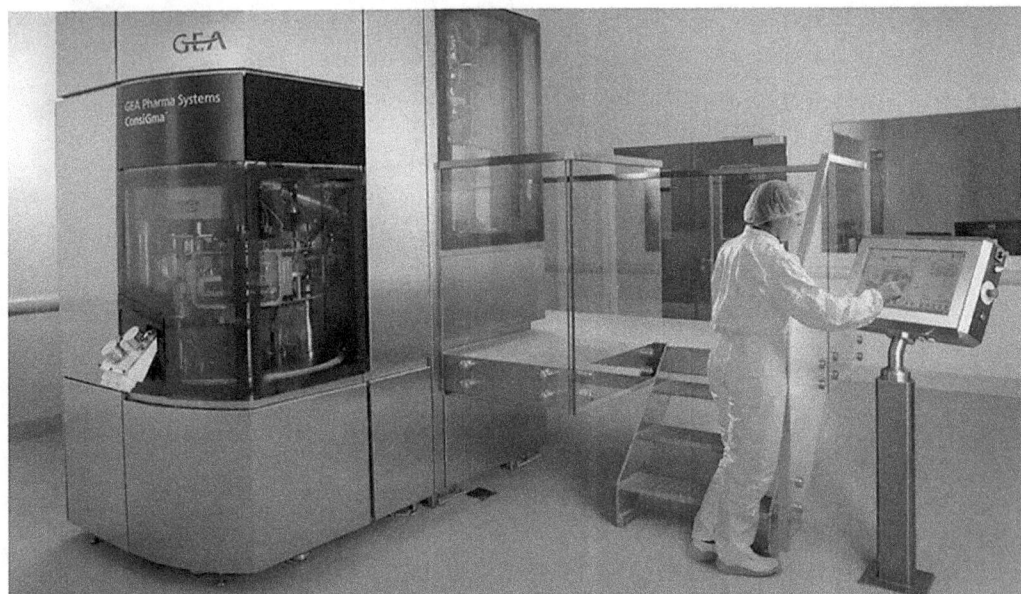

FIGURE 6.1   Mass CDC – GEA CDC 120LB2 – MS (previously known as CDC-50).

These materials are fed into a continuous blender with volumetric capacity in the order of 7–10 L. This gives a typical hold-up mass of 3.5–5 kg, and it is typically 5–7 kg of material 'in-flight' (when the volumetric capacity of material transfers is included). This represents the minimum mass required for the start-up phase. However, if we then factor in the intermixing between this material and adjacent powder (typically determined by RTD studies) it is not uncommon to find the mass required to start up is two to three times higher, that is, up to 15 kg. This means one requires 15 kg of blended powder to reach the point where the system is making material, with the required quality attributes, to manufacture just 1 kg of tablets for development or clinical supply. Obviously, this scale of equipment, whilst being better than batch (where one would need ~100 kg to be representative, at 1/10th commercial scale), is not efficient for QbD development because it still requires at least 14 kg (plus the mass required) for each experimental point, on a DoE. Furthermore, it heavily utilizes intermixing to achieve uniformity (and so product quality). The blender creates uniformity both in a radial dimension (mixing the different components added) and also axial dimension (removing any fluctuation/variance in the masses added over time). Mass scale often uses a control strategy reliant on 'funnel charts' to reflect whether an upstream deviation will result in a downstream non-conformance. Whilst this means it is very unlikely to manufacture non-conforming material, the large mass of material in-flight means large losses if there is an excursion (and materials need to be segregated). A secondary consideration is also significant. In general, with mass CDC, the mass in flight is similar to a batch CD. The acceptable materials space, therefore, does not benefit from the extended CDC regime map, and mass CDC can only typically be applied to materials which would also allow batch DC.

6.1.4.2 Macro CDC

The next scale of production is called macro-CDC (Figure 6.2, courtesy of L.B. Bohle) and has typical line rates in the order of 10–25 kg/h (Figure 6.2). It is particularly suitable for medium volume (75'000–200'000 kg/year) products and consists of continuous feeding/blending/compression. Using the same example as previously, this means API dosing rates of around 2 kg/h (assuming 10 kg/h total line rate), with approximately 8 kg/h total excipients but a lubrication addition rate of only around 100 g/h. This scale is reasonably efficient for QbD development with typically 2.5–3 kg of material in-flight and requiring around 4–5 kg to reach a steady state once the intermixed mass of around 1.5–2 kg intermixing is taken into account.

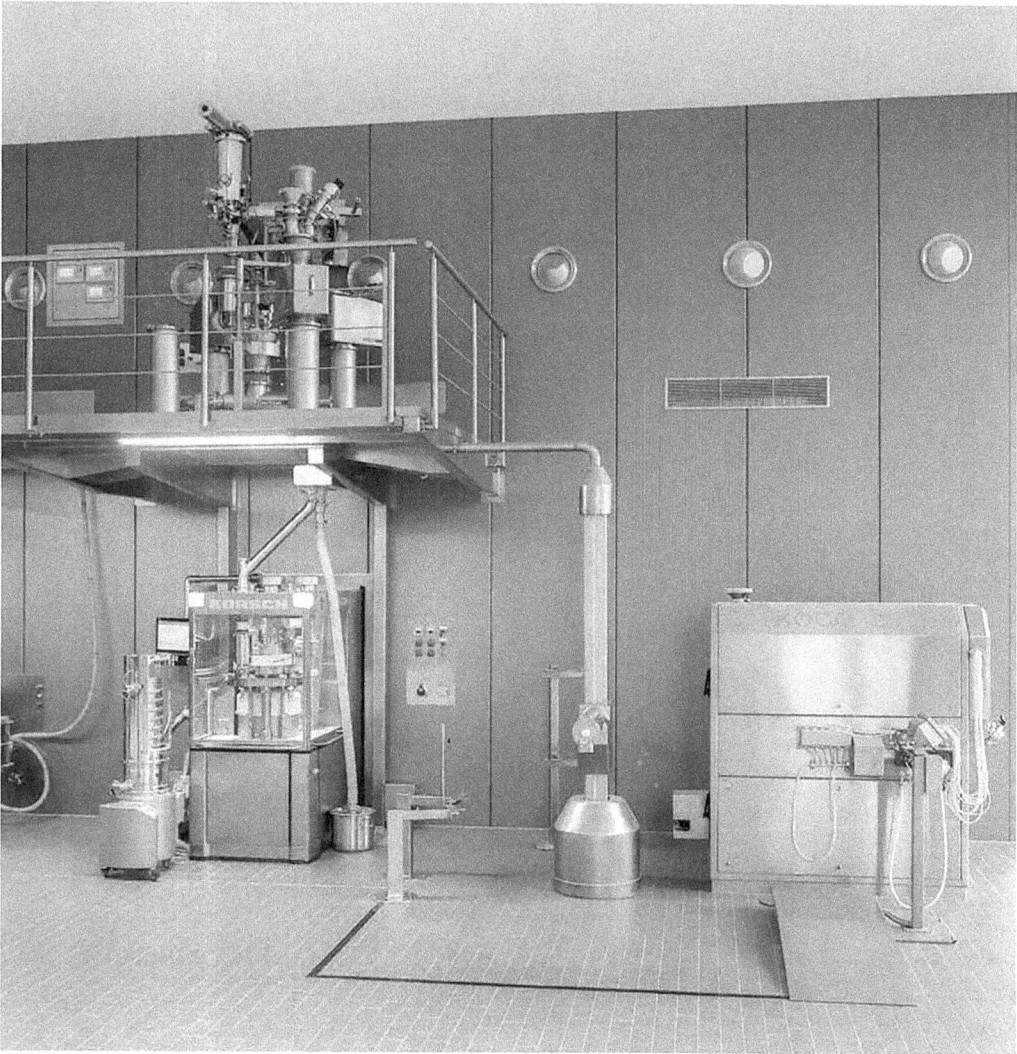

FIGURE 6.2   Macro CDC- LB Bohle QbCon 25.

Although the macro-CDC scale still utilizes intermixing to achieve uniformity (and so product quality), the reduced mass of material in-flight means it is much easier/responsive to process control. An analogy would be calling mass CDC a 'river' vs. macro-CDC being a 'stream'; the mini-batch CDC technology described in the next section would be a series on 'canal locks' in this analogy. As such, macro-CDC is better than mass CDC but still somewhat inefficient for QbD product development. Smaller mass in-flight/ intermixing also means reduced mass needs to be segregated in case of process deviation. However, the 'size' of the segregation is often dependent on the mass used to make a decision on the quality attribute. This means it is not uncommon to make a quality decision on the basis of 'mass of intermixing', that is, 1.5–2 kg in the case of macro-CDC. Thus, each non-conformance will be the mass on which the quality decision is made + the additional mass of intermixing, this approach is often called "waste by range".

6.1.4.3 Mini-Batch CDC

The smallest current production scale of CDC is called mini-batch CDC (Figure 6.3, courtesy of Gericke AG). It is particularly suited to low volume production (1–75,000 kg/year) and consists of small-scale

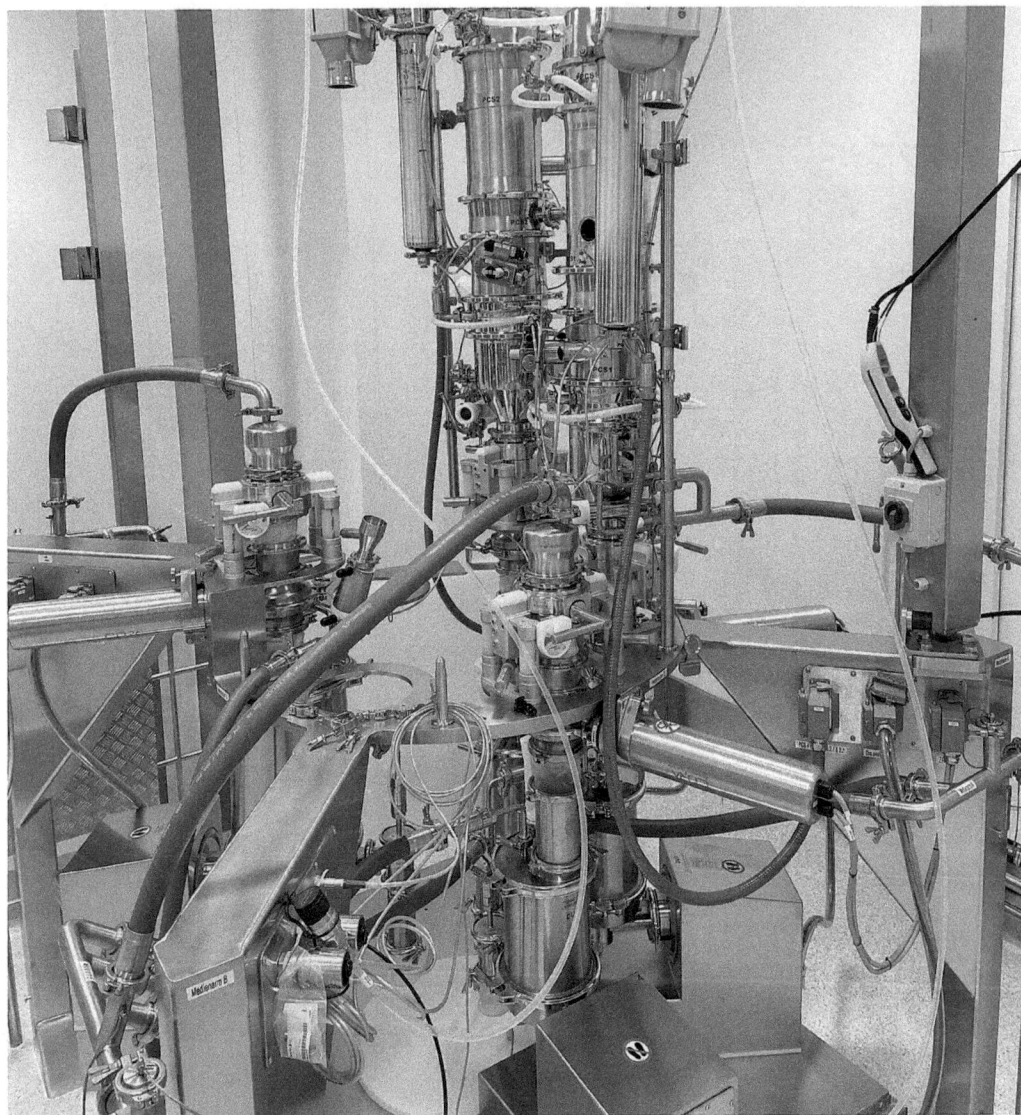

FIGURE 6.3	Mini-batch CDC – Glatt MBB.

batch feeding/ blending (1–2 kg plugs) operations, carried out repeatedly at a frequency to allow continuous compression, and thus achieve CM. As an example, the synchronized combination of a feeding/dosing time of 1 kg/2 min, a 2-min blend time, a 2-min period to discharge and transfer to the press, and the press running a 1 kg/6 min, altogether achieves a 10 kg/h line rate. This scale is very efficient for development as every plug is representative of the commercial process: literally, 1 kg of blend could ideally generate up to 950 g of tablets running at the commercial line rate (set at the press). Furthermore, because each repeating mini-batch is separate and identifiable from the adjacent mini-batch, a control strategy can be built around determining the quality of that specific mini-batch and a diversion point can be introduced for non-conforming material after blending and prior transfer to press. Mini-batch CDC does not rely on intermixing to achieve uniform character, instead, it relies on precise control of the dosing regimen/well-controlled blending operation. Mini-batch CDC also gives the possibility to compensate for excursions (by adjusting the addition of other components to reach the desired composition before starting blending). It, therefore, opens the opportunity for a simpler process with fewer process steps than batch DC and

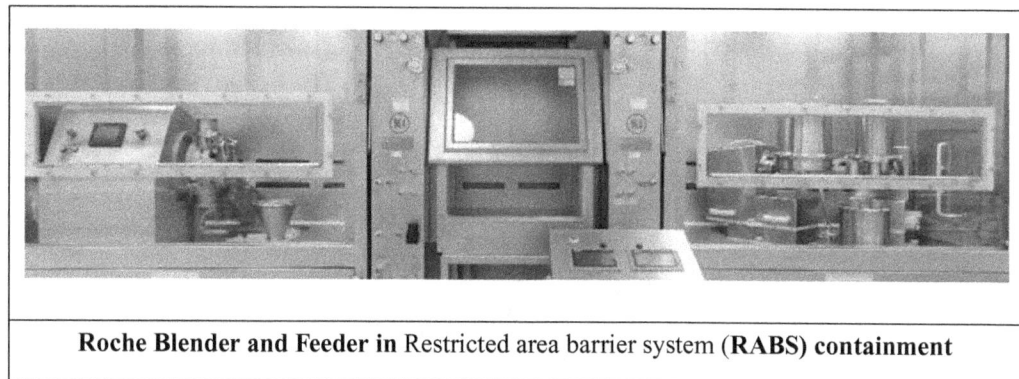

Roche Blender and Feeder in Restricted area barrier system **(RABS) containment**

FIGURE 6.4 Typical technical equipment used for development.

the possibility to apply a lean control strategy, where the material quality could be adjusted and confirmed after the blending steps and then further processed or isolated without intermixing with adjacent materials. Only material of known and confirmed quality would reach the tablet press. This fundamental process understanding removes the driver for control verification (e.g., parallel method) and even some primary controls. This scale offers the optimum efficiency for product development as the development, clinical supply, and commercial processes are all equivalent. A smaller mass in-flight than either mass CDC or macro-CDC, and discrete plug flow, means only the mass of excursion can go to waste, and only conforming material progresses to the next unit operation. Furthermore, mini-batch CDC enables the development of discrete unit operations on standalone 'technical' equipment at the commercial line rate and process dynamics of the commercial process (see Figure 6.4 for typical technical equipment used for development).

The mini-batch CDC scale also gives the ability to very quickly change dosage strength, and the future capability to target sub-populations (facilitating some degree of personalization of medicines). In addition, it gives the opportunity to accurately mimic (manually or automatically) material transfers between unit operations. This means even 'disconnected' unit operations with transfers can be equivalent to full integrated CM lines. It also introduces the term 'integrated processes' (where the unit operations are not continuous but the digital environment is used to align processes and materials) (Maurer, 2021). An integrated process is 'digitally continuous' and physically equivalent to an integrated CM process. Mini-batch CDC is particularly exciting as it not only offers flexible batch size (a batch is simply a number of mini-batches with uniform character, and that number can be changed within the approved range), but also opportunities for the supply chain to drive manufacturing on-demand.

We are actually now starting to see the ultimate deployment of mini-batch CDC, sometimes called Point of Patient (PoP) CDC (Figure 6.5, courtesy of PrivMed® GmbH). In PoP CDC, each mini-batch is specific for the patient, which opens possibilities for truly personalized dosing but also where the dosage strength is determined by the response of the patient, for example, via a sensor such as a wearable device. Here the wearable device is able to measure the response in real-time and inform the pharmacy of a need to change the dosage, which is then enacted in the next patient-specific 'mini-batch' – in effect, this is patient-centric feed-forward control (Bebinger, 2016).

6.1.4.4 *Inflexion Point between Continuous and Mini-Batch Operations (Strengths/Weaknesses of Both)*

In the earlier sub-sections, we have described the production scales of each type of CDC operation. Clearly, for high-volume products where the material properties are conducive to mass CDC, commercial operations benefit from the efficiencies of CM. This is especially important for legacy products (e.g., generic manufacturers). They may currently be running batch DC, and the transfer to continuous results in 85% equipment utilization rates vs. 25–30% for batch processes.

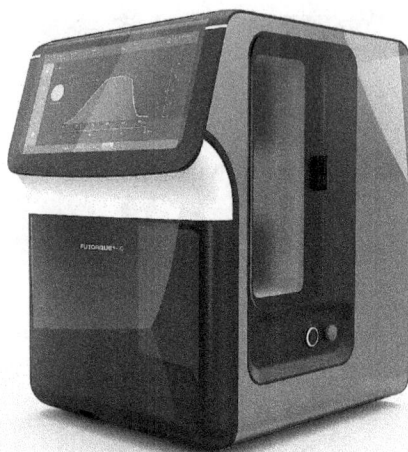

FIGURE 6.5   PoP CDC – UTP Futorque PrivMed® GmbH.

However, the drivers are more complex for new chemical entities (NCE). For NCE with a high patient population, and therefore requiring higher production volumes, there is a business decision to be made. Running development activities on a mass CDC equipment line is very inefficient (Thomas, 2012) but the costs may be worth absorbing to enable development to occur on the commercial scale equipment and at the commercial line rate. In doing so, the element of scale-up between development and commercial when running batch DC is removed. However, running the same process on a macro-CDC line (with its lower hold-up mass and line rate) would equate to an 80% reduction in API costs (to execute the same activities), but also an 80% reduction in the mass of API needed to execute the DSC runs. However, it has to be noted that this may still be more API than is available in early/mid-phase development and may mean the commercial process can only be locked in later phases. Considering that the macro-CDC line can run to 25 kg/h (only 50% of the line rate of the mass CDC throughput), there is an inflexion point where running a macro-CDC line for a longer time overlaps with the capabilities of running a mass CDC line. Of course, there is also the possibility to run parallel macro-CDC lines, although the more complex process dynamics (over, e.g., a mini-batch CDC line) mean it is much more challenging to claim equivalency between two parallel macro-CDC lines. Often the driver between a single mass CDC and multiple macro-CDC lines comes down to opportunities for distributed manufacturing vs. centralized sourcing.

Among the smaller scales, when should one choose macro-CDC vs. mini-batch CDC? There are two inflexion points that drive this decision. The first relates to formulation composition; in the example used so far (20% API composition), we are not challenging the feeder in terms of ability to dose with either approach. As previously stated, at 10 kg/hr (with a 20% API composition), the API feeder has to deliver 2 kg/h (a little over 33 g/min) for macro-CDC. This is achievable with the appropriate feeder configuration – even with cohesive materials. However, what happens if the API composition is lower, say 1%? Now the feeder would not only have to deliver API at 100 g/h (less than 1.7 g/min), but with an accuracy to allow the inherent intermixing of the blender to remove variability in that rate. Mini-batch CDC is advantageous in this case since it relies on total mass, and not mass flow, being tightly controlled. Consider further that there are periods where the feeder hopper will be topped-up, and so the loss-in-weight (LiW) feeders are not able to stay in gravimetric mode (the change in mass of material on the feeder balance triggers a reversion to volumetric mode). The general rule of thumb that can be applied is that LiW feeders do not perform well at less than 150 g/h, even with reasonably well-performing materials and often this threshold increases to 250–300 g/h for materials with low flowability/high cohesivity. If the combination of flow rate/composition requires feeder addition rates below the 300 g/h range, often macro-CDC is not viable and mini-batch CDC is the only option.

TABLE 6.3

Formulation Compositions for Equipment Evaluations

Excipient pack A		Excipient pack B	
Material	**Formulation [%]**	**Material**	**Formulation [%]**
Corn starch	15	Lactose	32
Mannitol	75	Microcrystalline cellulose	64
Croscarmellose sodium	5	Croscarmellose sodium	3
Sodium stearyl fumarate	3	Magnesium stearate	1
Fumed silica	2		

This effect was evaluated by Roche during the initial equipment evaluation work when equipment from all the main equipment vendors was tested using two common excipient packs (Table 6.3), and at three different API concentrations (1%, 10%, 30%). The trials also included different API material properties (micronized vs. non-micronized) to assess different flow properties.

This combination allowed an assessment of the following:

- Accuracy and precision of dispensing
- Impact of feed hopper material top-up
- Achieved uniformity (mass CDC, macro-CDC, and mini-batch CDC were evaluated)
- Time/mass required to reach a steady state
- Lubrication effects (impact of blend parameters on compression profile)

During these trials, the performance of the majority of MBB types was also established.

Acceptable precision was achieved when dosing both formulation types and all API concentrations using the non-micronized (good flowing) API, using all three equipment scales. Yet there were issues with many of the feeders (even though all were commercially available) when dosing the micronized API on both mass CDC and macro-CDC equipment. These issues ranged from:

- Inability to stay within the gravimetric mode. Here the flow properties of the material mean the on-board flow-factor calculation is not able to compensate for discrepancies between predicted/actual LiW. This triggers the feeders to switch from gravimetric into volumetric mode. Although the material is still being added, the addition is controlled simply by speed and not dosed weight/dosing rate. This change impacts both the assay and uniformity of the powder post blending. For such cases, variable assay/uniformity (above 4%) was observed, especially on macro-CDC where the feeder set-point was less than 150 g/h. In some cases, the only way to even conduct the trial of this equipment was to increase the API concentration from 1% to 3% and effectively move the experimental setting to the working range of the equipment.
- Poor flowing materials (both API and lubricant) also created significant issues during feeder top-up. Top-up is particularly important when dosing at a required rate, as the feed-factor used to predict mass dispensed/time will change based on the density within the hopper (Engisch, 2012), meaning the accuracy and precision of the dosing rate changes based on refill level. If the top-up regime is variable it leads to inconsistent dosing rates. In one case, using equipment that included an automated top-up using a mechanical valve, the micronized material simply bridged and even though the feeder was calling for top-up, and the valve was inverting, the material was not released from the rotating cup. This meant the feeder level would run low/variable but eventually the line simply stopped when the low-level alarm is reached.

In all cases, the issues were not seen when running mini-batch CDC, as the feeder is delivering a fixed mass, not a rate. Indeed, in the case of one feeder, the test exposed that when dosing a fixed mass, the onboard controller was configured to run at a dosing rate for a time to give a predicted mass dispensed, and less precise batchwise dosing. This required the feeder supplier to change the functionality of its onboard controller to simply dispense based on the change in weight of the hopper scale. This should be treated as a cautionary tale, as the mode of operation of that particular feeder had been changed by the vendor to improve the dosing rate, to the detriment of the fixed-dose operation. It is critical the equipment is appropriately configured for use.

6.2 Technology Aspects of Mini-Batch

In the following section, we will introduce the main mode of operations for both feeders and blenders used for mini-batch CDC. These are unit operations which differ technologically between batch, mass CDC, or macro-CDC. By contrast, for the compression step, the only special consideration is the line rate used. This means mini-batch CDC compression processes tend to have fewer stations, slower turret speeds, and so lower paddle speeds (lower levels of intermixing in the press feed-frame) than seen with higher line rates/throughputs found in the other operational scales. Typically, mini-batch CDC uses tablet presses more likely to previously be found in pilot plant/R&D settings.

6.2.1 Modes of Operation of Feeders When Running Mini-Batch

Unlike mass CDC and macro-CDC where the feeders are in a constant dosing mode, even during top-up, mini-batch CDC utilizes the LiW feeders in batch dosing mode. The control system thus ensures the feeder is never dosing during top-up and generates three distinct states for phase control.

6.2.1.1 Top-Up

Top-up is triggered at a low mass alarm; however, this alarm is itself set at a value which ensures the mass of material remaining in the feed hopper is more than required by the next feed operation. The top-up process is triggered after the end of the dosing state, whilst the feeder is paused and the blending step is underway. The maximum mass in the feed hopper is also set to ensure the weight of powder awaiting dispensing does not itself cause compaction in the feed hopper.

6.2.1.2 Feeding

The configuration of the feeder (screw diameter, screw pitch, screw speed) is determined by the material properties of the material being dispensed and the mass required within the blend time. Although the configuration is predetermined, the actual process of feeding is separated into two phases.

The first, or coarse, addition mode delivers the majority of the mass required at a high drive ratio/as quickly as practical. For example, if 500 g of a powder is required for a mini-batch CDC blend, one would typically set 475 g to be dispensed in the coarse mode.

Because of the speed of addition, one may slightly under or over-feed the 95% dispense mass. One then intentionally converts to a fine, or dribble mode to dose the remaining mass, with the dosing rate getting progressively slower as one approaches the desired end point (Figure 6.6). This reduces the possibility of power falling from the end of the feeder screws unless the screws are rotating; when the screw is set appropriately there should be little possibility of avalanching from the screws. Feeding of fine or micronized material can cause challenging electrostatic charging of the material at the exit point of the feeder. This can be prevented by the installation of an ionizer.

6.2.1.3 Sequential

The dosing phase of the feeder can also be configured to give sequential addition. In this mode, one may complete the API dosing before completing the excipient dosing, allowing the mass of excipients to be slightly adjusted to give the desired percent composition. This is particularly useful if the feeders are set

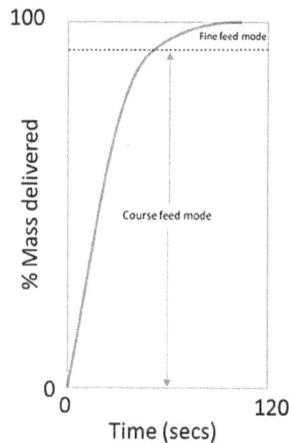

FIGURE 6.6 Typical mini-batch CDC feeding curve.

up to dose API, pre-mix of functional excipients (glidant, disintegrant, etc), a filler, and the lubricant. The filler can be used to give an exact composition of API without impacting the composition of the functional excipients. This is also very useful during product development where each individual mini-batch CDC blend can be a different composition as part of a QbD DoE.

The last but most significant advantage of sequential feeding relates to shear forces. Because one can dose API and excipients separately to lubricant, it has the ability to do multistage blending. This allows high shear conditions to be applied to API/excipients to break up any agglomerates that may have formed during feeding, and then add the lubricant with conditions suitable for micromixing without causing lubrication effects (Kushner, 2010).

Although this effect was witnessed during the equipment evaluation trials performed by Roche, this was primarily seen when using magnesium stearate as the lubricant. When using magnesium stearate within any high shear blender (even mini-batch CDC), the impact of the lubrication effect needs to be confirmed across the intended blend DSp (although the impact can be predicted using the calculation in the Kushner/Moore paper previously cited). More so because of the low shear nature of mass CDC, macro-CDC and some horizontal paddle design MBB, an under-lubrication effect has been experienced. In under-lubrication, the magnesium stearate forms soft agglomerates rather than being dispersed, and if inadequate shear force is applied, the resulting powder blend will have appropriate uniformity but contain large (larger than the primary particles) clumps of magnesium stearate. This can be confirmed either by the use of NIR chemical imaging (Koehler, 2002) or by applying NIR spectroscopy to the material collected by sieving, as was done in the Roche trials.

Critically, this effect was not seen when using sodium stearyl fumarate as a lubricant, with less criticality impact on tablet tensile strength from the blend conditions, which allows higher blend speeds/shear forces which removes the presence of the soft agglomerates of lubricant. It does have to be noted that typically a higher percent composition of lubricant is needed to achieve good powder flow/release during compression, but this is still under investigation.

6.2.2 Description of Types of MBB

Although there are several types of MBB deployed, they all have the same operating principle and scale-up and post-approval changes (SUPAC) equipment classification (convection mixers). Nonetheless, there are significant differences between the types.

6.2.2.1 Horizontal Paddle Mixers

The most common mixer type, found in the commercial equipment offerings from companies such as Glatt GmbH and Gericke AG (Figure 6.7), is a horizontal shaft paddle mixer. These blenders are in scope

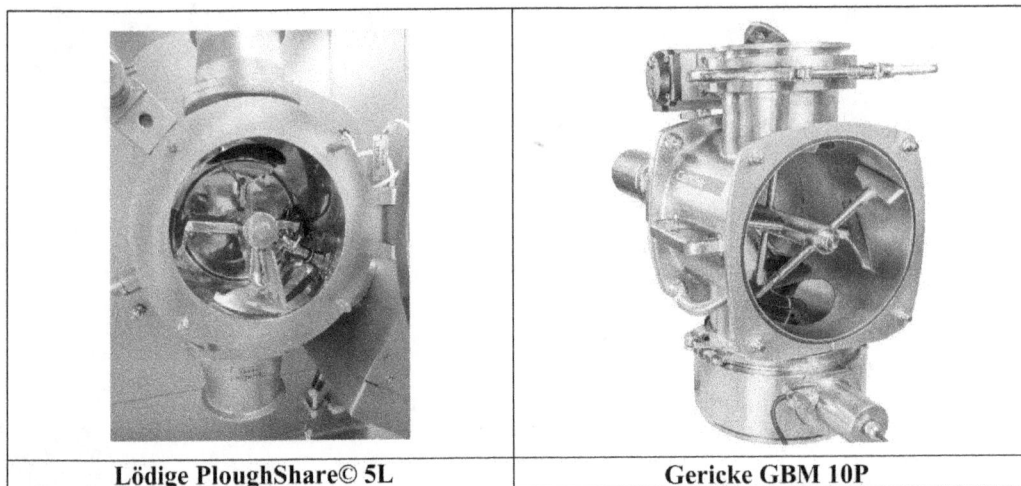

| Lödige PloughShare© 5L | Gericke GBM 10P |

FIGURE 6.7 Mini-batch CDC blenders.

to be integrated into a mini-batch setup. Although both of these units physically look very similar, they can be different in operation due to the shear energy imparted on the powder blend, a critical parameter to the blending operation.

Low shear energy is required to distribute the lubricant around the powder blend, so as not to cause lubrication effects during compression. Over-lubrication causes compression issues and impacts tablet hardness. However, higher shear is required to disperse/break up soft agglomerates that may form when cohesive materials run through the dosing feeders. Therefore, the blending process needs to be designed to provide the required dispersion to achieve uniformity whilst breaking up any soft agglomerates formed during dispensing and without causing over-lubrication. This is critical in a CDC process, since, in contrast to batch process, there is typically no sieving/deagglomeration operation step post feeding/prior to blending. To achieve this balance, often a chopper is added to the mixer, so that it can be used during an initial blend step, aimed specifically toward de-agglomeration.

Another critical aspect of the blender design, however, is easily overlooked. The blender has to not only achieve the desired uniformity, but also be designed to allow for optimal discharge, to prevent a significant residual mass from remaining in the blender. The following example illustrates the significance of residual mass: assuming a 1 kg mini-batch CDC mass, we would expect the discharged mass to be close to if not equal to the mass dispensed. If that correspondence is not achieved, then the retained mass gets carried over to the following mini-batch CDC blend. This will not only impact the assay of the subsequent blends, but also confirm that this residual mass is refreshed/replaced each mini-batch blend, and not simply held up until later mini-batches. To achieve this, the typical paddle design (whether low or high shear) has a scraper design with minimal clearance to the vessel wall, and it is typical to discharge with the paddle rotating slowly to clear material loosely attached to the wall. As a consequence, these blenders/paddles require high tolerances, typically precluding them from being jacketed.

As an example, the mini-batch CDC equipment evaluated by Roche during the initial equipment trials included a jacketed blender and a PloughShare© paddle design with a 5 mm gap (between the paddle and vessel wall). This resulted in a residual mass of between 6%–10% (dependent on the flow properties of the powder blend – better flow properties resulted in lower residual mass). These values were very consistent across repeated mini-batch blend, and by changing the percent composition of the API it was possible to confirm this was refreshed during repeated runs. In addition, in subsequent tests, the paddle was modified to reduce the gap to less than 1 mm which reduced the residual mass to 1% (10 g residual mass per 1 kg mini-batch).

The Roche mini-batch CDC equipment is specified for this reduced tolerance to ensure minimal residual mass which is refreshed by each subsequent mini-batch.

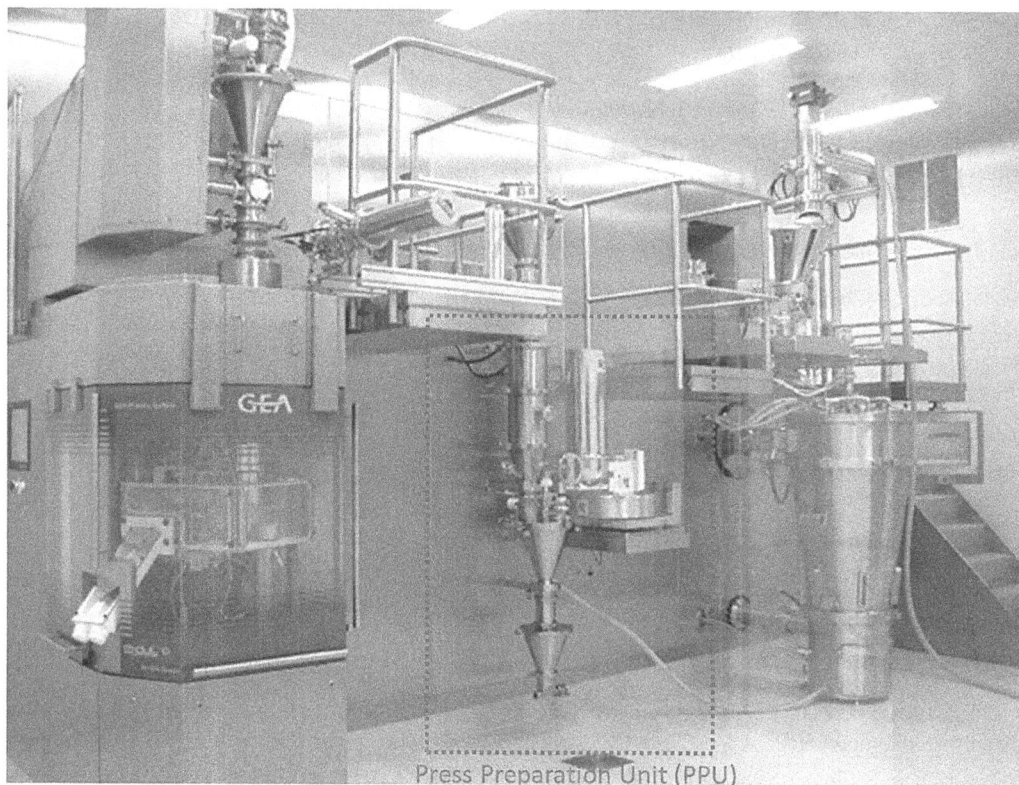

FIGURE 6.8 GEA press preparation unit (PPU).

6.2.2.2 Ribbon

Ribbon-type blenders have been in use on pharma CM lines for approximately 15 years. The versions that have so far been commercialized, however, tend to either be used within very high-volume mass CDC lines running continuously (powder in/powder out) or to provide mixing during a lubrication blend post granulation. A typical example of such equipment is provided by the GEA Press Preparation Unit (PPU), part of their ConsiGma® processing equipment line (Figure 6.8). The versions currently in use, are not suitable for the main blend steps, as they are designed to provide gentle dispersion of the lubricant to the granulated material phase. In operation, these units are very similar to Ekato Solidmix blenders used for agitated driers/mixers in other industries, and so they could be modified to provide adequate shear force.

6.2.2.3 Vertical

Vertical blenders are included in this section and whilst some equipment trains include this design, for example, the Portable Continuous Miniature Modular (PCMM) developed by Pfizer, GEA, and G-Con, they are not intended to solely run in mini-batch CDC mode. The PCMM includes a novel vertical mixing technology (Continuous Mixing Technology [CMT]) (Blackwood, Bonnassieux, & Cogoni, 2019). A novel aspect of this technology is that it 'starts' in mini-batch CDC (batchwise) mode, but then reverts to a macro-CDC mode (continuous). This means that it is possible to run small batch sizes for product development, then empty and do a step change to a new experimental condition, or simply continue at the same rate for routine production.

It is worth noting that this mini-batch to continuous transition is also possible on some macro-CDC equipment. The Gericke Continuous Mixer (GCM) used in that company's macro-CDC equipment train is able to run in an initial batch mode before reverting to continuous mode. It is not able to repeatedly run in a mini-batch CDC mode, however, due to the significant residual mass.

If considering the CMT blender, there are published examples demonstrating the impact of tip speed and hold-up mass on the extent of lubrication, and the illustrated operating ranges (Kushner, 2010). As explained previously, these ranges are specific to the lubricant (magnesium stearate) and can have an influence on which lubricant and lubricant percent composition are chosen.

6.2.2.4 Blending Modes: Thrusting vs. Turbulent vs. Intensify Mixer

When describing a horizontal paddle mixer operation, we typically use the Froude number (Fr) as a descriptor of the mode of operation. Fr is a dimensionless number defined as the ratio of the flow inertia to the external field (in the case of blending, gravity). It is named after engineer and naval architect William Froude. Fr can be represented for a horizontal mixer as:

$$Fr = R \, \omega^2 / g$$

where,

R = Radius of drum
ω = Angular velocity = $2\pi \cdot n$ (n = rps [s^{-1}])
g = Gravity acceleration (9.81 m/s^2)

Critically and dependent on the blender there is an ideal range of Fr where the paddle generates a fluidized bed and the blender acts as what is described as a *turbulent mixer*. At the lower end, the blender is described as being a *thrusting mixer*, mainly conveying the material forward with a folding action. At high Fr numbers, for example, at higher blending speeds, the blender is described as an *intensify mixer*, able to de-agglomerate any soft agglomerates.

A typical mini-batch CDC blends at ideal conditions to achieve uniformity through micro-mixing, but may include periods with high Fr, or application of a so-called chopper initially to de-agglomerate before the lubricant component is added, with a low Fr used during discharge to ensure a minimal hold-up mass.

Although the theoretical Fr range is quite wide, the Roche experience shows a narrower operating range is required to achieve the desired blend uniformity of better than 4% RSD. This operating range is typically established by DoE, and built upon correlations involving blend time, blend speed, and fill mass. However, these correlations will be dependent on material properties and so the response will need to be explored for the range of material properties likely to be experienced (e.g., the particle size range of the API).

6.2.3 Commercial Manufacturing

6.2.3.1 Batch Size

Because of the unique nature of mini-batch CDC, the batch size can be described simply in terms of the number and size of each mini-batch. There is nothing preventing the use of alternate descriptors such as line rate and run-time, or even the number of mini-batches that would be collectively coated – but the fundamental unit of manufacture is a mini-batch and any other indicator of batch size would be made up of the accumulative number of whole mini-batches.

6.2.3.2 Justifying Post Approval Changes in Batch Size

Because the inherent difference between consecutive mini-batches is measurable and, as previously described, used both in PPQ and CPV, mini-batch CDC offers a novel possibility for pre-approved, post-approval change to maximum batch size. Although the maximum batch size is set at the time of approval, it is supporting data to the approval and is managed under the PQS. This means if additional mini-batches fall within the same boundaries of acceptance and variability, as demonstrated under PPQ, the larger batch size (with additional mini-batches) could if justified subject to an annual report rather than a prior approval supplement. Of course, this approach would require that the PPQ determines typical variance between mini-batches, not simply that they all stay in a state of control, and that demonstration of maintenance of the same variance with additional mini-batches is accepted as part of the filing, however, this is possible.

6.2.3.3 Tech Transfer between 'Mirror' Equipment/Sites

Executing the tech transfer of a mini-batch CDC process between development (standalone technical equipment) and commercial manufacturing is very straightforward and relies on demonstrating the equivalence of the process. Furthermore, because the unit operations are the same (with the same DSp, CPP, and CQA), running on the same or equivalent equipment with well-characterized material transfers, it also opens the possibility of tech-transfer between equivalent mirror sites without re-execution of PPQ. There is even the possibility to reduce the significance of site-specific stability, with supporting stability data coming from the original process, and site-specific performance being confirmed once the process has moved. This hub (the main process location) and spokes (additional processing sites) also open the door for distributed manufacturing. At the time of writing, there is even ongoing public consultation by the regional health authorities (e.g., MHRA in the UK) to get feedback on Portable and Point of Care Manufacture of Medicines (including the hub and spokes model) (Rees, 2021).

6.2.3.4 Possibilities for Distributed Manufacturing

Although any individual mini-batch CDC line is constrained in terms of throughput, the technology is particularly suitable for distributed manufacturing. There are thus significant similarities to semi-conductor manufacturing, where silicon arrays are typically manufactured using a large number of manufacturing arrays repeating small-scale operations. These can be co-located in large manufacturing 'fabs' or act as micro-factories to local markets. Although mini-batch CDC was initially introduced to enable efficiencies in PD, it is clear that it suggests/can deliver a completely different (micro-factory) approach.

6.3 Safe, Compliant Operations

In this section, critical control strategy and PAT are first sketched out, followed by a systematic walk-through of the application of these concepts to the mini-batch CDC technology.

6.3.1 Control Strategy

The concept of control strategy is formally defined in ICH Q8 (R2), Section 2.5,

> A control strategy is designed to ensure that a product of required quality will be produced consistently. The elements of the control strategy discussed in Section P.2 of the dossier should describe and justify how in-process controls and the controls of input materials (drug substance and excipients), intermediates (in-process materials), container closure system, and drug products contribute to the final product quality. These controls should be based on product, formulation and process understanding and should include, at a minimum, control of the critical process parameters and material attributes. (ICH Q8 (R2), 2014)

However, not all control strategies are equal and one needs to consider what is called the control strategy complexity pyramid.

6.3.1.1 Complexity Pyramid

This concept has best been defined in the FDA whitepaper "Understanding Pharmaceutical Quality by Design" (Yu, 2014). It describes three levels of control strategy complexity represented as a pyramid (Figure 6.12, FDA control strategy complexity pyramid).

6.3.1.1.1 Recipe Control – Level 3

This level refers to a process that runs against set points where the control systems make actions to maintain set-point and product quality tested during processing (IPC) and end-line and used for product release and is widely used for batch processes. This level represents traditional approaches to manufacturing and a testing-to-compliance approach. It has been clearly articulated by the FDA in subsequent presentations and publications that they do not feel this level of control is viable for CM, simply because the level of scrutiny required to ensure any process perturbations able to impact product quality, do not go undetected, which in turn makes the level of testing unviable. Mini-batch CDC, however, provides a level of control (both in terms of control of the process and of prevention of non-conforming material progressing) that is far higher than previously achievable. The exact dispensed mass, and therefore, the percent composition is known (and assay can be calculated because the API potency is known before addition). This means the assay achieved is fundamental to the gravimetric data and more accurate/precise than a measure of blend assay. In addition, the small mass in-flight and automated control of the blend step ensures mechanistic control of the blend step, which is commonly operated well within the approved DSp. Going forward, it could yet be shown that a Level 3 control strategy is viable for mini-batch CDC, as the CPP are able to provide the necessary controls required under CFR 211.110.

6.3.1.1.2 Pharmaceutical Control – Level 2

A Level 2 control strategy requires an approved DSp and one ensures the process stays in a state of control using defined acceptance limits for CPP, critical material attributes (CMA), and IPC. An accumulation of the CPP, CMA, and IPC data replaces end-of-line testing for real-time release by predicting CQA. This is the typical level for companies operating QbD batch, mass/macro-CDC processes, and it is much easier to achieve with the mini-batch CDC technology due to the simplified process dynamics/material traceability and data alignment, which does not rely on mass flow/RTD process models".

6.3.1.1.3 Engineering Control – Level 1

A Level 1 control strategy also requires an approved DSp but also control models that allow the process to be driven to a specific process space with DSp. Mini-batch CDC is particularly amenable to Level 1 control simply because there is discrete plug flow during the feeding and blending steps. Furthermore, CPP, CMA, and IPC are all inputs to the process models used for control, and so the new process conditions are simply applied to the next iteration of that process operation causing a step change to the new process conditions.

Although a Level 1 control strategy can be applied to mass/macro-CDC, it requires process models to link intermediate CQA to final CQA thus allowing control decisions to ensure compliance of material produced, but complex vector-based control decisions to move from one location in DSp to another with moving outside the DSp during the movement.

The FDA viewpoint is that in both Level 1 and 2, there is a need to confirm the quality attributes of the material produced, with the expectation that this is achieved using timely measurements (either online, at-line, or using so-called soft-sensors [multivariate prediction models that predict quality attributes based on process data, i.e., a form of process model]). Agency representatives have also stated that they do not feel a Level 3 control strategy can be applied to CM as it would require a very high inspection rate for end-of-line testing.

However, because one has 100% measurements of the mini-batch quality attributes, only material with acceptable quality attributes is transferred to the compression process and the compression process is highly controlled (within the DSp), it gives the opportunity to set action limits for the process operations to ensure they cannot manufacture any non-conforming product. If the action limits prevent excursions and stratified sampling is applied to end-of-line testing, the final product quality can be ensured (using a Level 2 control strategy) and confirmed using a Level 3 approach (end-of-line testing). However, this approach has not yet been approved by global health authorities.

6.3.2 Application of PAT

As previously described, conversion from batch to CM, especially during development is seen as an opportunity for the use of PAT. Here it must be highlighted that PAT is not simply the application of online measurements (which is often the view taken by industry). In its fullest sense, PAT is the timely (both in frequency and scrutiny of scale) collection of data. Thus, PAT covers online, at-line, and even lab analysis of appropriate samples, as well as predictions using so-called soft sensors (where the process data are used in multivariate predictions of quality attributes). When viewed through this lens, PAT becomes an enabler for CM and not only to be used to confirm the quality attributes (PAT Implementation in Continuous Manufacturing, 2014). This means it is common to use PAT data to establish process understanding, but often a reduced level of PAT use is necessary for commercial manufacturing, and the ideal state would be "use the PAT data to build fundamental understanding, control the process using those fundamentals rather than commercial-scale PAT, and revert to the PAT tools to confirm the on-going basis of those fundamentals as things like raw material supply changes across the commercial life-cycle".

This means there are three separate paradigms of PAT use. The first is the use of PAT tools during development to establish process understanding. This paradigm typically revolves around acquiring data to support the development of correlations between process parameters and product attributes, which ultimately help decide which process parameters are CPP and which attributes CQA. Once the control limits are established for the CQA, the PAT systems provide the information to control the process within those limits, that is, verify the process stays in a state of control. One must not forget that the correlations that are built during PD, verified in PPQ, are 'historical', in so much that they are built on previous experience. It is essential that any lifecycle control strategy includes the third aspect; steps to ensure the maintenance of that historic process understanding as one goes forward, and includes CPV activities to ensure that the relationship between process performance and process understanding is maintained across the whole product lifecycle.

It is also critical to understand that each product quality decision has a different risk impact, and therefore, the PAT method will itself have, what is normally categorized as one of the three risk impact classifications (ICH Q8, Q9, & Q10 Questions and Answers – Appendix: Q&As from Training Sessions (Q8, Q9, & Q10 Points to Consider), 2012).

- Low-risk impact: This category is applied to PAT methods that are not making quality control decisions, that is, PAT used solely in development (although this category will be revised if later transferred to production) or to verify the quality decision that is made by another PAT method (and where non-verification will trigger a deviation and process investigation).
- Medium-risk impact: This category applies to PAT methods that make quality decisions that are verified downstream. A good example would be assay post blending, which is then verified in tablet assay downstream.
- High-risk impact: These are the PAT methods that make final quality decisions.

The control strategy is a combination of elements containing these different risk impact models. However, it has to include orthogonal (confirmatory) tests where there is a possibility of non-observed/misprediction within the primary method. This means that the control strategy takes into consideration both the risk impact of the decision and the risk of the method (used to make the decision) being 'misprediction'. Once, process performance is established, the ongoing frequency could be determined by the state of the process and set at different rates to cover the start-up, routine operation, and shut-down phases.

Let us now consider which PAT methods are available for the mini-batch CDC technology.

6.3.2.1 Blend Assay

In mini-batch CDC, the determination of BA is very robust and straightforward. The actual value that we need to confirm is the mean BA for an individual mini-batch. In reality, this is simply the achieved dose weight of API relative to the achieved dose weight of all the other components, represented as a weight/weight. Using the previous case of a 20% API composition and a 1 kg target mini-batch mass, if 200.01 g of API is dispensed vs. a total weight of 800.10 g for the other components (excipients), the total weight of the mini-batch CDC blend is 1000.11 g of which 200.01 g is API, or 20% in composition (once rounded) or 200.03 g/kg. These values are generated from the (calibrated) balances that form part of the dosing feeders, and so the precision of the soft-sensor method is simply the precision of those balances. This means one can set action limits, not only on the required specification for BA, but also on one's ability to determine that value. Using the same example of a target blend assay of 20%, the API dosed mass set-point would be 200 g/kg. Let us assume a +/− 10% acceptance range (also known as the control limit), and factor in the typical precision of the feeder (e.g., 2%). One can see, that whilst the blend assay needs to be within 180–220 g/kg, the feeder action limits would then be set at 2% within those limits. This ensures one stays within the control limits (that determine the product is of acceptable quality). The lower and higher action limits are then 180 + 2%, that is, 183.6 g/kg and 220 − 2%, that is, 215.6 g/kg, respectively.

In practice, other considerations may also apply. If the carry-over mass is significant between mini-batch CDC blends, these values may need to be adjusted, with the carry-over mass (and composition of the mass carried over) being added into this calculation.

6.3.2.2 Determining Blend Uniformity

Although the determination of BA is straightforward, this is not the case with BU. Here we are referring not to the BU of the entire batch, but to the uniformity of the individual mini-batch. To be specific, the BU is the deviation/variance in assay relative to the mean BA for that mini-batch. The three ways to achieve this are discussed in the following sections.

6.3.2.2.1 At-Line/Off-Line Analysis

One can take samples from the blend and determine the variance around the mean using either traditional wet chemistry techniques (such as HPLC) or faster at-line (samples are removed but analysis typically occurs on the manufacturing shop floor) techniques (such as at-line near-infrared (NIR) or Raman). Because of the challenges in acquiring samples from the blender, this approach is typically applied after blending has occurred. This means if different blend types are to be investigated, separate experiments are needed for each blend time. In addition, one then needs to collect representative samples across the mass of the mini-batch, and so typically the blend is sampled during discharge (so that the spatially resolved differences within the blender become temporally resolved/stratified samples of the discharge).

Although this is viable and valuable to support development activities, or even as a verification method (e.g., parallel method), it is not viable to collect multiple samples (needed to determine variance) on each mini-batch when running commercially. Faster methods are required to decide if the BU is acceptable to allow the mini-batch to progress to compression – in other words, alternatives are necessary.

6.3.2.2.2 Soft-Sensor/Process Models

The first alternative to sampling is to predict the BU based on a process model. This approach builds on the QbD DoE activity that is used to define the DSp for blending. Here, instead of simply setting the boundary/control limits for blend CPP (typically a multivariate process model consisting of blend time, blend speed, blend mass, etc), one uses the surface response curve (within the control limits) to predict what the BU would be if measured, based on the co-ordinates (achieved values) obtained. This approach of using the same DoE model that sets the control limits for DSp is often called a soft-sensor but is, as previously indicated, still regarded as a PAT, and so is sometimes called a PAT soft-sensor.

It is important to understand that these process models are generated by the QbD DoE activity, and therefore a consequence of product development. This means one would rely on alternate ways to measure

BU in development, which could be the off-/at-line methods mentioned above but also could be the last option of online spectroscopy.

6.3.2.2.3 Online Spectroscopy

The use of online spectroscopy, in particular NIR, to determine uniformity is now common during batch blending. In the batch blending application, a specialist 'portable' NIR is attached to the lid of the intermediate bulk container (IBC) and a spectrum is acquired each time the IBC inverts. The trigger to collect data comes from accelerometers built into the spectrometer. Whilst the IBC continues to rotate, the powder is stationary on the lid and so a high-quality/static spectrum can be acquired. The spectra collected can be used to determine the progression of the blend process, and also to quantify the homogeneity of the blend once that end point is reached. In the same way, one could consider using NIR via a probe inserted through the wall of the MBB. Here the powder is in motion past the end of the probe, and the location needs to be selected to ensure it is totally covered by powder when acquiring the spectra. This approach only works for non-adhesive materials which prevent material build-up on the probe window and fouling over the intended process time.

Providing a location can be found that ensures constant power coverage and the spectral acquisition time can be chosen to determine the mass of material that will be measured. This calculation starts by calculating the measured volume. This is the surface area of a static measurement spot multiplied by the distance travelled during data acquisition (linear velocity × time) and the depth of penetration of the NIR light into the sample. By multiplying the measured volume by the powder density at the time of measurement, one can calculate the measured mass. Because the acquisition time can be varied, one can select a time that gives a measured mass which is indicative of the intended unit dose (e.g., a tablet). One can also choose the repeating frequency to allow the progression of the blending process (typically an exponential decay curve) and/or the uniformity at the end of the blending process.

Using NIR to monitor the progression of blending is a very powerful tool in determining the endpoint. Here one can use a qualitative approach and use trend plots to visualize change (in the unique spectral regions) over time. During development, this approach is also a powerful tool to determine uniformity at the end of blending, by applying a quantitative model to predict API concentration, and by looking at the change/trend in API predictions across repeated acquisitions (very similar to the approach used in batch blending). However, if this same method is to be used as part of a control strategy, the methods will need to be appropriately validated. For GMP use, the blend uniformity method is categorized as medium risk impact. This means that one is making a control decision (to keep or discard that specific mini-batch), but that the control decision will be later verified downstream, either by end-of-line testing or analysis of tablet cores if following a real-time release testing (RTRT) strategy. A medium-risk impact method requires validation as defined in ICH Q2 (R1). The prediction models will have been developed using previously collected data (which would have included model calibration and validation steps) but those models need to be validated by the execution of a pre-approved validation protocol (maintained under the PQS). Typically, this means collecting new spectra of known concentration, verifying that the new predictions meet expected prediction performance, so that the method can be approved for GMP use.

Although challenging to determine BU in the blender, it is much more straightforward to determine uniformity post blending. One can manage/control the powder flow as the blender discharges via what is typically called a sample interface. Using a sample interface, one can present that powder sequentially to an NIR (or Raman) probe, and if the powder flow is controlled with a known flow rate, the concentration can be determined (amount per mass). This approach (using the sample interface) also allows multiple (stratified) measurements from each mini-batch. These sample interfaces are commercially available, and an example is the Spectrum from Expo Pharma Engineering Services (Figure 6.9). Because these devices manage the flow of powder across the PAT probe, it is possible to build a mimic of that section of the production equipment, which means the PAT data can be collected to allow calibration/validation of the prediction model, as well as validation of the method (against the criteria laid out in ICH Q2 (R1), before transferring the method onto the production equipment).

There remains in all cases a significant burden to using online methods to confirm quality attributes (i.e., to use online methods as the primary method) and this endeavor should not be undertaken lightly. A far leaner approach is to use the online techniques to establish process understanding and support

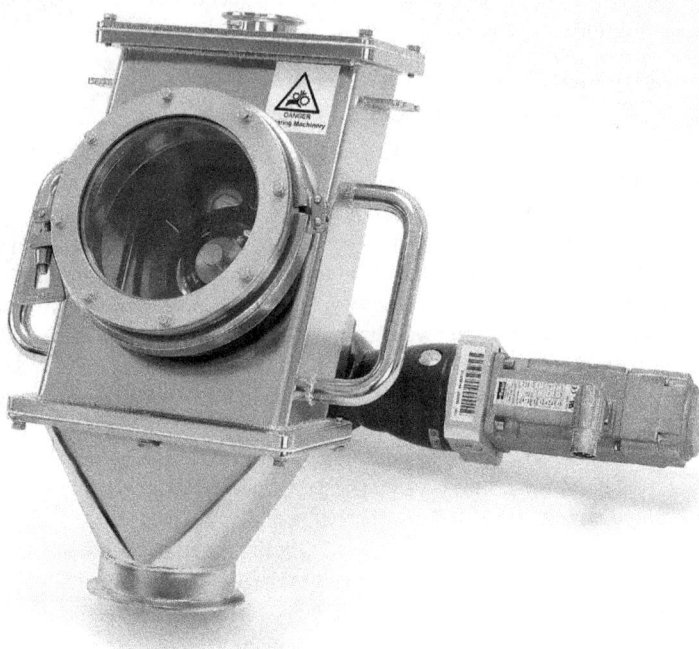

FIGURE 6.9 Spectrum from expo pharma engineering services.

development, then decide if a soft-sensor approach is appropriate to confirm the quality attributes, whilst using the at-line analysis to verify that there has not been a change in underlying process understanding over the life-cycle of the product.

6.3.2.2.4 BA/BU at Point of Compression

Although per CFR 211.110, one needs to ensure the mini-batch CDC process has stayed in a state of control (BA/BU needs to be confirmed for each mini-batch), it is also possible to achieve this assurance using data collected during the compression step. In this case, one measures tablet assay/CU, as a surrogate to BA/BU but with a sampling frequency able to observe any perturbations in the upstream process. Much like batch and other CDC scales, during mini-batch CDC, one can install a PAT measurement (either NIR, Raman, or fluorescence) into the press feed-frame. Typically, this installation is immediately above the press tooling to ensure the measured powder characteristics (BA/BU) are representative of the tablet cores (i.e., no subsequent mixing occurs) (Figure 6.10, Sentronic NIR mounted in Fette feed-frame, courtesy of Fette Compacting). Assuming adequate modification of the feed-frame paddles to minimize the effect caused by the rotation of the paddles, one can calculate the mass measured by factoring in the diameter of the PAT measurement spot, the depth of penetration of the light, and the linear velocity of the powder under the probe, to quantitatively predict the assay and variance in the assay at the point of compression. Although the methodology is similar to that used in batch mass/macro-CDC, the application is better suited to mini-batch CDC as the press turret speed is reduced and a lower number of tablets per hour is produced. This means, unlike when used for batch/macro-CDC, where the NIR is often configured to the highest possible rate, not necessarily reflective of the unit dose size, in mini-batch CDC, we have more time/flexibility to configure the data acquisition time to give a specific 'sample mass' ((Hetrick, 2021).

As with the previous example of online spectroscopy to measure BU post blending, it is possible to set up a mimic of the manufacturing process (a standalone replica of the press feed-frame). This allows model calibration/validation and method validation to happen without running the process. Once validated, the method can be transferred to the running process as a tech transfer activity (Shi, 2017) (Figure 6.11, example feed-frame table used for offline model calibration/validation).

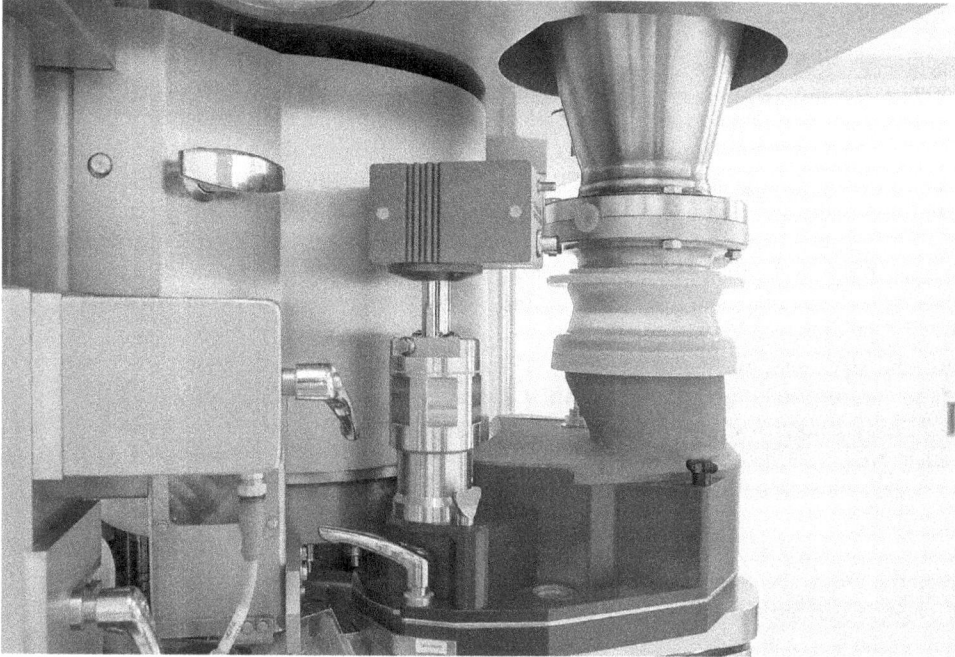

FIGURE 6.10 Sentronic NIR mounted in Fette feed-frame.

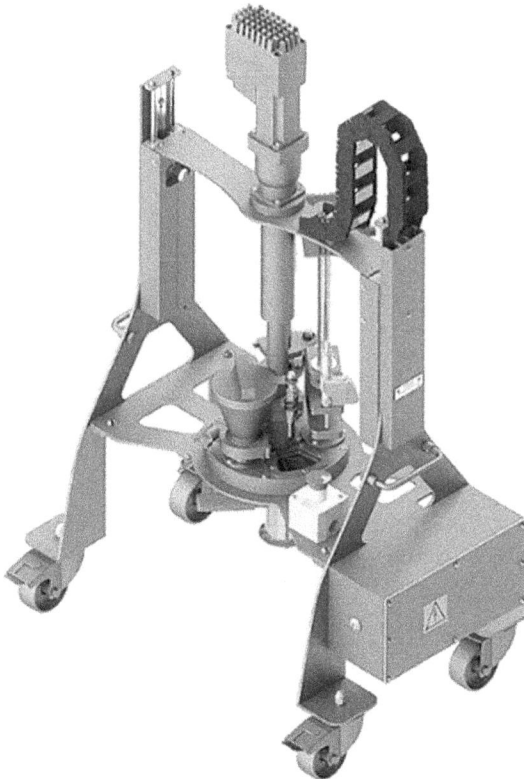

FIGURE 6.11 Expo pharma engineering – feed frame table used for offline model calibration/validation.

6.3.2.3 Tablet Weight, Tablet Assay, and Content Uniformity

As with most other QbD tablet formulations, the process parameters for compression will be set to ensure CQA are met, including tablet weight and hardness. To do so, the tablet press controls parameters such as compression force are set up, but those values are set based on the correlation of compression force (main compression force [MCF]) to tablet weight. An acceptable range is set for those process parameters and used as the control limits for CPP. However, just like the previous blend example, the process model can not only be used to determine the CPP boundaries, but also to confirm the quality attributes. The surface response curve can be used as a soft sensor to calculate/ predict the tablet weight (Manley, 2019). This prediction of tablet weight by MCF is not typically available during development, since it is a consequence of the compression PD. Because the model is calibrated both before and during the compression process using an automated tablet tester checking weight, thickness, and hardness, the MCF model is categorized as having a low risk of non-observed variance and it is typically qualified and part of the tablet press automation and calibrated in use. This means that even though the PAT method for tablet weight is categorized as high-risk impact, verification via an orthogonal method is not required; although the automated tablet tester could be described as both, a calibration tool for the MCF and a verification test for predicted tablet weight if needed.

Despite the compression step itself being identical to that for a batch process, in mass/macro-CDC, the material fed to the compression step is not equivalent. In batch DC the entire mass of the batch would have experienced the same process conditions/at the same time, and so BA/BU can be demonstrated for the whole mass of material. In mass/macro-CDC there is a flow of material from the feeder, through the blender. This means although there is variability in that flow (the set-point is constant but the value achieved can fluctuate) – the actual dosing and blending process is not constant and the process experience changes over time. Indeed, one can use residence time/RTD to calculate the mass of the blend which would have been mixed and the blend is often described as having a variance reduction ratio (VRR) (Vanarase & Muzzio, 2011). In mini-batch CDC, each mini-batch is a distinct discrete plug flow from the feeder and blender to the press. As a consequence, the sampling frequency needed

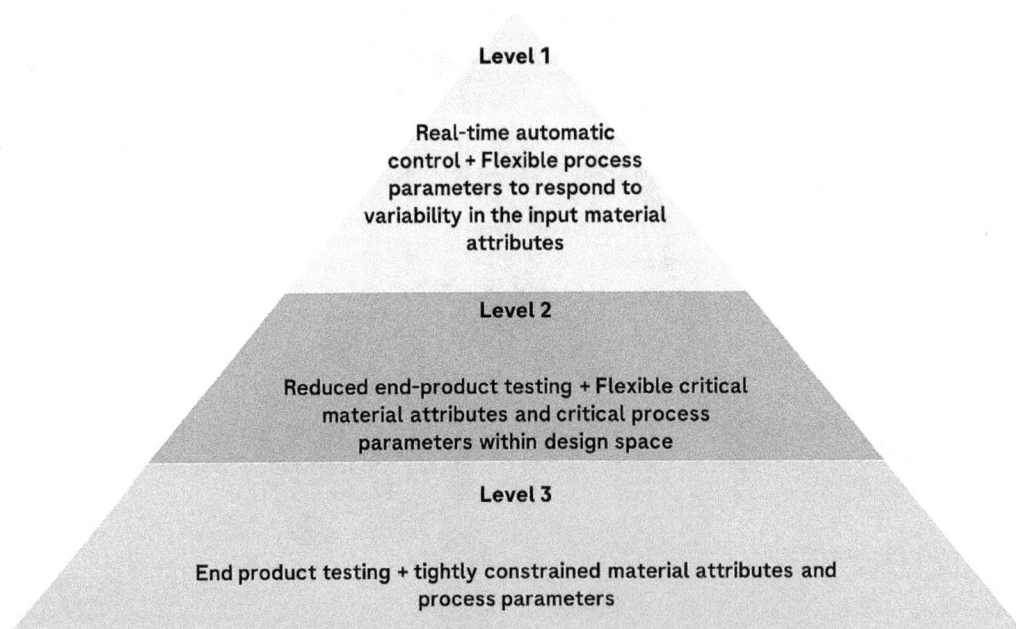

Level 1

Real-time automatic control + Flexible process parameters to respond to variability in the input material attributes

Level 2

Reduced end-product testing + Flexible critical material attributes and critical process parameters within design space

Level 3

End product testing + tightly constrained material attributes and process parameters

FIGURE 6.12 FDA control strategy complexity pyramid (adapted from (Xu et al., 2014).

for tablet assay and CU verification is based on the scale/frequency of the blending step. That said, it is possible to take the applicable values for tablet weight and blend assay at the point of compression to calculate the tablet assay and variance around the mini-batch average tablet assay, to give a CU for each mini-batch.

A mini-batch CDC line may not be equipped with PAT, either for measuring blend assay/blend uniformity, measurement of assay in the feed-frame, or in-line measurement of tablet assay/uniformity. The data required for product development could be acquired with appropriate sampling and therefore, the equipment would have to have the ability to pull stratified samples post blending and post compression. This means during development, a DoE would be designed to leverage this capability. As an example, the blend DoE would include separate experimental points for increasing blend time, not relying on the PAT measure as blend time increases. The reasoning behind this approach is simple: any PAT method used in development will be validated across the entire range of compositions that could be experienced as moving from 'unblended' to uniform blends. Samples collected and analyzed either at-line or by wet-chemistry (the reference method), would have considerably higher accuracy and precision when analyzing unknown mixes. Although the requirement to confirm the quality attributes during commercial manufacturing is very well understood and recognized, the provision of tight CPP action limits and the ability to 'pull a sample' to verify at-line/off-line by the inclusion of the sampler address this requirement.

6.3.3 Impact of Material Transfers

Although the feeding and blending operations of a mini-batch CDC process are discrete plug flow, with no opportunity for mixing or segregation, these phenomena can potentially take place during material transfers. If so, these phenomena would lead to inhomogeneity. A good understanding of the process dynamics is therefore critical. Such effects have been evidenced in studies on dead mass on blending efficiency and RTD (Kauppinen, Karhu, & Lakio, 2019).

6.3.3.1 Segregation

The opportunity to segregate occurs when a mass of mixed powder is subjected to a process operation (e.g., a material transfer) that overcomes the segregation potential of the powder (Jakubowska & Ciepluch, 2021). Practically this means that differences in material properties of individual components of the mixture (e.g., different flowabilities or cohesivity) result in the transfer happening at different rates for different components. These differences may be caused by chemical differences but could just be morphology or physical differences of a powder population that is chemically the same. A simple analogy is massing a mixed powder population through a sieve; particles with a size larger than the mesh get retained and particles smaller than the mesh pass through. As this is an example of categorical segregation and so easily visualized, if the sieve is replaced with a different resistive force (e.g., a countercurrent air flow) the powder is not split into two categories but rather 'rank ordered' with particles less impacted by the resistive forces arriving at the next process step before particles impacted to a greater extent. Preventing segregation is particularly important if the previous process step aims to generate uniformity. For this reason, it is essential that all material transfers (discharge from the blender, passage through PAT sample interfaces, and between unit operations) are designed to minimize the impact of segregation – and also that this is verified on a product-by-product basis.

6.3.3.2 Intermixing

In the present context, 'intermixing' refers to processes whereby mini-batches do not stay perfectly distinct. Although the majority of unit operations and material transfers in mini-batch CDC occur as discrete plug flow, it is critical to understand the impact of intermixing at any point where the adjacent mini-batches can come into contact. This applies to sections of the process where we revert from discrete plug flow to continuous flow, namely after the press inlet tube/chute. Because the intention is to run the press continuously, the inlet tube acts as a surge hopper. Using the example of a mini-batch CDC line running at 10 kg/h, a 1 kg mini-batch is made every 6 minutes. However, feeding takes up to 2 minutes, blending takes up to 2 minutes, and discharge and transfer to the press can take up to 2 minutes, so the entire feeding/blending step takes 6 minutes. The tablet press receives a discrete mass of 1 kg every 6 minutes, even though it discharges at a constant rate of 10 kg/hr. Therefore, the mass in the inlet chute fluctuates, or rather pulses, being topped up by 1 kg each time a new mini-batch arrives. Typically, the inlet contains between one and two mini-batches. Although the flow of material in the inlet tube is plug flow, the drag of material on the walls creates a localized resistive force. However, this time the impact is not seen in segregation but rather in intermixing as the 'tail' of one mini-batch has the opportunity to mix with the 'front' of the next.

Although generally not significant, it is not unknown for these transfers to happen within a positive pressure environment (part of the containment system), and if accompanied by a pressure equalization/ airflow that can easily fluidize all the material in the inlet tube and give a very high degree of intermixing (not just the tail of a mini-batch mixing with the front of the next). Left unmitigated, such phenomena can severely impact the ability to trace material and align CQA data generated at one location to calculate downstream CQA data, for example, using BA data calculated prior to blending to calculate tablet assay data, if adjacent mini-batches with different BA values could have mixed.

6.3.3.3 Impact of Passage Through the Tablet Press

The degree of intermixing as material passes through the press is a function of the design of the press. It can thus differ significantly depending on the equipment geometry. Some tablet presses have low hold mass and paddle design to minimize intermixing (the feed-frame acts as a conveyer from the inlet tube to tooling). These press designs have a lower RTD as can be visualized by spiking colored dye into the blend powder and watching how quickly the tablet cores change from white to colored; however, this requires precise alignment between the turret and feed-frame rpm. To compensate, the blade design of the feed-frame paddle is often exchanged for a 'rod' or 'spaghetti' paddle to prevent pre-compression in the feed-frame, especially if the material has a cohesive nature. However, this is not the case with conventional rotary tablet presses and several actually have feed-frames designed with high intermixing specifically to ensure homogeneity of blend at the point of compression. These feed-frame designs act as mixers and significantly impact the ability to ensure material traceability. This precludes the use of such feed-frames in control strategies which rely on pairing data (e.g., blend assay × tablet weight = tablet assay). Indeed, because the benefit of mini-batch CDC comes from minimizing the mass of material in-flight, tablet presses with high feed-frame volumes often require inserts and alternate paddle wheels with an in-filled design to be fitted to effectively reduce their hold-up mass. Of course, this increased traceability correlates with a lower ability to ensure powder is mixed right up to the point of compression.

6.3.3.4 Control Strategy Consideration

In the ideal state, the mini-batch technology utilizes and benefits most from a completely discretized plug-flow behavior. Deviations from this ideal behavior lead to additional considerations in the control strategy to ensure a state of control. Specifically, segregation and intermixing, even when intentionally part of the equipment design, reduce the ability to use upstream data to predict downstream performance. This effect can be mitigated by the use a complex mass flow/RTD compensating process models. In general, the higher the complexity of the process dynamics, the more complex the control strategy, and the less benefit from running discrete plug flow feeding/blending unit operations.

If a process is developed using a mini-batch CDC feeding/blending unit, combined with a conventional rotary tablet press with a certain level of intermixing, it may require a different approach for a control strategy in order to maintain the benefit of the mini-batch concept. One could consider the following:

The blend assay is very accurately controlled by the CPP of the feeders and the individual weight dispensed. The percent composition of each component (including API) is calculated from the dispensed mass. In addition, the blend assay is calculated based on the potency of the API. This calculated blend assay serves as a confirmation of the quality attribute, even though there are action limits set for the CPP to ensure the blend assay cannot cross the control limits set to ensure product quality.

During development, a blend DoE is carried out to establish the multivariate DSp and CPP action limits to ensure blend uniformity stays within the control limits. These blend uniformity action limits are set based on confidence limits, making sure that the blend uniformity would conform if tested.

These values would be verified by stratified sampling of the blend and at-line analysis at a statistically justified frequency. This frequency would be chosen to ensure the process understanding built during the development of DoE is still valid, and/or if the DoE process model needs updating.

The residual mass of each mini-batch would be confirmed post discharge by weight verification with a gain-in-weigh hopper and CPP action limits would be set for mass not discharged (using the dosed weights and the discharged weight data to calculate residual mass).

The system would be capable of feeding forward the residual mass/assay of the residual mass to be taken into consideration in the next percent composition calculation.

This would mean that CPP for mass not discharged could be used to trigger a non-conformance of the mini-batch, based on specific action limits and/or an input into the percent composition calculation for the next. That said the intention is to develop robust processes, with minimal carryover so that the CPP action limit for mass, not discharge, would only be used along with other CPP action limits, to trigger the segregation of the mini-batch just produced. Only conforming mini-batches would be fed forward to the press.

Not all equipment is specifically designed for mini-batch plug flow – in particular, if originally intended (or still used in parallel) for batch operations, equipment may be demonstrated or potentially susceptible to intermixing. Intermixing can actually be difficult to detect/demonstrate upfront. The Roche implementation was therefore designed to be independent of intermixing, that is, offer maximum flexibility while the equipment was still being developed, and accepting the necessity to adapt the control strategy accordingly. In this case, the tablet assay/intra-mini-batch content uniformity, using the blend assay × tablet weight could not be used. Although the blend assay at the point of compression would be acceptable, intermixing in the press feed-frame would mean that the actual value is not known and cannot be used to calculate tablet assay. There would be two considerations for ensuring the tablet quality attributes: (i) The blend assay/blend uniformity CPP action limits would be set significantly within the control limits to ensure the material would conform if tested (based on the confidence limits of the process model); (ii) CPP action limits for the press process parameters would be set to ensure the tablet weight would also conform if tested.

This would mean that during blending, the quality attributes of the uncoated tablet core would be confirmed as part of end-of-line testing. It is accepted that the frequency of verification would be higher earlier in the product life-cycle, and the intention could be to build on the increased knowledge/demonstration of process robustness, to reduce this frequency during the product life-cycle, including changing to RTRT once confidence in the approach can be proven.

6.3.4 Mini-Batch CDC Validation Approaches

Although efficiencies during development are often flagged as drivers for CM and mini-batch CDC in particular, there are significant possibilities during other stages of PV (Guidance for Industry Process Validation: General Principles and Practices, 2011). The first stage of PV is PD. Typical PD is the QbD development for a new product, built on process understanding/knowledge for existing products, including the development of a control strategy. The next stage is PPQ. During PPQ one demonstrates the control strategy is able to keep the process in a state of control. Lastly, there is PM as part of CPV. This is also known as ongoing process verification and ensures the process remains in a state of control on an ongoing basis (Figure 6.13).

6.3.4.1 Process Performance Qualification

PPQ replaces traditional PV and is used to demonstrate that the control strategy keeps the process in control during all phases/states of operation. But what are those process phases?

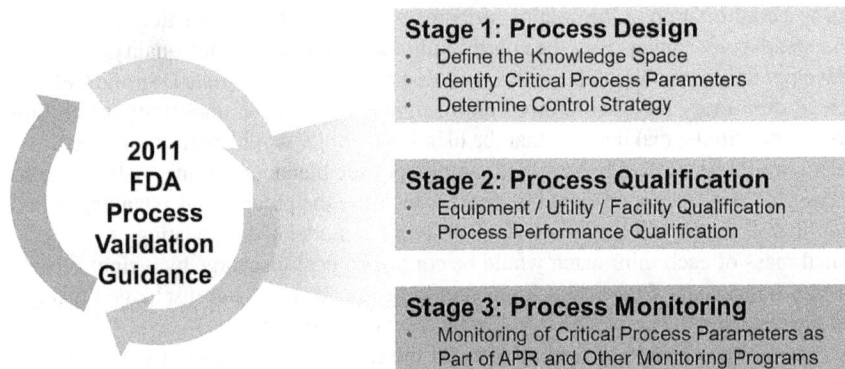

Stage 1: Process Design
- Define the Knowledge Space
- Identify Critical Process Parameters
- Determine Control Strategy

Stage 2: Process Qualification
- Equipment / Utility / Facility Qualification
- Process Performance Qualification

Stage 3: Process Monitoring
- Monitoring of Critical Process Parameters as Part of APR and Other Monitoring Programs

FIGURE 6.13   FDA stages of process validation.

6.3.4.1.1 Understanding Start-Up, Run, Pause, and Shut-Down States

Typically, a process will experience three phases; start-up, run, and shut down. The start-up phase typically represents the time to reach not only a state of control but also a steady state of operation. The run phase represents a period of return operation during which all the typical process events are experienced (vessels filling, feeders being top-up, etc.). The shut-down phase is the processing period where the line is emptying up to the point the process is no longer maintaining a state of control and the process is stopped. The process could also experience an interruption in the run state if there is a line pause. The process can also experience multiple repeating cycles of the run state (Figure 6.13, diagram of process states).

Although these phases are useful in describing a typical CM process such as mass/macro-CDC and PPQ runs typically demonstrate the control strategy across the three phases, each mini-batch of a mini-batch CDC run is autonomous: there is no start-up or shut-down phase and each mini-batch represents the run phase. This means that although typically PPQ will be executed against using the number of mini-batches expected to make up a batch (and batch size can be defined by the number and size of each mini-batch – e.g., a batch could be defined as 100 mini-batches each of 1 kg, i.e., 100 kg), but in addition to ensuring the process is kept in a state of control for the batch, one can observe what is the typical variance between each mini-batch. Why would one do that?

6.3.4.2 Process Monitoring

PM ensures the process remains in a state of control on an ongoing basis. However, it is more than that: it is the basis for process trending.

6.3.4.2.1 Ongoing Process Trending

Typically process trending plots the achieved process performance (categorized as the CPP, CQA, and other important process indicators) over time, and correlates any disturbances to process events (e.g., change of raw material supply) to capture the impact of those events as additional process understanding. However, with mini-batch CDC, each batch has a separate identity. One is thus able to not only trend process performance for operational purposes, but also use multivariate approaches to demonstrate how each mini-batch compares to other mini-batches, best described as a step-wise multivariate statistical process control (with each mini-batch being a step).

6.4 Mini-Batch CDC Technology: Formulation Composition and Development Consideration

A tablet composition intended for a mini-batch CDC process could look rather similar to a formulation for a conventional batch DC process. Independent of development stage or commercial demands, a mini-batch CDC process runs at low line rates and the actual mini-batch size remains small (~1 kg). Therefore, mini-batch CDC is likely to be more forgiving in terms of powder flow requirements and overcoming an unfavorable compression performance (Karttunen, et al., 2019).

Still, there are three important mini-batch CDC-related formulation aspects to be considered: (i) segregation prevention, (ii) technical restrictions in terms of number of feeders, and (iii) inappropriate API properties and/or variability, leading to an increased emphasis on particle engineering.

i. Mini-batch CDC technology inherits specific process dynamics and a constant product flow between unit operations needs to be maintained. For instance, a discretely blended mini-batch moves from the blender outlet into the gain-in weight hopper and further through the material diversion point into the press. Therefore, it is essential to investigate the segregation potential of a target composition and gain an understanding of beneficial particle properties when selecting excipients for a CDC composition (Deng, Garg, Salehi, & Bradley, 2021). A fundamental understanding is essential since a significant change of blend uniformity between material diversion and the tableting process has to be avoided.

ii. API and excipients are simultaneously fed into the blender, and the technology benefits from the avoidance of additional production steps in order to make physical pre-blends. This comes with a major disadvantage. Due to design restrictions and containment requirements, only limited space is available to install LiW feeders above the blending unit. A conventional DC composition typically consists of an API, a filler–binder combination of lactose, microcrystalline cellulose, mannitol, isomalt and/or corn starch, disintegrants like crospovidone or croscarmellose sodium, glidants like fumed silica, and lubricants like magnesium stearate or sodium stearyl fumarate. In addition, the formulation may also require additional components like acidifiers, sweeteners, wetting agents, or a flavor. At least six individual compounds are usually present. Therefore, a formulation intended for all scales of CDC has to be simplified in order to match the available number of feeders. This can be achieved by using commercially available co-processed excipients. Co-processed excipients consist of two or more compounds of compendial grade which, unlike simple powder blends, cannot physically be separated anymore. They basically act as single excipients with multiple functionalities. A good example is silicified microcrystalline cellulose (Prosolv® etc.), where the filler is combined with a glidant, providing a filler/binder with improved flow properties (Komersová, Lochař, Myslíková, Mužíková, & Bartoš, 2016). Microcelac® is another binary excipient, which consists of microcrystalline cellulose and lactose. Combilac® additionally contains starch to improve the disintegration behavior (Dominik, et al., 2021; Bekaert, et al., 2021). Ludipress® provides similar functionality by combining lactose, crospovidone, and povidone. There are even multifunctional ready-to-use compositions commercially available (e.g., Prosolv® Easytab) providing the option to add even more additional excipients.

iii. In DC processes, especially in the case a high drug loading is required, the API particle properties become critical and may directly impact the final bulk properties (flowability) and compression behavior (Van Snick, et al., 2018). This effect can be further amplified, in case biopharmaceutical considerations lead to fine milling of the API (micronization) which often results in low bulk density and increased cohesiveness and related poor flow properties. In addition, during the different DP development stages, also the DS process is further optimized. This can cause variability in the API properties, directly impacting the DP manufacturing process performance and quality. For such cases, formulators so far took the opportunity to switch to a wet or dry granulation process, in order to compensate for possible negative effects caused by the API particles (Leane, Pitt, & Reynolds, 2015). It has to be considered that DC inherently is the simplest tablet manufacturing process with the smallest number of potential CPP. This simplicity makes DC the preferred technology to maintain short development timelines and minimize transfer and scale-up efforts. It is also attractive for CM applications, without complex granulation and/ or drying unit operations. In order to overcome the aforementioned particle property-related limitations, a very early collaboration between DS and DP is mandatory, in order to explore if the API properties can be further optimized and specified. Particle properties can be improved by optimizing the crystallization and/or milling process or achieved by more advanced technologies like dry or polymer coating, spherical agglomeration, or usage of carrier particles.

6.5 Conclusion

In summary, the progression in paradigm over the last 20 years has been a huge challenge for the pharmaceutical industry. The earlier testing-for-compliance behavior is giving way to a situation where process understanding is developed in PD, verified in PPQ, and then further maintained via PM. Partly this challenge has been a need for a cultural change, but partly the way we previously developed products has had to change from developing processes that worked, to establishing why those processes worked.

Pharmaceutical developers have had to find ways to establish what attributes of the process are critical, the acceptable process space in which to operate, and how to establish controls to ensure process and product quality, and also to maintain these learnings over the lifecycle of the product.

Traditional batch approaches simply prevented this (because of cost and availability of API, coupled with the large API amounts required for batch development) and CM enabled the paradigm shift to happen, but still required us to establish knowledge and understanding of complex processes. One of the most significant learnings was that we could manufacture the products at the volumes required, for the patient populations with much simpler processes, and vastly reduced mass of material in-flight, making possible both lean processes and lean control strategy. As we reduce scale, we establish higher levels of fundamental understanding. Mini-batch CDC offers the current best combination: greatest reduction in manufacturing scale, lowest complexity of unit operations, simplest process dynamics, and highest yield. It allows us to leave behind the fundamental limitations of batch processing even for small volume molecules – thus offering a truly transformational technology for DP development and manufacture. With mini-batch CDC, the commercial process can be locked earlier in development, without the need for scale-up, and also the control strategy can be very lean with appropriate process control and quality attributes confirmed by soft-sensor predictions, using at-line/offline analysis to confirm the state of process understanding and PAT methods used for PM.

As outlined above, the mini-batch CDC process has intrinsic advantages compared to a batch process. On the other hand, it requires the need to simplify the composition and optimize the API particle properties in order to make the technology broadly applicable.

REFERENCES

Badman, C., Cooney, C., Florence, A., Konstantinov, K., Krumme, M., Mascia, S., ... Trout, B. (2019). Why we need continuous pharmaceutical manufacturing and how to make it happen. *J. Pharm. Sci.*, *108*, 3521–3523.

Bebinger, M. (2016, May 23). *Inventing a Machine That Spits Out Drugs in a Whole New Way*. Retrieved from NPR – All Things Considered: https://www.npr.org/sections/health-shots/2016/05/23/478576727/inventing-a-machine-that-spits-out-pills-a-whole-new-way?t=1637572958155

Bekaert, B., Penne, L., Grymonpré, W., Van Snick, B., Dhondt, J., Boeckx, J., ... Vanhoorne, V. (2021). Determination of a quantitative relationship between material properties, process settings and screw feeding behavior via multivariate data-analysis. *Int. J. Pharm.*, *602*, 120603.

Blackwood, D., Bonnassieux, A., & Cogoni, G. (2019). Continuous Direct Compression Using Portable Continuous Miniature Mdular & Manufacturing (PCM&M). In M. Am Ende, & D. Am Ende, *Chemical Engineering in the Pharmaceutical Industry: Drug Product Design, Development, and Modeling*, 2nd Edition. Wiley.

Deng, T., Garg, V., Salehi, H., & Bradley, M. S. (2021). Correlations between segregation intensity and material properties such as particle sizes and adhesions and novel methods for assessment. *Powder Technol.*, *387*, 215–226.

Dominik, M., Vraníková, B., Svačinová, P., Elbl, J., Pavloková, S., Prudilová, B., ... Franc, A. (2021). Comparison of flow and compression properties of four lactose-based co-processed excipients: Cellactose® 80, CombiLac®, MicroceLac® 100, and StarLac®. *Pharmaceutics*, *13*, 1486.

Engisch, W. E. (2012). Method for characterization of loss-in-weight feeder equipment. *Powder Technol.*, *228*, 395–403.

FDA. (2011). *Guidance for Industry Process Validation: General Principles and Practices*.

FDA. (2012). *ICH Q8, Q9, & Q10 Questions and Answers – Appendix: Q&As from Training Sessions (Q8, Q9, & Q10 Points to Consider)*.

Gordon, L. (2018). Continuous OSD in the field. Pharma Engineering, Nov/Dec, 52–57.

Hetrick, E. M. (2021). Sample mass estimate for the use of near-infrared and raman spectroscopy to monitor content uniformity in a tablet press feed frame of a drug product continuous manufacturing process. *Appl. Spectrosc.*, 75(2) 216–224.

Holman, J., Tantuccio, A., Palmer, J., van Doninck, T., & Meyer, R. (2021). A very boring 120 h: 15million tablets under a continuous state of control. *Powder Tech.*, *382*, 208–231.

ICH Q8 (R2). (2014). *International Conference on Harmonisation of Technical Requirements for Registration of Pharmaceuticals for Human Use considerations (ICH) guideline Q8 (R2) on pharmaceutical development*.

Jakubowska, E., & Ciepluch, N. (2021). Blend segregation in tablets manufacturing and its effect on drug content uniformity—A review. *Pharmaceutics*, *13*, 1909.

Karttunen, A.-P., Wikström, H., Tajarobi, P., Sparén, A., Marucci, M., Ketolainen, J., … Abrahmsén-Alami, S. (2019). Comparison between integrated continuous direct compression line and batch processing – The effect of raw material properties. *Eur. J. Pharma. Sci.*, *133*, 40–53.

Kauppinen, A., Karhu, H., & Lakio, S. (2019). Dead mass in continuous blending. *Powder Tech.*, *355*, 67–71.

Koehler, F. W. (2002). Near infrared spectroscopy: the practical chemical imaging solution. *Spectrsc. Eur.*, *14*(3), 12–19.

Komersová, A., Lochař, V., Myslíková, K., Mužíková, J., & Bartoš, M. (2016). Formulation and dissolution kinetics study of hydrophilic matrix tablets with tramadol hydrochloride and different co-processed dry binders. *Eur. J. Pharm. Sci.*, *95*, 36–45.

Kushner, J. (2010). Scale-up model describing the impact of lubrication on tablet tensile strength. *Int. J. Pharm.*, *399*, 19–30.

Leane, M., Pitt, K., & Reynolds, G. T. (2015). A proposal for a drug product manufacturing classification system (MCS) for oral solid dosage forms. *Pharm. Dev. Technol.*, *20*, 12–21.

Manley, L. (2019). Tablet compression force as a process analytical technology (PAT): 100% inspection and control of tablet weight uniformity. *J. Pharm. Sci.*, *108*(1), 485–493.

Maurer, R. (2021). Mini-batch technology: equivalence between integrated process and integrated line. *IFPAC 2021, Portable and Point of Patient Manufacturing*.

Miggliaccio, G. (2004). The case for manufacturing science. *Arden House Conference March 23, 2004*.

Rees, I. (2021). Mobilizing manufacturing: portable and point of care manufacture of medicines. *DIA 2021 Global Annual Meeting*.

Shi, Z. (2017). Development of near infrared (NIR) spectroscopy-based process monitoring methodology for pharmaceutical continuous manufacturing using an offline calibration approach. *Anal. Chem.*, *89*(17).

Thomas, H. (2012). Utilizing continuous processing for streamlined and efficient development of QbD products. *IFPAC*, Cortona.

Van Snick, B., Grymonpré, W., Dhondt, J., Pandelaere, K., Di Pretoro, G., Remon, J., … Vanhoorne, V. (2018). Impact of blend properties on die filling during tableting. *Int J Pharma.*, *549*, 476–488.

Vanarase, A. U., & Muzzio, F. J. (2011). Effect of operating conditions and design parameters in a continuous powder mixer. *Powder Technol.*, *208*, 26–36.

Vanhoorne, V., & Vervaet, C. (2020). Recent progress in continuous manufacturing of oral solid dosage forms. *Int. J. Pharma.*, *579*, 119194.

Xu, L., Amidon, G., Khan, M., Hoag, S., Polli, J., Raju, G., & Woodcock, J. (2014). Understanding pharmaceutical quality by design. *AAPS J.*, *16*, 771–783.

Yu, L. X. (2014, July). Understanding pharmaceutical quality by design. *AAPS J.* *16*(4), 771–783.

Warman, M., PAT Implementation in Continuous Manufacturing, *IFPAC Conference* 22 Jan 2014.

7

Predictive In-Vitro Dissolution for Real-Time Release Test (RTRT) for Continuous Manufacturing Process on Drug Product

Zhenqi Shi
Small Molecule Pharmaceutical Sciences, Genentech, South San Francisco, CA, USA

Stan Altan and Dwaine Banton
Janssen Pharmaceutical LLC, Spring House, PA, USA

Sarah Nielsen
Janssen Supply Chain, Spring House, PA, USA

Martin Otava
Janssen-Cilag s.r.o. Janssen Pharmaceutical Companies of Johnson & Johnson, Praha, Czechia

Aaron Garrett
Global Quality Laboratory, Eli Lilly and Company, Indianapolis, IN, USA

Matthew Walworth
Small Molecule Design and Development, Eli Lilly and Company, Indianapolis, IN, USA

CONTENTS

DOI: 10.1201/9781003149835-8

7.1 Introduction

With the rapid adoption of continuous manufacturing (CM) in development and manufacturing operations, it is commonly acknowledged that end-to-end data integration is critical for success. End-to-end data integration refers to the consolidation of data related to raw material attributes, process parameters, and intermediate and finished drug product quality attributes. The increasing use of automated data historian and process analytical technology (PAT) data warehousing IT packages in CM enables data integration, sometimes in a real-time fashion. Holistic data integration plays an important role in establishing development understanding and robust deployment of the CM process, but it also provides a good opportunity to link all the relevant material attributes and process parameters to predict *in vitro* drug product performance. The intent of this chapter is to document best practices for developing predictive dissolution models for CM DP to fulfill its intended purpose as a real-time release test (RTRT).

Oral solid dosage forms (tablets and capsules) constitute a large fraction of pharmaceutical products. Dissolution testing is an *in vitro* laboratory performance test that assesses how efficiently a drug is released from its dosage form. In drug development, dissolution profiles have been used to investigate the impact of formulation composition and process parameters on the *in vitro* release of API, as a surrogate to evaluate its bio-performance, that is, *in vivo* release of API. In manufacturing, *in vitro* dissolution has been used routinely as a quality control (QC) test to ensure batch-to-batch manufacturing consistency and quality. Thus, it has become an integral part of regulatory filings worldwide, with the expectation to serve as a QC tool to detect any chemical or physical property deviations that could affect *in vitro* release leading to its *in vivo* exposure (i.e., bio-performance).

Predictive dissolution modeling is an emerging mathematical and statistical methodology used to generate a time profile of the dissolved amount of an API based on information associated with material physical properties, dissolution method conditions, formulation composition, and/or process parameters. While both *in vivo* and *in vitro* dissolution can be simulated and predicted, the focus of this paper is to document best practices for *in vitro* predictive dissolution modeling. *In vivo* predictive dissolution (an important part of drug product bio-performance), the integration of dissolution profiles into physiology-based pharmacokinetic (PBPK) models, and the demonstration of the clinical relevance of the *in vitro* dissolution method are outside the scope of this chapter and have been documented elsewhere [1, 2].

In pharmaceutics, *in vitro* dissolution modeling has primarily been used for (i) early-stage formulation and process development and (ii) late-phase predictive dissolution development for RTRT in manufacturing [3]. The dissolution working group under the International Consortium for Innovation and Quality in Pharmaceutical Development (IQ) recently published a white paper on the use of such a phase-dependent predictive modeling approach for *in vitro* dissolution [3]. During early-phase formulation and process development, first-principle and mechanistic modeling combined with targeted experimentation has been used to identify critical material attributes (CMAs) and critical process parameters (CPPs). Subsequent screening studies lead to the development of a robust formulation design space. The use of dissolution models can facilitate the formulation and process development, as well as significantly reduce laboratory dissolution testing during early-phase development, thereby minimizing the amount of API that would otherwise be required for traditional testing. As development advances and the amount of product and process data increases, dissolution modeling approaches are refined, resulting in enhanced predictive capability. In late-phase development, empirical models are frequently used to develop data-driven predictive models to enable RTRT and QC testing. It enables commercial release via leveraging offline and real-time process data throughout a manufacturing process to predict a dissolution profile, rather than basing the release decision on product testing conducted after completion of the manufacturing process. Thus, it can minimize or eliminate destructive testing on tablets/capsules in a QC environment and speed up the product release. The aforementioned white paper provided a very well-rounded overview of different modeling approaches, but with a limited case study illustrating how empirical approaches have been used in industrial settings to develop an RTRT method for QC batch release under CM. The purpose of this chapter is to showcase recent progress, with the addition of the most recent literature since the publication of the IQ white paper, in the field of *in vitro* predictive dissolution modeling for RTRT and QC testing, as well as to provide case studies that highlight recommended approaches to develop *in vitro* predictive dissolution models for batch release. It is the authors' intention to leverage this chapter to increase communication with regulatory authorities, working toward establishing an appropriate framework and/or acceptance criteria for the use of dissolution models in future regulatory submissions.

7.2 Model Development

7.2.1 Reference Dissolution Method Development

A successful strategy for implementation of *in vitro* predictive dissolution starts with the Quality Target Product Profile (QTPP) in mind. The QTPP helps define the CQAs that define the product quality, including a target for how the drug is to be released *in vivo*. The QTPP informs formulation and process development as well as dissolution method development. Before performing any modeling exercises, it is important to identify the CMAs and CPPs that are based upon the physical and chemical properties of the API and of formulation and process conditions, which, in turn, can be linked to dissolution performance. For immediate release (IR) drug products, the Biopharmaceutics Classification System (BCS) provides high-level guidance for CMAs based on API properties [4]. For drug products of BCS class I and III with high solubility, the rate and extent of drug absorption are unlikely to be dependent on drug dissolution and/or GI transit time. Consequently, according to the International Conference on Harmonization (ICH) procedure Q6a [5], surrogate methods such as disintegration and/or models used to predict disintegrations can replace dissolution to guide formulation development. For those drug products of BCS class I and III that do not meet the above criteria, or for drug products of BCS class II and IV drug substances, that is, characterized as poorly soluble, the dissolution profile must be carefully determined, as it could be the rate-limiting step for absorption [6]. Thus, for these compounds, it is essential to thoroughly understand the factors that affect *in vitro* release. The factors chosen for the predictive modeling exercise can originate from either a risk-based approach or experimental data illustrating the impact of CMAs and CPPs on dissolution profiles. Experimental approaches often use a scientifically rigorous design of experiment (DoE) and statistical analysis tools to screen for the CMAs and CPPs. A fishbone diagram is often used to facilitate the identification of CMAs and CPPs regardless of a risk-based approach or an experimental approach [3].

Development of a predictive dissolution model requires the availability of a reference dissolution method against which the model can be calibrated/trained. A reference dissolution method should be designed to discriminate for those CMAs and CPPs that impact the rate-limiting processes contributing to dissolution. Discriminating capability of the dissolution method is an important element of new drug applications (NDA) that health authorities seek during CMC review. If the discriminating capability of the method is demonstrated on the most relevant CMAs and CPPs, the method can be considered a QC tool to be used in commercial and stability testing to ensure the consistency and quality of drug product release profiles. Thus, the fact that a predictive model is calibrated against a dissolution method makes the discriminating ability of the predictive model dependent upon that of the dissolution method. In other words, a less discriminating dissolution method is expected to result in a less capable predictive dissolution model.

7.2.2 Model Calibration

Because this predictive modeling approach is data-driven and matures as it progresses through drug product development, the "fit-for-purpose" model development exercise typically occurs during late-phase development and follows the "Lifecycle Approach", where the development of a dissolution model is concurrent with formulation development and process optimization. The details of applying a lifecycle approach to develop a sensitive and robust chemometric model for dissolution are consistent with the general guidelines for developing a chemometric model, which can be found elsewhere [7, 8]. Exploring the formulation and process knowledge space provides an opportunity to understand the impact of various formulation and process variables on dissolution, which also establishes a foundation for the subsequent model-building exercise. Generally, it is recommended to demonstrate enough dissolution variability from model training data to allow subsequent modeling algorithms to provide sufficient discriminating power. The predictive model is then expected to serve as a surrogate for product dissolution testing within the space explored during formulation/process optimization. In that case, a predictive model can be leveraged as a release test to directly support the control strategy. However, the use of the predictive model as a test surrogate in a regulatory filing is not always the end goal of such a modeling exercise. Modeling efforts could also be leveraged to improve process understanding and to support regulatory filings.

Given the empirical nature of dissolution models intended for release testing, the clinical relevance of the QC release method needs to be evaluated on a case-by-case basis based on the physical, chemical, and physiological properties of the drug product. The key is to understand the relationship between dissolution and clinical relevance, which is often carried out via dedicated PBPK modeling and/or *In Vivo-In Vitro* Correlation (IVIVC) and pharmacokinetics (PK) studies. In cases when a dissolution method is found to be clinically relevant, a QC release method is expected to reject non-bioequivalent batches. In such cases, dissolution is considered the critical *in vivo* surrogate sensor as it is the only *in vitro* performance test that probes the extent and rate of *in vivo* release. For cases when no clinical relevance is observed for dissolution (e.g., dissolution is not the rate-limiting step of drug absorption), it is possible to establish a normal operating range (NOR) of the formulation and process conditions well within the design space explored during the formulation and process development. In those cases, a dissolution model (if established) can predict with confidence that every batch of product manufactured within that space would pass dissolution specification. The increasing adoption of CM provides additional assurance compared to a traditional batch process that a NOR could be achieved within a state-of-control in a consistent manner. In that scenario, it may not matter whether the predictive dissolution model leverages real-time data, since at that point real-time collected data would only verify the entire manufacturing process as it would no longer be a decision-making point. In such a case, the dissolution test shall be considered low/medium risk. Thus, instead of developing a predictive dissolution model, mapping out a dissolution safe space is expected to provide regulatory flexibility and can potentially justify setting a wider specification given the safe space identified through formulation/process development and optimization and supported by justifiable PBPK evidence.

7.2.2.1 Independent Data

Two types of data sources are often used in the empirical approach for dissolution modeling. The first type is off-line set-points and characterization data, such as formulation parameters (e.g., composition, component particle sizes, and bulk density of the process intermediate) and/or process conditions (e.g., compression force, blending time, granulation endpoint moisture content). The use of these parameters in building quantitative models of dissolution profiles/parameters has been a common practice during formulation and process optimization for the desired release profile for both immediate release (IR) and modified release (MR) products [9–17]. Multiple linear regression and response surface methodology have been reported for that purpose. The second type is real-time data, often via the use of non-invasive analytical tools, collected at-line, online, and/or in-line during the manufacturing process. Examples include tablet weight and thickness, blend or tablet spectroscopy profiles (such as near-infrared spectroscopy [NIRS] and Raman spectroscopy), or final product visual imaging. Since the issuance of the PAT guideline by the United States Food and Drug Administration (FDA) in 2004 [18], the use of these tools (especially spectroscopy) has gained popularity. The most used spectroscopic data is from NIRS, given its sensitivity to both chemical and physical properties and its versatility to analyze samples of powder, granules, ribbons, and tablets [19–35]. Recently, the combinational uses of both types of data have gained popularity, especially with the use of machine learning and artificial intelligence [36–38]. Case studies in the later section of this chapter are good examples of these different independent data sources.

7.2.2.2 Dependent Data

Literature surveys suggest that dissolution models are typically used to forecast either (i) dissolution percentage at a specific time point (or the converse: time required to reach a specific percentage of release), or (ii) a mathematical description of dissolution profiles with calculated or fitted coefficients (kinetics-driven exponential decay, Weibull profile, etc.). Each approach is valid and is best applied at different phases of product development. For a target time point/release level coordinate, both measured and predicted values have been reported. This is the most common release specification type and the easiest to evaluate and apply in a QC environment and under a manufacturing setting. However, it potentially ignores valuable information found by evaluating the entire profile. By contrast, the fitted or predicted full-profile target demonstrates a systematic understanding of the relationship between fitted coefficients and the formulation and process variables, since these profile-defining parameters/coefficients are metrics containing aggregate information on the entire dissolution time profile. With a proper DoE and statistical analysis to account for multiple sources of error, full dissolution profile prediction can be used to discriminate for design variables across multiple unit operations. Although a release specification on a fitted or calculated coefficient is not a typical regulatory-approved approach, it can provide guidance and flexibility in a post-approval change setting to justify which time point is to be used as the univariate release spec, even for interpolated time points. For instance, the highest discrimination power across a dissolution profile within a DoE may not be at a pre-defined time point, for example, 41.4 minutes. The use of interpolated dissolution profiles based upon fitted/calculated parameters allows the release spec to be set at the time point with the highest discriminating ability if that meets the intended purpose.

7.3 Model Validation

A predictive *in vitro* dissolution model is dependent upon a traditional dissolution method. Thus, it is imperative that the reference method is validated and is sufficiently discriminating to changes in the CMAs and/or CPPs. Additionally, a predictive dissolution model that includes data from multiple upstream in-process methods (e.g., granule PSD and moisture) is also expected to ensure that those in-process methods/models themselves be fitfully validated according to their intended purposes.

Predictive *in vitro* dissolution method development is multifaceted, given that calibration samples could be either manufactured or prepared in a laboratory, spanning anticipated sources of variation. It is of utmost importance that an independent validation set that spans the operational space defined by the calibration set be used for model validation. Achieving all these requirements in a single manufacturing campaign is improbable. Thus, it is likely that a combination of manufacturing campaign samples and development samples will be required.

Validation of a predictive dissolution model used as a surrogate for traditional dissolution testing (i.e., RTRT) is similar to the validation of a spectroscopy-based model for content uniformity release testing [39]. Validation elements specific to a predictive dissolution model primarily include accuracy relative to the reference method and robustness. First, linearity and accuracy can be demonstrated by the correlation coefficient R [40], and the root mean square error, respectively, for an observed versus predicted fit of either (i) percentage dissolved at a specific time point or (ii) dissolution profile reconstructed by those fitted coefficients. To gauge model accuracy, a comparison of passing/failing acceptance criteria, the root mean square error of calibration and/or cross-validation, and the root mean error of prediction (using an independent validation set) can be reported. Furthermore, if the entire dissolution profile is predicted, an observed versus predicted similarity metric (e.g., f_1, f_2, or Mahalanobis' distance) can be presented to indicate equivalency to the reference method [25, 30, 41]. Second, demonstration of model robustness should leverage data collected throughout the process and model development with designed sources of variability. Variations studied can be deemed "no practical impact" to model performance (i.e., robust) using statistical probability testing in a Bayesian framework. Material, process, and/or equipment variations that have a significant effect on the model should be rigorously managed via a defined model operating space and the development of model outlier diagnostics sensitive to such variations. Outlier detection methods are a common risk mitigation strategy in multivariate regression models. These are statistical tests (e.g., Hotelling's T^2 and residual variance) conducted to determine whether the analysis of a multivariate response using a calibration model represents a result outside the calibration space. Further details on validation can be found within the referenced FDA guidance for industry [42]. Third, the specificity of a predictive dissolution model can be addressed by either checking the validity of those CMA and CPPs included as independent variables for the model or checking the consistency of the model loading plot against pure API spectrum if a spectroscopy signal is used as the model input.

7.4 Lifecycle Management

Two different deployment approaches are common in the field after a predictive dissolution model passes its validation for the purpose of RTRT. One approach is to use the validated model for batch release immediately from the first commercial campaign. The other is to perform, in parallel, both traditional dissolution testing and predictive dissolution modeling. After a consistent agreement between the two methods, evaluated by appropriate statistical means, the pharmaceutical manufacturer has the option to use the predictive dissolution model exclusively for the purpose of real-time batch release. Based upon prior successful experiences with predictive models for RTRT for assay and content uniformity, it is highly recommended to gain pre-alignment with regulatory agencies regarding the choice of deployment approach.

A predictive dissolution model used for RTRT requires model maintenance and ongoing verification, regardless of whether it is deployed for batch or continuous process. Current good manufacturing practices (cGMP) must be in place to determine the triggers for model updates and the frequency of ongoing verification. CM may offer earlier and more sensitive detection of such variations for model updates compared to batch processes, especially when upstream in-process method/model outputs are used as inputs for the predictive dissolution model. In this case, the model update on an upstream in-process method/model is likely triggered earlier than the downstream predictive dissolution model. Thus, it is foreseeable that the use of predictive dissolution modeling for RTRT under CM may experience less frequent model updates relative to batch processes. Nevertheless, periodic verification against a reference dissolution method as a routine exercise for ongoing verification is highly recommended to assure the validity of common causes of variation. Protocols are recommended to be put in place to differentiate special cause variation from common cause variation and the associated control actions. Special-cause-triggered verification may take place on an as-needed basis, such as a change in excipient vendor. The trigger for model update often relies on multivariate diagnostics values (such as Hotelling T^2 and residual values) indicating that the process or material changes have a significant potential to impact drug product dissolution. Control limits must be in place for these diagnostic values to ensure the method remains in a validated state. If a model update is needed, a risk-based revalidation protocol must be executed to bring the predictive model back to its validated state.

Post-approval changes can be aided by dissolution modeling as well, especially if validated dissolution models were part of the original submission. The modeling approach and utility of dissolution modeling for post-approval changes are highly dependent on the nature and level of the change. Mechanistic understanding of the dissolution phenomena that is used in early-phase development and formulation selection can also be used to predict the effects of post-approval changes with minimal, targeted experimentations.

For manufacturing release and QC, validated dissolution models for batch release or RTRT and/or model-based *in vitro* dissolution methods can be used following post-approval changes if it can be shown that the model space encompasses the process post-change. If the change positions the process outside the limits of existing release models or methods, then the process understanding gained through establishing the models can also be used to guide experiments for reestablishing and revalidating the models/methods with a minimal experimental burden. In these cases, dissolution models can be powerful tools to minimize *in vivo* and *in vitro* experimental burdens to support post-approval changes.

7.5 Janssen's Case Study – A Statistical Approach to the Development of a Real-Time Release Testing Surrogate Model for Dissolution [43]

7.5.1 Introduction

The full realization of RTRT of solid dose products in either CM or traditional batch manufacture applying PAT must include the development of a surrogate model for dissolution testing (*in vitro* release). It is both a scientific and commercial challenge. We propose a statistical approach to a surrogate model permitting the prediction of the full dissolution profile and studying its properties. A case study of a fluid bed granulated BCS Class 4 batch manufactured product is given. Base SAS® software [58] and SAS/STAT® code are included to permit the interested reader to implement the approach with minimal adaptation. Our goal will be to provide a roadmap to an evidentiary framework which can establish statistical assessment and qualification of the proposed surrogate model.

The proposed surrogate dissolution model relies on a comprehensive experimental design to identify CPPs, leading to a "process" model in the first step. The process model relates the full dissolution profile and API content by NIR measurements as a multivariate response to the experimental design factors as independent predictors. One advantage of a formal and data-rich experimental design is that it carries causal predictive ability.

The dissolution response could also be a partial profile, say specifically selected time points, for example, 20- or 30-minute release, or it could be the parameters of a parametric nonlinear function describing the full profile. In the former, it is a specific time point(s) model, whereas, in the latter, it is a full dissolution profile prediction model.

Following the definition of the response as a multivariate vector, in the second step, a conditional regression [50] method is applied to the process model to develop a population average predictive surrogate model. Consequently, comparison across run averages rather than at individual tablet levels will be the standard comparison approach. Placing this statistical approach into a Bayesian context permits simulations that can characterize its analytical performance metrics.

We recommend that the experimental manufacturing protocols be coupled with *in vitro* dissolution testing that orthogonalizes dissolution/HPLC run effects with apparatus vessel and experimental batch effects. This aspect of the surrogate model development will not be discussed in this chapter.

Figure 7.1 lays out a schematic for the steps, principles, and concepts important to the surrogate model development approach. The subsequent sections of this chapter will closely follow these steps. The discussion will stay at a conceptual level as much as possible, and minimize the use of statistical and mathematical notation in the main text except where it is unavoidable. We will direct attention to the case study, where the approach will be laid out step by step including Base SAS® software code, with additional mathematical and statistical detail to explicate the approach. The simulated raw data for the case study are shown in Appendix 1.

7.5.2 The Three-Step Surrogate Model Development Paradigm

7.5.2.1 Step 1: Experimental Design

It would be difficult to overestimate the importance of a comprehensive experimental design to set the stage for the subsequent steps leading to the surrogate model. This is a consequence of the necessity

Principle   **Step**   **Considerations**

- Randomize
- Orthogonalize
- Blocking
- Factorial vs
  Split-Plots

Experiment
Design

- New CM Process
- Legacy Product Conversion to CM
- Legacy Product RTRT Conversion

| Parameter Selection |
| Parameter Ranges |
| Scale |

- Process Model
  driven by design
  relating dissolution
  to CPPs

Statistical
Process
Model

- Parameter Criticality Criteria
- Bayesian vs Frequentist Model

- Multivariate response
- Population Average
- Batch and Tablet
  level correlations
- Conditional Regression
  to construct surrogate
  model

Surrogate
Model

- Single Time Point
- Complete Dissolution Profile
  3-parameter Weibull

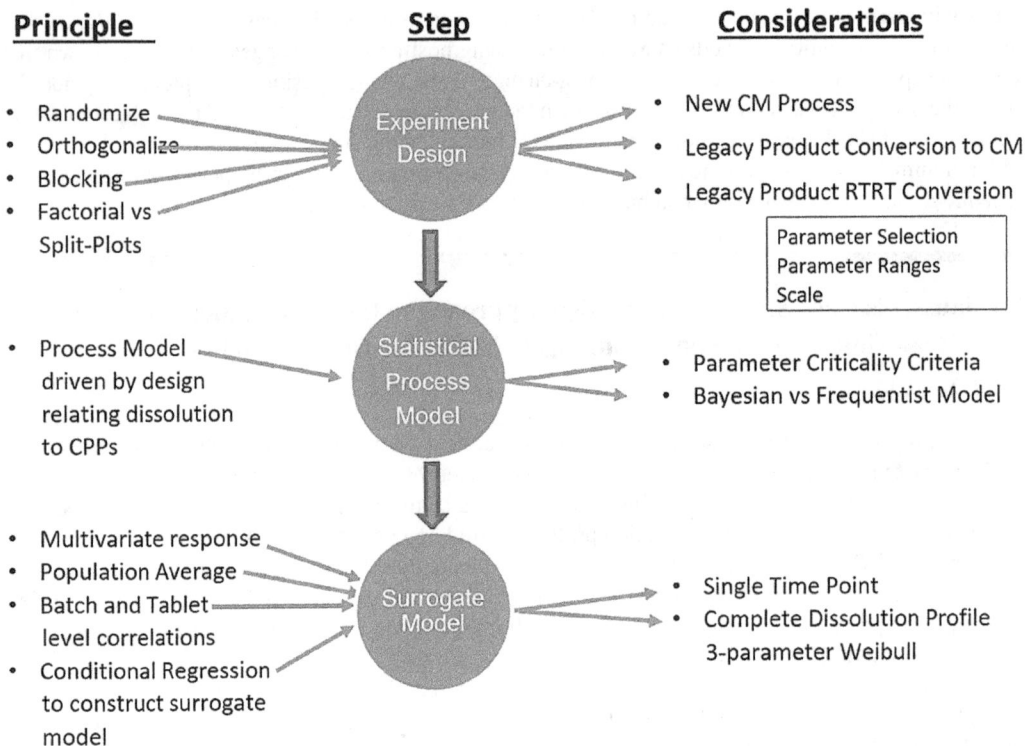

FIGURE 7.1   Overview of statistical surrogate modeling steps.

to identify the CPP in relation to critical quality attributes (CQA). This is part of a Quality-by-Design framework for process and product understanding. The choice of factors to include in the experiment can follow a criticality analysis, combined with scientific judgment and experience. A range of API concentrations is advisable as one of the factors in the design, for example, varying API concentration over the range of 90% to 110%. This would serve to establish a strong regression relationship to NIR in the surrogate model since API Content by NIR would be one of the predictors in the surrogate model. By including API concentration as an independent factor, API content free of tablet level variation would be linked directly to the NIR readings. In addition, it would permit a statistical inference on linearity in the analytical performance assessment. At the same time, the need for respecting good experimental design principles related to randomization, blocking, and orthogonalization is especially crucial in this context. A good discussion of statistical design principles and standard designs, their statistical analyses, and interpretations can be found in the literature [51, 47].

In the case study, a factorial design combined with a "split-plot" factor was used to identify the CPPs as the basis for developing a process model, that is, a model that relates CQAs to CPPs. A split-plot factor is a term used to describe a factor when it requires a given experimental run to be sampled repeatedly and each sample of that run is subjected to a different level of the split-plot factor (the term "treatment" is synonymous with factor in the statistical literature). An example of a split-plot factor is compression force, studied at three levels – typically low, mid, and high for each experimental run – to determine its effect on tablet properties. The responses for these three levels would be correlated by virtue of sharing a common set of experimental conditions and materials. Ideally, each run would be subjected to the levels of the split-plot factors in a random fashion; for example, run 1 might be studied at compression force levels in the order Mid, High, Low, and run 2 might be studied in the order Low, Mid, High, and so on. The randomization principle in experimental design is necessary to confer statistical validity on the subsequent analysis and inferences.

The choice of experimental design, for example, a definitive screening [52], factorial, response surface design, or one based on optimality criteria is an important consideration. It is beyond the scope of this chapter to discuss design selection in detail, other than to say that the choice of design should be driven by both practical considerations related to cost, time and material, and statistical objectives. Part of the design consideration is the number of tablets that should be studied at each factor combination, respecting both practical limitations as well as statistical uncertainty. We will not address this question in detail in this chapter, but it is advisable to consider the a priori tolerance to uncertainty of critical quantities in guiding the choice of sample size. We answer this question in general terms by requiring full dissolution profiles be collected from "n" tablets per experimental run. In the case study, $n = 6$, but this may vary in different experiments depending on the specific needs of the experimental program, possible power considerations, and downstream objectives.

It is necessary to keep in mind the possibility of "blocking" the runs. For example, if some runs share common starting materials, such as drug substance lots, then those experimental runs arising from common drug substance lots would be correlated and can be considered a "block". The way the blocking affects the order of the runs needs to be considered at the design selection stage and has implications for later modeling.

Understanding the sources of variability in the experimental design is another important consideration. Typically, manufacturing variability or batch-to-batch variability is a separate source of variability from analytical uncertainty. It is also known that for solid dose products such as tablets, no two tablets can be assumed to be identical with respect to physical and chemical characteristics, for example, API content. Thus, tablets can represent another level of variability, which is generally confounded with analytical uncertainty. However, with modern NIR technology, under certain conditions, tablet–tablet variability can be estimated free of analytical uncertainty. These different sources of variability, individually referred to as variance components, must be clearly understood and accounted for in any experimental plan, and is critical in the case of surrogate model development because some part is included in the surrogate model construction.

Finally, the ability to extrapolate the experimental results to full-scale commercial production requires a clear understanding. This question is one of the most crucial in surrogate model development. The factors studied in the development experiment must be directly comparable to the same factors in the commercial scale environment. For example, if compression force is studied with a certain tablet press in the experiment, then we must require the ability to extrapolate experimental results to the corresponding equipment at a commercial scale. Attentive due diligence is required in establishing that the experimental conditions at the development scale are comparable to the commercial environment where the surrogate model predictions will be carried out subject to regulatory rules.

7.5.2.2 Defining the Multivariate Response – The Three-Parameter Weibull Function

Once the dissolution profiles are collected, following the experimental plan decided on in the first step, then a three-parameter Weibull function is fitted to the dissolution profiles, with each tablet yielding estimates of the three parameters. The Weibull function was selected to represent dissolution profiles for its ability to capture a range of profile shapes [48], and to allow for a tablet-specific estimate of tablet API content. In practice, any parametric nonlinear model thought to be an appropriate descriptor of the dissolution profile could be applied as well. Heterogeneity across time points should be investigated at this stage.

The three-parameter Weibull can be written as follows:

$$(Y_{it} \mid t, b_1, b_2, b_3) = b_1 * \left[1 - e^{-\left(\frac{t}{b_2}\right)^{b_3}} \right] + \varepsilon_{it}$$

where Y_{it} – Dissolution of Tablet i at Time t, b_1 – Dissolution Extent Parameter (upper bound, $b_1 = 100$ in Figure 7.2), b_2 – Rate Parameter, time to achieve, 62.5% (here, $b_2 = 10$), and b_3 – Shape Parameter.

A graph of the three-parameter Weibull function is shown in Figure 7.2 indicating the effect of three values of the shape parameter.

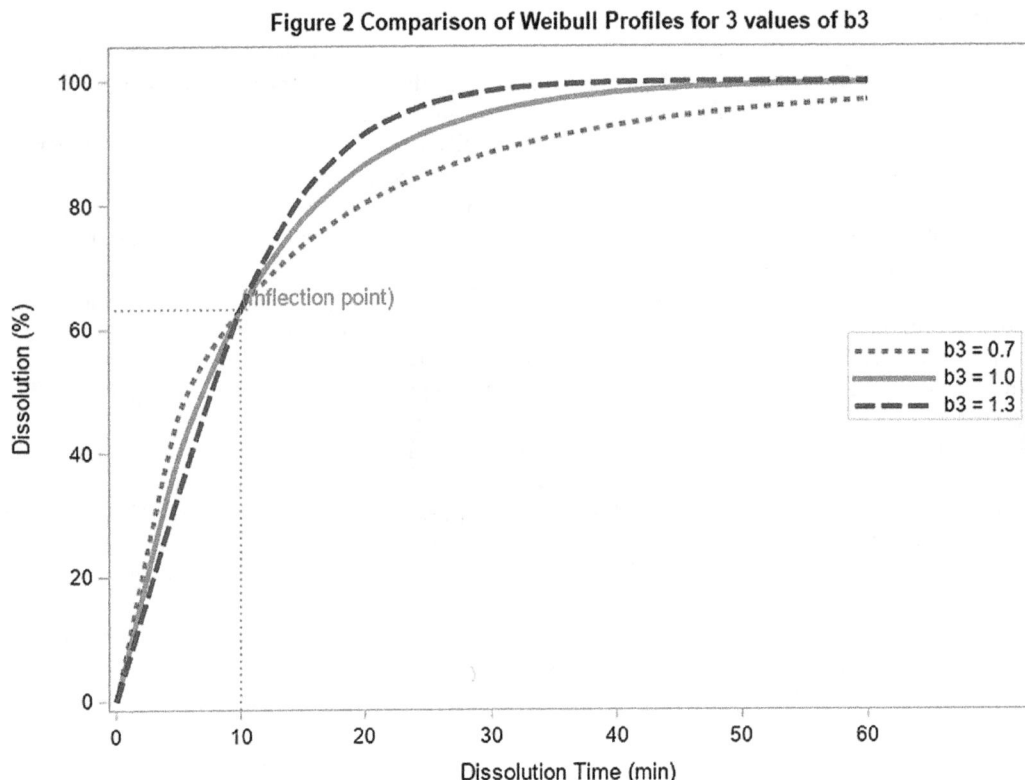

FIGURE 7.2 Comparison of Weibull profiles for three values of b3.

7.5.2.3 Step 2: Development of the Process Model

The three Weibull parameters, augmented with the API content by NIR for each tablet, are modeled as a multivariate response against the experimental factors to identify the CPPs leading to a final process model. Note that API content needs to be used as one of the responses and not as a covariate in the model, due to inherent measurement error in the NIR procedure. The modeling typically is an iterative process, proceeding in stages, where the early stages can be considered exploratory in nature, and the later stages arrive at the final process model. The model building or model selection process entails concepts described by Box et al. [44]. An important aspect of this process is the practical and statistical criteria used to aid model selection. These criteria are used to arrive at the final process model. The choice of model selection criteria is beyond the scope of this chapter, but one can consider, for example, the Akaike Information Criterion corrected (AICc) for bias, reduction in variance components or residual error, and the p-value combined with the meaningful magnitude of factor effects based on scientific considerations. Over-emphasis on p-values should be avoided [43]. A good discussion of selection methods is given in Kadane and Lazar [53]. In the end, we arrive at a process model relating dissolution and API content by NIR to the CPPs. Note that at this point, the process model alone is not capable of predicting dissolution as a surrogate prediction, since the API content is still represented as a response here. It will be the goal of the next section to show how the NIR measurement is used to help predict dissolution.

7.5.2.4 Step 3: Surrogate Model

In the final step, a conditional regression model is derived leading to the surrogate model itself. The conditioning procedure described in this section permits prediction with the measured NIR API content.

Hence, the Weibull parameters are conditionally regressed on the NIR reading (and CPP levels as covariates). The statistical details of this step are described in Appendix 2 and will be elaborated on in the case study.

In summary, we outline the three steps as follows:

Step 1: Experimental Design Selection and Multivariate Response
- Choose an appropriate experimental design
- Fit the Weibull model to each tablet's dissolution profile, three Weibull parameters are associated with each tablet

Step 2: Process Model
- Fit multivariate response (three Weibull parameters and API Content by NIR) against the DoE factors
- Identify the CPPs and fit the final model

Step 3: Surrogate Model
- Conditional regression of Weibull parameters on API Content by NIR and CPPs.
- Model fit, assessment of accuracy, and precision

We have described the first two steps with a minimal amount of statistical and mathematical notation. However, for step 3, the derivation of the surrogate model is difficult to describe without technical language. We will use some mathematical notation to explain the method in the case study. We can understand step 3 as an algebraic technique, known as conditional regression, for deriving a predictive model of three of the elements of the response vector (Weibull parameters), against the remaining element of the response vector (API Content by NIR) and given knowledge of the CPP levels used to manufacture the sample of tablets being measured. The conditional regression model then allows predictions of these Weibull parameters given a measured NIR value combined with the known levels of the CPPs. We ask the reader to consider the detailed sequence of steps we advocate in developing a surrogate model for dissolution, as laid out in the case study.

Finally, we hasten to add that there are various computing tools that one might consider for carrying out the statistical calculations laid out in the case study. We will use SAS® 9.4, as the primary computing tool in this chapter and give examples of SAS software code and output to steer the reader along the steps that we recommend for the development of a surrogate model. SAS software is a record-oriented computing language, that carries out calculations sequentially through each record, or data line in the dataset. Therefore, it's important to pay attention to the layout or data structure in preparation for data processing. The format of the SAS datasets will be part of the discussion in following the steps to the surrogate model development. We will separately publish R code to carry out similar calculations as the subject of another publication, which offers substantial statistical computing benefits as well. We turn now to the practical implementation of the approach being proposed through a case study.

7.5.3 Case Study

We begin with a description of the experimental design. Table 7.1 shows the factorial design with the split-plot factor; the levels of the factors are shown on a coded scale (-1, 0, $+1$). The factorial design consists of three factors arranged according to a 2^3-factorial design, with two center-point runs, and replications for two extreme runs giving a total of 13 runs. This provides a minimum of four degrees of freedom to estimate batch-batch (manufacturing) variability. Each experimental run (Exptal Run) is then studied at three levels of the split-plot factor, designated Factor 4. All four factors are continuous. The column headed by "Rep" indicates the replication number of the given experimental factor combination. The column designated "Run Order" gives the randomization for the order of carrying out the given factor combinations. Each of these runs can also be referred to as the main plot factor. Note that six tablets were studied for each combination of the four factors, thus yielding a total of 234 tablets (13 runs, 3 Factor

TABLE 7.1

Experimental Design Layout

Exptal Run	Rep	Run Order	Factor 1	Factor 2	Factor 3	Factor 4 Low	Mid	Hi
Run01	1	9	−1	−1	−1	−1	0	1
Run02	2	12	−1	−1	−1	−1	0	1
Run03	1	8	−1	−1	1	−1	0	1
Run04	1	5	−1	1	−1	−1	0	1
Run05	1	10	−1	1	1	−1	0	1
Run06	1	6	0	0	0	−1	0	1
Run07	2	13	0	0	0	−1	0	1
Run08	1	1	1	−1	−1	−1	0	1
Run09	1	3	1	−1	1	−1	0	1
Run10	1	4	1	1	−1	−1	0	1
Run11	1	2	1	1	1	−1	0	1
Run12	2	7	1	1	1	−1	0	1
Run13	3	11	1	1	1	−1	0	1

4 levels, six tablets, 13*3*6 = 234). A full dissolution profile at seven time points (5, 10, 15, 20, 30, 45, and 60 minutes) is collected according to a design partially balancing for dissolution vessel, experimental run, and dissolution run. These profiles constitute the essential response for the purpose of calculating a set of Weibull parameter estimates associated with each tablet.

7.5.3.1 Step 1: Weibull Fit by Tablet

The first step fits the Weibull function to each tablet's dissolution profile. The data shown in Appendix 1 requires a transposition of the dissolution profile prior to SAS software processing. For example, the first experimental run, designated Run01, has 18 tablets in 18 rows. Table 7.2 shows the row-wise data for the first two tablets.

The estimation of the Weibull parameters requires the data to be transposed to look as follows for the first tablet (Table 7.3).

The transposed dataset can be input to SAS/STAT® PROC NLIN to calculate the Weibull parameter estimates by tablet. The below SAS macro, WEIBULLPARAMS, can be called to carry out the calculations for each tablet in the dataset. A macro is a code that is specified with a notation that permits it to be repeatedly called to avoid extensive lines of code for calculations that require multiple executions, for example, for each tablet. The arguments to the macro are the name of the transposed dataset, and starting values for the Weibull parameters referred to as t1, t2, and t3. The Marquardt numerical method was specified because of the correlated nature of the parameters b1 and b2. This is a consequence of the tendency of the location parameter b2 to increase as the asymptote increases.

TABLE 7.2

Partial Listing of by Tablet Dataset

Exptal Run	Tablet Number	Content NIR	Dissolution Time (min) 5	10	15	20	30	45	60
Run01	1	93.1	47.1	71.8	81.9	87.9	94.9	95.7	93.5
Run01	2	94.4	47.8	78.7	86.9	90.4	96.0	96.4	97.4

TABLE 7.3

Partial Listing of Transposed Dataset

Exptal Run	Tablet Number	Time	Content NIR	Dissolution (%)
Run01	1	5	93.2	47.1
Run01	1	10	93.2	71.8
Run01	1	15	93.2	81.9
Run01	1	20	93.2	87.9
Run01	1	30	93.2	94.9
Run01	1	45	93.2	95.7
Run01	1	60	93.2	93.5

SAS code 1 – Weibull Model Fit by Tablet

```
%macro weibullparams(dat,t1,t2,t3);

    proc nlin data=&dat method=marquardt outest=out;
    by Run tabletnum;
    parms b1=&t0 b2=&t1 b3=&t2;
    model y = b1*(1-exp(-((time/b2)**b3)));
      output out=pred&dat R=RESID P=PRED
        student=res_stud stdi=se;
    ods output parameterestimates=parout&dat ;
    title1 "Weibull Model parameter Estimates by Tablet";
    run;

%mend weibullparams;

%weibullparams(a2, t1 = 100, t2 = 7, t3 = 1.1);
```

A partial sample output of Proc NLIN for the first tablet is given in Output Listing 1.

Output Listing 1 – Weibull model fit by tablet

The NLIN Procedure

Iterative Phase				
Iter	**b1**	**b2**	**b3**	**Sum of Squares**
0	100.0	7.0000	1.1000	246.9
1	94.9181	7.2266	0.9809	7.8371
...				
5	95.0298	7.2814	0.9882	7.6948

Note: Convergence criterion met.

Parameter	Estimate	Approx Std Error	Approximate 95% Confidence Limits	
b1	95.0298	0.9319	92.4426	97.6170
b2	7.2814	0.2448	6.6016	7.9612
b3	0.9882	0.0568	0.8307	1.1458

The Weibull parameter estimates are then collected and merged into another dataset containing the experimental factor identifiers, the tablet number, and the content by NIR. The first two tablets in that dataset are shown in Table 7.4. This dataset is the input for the next step, building the process model.

TABLE 7.4

Partial Listing of Dataset with Weibull Parameters by Tablet

Exptal Run	Factor				Tablet Num	Content NIR	Parameters		
	1	2	3	4			b1	b2	b3
Run01	−1	−1	−1	−1	1	93.1	95.03	7.28	0.99
Run01	−1	−1	−1	−1	2	94.4	96.15	6.76	1.14

7.5.3.2 *Step 2: Building the Process Model*

The previously described dataset in Table 7.4 is used to build the process model. The response vector is the Weibull parameter estimates augmented with the content by NIR measurement. The experimental factors are on the right side of the equality sign as the independent predictors. We begin in a univariate way and model the three Weibull parameters and NIR (individually referred to as elements of the response vector) separately. A model selection algorithm that we will apply is AICc, combined with a meaningful effect criterion and the p-value. We will apply it in successive steps in driving us to a final reduced model. The detailed steps of the model selection process and the SAS/STAT® code followed in arriving at a final reduced model are described in Appendix 3.

Following the model selection process as discussed, we arrive at this final summary of meaningful terms by element shown in Table 7.5.

The next part of the process model development is to construct the matrix of independent predictors by element in a way that acknowledges that different sets of predictors are needed for each element of the response vector (i.e., multivariate model with element-wise disparate effects). To do this in a concise way in SAS (approach may differ for other software packages), the dataset defined in Table 7.4 must be transposed, and indicator variables added as columns to define the multivariate nature of the response. Another set of indicator columns is added to assign the proper factors to each element. This allows us to then model element-wise disparate inputs for each element. The transposed dataset with indicator variables (t1, t2, t3, t4) associated with the four elements in the response vector for the first tablet is shown in Output Listing 2. The indicator variables assigning the correct model terms to the element are designated (f1r, f3r, f1_2r, f4r, f14r, f34r, f4_2r), y is the response for the element given in the column headed par.

Output Listing 2: Partial Dataset in Preparation for Multivariate Process Model

Exptal Run	Rep	Tab num	y	par	t1	t2	t3	t4	f3r	f1_2r	f14r	f34r	f4_2r
Run01	1	1	95.03	b1	1	0	0	0	1	1	1	0	0
Run01	1	1	7.28	b2	0	1	0	0	0	0	0	1	0
Run01	1	1	0.99	b3	0	0	1	0	1	1	1	1	1
Run01	1	1	93.10	NIR	0	0	0	1	0	0	0	0	1

TABLE 7.5

List of Active Terms in Final Reduced Model by Element

Element	AICc			f1	f3	f1_2*	f4	f1*f4	f3*f4	f4_2*	Terms
	Full	Final	Δ								
b1	762.9	754.4	−18.5	x	x	x	x	x			5
b2	758.1	738.8	−19.3	x			x		x		3
b3	−191.4	−229.8	−38.6	x	x	x	x	x	x	x	7
NIR	781.6	783.6	2.0	x			x			x	3

* Curvature term for f1 or f4

The transposed dataset as described in Output listing 2 is ready now to be modeled as a multivariate response in relation to the element-specific factors described. Note that Factors 1 and 4 do not require indicator columns since these two are common to all four elements. At this point, thinking slightly ahead, we consider a Bayesian approach for the calculation of the multivariate coefficients and multivariate random effects, acknowledging the hierarchical structure of the data arising from the experimental design. Part of the exercise of developing a surrogate model also requires the ability to assess in some sense the uncertainty in predictions. This aspect of the problem is best addressed through a Bayesian approach, which allows us to simulate directly future observations under certain conditions, and to study these predictions with known parameter values. We will cover this in more detail in Section 7.5.3.5. For the moment, we are setting the stage now for the Bayesian analysis.

SAS/STAT® PROC BGLIMM is a flexible program that allows Bayesian analysis of general mixed linear models as we have here. SAS Code 3 is a sample code that sets up the model we wish to estimate indicating the fixed and random terms of the model.

SAS code 3 – Proc BGLIMM

```
ods graphics on ;
proc bglimm data = out3 nmc=100000 nbi=2000 seed=144672053 STATS=sum
      outpost=post1 thin=10 plots = ALL diag=all nthread=4 ;
 class par runx dosenum rep / order=internal ;
 model y = par par*f1 par*f4 par*f3*f3r par*f1_2*f1_2r
          par*f1*f4*f14r par*f3*f4*f34r par*f4_2*f4_2r / noint ;
 random t1 t2 t3 t4/subject=runx type=un G gcorr
 COVPRIOR=IGamma(scale=0.0001 shape=0.0001) ;
 repeated par/subject=dosenum type=un r rcorr
 COVPRIOR=IGamma(scale=0.0001 shape=0.0001) ;
 ods output G = G8 gcorr=gcorr8 R=R8 rcorr=rcorr8 postsummaries = Postsum8 ;
 title5 "Multivariate Mixed model Bayesian simulation" ;
 title6 "Vague priors on fixed and random effects" ;
run;
ods graphics off ;
```

The critical output of the BGLIMM analysis is the covariance matrices and the coefficient matrix of fixed effects. Appendix 6 shows the full results along with a graph of the posterior and prior distribution of parameter b1 and its corresponding variance term at the batch level. We show the estimates for element b1 in Output Listing 3 for comparison purposes with the univariate results shown in Output Listing 3.

Output Listing 3 Partial Proc Mixed Listing Reduced Model

			Posterior Summaries			
				Percentiles		
Parameter	N	Mean	Standard Deviation	25	50	75
Intercept	10000	100.1	0.5234	99.7360	100.1	100.4
F1	10000	0.5435	0.2893	0.3666	0.5476	0.7194
F4	10000	4.8060	0.0917	4.7452	4.8052	4.8676
F3	10000	−0.4043	0.2104	−0.5342	−0.4050	−0.2761
F1_2	10000	−0.9032	0.5410	−1.2421	−0.8998	−0.5711
F1*F4	10000	−0.2045	0.0788	−0.2572	−0.2045	−0.1515

At this point, it is necessary to discuss some basic introductory Bayesian concepts. As opposed to classical statistical methods, which rely on a frequentist notion of probability as an estimation approach, the Bayesian approach relies on Bayes' rule to integrate information as currently observed, with prior information to produce a posterior probability distribution for the parameters in the statistical model. The posterior distribution's mean or median serves as a point estimate of the parameter if needed, but the full posterior distribution contains all the current information on the parameter. The estimates given in Output Listing 3 for b1, for example, are headed by the term "Posterior Summaries" followed by the posterior mean. Prior information and how it is integrated into the Bayesian analysis requires that it be expressed through a probability distribution statement. In the case of the data at hand, a "flat" prior distribution is proposed, reflecting the relative lack of knowledge available regarding the parameters of interest before data from the experiment are collected. In those cases where substantial prior information is available about the parameters, distributions can be chosen to reflect the greater level of knowledge. This can, for example, be useful during subsequent model maintenance.

Another important requirement of Bayesian modeling relates to the convergence properties of the posterior distribution when a numerical method, such as MCMC sampling, is used for this purpose. It is outside the scope of this chapter to delve into this question in detail, other than to say that checking for convergence is critical to the validity of the Bayesian analysis. There are several diagnostics that provide support for convergence; however, there is no generally accepted single way to make this determination. Examination of the trace plots, the autocorrelation, the expected sample size, and tests such as the Heidelberger-Welch test and Raftery-Lewis test are useful ways to address this question. For a good discussion on Bayesian methods, see Gelman et al. [49].

We have now arrived at the final multivariate process model. The response is the vector of four elements: the three Weibull parameters, b1, b2, b3, and API content by NIR measurement for each tablet. The predictors are the seven terms F1, F3, F4, F1_2 (curvature F1), F14 (interaction of F1 and F4), F34 (interaction of F3 and F4), and F4_2 (curvature F4). These terms are associated with levels ranging on the coded scale from −1 to +1, or 0 to +1, and their effects on the elements of the response vector are defined by a coefficient matrix including the means. The full coefficient matrix and the run and tablet level covariance matrices, calculated from PROC BGLIMM, are shown in Output Listing 4 and 5, respectively. The coefficient matrix is of dimension 4 × 8 and the covariance matrices are of dimension 4 × 4.

Output Listing 6 Coefficient Matrix

Par	Mean	Model Term						
		f1	**f4**	**f3**	**f1_2**	**f14**	**f34**	**f4_2**
b1	100.1	0.5435	4.8060	−0.4043	−0.9032	−0.2045	0	0
b2	8.0473	−0.9044	1.9517	0	0	0	−0.2583	0
b3	0.9924	−0.0458	0.2070	0.0361	0.1086	0.0729	−0.0630	0.0401
NIR	99.0050	0.5424	4.8457	0	0	0	0	−0.2260

Output Listing 7 Covariance Matrix at run level (Σ_λ)

Par	b1	b2	b3	NIR
b1	0.8187	0.1547	0.0212	0.7390
b2	0.1547	0.0669	0.0028	0.2739
b3	0.0212	0.0028	0.0016	0.0123
NIR	0.7390	0.2739	0.0123	2.0153

Covariance Matrix at tablet level (Σ_ε)

Par	b1	b2	b3	NIR
b1	1.3079	0.3077	−0.0515	0.8059
b2	0.3077	1.3218	−0.0320	0.2246
b3	−0.0515	−0.0320	0.018	0.0061
NIR	0.8059	0.2246	0.0061	1.4314

The full multivariate process model can be described more clearly as follows:

Vector of Weibull parameters and NIR is a function of 8 terms whose effects on the response vector are given by the coefficient matrix **B**, with dispersion in the response vector from 2 sources, at the run level (Σ_λ), and at the tablet level (Σ_ε).

This is written in the compact statistical form in Appendix 2, step 2. We can also write the full model out as follows:

$$\underline{y}_{j(i)} = BX_{j(i)} + \underline{\lambda}_{j(i)} + \underline{\varepsilon}_{j(i)}$$

where

$\underline{y}_{j(i)}$ = *response from the jth tablet and i^{th} run* = $(b_1\ b_2\ b_3\ NIR)^t_{j(i)}$, dimension 4 × 1,
B = *coefficient matrix*, dimension 4 × 8,
$X_{j(i)}$ = *Levels of the terms*: Mean, F1, F4, F3, F1_2, F14, F34, F4_2, dimension 8 × 1,
$\underline{\lambda}_{j(i)}$ = *vector of random run level dispersion*, dimension 4 × 1,
$\underline{\varepsilon}_{j(i)}$ = *vector of random tablet level dispersion*, 4x1., dimension 4 × 1.

The process model estimated through the SAS BGLIMM procedure is then later used to carry out Bayesian simulations to study the properties of the surrogate model. We will come back to this in Section 7.5.3.5.

7.5.3.3 Step 3: Building the Surrogate Model

Given the process model and the associated coefficient matrix, B, and the covariance matrix, Σ_λ, we turn to the construction of the surrogate model, following the conditional regression method. The batch level covariance matrix is chosen because it is consistent with the population average inferential approach. As shown in Appendix 2, step 3, this is an algebraic approach that conditions the three elements of interest in the response vector, the three Weibull parameters, b_1, b_2, b_3, on API content by NIR, and incorporates the CPPs as independent predictors. This is equivalent to a way of regressing the three Weibull parameters on the NIR measurement acknowledging the uncertainty in the NIR measurement. SAS PROC IML code shown in Appendix 7 carries out the calculations required to make the surrogate predictions. The surrogate model calculations are described succinctly by the following expression, resorting to mathematical notation to show the algebraic details of how the calculations proceed. In this formulation, $x_{\mathbf{pred}}$ is a 1 × 6 row vector of intercept and process factors corresponding to the process terms previously defined in the model, representing the manufacturing conditions on a coded scale, and **NIR** is a given Content-by-NIR value from the tablet for which a predicted dissolution value is needed. The equation(s) below involves two steps. The first part represents the prediction of the Weibull parameters at the process level, while the second part adjusts this prediction on the difference between measured NIR and its process prediction. The degree of adjustment is proportional to the correlation between the NIR and the respective Weibull parameter.

Conditional Weibull Parameters	An observed API Content by NIR	An observed API Content by NIR

$$\left(\boldsymbol{b}\,|\,\mathrm{NIR}=\mathrm{nir},\boldsymbol{x}_{\mathrm{pred}}\right)=\left(\boldsymbol{x}_{\mathrm{pred}}*B[,1:3]\right)^{T}+\left(\!\left(\frac{\Sigma_{\lambda}[1:3,4]}{\Sigma_{\lambda}[4,4]}\right)\!\right)*\left(\mathrm{nir}-\boldsymbol{x}_{\mathrm{pred}}*B[,4]\right)=\boldsymbol{b}^{*}$$

Model	B[,1:3]				0.3667	B[,4]
Term	b1	b2	b3		0.1359	NIR
Mean	100.06	8.0473	0.9924		0.0061	99.0050
f1	0.5435	-0.9044	-0.0458			0.5424
f4	4.8060	1.9517	0.2070			4.8457
f3	-0.4043	0	0.0361			0
f1_2	-0.9032	0	0.1086			0
f14	-0.2045	0	0.0729			0
f34	0	-0.2583	-0.0630			0
f4_2	0	0	0.0401			-0.2260

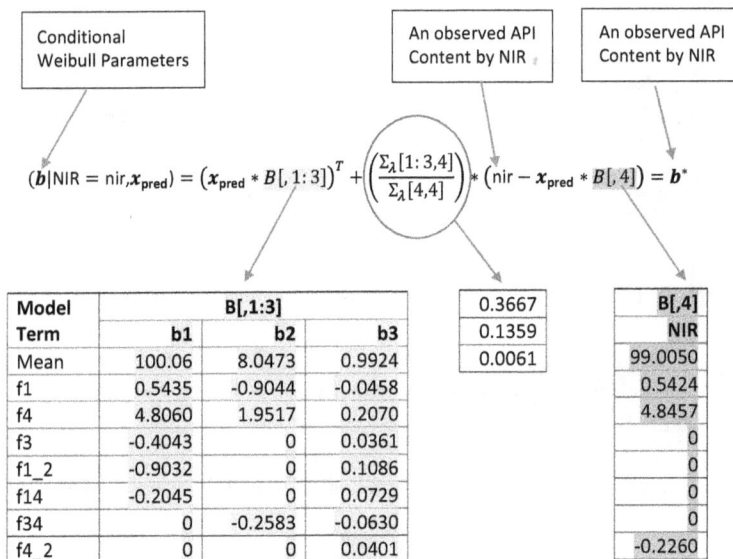

The above expression reduces to the following three equations at the center point of the experimental space (i.e., where all factor settings equal zero on the coded scale), corresponding to the anticipated manufacturing conditions at full scale (rounded to two decimal places):

$$b1^{*}=100.06+0.37^{*}\,(\mathrm{nir}-99.01),$$

$$b2^{*}=8.05+0.14^{*}\,(\mathrm{nir}-99.01),$$

$$b3^{*}=0.99+0.01^{*}\,(\mathrm{nir}-99.01).$$

These three equations provide Weibull parameter predictions for center point conditions. These can then be substituted into the Weibull model given in Section 7.5.2.2, and surrogate dissolution predictions are calculated for any desired time point.

As an example of the application of conditional regression, given the process model, we apply surrogate model predictions to the data in Appendix 1, using the PROC IML code shown in Appendix 7. The output gives the surrogate predictions of the Weibull parameters for each tablet, using its measured API content by NIR and its experimental factor levels. The output of PROC IML can then be merged into the dataset described in Table 7.4 to create a combined dataset as shown in Output Listing 6 showing both the empirical Weibull parameters calculated earlier for modeling purposes, along with the surrogate model predicted Weibull parameters at each of the levels of F4 for the center point run, Run08. Although this is useful for evaluating the predictions at the level of the parameters, the main interest is not so much on the Weibull parameters themselves, but the subsequent dissolution estimates at desired time points, as we will see in the next section.

Output Listing 8 Partial Listing of PROC IML run

Run	Tab Num	Factor					Empirical			Surrogate		
		1	2	3	4	nir	b1	b2	b3	b1	b2	b3
Run08	127	1	-1	-1	-1	94.6	94.7	6.0	0.8	95.5	4.9	0.7
	133	1	-1	-1	0	99.8	100.6	8.2	0.9	100.2	7.2	1.0
	139	1	-1	-1	1	103.3	102.6	10.2	1.1	104.4	9.2	1.4

7.5.3.4 Model Fit Assessment

Once the surrogate model has been established, it is important to assess the model fit before proceeding to the next section on model assessment for accuracy and precision. There are two aspects that we consider:

1. How close are the predicted Weibull parameters to the fitted Weibull parameters,
2. How close are the surrogate model predictions at the important Q-spec timepoint(s) to the fitted and empirical measurements.

We begin by examining the congruence between the Weibull fitted and surrogate parameters graphically at the run mean level. These are shown in Appendix 8, Figures A1, A2 and A3, for the three Weibull parameters. The ellipse is an approximate 95% confidence region, and the red dashed line represents a 45° line to aid the interpretation for accuracy. All three congruence plots corresponding to the three parameters indicate an average line close to the ideal line, and no systematic or unusual patterns or departures.

Lin's concordance correlation coefficient (CCC) [40] is also useful as a formal assessment of congruence. The CCC [56, 57] is commonly used in the comparison of analytical methods. Table 7.6 gives a summary of the Weibull parameter of the CCC. Note that the means and the high CCC support a claim of good agreement on average.

Another fit assessment examines the differences between the fitted and surrogate predictions by time point. We can make this comparison in two ways: (i) with respect to a fitted estimate, that is the Weibull model predicted value, and (ii) the observed empirical value. If the three-parameter Weibull is the appropriate descriptor for the dissolution profile, then we would expect the fitted values to be less biased in general than the empirical observed values, that is the actual observed measured values. A summary of these two sets of differences is given in Table 7.7.

TABLE 7.6

Lin's Concordance Correlation Coefficient (CCC) between Fitted Empirical and Surrogate Prediction

Parameter	Method Mean (SD)		CCC (95% Conf.)
	Empirical	Surrogate	
b1	99.3 (4.1)	99.3 (4.0)	0.99 (0.98–0.99)
b2	7.98 (1.85)	7.98 (1.82)	0.98 (0.96–0.99)
b3	1.11 (0.20)	1.11 (0.19)	0.97 (0.95–0.99)

TABLE 7.7

Average Differences and Range between Fitted/Observed and Surrogate Predictions by Time Point

Time (min.)	Empirical-Surrogate			Fitted-Surrogate		
	Mean Difference	Range Min	Max	Mean Difference	Range Min	Max
5	−0.6	−3.7	3.2	−0.6	−3.6	3.0
10	−0.3	−4.2	3.3	−0.3	−3.7	3.7
15	0.2	−4.3	3.8	0.2	−3.2	3.6
20	0.8	−2.7	3.4	0.5	−2.6	2.9
30	0.2	−1.9	1.8	0.4	−1.4	2.3
45	0.0	−1.9	1.7	0.2	−1.5	1.7
60	0.1	−1.3	1.7	0.0	−1.7	1.4

Histograms of the differences observed in Table 7.7 for the 20- and 30-minute dissolution time points are shown in Figures 7.3 and 7.4.

Finally, the "goodness" and consistency of the surrogate model predictions can be visually assessed by graphing the surrogate predictions of the seven-point dissolution profile overlaid on the empirically observed fits. We emphasize that the covariance matrix at run level was used for building the surrogate model, which suggests that profiles at the run average level should be compared. Comparing at the individual tablet level introduces additional sources of variability that cannot be accounted for in the model. The profiles are shown in Appendix 9. Systematic biases and unusual lack of congruence would be obvious from such graphics. The visual inspection does not indicate systematic biases or unusual differences.

7.5.3.5 Bayesian Model Assessment for Accuracy and Precision

We turn to the question of accuracy and precision, having satisfied ourselves that the surrogate model fit is acceptable and can be regarded now as provisionally qualified.

We continue the model assessment by investigating how the model might perform in future applications, given certain conditions. This can be addressed through a Bayesian simulation of predicted future outcomes at any point in the experimental space, but for convenience, we will choose the center point. We touched briefly on the notion of posterior distributions of the parameters in Section 7.5.3.2. Based on those, we can simulate a posterior predictive distribution of future outcomes. The simulation of future outcomes generates random realizations of the "true" process mean, and simultaneously a covariance matrix at the batch and tablet levels. For each random generation, or "draw" from the posterior, we can then simulate a random batch, and a random sample of tablets from that random batch, which provides a simulated batch average measurement. We then apply the surrogate model to the simulated "measured" NIR to generate a surrogate outcome, and compare the surrogate predictions with both the known "true" batch mean, as well as the simulated "measured" batch mean. These predictions of future outcomes provide a way to quantify the analytical performance of the surrogate model in terms of accuracy and precision.

In Section 7.5.3.2, we discussed the building of the process model. The process model was used to estimate important parameters for the later construction of the surrogate model. But in addition, the Bayesian

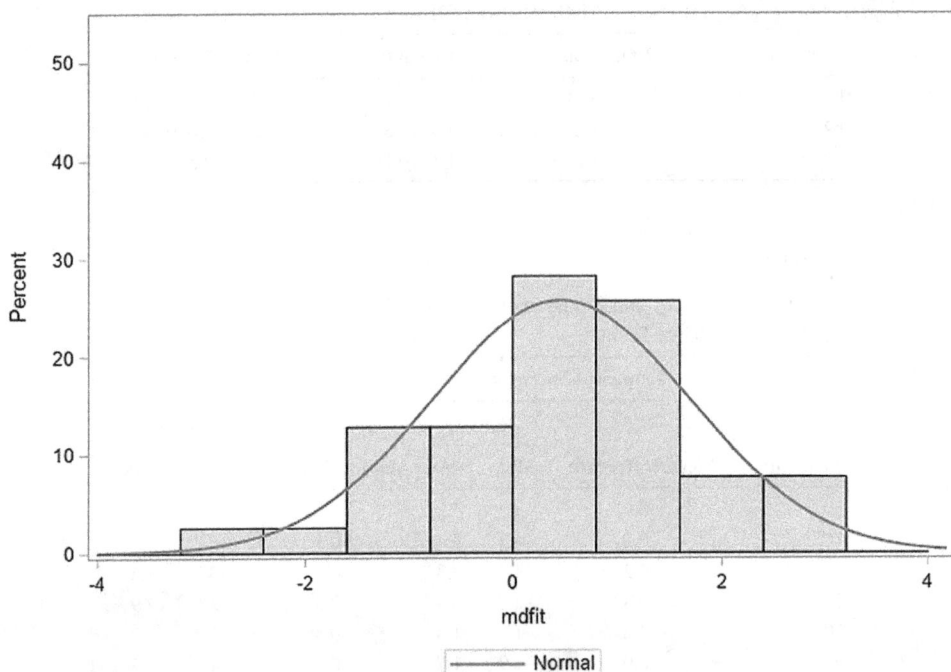

FIGURE 7.3 Histogram of differences between fitted and surrogate predictions time (minutes) = 20.

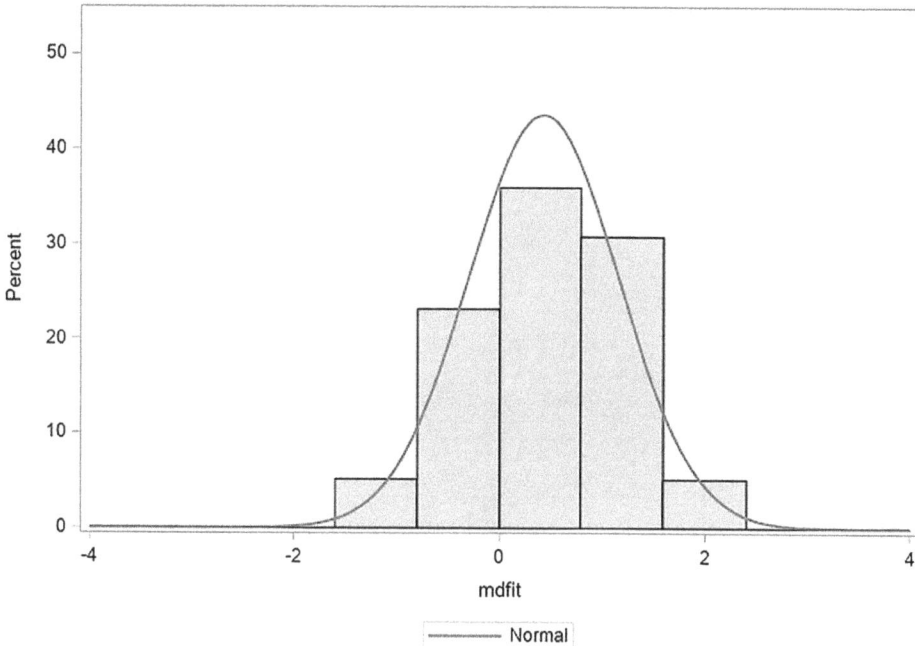

FIGURE 7.4 Histogram of differences between fitted and surrogate predictions time (minutes) = 30.

process model generated the posterior parameter distributions, consisting of 10000 future outcomes of the full set of parameters in the model. These distributions are used to simulate future outcomes of a random future batch, and measurement error associated with a random sample of future tablets from that batch. SAS macro SIM1, shown in Appendix 10, can be used to generate these simulated outcomes. The macro call takes the posterior parameter estimates contained in a dataset called POST2. The format of POST2 consists of 95 columns as follows: an iteration counter column, 20 columns of covariances at batch and tablet levels, 22 fixed effects, and four sets of 13 columns of random batch effects, corresponding to the four parameters in the response vector (b1, b2, b3, nir). The three arguments in the macro call are n1 = starting point in the simulation, for convenience 1, n2 = end point in the simulation, for convenience, 10000, and n0, the number of tablets used to estimate the batch mean. It had been previously decided to use a sample size of 30 tablets to estimate the batch mean. The macro cycles through each of the posterior simulations, draws a random process mean, generates a random batch from that process mean, and samples error associated with 30 tablets to simulate a measured batch mean. Based on the simulated measured NIR value, the surrogate predictions are generated. For the purposes of this discussion, 20-minute and 30-minute dissolution values are generated from the three sets of parameters, yielding "true" values, "measured" values, and surrogate predicted values. The statistical validation entails a comparison of the surrogate predictions with the true and measured values. The mean differences and 99% range of differences are given in Table 7.8.

Histograms of the differences are shown in Figures 7.5 and 7.6.

TABLE 7.8

Mean Differences Surrogate – True/Measured Batch Means at 20 and 30 Minutes

Dissolution Time	True			Measured		
	Mean (SD)	90% Range	99% Range	Mean (SD)	90% Range	99% Range
20 minutes	−0.2 (1.2)	(−2.0, 1.7)	(−3.4, 3.0)	0.1 (1.2)	(−1.8, 2.0)	(−3.3, 3.9)
30 minutes	−0.1 (0.9)	(−1.6, 1.5)	(−2.7, 3.0)	0.0 (1.0)	(−1.6, 1.6)	(−2.9, 3.3)

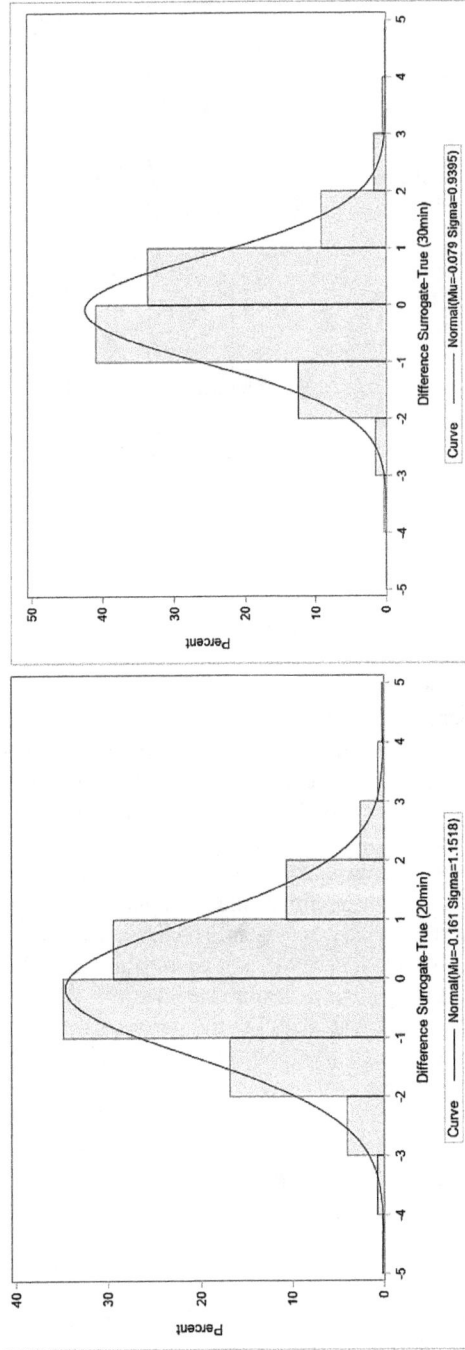

FIGURE 7.5 Histograms of Surrogate – True mean Batch differences at 20 and 30 minutes.

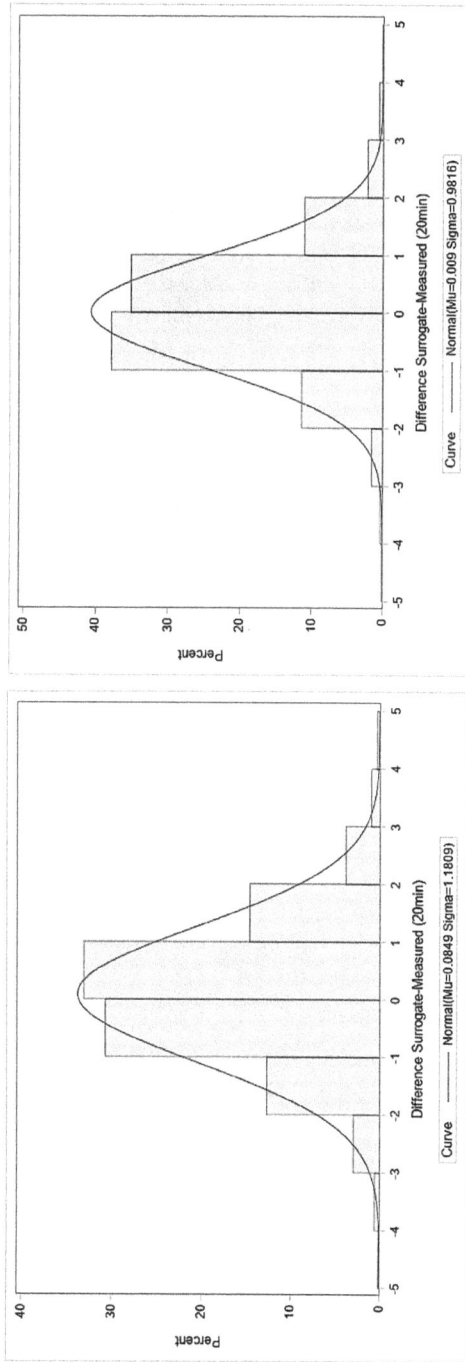

FIGURE 7.6 Histograms of Surrogate – Measured mean Batch differences at 20 and 30 minutes.

It had previously been discussed that given the mean dissolution values at both 20 and 30 minutes are more than 90% on average, and the regulatory Q-specification was Q = 80%, a fit-for-purpose requirement would be to see the differences fall close to 0 on average, and an expectation that few differences would fall outside of a 6% difference margin. The results shown in Table 7.6 indicate good accuracy of the surrogate predictions, and the 99% range of differences fell well within the fit-for-purpose margin of 6%. The histograms shown in Figures 7.5 and 7.6 indicated a good central tendency with 90% of the differences expected to fall within 2% of the true value on average.

7.5.4 Surrogate Model Validation

Surrogate model validation is a critical part of the development plan. To a large extent, it must be designed as a separate exercise based on the results of the surrogate model development process itself, and necessarily involve external and independent data from a separate experiment. The independent data validation would follow the statistical assessment, and will not be discussed in this chapter. We emphasize that the external data component is necessary for conferring final validity to the surrogate model.

7.5.5 Summary

Surrogate model development in the context of RTRT was approached from a statistical modeling perspective, relying on the conditional regression method to account for measurement errors in the API content by NIR measurement as a predictor. A comprehensive experimental design was shown to be essential to the development of a surrogate model. Model fit, qualification, and validation were shown to be essential parts of the exercise, enhanced by a Bayesian approach to characterizing the performance of the surrogate model. Important aspects of the model development related to design considerations and independent data validation were touched upon but require further elaboration.

APPENDIX 1: RAW DATA LISTING ARRANGED BY EXPERIMENTAL RUN (EXPTAL RUN)

TABLE A1

Raw Data Listing for Experimental Run 1

Exptal Run	Factor 1	2	3	4	Tablet Number	Content NIR	5 min.	10 min.	15 min.	20 min.	30 min.	45 min.	60 min.
Run01	−1	−1	−1	−1	1	93.1	47.1	71.8	81.9	87.9	94.9	95.7	93.5
					2	94.4	47.8	78.7	86.9	90.4	96.0	96.4	97.4
					3	94.2	48.0	69.9	80.8	90.2	95.1	94.3	94.9
					4	95.2	40.5	69.0	80.6	87.8	94.2	95.6	94.7
					5	95.7	44.3	68.1	83.7	90.9	95.2	96.1	95.6
					6	93.9	47.9	67.8	77.9	83.9	92.9	95.1	95.5
			0		7	99.5	43.7	65.2	80.3	90.4	97.2	99.8	100.0
					8	100.5	40.1	67.7	85.3	93.1	99.2	100.6	101.0
					9	100.1	36.8	71.8	85.9	93.9	99.7	100.2	100.0
					10	99.8	42.7	73.4	87.0	95.0	97.2	101.2	100.6
					11	100.1	40.3	68.0	82.9	93.9	99.9	100.1	100.7
					12	99.3	40.8	72.3	874	94.2	97.8	98.9	99.0
			1		13	101.3	27.9	59.2	84.2	94.5	104.0	105.0	104.7
					14	102.7	29.1	56.0	80.3	89.9	100.0	103.6	104.8
					15	103.1	32.4	59.4	81.4	90.8	100.7	105.1	106.0
					16	102.9	26.7	56.2	80.3	91.1	103.3	108.1	107.3
					17	103.0	26.7	53.8	74.1	86.9	101.9	105.3	104.9
					18	102.1	35.8	60.5	80.9	90.2	102.0	104.2	104.1

TABLE A2

Raw Data Listing for Experimental Run 2

Exptal Run	Factor 1	2	3	4	Tablet Number	Content NIR	5 min.	10 min.	15 min.	20 min.	30 min.	45 min.	60 min.
Run02	−1	−1	−1	−1	19	90.6	52.0	73.7	82.5	85.8	90.5	91.5	90.9
					20	91.0	52.3	72.8	81.7	87.0	91.4	91.0	91.4
					21	89.8	52.9	72.6	79.0	84.0	88.9	90.0	90.3
					22	90.4	48.1	63.8	77.0	87.4	90.9	92.4	91.6
					23	92.7	46.0	66.6	76.2	80.7	88.0	92.0	91.1
					24	93.7	46.3	69.6	79.9	87.2	92.3	92.8	92.9
			0		25	97.3	40.7	74.2	86.1	92.7	96.6	97.4	96.7
					26	100.3	42.0	66.2	81.0	87.6	94.8	99.2	99.3
					27	98.8	40.1	68.9	81.8	88.7	96.7	99.4	99.0
					28	99.7	39.7	68.0	82.9	91.3	97.7	100.0	98.9
					29	96.9	40.2	65.0	79.0	87.5	95.5	97.3	96.9
					30	96.8	40.8	66.2	80.8	87.4	95.8	96.0	97.6
			1		31	102.2	34.7	68.1	90.9	97.4	102.0	103.4	103.1
					32	101.3	30.2	60.3	82.6	93.0	102.1	102.0	102.2
					33	101.8	34.6	63.3	78.9	90.0	100.4	103.0	102.2
					34	103.5	30.9	60.8	84.2	94.9	105.0	105.2	104.3
					35	103.0	29.7	57.7	77.4	89.1	99.6	102.8	102.8
					36	102.1	32.0	61.0	82.9	92.8	100.0	101.9	101.5

TABLE A3

Raw Data Listing for Experimental Run 3

Exptal Run	Factor 1	2	3	4	Tablet Number	Content NIR	5 min.	10 min.	15 min.	20 min.	30 min.	45 min.	60 min.
Run03	−1	−1	1	−1	37	95.7	53.7	83.3	90.1	92.0	94.3	93.6	94.3
					38	95.6	43.0	66.6	80.0	88.0	94.4	93.2	94.4
					39	93.1	42.1	79.9	88.3	89.5	92.2	92.7	93.0
					40	93.7	46.4	77.7	86.1	90.3	92.3	92.9	92.9
					41	94.4	49.2	72.6	83.2	88.4	93.1	94.1	93.9
					42	94.5	41.6	68.6	81.1	88.1	93.5	93.0	92.9
				0	43	98.3	52.0	78.9	93.5	97.3	98.2	98.5	98.5
					44	96.0	38.7	58.9	75.0	84.3	93.0	98.2	98.0
					45	97.4	43.0	68.1	88.9	94.4	95.6	96.7	97.2
					46	97.5	38.9	73.3	85.6	93.4	97.4	98.0	98.1
					47	98.3	39.1	59.7	77.9	87.0	94.9	97.3	98.6
					48	98.2	41.0	67.2	80.3	88.0	94.5	99.5	98.9
				1	49	103.6	44.3	78.4	98.9	103.5	102.9	103.0	102.9
					50	103.5	39.5	71.1	88.8	96.9	103.0	104.1	103.5
					51	104.8	30.8	58.6	75.9	88.2	99.2	103.1	102.7
					52	103.1	27.4	57.4	91.7	94.1	99.9	102.7	103.2
					53	102.5	31.6	59.0	76.1	87.3	97.8	101.6	101.7
					54	102.5	35.4	65.9	83.5	94.3	102.0	103.2	102.7

TABLE A4

Raw Data Listing for Experimental Run 4

Exptal Run	Factor 1	2	3	4	Tablet Number	Content NIR	5 min.	10 min.	15 min.	20 min.	30 min.	45 min.	60 min.
Run04	−1	1	−1	−1	55	93.5	58.5	78.9	87.1	90.9	94.9	94.7	94.8
					56	95.4	42.8	67.3	77.8	85.5	92.2	95.1	95.1
					57	91.8	57.1	76.7	85.2	88.3	92.1	93.2	93.6
					58	92.6	46.0	67.9	78.9	84.9	90.8	92.7	92.7
					59	95.1	47.7	70.1	82.1	89.0	93.0	95.1	94.8
					60	92.3	58.0	74.4	83.8	90.0	92.7	93.1	93.1
				0	61	98.1	40.0	63.9	81.7	88.8	96.0	99.0	99.1
					62	97.3	36.1	62.7	79.8	87.6	95.5	97.5	98.3
					63	99.0	42.0	67.1	80.8	90.7	98.8	99.5	99.4
					64	98.0	47.0	68.1	85.2	91.9	97.6	98.4	98.2
					65	95.9	38.9	69.0	79.5	89.7	95.7	95.6	96.0
					66	98.2	41.4	64.8	77.9	86.8	95.9	97.8	97.9
				1	67	103.3	28.0	59.2	78.0	89.1	100.3	104.9	104.3
					68	102.7	30.3	58.9	77.9	89.0	98.9	104.1	104.2
					69	102.5	36.0	66.9	84.9	92.6	100.0	102.7	103.2
					70	104.7	28.9	57.2	79.5	91.8	102.2	105.1	105.3
					71	102.6	29.3	56.5	74.9	86.4	97.4	102.6	102.7
					72	103.2	33.1	65.3	83.2	93.4	102.8	103.8	103.0

TABLE A5

Raw Data Listing for Experimental Run 5

Exptal Run	Factor 1	2	3	4	Tablet Number	Content NIR	5 min.	10 min.	15 min.	20 min.	30 min.	45 min.	60 min
Run05	−1	1	1	−1	73	91.5	46.5	72.9	83.0	87.0	91.2	91.8	92.0
					74	90.7	37.4	66.6	79.9	85.3	90.2	93.3	91.7
					75	95.3	50.3	70.3	84.2	88.5	92.7	95.3	94.8
					76	92.1	42.9	70.8	81.3	85.4	90.6	91.5	92.1
					77	95.5	37.9	62.2	76.9	84.6	91.8	94.0	95.6
					78	92.7	41.0	66.9	78.6	84.0	90.6	91.0	91.7
				0	79	96.3	43.7	63.0	79.2	88.3	96.9	98.2	98.0
					80	96.9	42.7	62.5	78.3	86.9	95.6	96.9	96.9
					81	96.3	42.7	81.7	87.1	91.4	94.0	95.2	94.9
					82	96.6	38.9	66.9	85.2	92.0	95.8	97.4	97.2
					83	99.3	38.2	67.7	87.1	94.1	98.2	99.6	99.3
					84	95.3	34.2	68.4	80.9	89.5	93.7	95.8	96.1
				1	85	105.1	28.8	58.9	76.0	87.0	96.9	103.9	104.3
					86	104.3	32.4	65.5	84.7	97.4	102.4	103.2	104.3
					87	105.9	30.0	57.4	74.8	86.1	100.8	104.9	103.5
					88	101.5	30.2	56.6	75.8	87.8	97.7	102.3	102.1
					89	104.6	28.8	58.2	77.8	90.4	100.1	103.1	103.5
					90	103.5	36.2	65.6	84.8	95.3	100.5	102.3	101.9

TABLE A6

Raw Data Listing for Experimental Run 6

Exptal Run	Factor 1	2	3	4	Tablet Number	Content NIR	5 min.	10 min.	15 min.	20 min.	30 min.	45 min.	60 min.
Run06	0	0	0	−1	91	96.6	52.1	69.1	83.4	91.7	97.0	96.9	96.9
					92	96.6	53.1	72.0	82.6	89.2	95.2	96.1	96.3
					93	95.4	64.2	79.3	86.4	91.6	95.7	95.1	95.0
					94	94.3	55.5	72.5	80.9	86.3	93.7	94.0	94.0
					95	96.1	55.9	71.3	83.1	90.7	94.7	94.7	95.1
					96	96.7	53.8	70.9	83.1	89.8	95.4	96.0	96.0
				0	97	100.6	49.0	73.9	84.9	90.0	98.1	99.5	98.9
					98	101.0	45.2	70.9	83.1	90.4	98.4	99.8	99.8
					99	100.8	48.8	73.5	86.3	91.0	99.0	100.2	99.6
					100	100.9	44.7	67.1	80.5	88.3	97.9	99.8	99.1
					101	102.0	41.1	75.1	86.6	93.7	99.7	99.9	100.5
					102	102.0	50.6	70.9	82.9	91.0	98.4	99.0	99.4
				1	103	106.3	31.0	62.2	82.0	92.9	100.9	105.1	106.3
					104	104.9	35.8	65.1	81.8	91.3	103.5	103.7	104.2
					105	105.2	39.0	74.7	90.3	98.4	103.9	105.0	105.0
					106	107.6	29.8	59.7	78.4	89.2	100.5	105.9	106.0
					107	106.7	32.1	62.7	81.0	92.7	103.1	105.5	104.9
					108	106.9	35.3	70.6	92.5	101.4	105.5	104.7	105.4

TABLE A7

Raw Data Listing for Experimental Run 7

Exptal Run	Factor 1	2	3	4	Tablet Number	Content NIR	5 min.	10 min.	15 min.	20 min.	30 min.	45 min.	60 min.
Run07	0	0	0	−1	109	92.8	59.7	76.1	85.0	90.1	94.1	94.3	93.5
					110	94.7	61.4	78.3	88.9	91.6	96.2	95.8	94.8
					111	93.4	47.2	67.4	75.2	81.9	91.1	94.2	93.9
					112	93.8	54.0	71.4	80.7	88.7	94.5	94.4	93.5
					113	94.4	52.7	70.8	82.2	88.1	94.1	95.4	94.4
					114	95.2	55.0	72.4	80.8	87.1	94.0	95.5	95.1
				0	115	98.9	57.2	78.8	89.5	93.8	100.5	99.9	99.9
					116	98.3	43.7	71.3	85.1	92.9	99.7	100.3	99.7
					117	98.8	44.6	69.1	80.9	89.3	98.9	99.9	99.5
					118	97.6	55.3	76.8	88.2	93.9	99.5	101.2	99.3
					119	99.7	45.9	76.6	89.2	96.6	99.7	101.4	100.9
					120	97.3	43.3	66.8	80.9	88.9	97.0	98.1	98.7
				1	121	102.2	36.2	71.9	88.5	96.1	103.0	103.9	104.1
					122	102.5	34.8	68.0	86.2	93.9	102.7	103.9	104.9
					123	102.2	35.8	67.2	84.6	93.6	104.3	105.2	104.7
					124	103.0	35.6	71.5	86.3	95.2	104.1	104.5	105.1
					125	102.5	33.9	69.6	84.2	93.1	103.2	104.2	104.5
					126	100.3	41.9	72.8	87.2	95.7	101.7	103.3	103.1

TABLE A8

Raw Data Listing for Experimental Run 8

Exptal Run	Factor 1	2	3	4	Tablet Number	Content NIR	5 min.	10 min.	15 min.	20 min.	30 min.	45 min.	60 min.
Run08	1	−1	−1	−1	127	94.6	55.0	73.1	82.9	89.2	91.7	94.2	93.9
					128	94.3	51.1	68.3	77.8	84.0	91.0	93.6	94.1
					129	93.8	74.9	85.8	91.1	93.0	94.6	95.7	94.9
					130	94.2	66.9	83.2	89.6	93.6	94.5	95.6	94.9
					131	95.2	56.4	75.0	82.5	88.1	93.9	94.7	95.3
					132	94.8	57.6	74.9	86.1	89.7	94.1	94.0	94.0
				0	133	99.8	48.0	69.8	81.7	88.8	95.9	99.1	100.2
					134	99.6	54.7	77.1	86.5	92.7	98.0	99.2	100.2
					135	101.1	51.7	84.3	95.1	99.1	100.5	101.3	102.9
					136	101.3	59.7	89.0	95.9	98.8	101.1	101.4	102.1
					137	101.4	49.7	72.4	84.9	93.5	100.5	101.0	101.1
					138	101.4	48.8	81.2	91.9	97.9	101.3	100.8	100.6
				1	139	103.3	36.2	65.4	82.0	90.1	97.5	101.2	103.1
					140	103.1	27.0	56.2	80.5	91.9	99.9	104.0	103.9
					141	103.3	41.4	75.6	96.4	100.2	104.3	105.9	106.0
					142	103.5	40.2	71.8	91.3	97.8	103.3	103.9	105.1
					143	103.8	33.8	71.1	93.9	100.0	104.3	105.4	104.9
					144	103.7	33.9	67.9	95.6	100.1	103.6	105.1	103.9

TABLE A9

Raw Data Listing for Experimental Run 9

Exptal Run	Factor 1	2	3	4	Tablet Number	Content NIR	5 min.	10 min.	15 min.	20 min.	30 min.	45 min.	60 min.
Run09	1	−1	1	−1	145	95.4	55.8	79.1	87.1	91.7	95.3	95.6	94.9
					146	95.0	63.2	83.9	90.2	92.4	95.0	94.8	96.3
					147	95.1	52.6	70.1	80.8	87.1	93.6	93.6	93.8
					148	96.4	56.0	73.1	83.0	88.5	93.7	95.4	94.9
					149	96.4	55.5	74.6	85.2	90.3	94.8	95.3	95.5
					150	94.8	62.7	83.9	87.9	89.7	92.4	94.2	93.9
				0	151	99.0	43.6	74.4	88.3	93.9	98.0	99.5	98.0
					152	100.4	55.1	84.8	94.6	97.3	99.2	100.4	100.0
					153	100.9	54.2	86.4	93.8	97.4	98.9	100.0	99.1
					154	101.7	55.4	74.8	85.1	91.6	98.3	99.9	100.0
					155	101.0	51.8	78.0	91.8	97.5	98.9	99.6	99.2
					156	100.2	42.2	65.1	80.5	90.1	98.5	101.3	100.6
				1	157	106.3	30.5	58.9	80.2	94.4	102.9	103.7	105.0
					158	104.9	40.3	79.0	94.5	100.0	103.0	105.3	104.9
					159	107.1	31.8	62.7	82.1	92.4	100.2	104.9	104.8
					160	105.0	31.0	63.3	80.6	92.5	101.8	104.2	105.2
					161	104.0	41.9	77.8	97.1	99.9	102.7	103.9	105.0
					162	106.3	36.1	66.2	84.9	94.9	102.7	103.7	105.2

TABLE A10

Raw Data Listing for Experimental Run 10

Exptal Run	Factor 1	2	3	4	Tablet Number	Content NIR	5 min.	10 min.	15 min.	20 min.	30 min.	45 min.	60 min.
Run10	1	1	−1	−1	163	96.0	49.0	69.5	80.0	86.1	92.8	94.8	96.0
					164	94.8	77.7	87.3	90.5	92.6	94.1	94.5	95.4
					165	95.2	51.7	70.3	78.7	84.9	91.8	94.1	95.0
					166	93.7	73.0	88.2	93.5	94.2	93.8	94.2	93.0
					167	96.1	68.0	82.9	90.0	92.3	93.5	94.9	96.2
					168	95.0	65.2	81.8	91.7	94.0	94.5	94.9	94.6
				0	169	102.0	50.0	74.0	85.2	92.3	99.3	100.3	99.8
					170	98.9	55.3	77.6	88.4	93.8	103.1	99.2	100.7
					171	98.3	41.2	67.2	79.8	88.4	95.5	97.1	97.1
					172	100.7	50.9	75.1	86.3	92.8	98.0	100.3	99.7
					173	101.0	61.7	77.7	88.1	93.9	98.7	99.9	100.4
					174	100.1	49.8	75.8	87.8	94.8	99.1	98.7	100.0
				1	175	105.7	25.0	54.0	73.7	87.5	101.1	103.7	103.9
					176	104.8	33.8	70.2	89.4	96.8	101.6	102.6	104.1
					177	104.5	28.6	59.9	84.1	94.2	101.8	104.2	103.2
					178	104.3	38.3	72.8	92.8	100.9	103.7	104.2	103.9
					179	104.3	40.5	80.7	97.3	100.9	104.8	104.9	105.1
					180	103.5	42.5	81.5	102.1	104.8	104.3	103.7	105.4

TABLE A11

Raw Data Listing for Experimental Run 11

Exptal Run	Factor 1	2	3	4	Tablet Number	Content NIR	5 min.	10 min.	15 min.	20 min.	30 min.	45 min.	60 min.
Run11	1	1	1	−1	181	94.3	56.4	69.9	80.9	88.0	93.0	94.3	94.0
					182	94.5	49.2	80.8	88.8	90.2	93.3	93.2	93.7
					183	92.9	55.6	74.7	84.1	87.7	92.0	95.3	94.9
					184	93.2	63.1	84.6	89.8	91.6	93.7	94.0	93.6
					185	92.8	56.1	75.6	85.1	88.7	91.3	93.0	93.2
					186	93.7	67.0	82.9	89.3	90.5	94.2	93.7	93.1
				0	187	98.6	36.4	63.4	76.9	84.8	93.9	98.3	99.0
					188	99.2	35.0	65.5	81.5	88.1	95.8	99.1	98.6
					189	99.5	63.6	87.6	96.0	99.0	100.9	100.4	100.9
					190	98.8	46.6	75.0	87.0	92.0	97.7	100.4	100.8
					191	100.9	47.6	75.0	87.8	94.1	99.1	100.1	99.5
					192	99.0	49.1	75.9	89.9	94.6	98.0	99.2	98.7
				1	193	103.1	37.8	68.8	85.7	93.9	99.8	102.6	103.4
					194	103.9	37.0	67.0	83.8	91.0	101.2	104.3	105.3
					195	103.5	39.9	75.3	95.9	101.5	104.9	106.4	105.8
					196	103.1	39.6	70.1	89.1	98.2	102.9	105.7	104.0
					197	104.2	39.6	72.1	93.8	100.0	103.2	104.3	105.1
					198	103.6	43.0	73.9	94.8	100.4	103.4	104.4	104.3

TABLE A12

Raw Data Listing for Experimental Run 12

Exptal Run	Factor 1	2	3	4	Tablet Number	Content NIR	5 min.	10 min.	15 min.	20 min.	30 min.	45 min.	60 min.
Run12	1	1	1	−1	199	93.2	60.1	77.3	83.9	87.6	92.1	93.5	93.0
					200	93.1	56.3	78.6	86.6	90.4	91.7	92.9	93.2
					201	93.9	63.5	84.1	90.1	92.0	93.2	93.2	92.8
					202	93.7	61.2	82.5	88.2	91.6	93.0	93.0	93.2
					203	92.9	56.9	72.4	80.9	85.6	93.1	93.9	94.3
					204	94.5	50.2	70.0	78.9	84.4	90.9	94.1	94.1
				0	205	99.2	47.0	75.2	87.6	92.0	98.4	99.1	98.7
					206	99.7	48.1	71.5	84.8	91.1	98.1	100.3	99.5
					207	98.9	48.9	74.2	87.5	92.2	95.7	96.9	98.0
					208	100.1	58.8	86.4	95.1	98.3	99.0	98.5	99.5
					209	99.9	48.1	71.7	84.4	92.1	98.1	98.7	99.2
					210	97.7	51.8	73.6	84.9	91.2	97.7	98.7	99.2
				1	211	105.7	45.5	83.1	98.7	103.1	105.0	104.8	105.4
					212	105.6	34.5	68.2	88.9	97.6	103.1	105.0	105.0
					213	106.0	38.9	68.6	86.6	96.3	105.6	105.9	107.2
					214	104.7	49.9	87.0	99.9	102.7	103.9	103.9	104.3
					215	104.8	39.2	67.0	82.7	93.3	101.5	104.6	103.8
					216	105.4	35.7	69.0	87.7	97.1	103.3	103.9	104.0

TABLE A13

Raw Data Listing for Experimental Run 13

Exptal Run	Factor 1	2	3	4	Tablet Number	Content NIR	5 min.	10 min.	15 min.	20 min.	30 min.	45 min.	60 min.
Run13	1	1	1	−1	217	90.2	50.2	72.1	85.3	91.7	94.0	94.8	95.2
					218	92.7	72.5	89.1	91.9	93.4	93.8	93.8	93.9
					219	93.9	50.5	80.3	86.7	90.3	93.5	94.1	94.9
					220	93.8	55.7	74.1	85.4	92.7	94.9	96.1	96.0
					221	93.1	59.3	81.3	89.6	92.2	94.3	93.7	93.9
					222	93.7	72.3	88.6	92.3	93.7	94.7	94.7	93.9
				0	223	98.3	53.3	79.7	91.2	95.4	99.2	100.3	100.1
					224	96.9	43.3	72.9	84.8	94.7	97.6	98.6	99.1
					225	99.9	46.4	72.3	85.9	92.8	98.9	99.9	100.4
					226	97.3	51.5	78.9	89.4	93.8	96.8	98.3	99.2
					227	97.6	58.8	90.1	96.1	96.8	98.0	97.9	98.1
					228	97.6	52.2	70.0	82.9	90.1	96.6	98.1	97.7
				1	229	101.2	40.0	77.0	94.6	100.1	102.7	102.3	102.8
					230	99.5	41.4	72.2	88.3	96.1	102.1	102.8	103.3
					231	102.7	43.5	70.4	85.9	95.7	102.8	104.2	104.3
					232	100.8	39.6	75.5	90.9	98.2	101.3	101.7	102.9
					233	101.7	46.5	81.2	96.2	100.7	103.0	102.7	102.8
					234	102.7	46.6	81.0	93.4	98.9	104.3	103.6	104.2

APPENDIX 2: STATISTICAL DESCRIPTION OF SURROGATE MODEL DEVELOPMENT STEPS

Step 1: Define Multivariate Response

- **Fit Weibull model to each tablet's dissolution** profile

- $y \mid t, \boldsymbol{b} \sim N\left(b_1 * \left[1 - e^{-\left(\frac{t}{b_2}\right)^{b_3}} \right], \sigma_d \right)$

    y = dissolution %, $\boldsymbol{b} = (b_1, b_2, b_3)$

    $\underline{r}'$ = calculated $\boldsymbol{b}$ per tablet

Step 2: Process Model

Fit Multivariate response r augmented with API Content by NIR measurement against DoE factors

$$\text{r}, \text{y}_{\text{NIR}} \mid X, B \sim MVN(XB, \Sigma_\lambda, \Sigma_\varepsilon)$$

X = design matrix, B = regression coefficients,

Σ_λ, Σ_ε = covariance matrices at Experimental run (Batch), and Tablet levels

Step 3: Conditional regression of API Content by NIR on θ

$$E(\theta \mid \text{NIR}, x_c, B, \Sigma) = (x_c * B[,1:3]) + \left(\frac{\sum_\lambda [,1:3,4]}{\sum_\lambda [4,4]} \right) * (\text{NIR} - x_c * B[,4])$$

$$= \theta^s, x_c = \text{design factor combination of interest}$$

APPENDIX 3: MODEL SELECTION PROCESS

The initial exploratory model includes all main plot factorial effects (3 terms), all 2- way interactions and one 3-way interaction (4 terms) and 1 curvature term, a total of 8 terms. This leaves 4 degrees of freedom (13 run – 8 model terms – 1 intercept) to estimate manufacturing variability and test the factorial effects F1, F2 and F3. If the design had not included replication of 3 of the runs, this model would have been completely saturated, meaning no degrees of freedom left over for calculating uncertainty. If that were the case, half normal probability plots, or Lenth's method [54] would be useful for identifying active factors to continue the model building process. The split-plot factor F4 and its interactions with the main plot effects F1, F2, and F3 add an additional 4 terms to the model, and a curvature term, so a total of 5 additional terms. These would be tested against the residual error term which we previously discussed is mainly driven by tablet-tablet and analytical uncertainty.

Example Base SAS® software code analyzing the model we just described acknowledging both the fixed continuous effects F1, F2, F3, F4 and the random effects attributable to batch-to-batch manufacture and residual error are estimated using the SAS/STAT procedure PROC MIXED. Note that the univariate models are part of the exploratory phase to identify CPPs for each element of the response vector individually, since it's not likely that each element will have the same relationships to the experimental factors. Once these are identified individually, then the final step is the formation of the multivariate model with element wise disparate effects (i.e., each response element may depend on different factors) to reflect the knowledge learned from the univariate analyses. Sample code follows a similar idea as before, where we embed the code into a macro called Expmodel. It can be called repeatedly for each of the elements to carry out a set of univariate analyses.

SAS code 2 – Mixed Model Code

```
%macro Expmodel (ct, px, fx, modx) ;

        proc mixed data=&fx ;
        class  run ;
        model y = &modx
            / solution outp=xpred&ct ddfm = KR ;
          random run ;
        title "Univariate Mixed model ";
        run;

%mend Expmodel ;
```

The first call for the first element of the response vector, b1, would be specified as follows:

%*Expmodel*(**1**,b1,out21,f1 f2 f3 f1*f2 f1*f3 f2*f3 f1*f2*f3 f1*f1 f4 f4*f1 f4*f2 f4*f3 f4*f4);

where the arguments to the macro call are *ct* = an index referring to the element number in the vector, *p* = parameter name, *fx* = dataset name, modx = terms in the model. At this first call, we simply specify all 13 terms discussed previously. The PROC MIXED OUTPUT of this macro call is shown in Appendix 4. The relevant part is the random and fixed effects estimates abstracted here for illustrating the model building process. First we have the random effects or variance components corresponding to manufacturing batch-to-batch variability designated run, and residual error:

Covariance Parameter Estimates	
Cov Parm	**Estimate**
Run	0.94
Residual	1.29

The AICc is a fit statistic useful for model selection. The AICc for this model was 762.9. We will refer to this value later in arriving at a final model.

The fixed effects estimates are given in the Output Listing 9.

Output Listing 9 – Partial Proc Mixed Listing Full Model

Solution for Fixed Effects

Effect	Estimate	Standard Error	DF	t Value	Pr > |t|
Intercept	100.32	0.72	4.17	139.25	<.001
f1	0.61	0.33	4	1.85	0.137
f2	−0.21	0.33	4	−0.63	0.564
f3	−0.43	0.33	4	−1.29	0.266
f1*f2	−0.029	0.33	4	−0.09	0.933
f1*f3	0.10	0.33	4	0.31	0.771
f2*f3	−0.08	0.33	4	−0.24	0.823
f1*f2*f3	−0.002	0.33	4	−0.01	0.996
f1*f1 (curvature)	−1.16	0.79	4	−1.48	0.213
f4	4.80	0.09	216	52.46	<.001
f1*f4	−0.22	0.11	216	−2.10	0.037
f2*f4	0.003	0.11	216	0.02	0.981
f3*f4	0.14	0.11	216	1.35	0.179
f4*f4 (curvature)	−0.03	0.16	216	−0.20	0.842

The task now is to continue the model building process to identify a parsimonious model. Such a model will have a smaller estimate of the manufacturing variance component compared to the full model, while removing model terms with little impact and preserving factors with high impact. For b1, the Weibull parameter describing the upper asymptote of the dissolution profile, one can choose a criterion for effect, such as 0.25% (dissolution) to separate meaningful effects from less meaningful effects as an example of a practically meaningful effect criterion. Recall also that we have only 4 degrees of freedom for testing the factorial effects against incipient manufacturing variability. This would not be regarded as a sensitive test, so for these factors, one can use a higher p-value criterion to select effects, say p=0.25 or thereabouts to suggest active factors in combination with the effect criterion. For the split plot factor (Factor 4), because these are 3 levels within each experimental run, we have 216 degrees of freedom, so we can be more stringent, and use a criterion of p=0.05 for these terms.

Based on these criteria, we can fit a reduced model with only the terms that we believe at this stage exhibit a meaningful effect. Having identified those potentially meaningful effects, we would change the model specification to reflect only these terms as follow:

$$\%\textbf{Expmodel}(\textbf{1}, b1, out21, f1 \; f3 \; f1*f1 \; f4 \; f1*f4);$$

The detailed results of this macro call are given in Appendix 5. The relevant results are abstracted in Output Listing 10, first the variance components and then the fixed effects estimates.

$$AICc = 754.4,$$

The goal of the model selection process is to arrive at a model that explains the maximum amount of variation with the least number of explanatory terms in the model. In this example, we have reduced the model from 14 terms to 6 terms. The AICc decreased from 762.9 to 754.4, and the estimate of manufacturing variance reduced from 0.94, to 0.44. It's important to note that model selection is not a completely objective procedure. There are various approaches one might consider which are outside the scope of this chapter to delve into. Whichever method one uses to arrive at a final reduced model, it represents a balance between parsimony and explanatory power. We emphasize that the goal is to find a reduced model that preserves as much of the explanatory power of the full model with the fewest number of model terms subject to scientific judgment and practicality. A good discussion of model selection using the AICc is by Portet [55]. Box and Meyer [45, 46] in two publications, have proposed a Bayesian approach to model selection. However, their method involves a prior distribution assumption which may need some adjustment to fit the experience of pharmaceutical manufacturing and engineering experimenters. Therefore, this method should be approached with caution and adaptation.

APPENDIX 4: EXPLORATORY MODEL LISTING FOR ELEMENT B1

The Mixed Procedure

Model Information

Data Set	WORK.OUT21
Dependent Variable	y
Covariance Structure	Variance Components
Estimation Method	REML
Residual Variance Method	Profile
Fixed Effects SE Method	Kenward-Roger
Degrees of Freedom Method	Kenward-Roger

Class Level Information

Class	Levels	Values
runx	13	Run01 Run02 Run03 Run04 Run05 Run06 Run07 Run08 Run09 Run10 Run11 Run12 Run13

Dimensions

Covariance Parameters	2
Columns in X	14
Columns in Z	13
Subjects	1
Max Obs per Subject	234

Number of Observations

Number of Observations Read	234
Number of Observations Used	234
Number of Observations Not Used	0

Iteration History

Iteration	Evaluations	–2 Res Log Like	Criterion
0	1	795.58433110	
1	1	758.80238395	0.00000000

Convergence Criteria met.

Covariance Parameter Estimates

Cov Parm	Estimate
runx	0.9445
Residual	1.2857

Fit Statistics

−2 Res Log Likelihood	758.8
AIC (Smaller is Better)	762.8
AICC (Smaller is Better)	762.9
BIC (Smaller is Better)	763.9

Solution for Fixed Effects

Effect	Estimate	Standard Error	DF	t Value	Pr > |t|
Intercept	100.32	0.7204	4.17	139.25	<.0001
f1	0.6106	0.3294	4	1.85	0.1373
f2	−0.2069	0.3294	4	−0.63	0.5639
f3	−0.4250	0.3294	4	−1.29	0.2664
f1*f2	−0.02934	0.3294	4	−0.09	0.9333
f1*f3	0.1028	0.3294	4	0.31	0.7706
f2*f3	−0.07865	0.3294	4	−0.24	0.8230
f1*f2*f3	−0.00178	0.3294	4	−0.01	0.9959
f1_2	−1.1611	0.7851	4	−1.48	0.2133
f4	4.7951	0.09141	216	52.46	<.0001
f1*f4	−0.2204	0.1052	216	−2.10	0.0373
f2*f4	0.002534	0.1052	216	0.02	0.9808
f3*f4	0.1417	0.1052	216	1.35	0.1792
f4_2	−0.03147	0.1572	216	−0.20	0.8416

Type 3 Tests of Fixed Effects

Effect	Num DF	Den DF	F Value	Pr > F
f1	1	4	3.44	0.1373
f2	1	4	0.39	0.5639
f3	1	4	1.67	0.2664
f1*f2	1	4	0.01	0.9333
f1*f3	1	4	0.10	0.7706
f2*f3	1	4	0.06	0.8230
f1*f2*f3	1	4	0.00	0.9959
f1_2	1	4	2.19	0.2133
f4	1	216	2752.08	<.0001
f1*f4	1	216	4.39	0.0373
f2*f4	1	216	0.00	0.9808
f3*f4	1	216	1.82	0.1792
f4_2	1	216	0.04	0.8416

APPENDIX 5: FINAL PROC MIXED FINAL REDUCED MODEL LISTING FOR B1

The Mixed Procedure

Model Information

Data Set	WORK.OUT 21
Dependent Variable	y
Covariance Structure	Variance Components
Estimation Method	REML
Residual Variance Method	Profile
Fixed Effects SE Method	Kenward-Roger
Degrees of Freedom Method	Kenward-Roger

Class Level Information

Class	Levels	Values
runx	13	Run01 Run02 Run03 Run04 Run05 Run06 Run07 Run08 Run09 Run10 Run11 Run12 Run13

Dimensions

Covariance Parameters	2
Columns in X	6
Columns in Z	13
Subjects	1
Max Obs per Subject	234

Number of Observations

Number of Observations Read	234
Number of Observations Used	234
Number of Observations Not Used	0

Iteration History

Iteration	Evaluations	-2 Res Log Like	Criterion
0	1	782.61063366	
1	1	750.31883260	0.00000000

Convergence criteria met.

Covariance Parameter Estimates

Cov Parm	Estimate
runx	0.4424
Residual	1.2795

Fit Statistics

−2 Res Log Likelihood	750.3
AIC (Smaller is Better)	754.3
AICC (Smaller is Better)	754.4
BIC (Smaller is Better)	755.4

Solution for Fixed Effects

Effect	Estimate	Standard Error	DF	t Value	Pr > |t|
Intercept	100.30	0.5067	9	197.93	<.0001
f1	0.5664	0.2251	9	2.52	0.0330
f3	−0.4692	0.2251	9	−2.08	0.0668
f1_2	−1.1734	0.5514	9	−2.13	0.0622
f4	4.8033	0.09088	219	52.85	<.0001
f1*f4	−0.1818	0.09880	219	−1.84	0.0671

Type 3 Tests of Fixed Effects

Effect	Num DF	Den DF	F Value	Pr > F
f1	1	9	6.33	0.0330
f3	1	9	4.34	0.0668
f1_2	1	9	4.53	0.0622
f4	1	219	2793.15	<.0001
f1*f4	1	219	3.39	0.0671

APPENDIX 6: PROC BGLIMM LISTING OF MULTIVARIATE BAYESIAN PROCESS MODEL

TABLE A14

Priors for Scale and Covariance Parameters

Parameter	Prior
Residual Cov (Diag)	Inverse Gamma (Shape=0.0001, Scale=0.0001)
Residual Cov (Off-Diag)	Constant
Random Cov (Diag)	Inverse Gamma (Shape=0.0001, Scale=0.0001)
Random Cov (Off-Diag)	Constant

TABLE 15

Posterior Summaries

Parameter	N	Mean	SD	Percentiles		
				25	50	75
par b1	10000	100.1	0.5234	99.7360	100.1	100.4
par b2	10000	8.0473	0.1038	7.9799	8.0485	8.1143
par b3	10000	0.9924	0.0360	0.9693	0.9920	1.0159
par NIR	10000	99.0050	0.4090	98.7578	99.0137	99.2605
f1*par b1	10000	0.5435	0.2893	0.3666	0.5476	0.7194
f1*par b2	10000	−0.9044	0.1122	−0.9748	−0.9031	−0.8313
f1*par b3	10000	−0.0458	0.0158	−0.0559	−0.0458	−0.0359

Posterior Summaries

Parameter	N	Mean	SD	Percentiles		
				25	50	75
f1*par NIR	10000	0.5424	0.4246	0.2702	0.5380	0.8108
f4*par b1	10000	4.8060	0.0917	4.7452	4.8052	4.8676
f4*par b2	10000	1.9517	0.0924	1.8886	1.9512	2.0122
f4*par b3	10000	0.2070	0.0107	0.1998	0.2071	0.2140
f4*par NIR	10000	4.8457	0.0957	4.7811	4.8461	4.9111
f3*f3r*par b1	10000	−0.4043	0.2104	−0.5342	−0.4050	−0.2761
f3*f3r*par b2	0	.	.	.	.	.
f3*f3r*par b3	10000	0.0361	0.0144	0.0269	0.0361	0.0452
f3*f3r*par NIR	0	.	.	.	.	.
f1_2*f1_2r*par b1	10000	−0.9032	0.5410	−1.2421	−0.8998	−0.5711
f1_2*f1_2r*par b2	0	.	.	.	.	.
f1_2*f1_2r*par b3	10000	0.1086	0.0370	0.0854	0.1089	0.1320
f1_2*f1_2r*par NIR	0	.	.	.	.	.
f1*f4*f14r*par b1	10000	−0.2045	0.0788	−0.2572	−0.2045	−0.1515
f1*f4*f14r*par b2	0	.	.	.	.	.
f1*f4*f14r*par b3	10000	0.0729	0.0118	0.0649	0.0728	0.0806
f1*f4*f14r*par NIR	0	.	.	.	.	.
f4*f3*f34r*par b1	0	.	.	.	.	.
f4*f3*f34r*par b2	10000	−0.2583	0.0975	−0.3222	−0.2589	−0.1937
f4*f3*f34r*par b3	10000	−0.0630	0.0108	−0.0701	−0.0629	−0.0558
f4*f3*f34r*par NIR	0	.	.	.	.	.
f4_2*f4_2r*par b1	0	.	.	.	.	.
f4_2*f4_2r*par b2	0	.	.	.	.	.
f4_2*f4_2r*par b3	10000	0.0401	0.0173	0.0283	0.0400	0.0518
f4_2*f4_2r*par NIR	10000	−0.2260	0.1336	−0.3164	−0.2256	−0.1362
Residual UN(1,1)	10000	1.3079	0.1269	1.2198	1.3011	1.3871
Residual UN(2,1)	10000	0.3077	0.0922	0.2458	0.3061	0.3673
Residual UN(2,2)	10000	1.3218	0.1261	1.2345	1.3122	1.4020
Residual UN(3,1)	10000	−0.0515	0.0110	−0.0587	−0.0510	−0.0438
Residual UN(3,2)	10000	−0.0320	0.0107	−0.0389	−0.0316	−0.0248
Residual UN(3,3)	10000	0.0180	0.00174	0.0168	0.0179	0.0191
Residual UN(4,1)	10000	0.8059	0.1090	0.7302	0.8015	0.8758
Residual UN(4,2)	10000	0.2246	0.0956	0.1618	0.2235	0.2877
Residual UN(4,3)	10000	0.00612	0.0110	−0.00122	0.00601	0.0134
Residual UN(4,4)	10000	1.4314	0.1390	1.3329	1.4241	1.5201
Random UN(1,1)	10000	0.8187	0.6776	0.4256	0.6373	0.9874
Random UN(2,1)	10000	0.1547	0.1742	0.0547	0.1182	0.2091
Random UN(2,2)	10000	0.0669	0.0742	0.0220	0.0451	0.0859
Random UN(3,1)	10000	0.0212	0.0261	0.00735	0.0159	0.0288
Random UN(3,2)	10000	0.00277	0.00708	−0.00031	0.00199	0.00521
Random UN(3,3)	10000	0.00163	0.00185	0.000600	0.00110	0.00201
Random UN(4,1)	10000	0.7390	0.7670	0.3093	0.5687	0.9493
Random UN(4,2)	10000	0.2739	0.2760	0.1143	0.2125	0.3624
Random UN(4,3)	10000	0.0123	0.0357	−0.00430	0.00913	0.0256
Random UN(4,4)	10000	2.0153	1.4167	1.1537	1.6342	2.4015

Comparison of Posterior Distribution with Prior distribution for fixed effect parameter b1 and Batch covariance term $\Sigma_\lambda(1,1)$

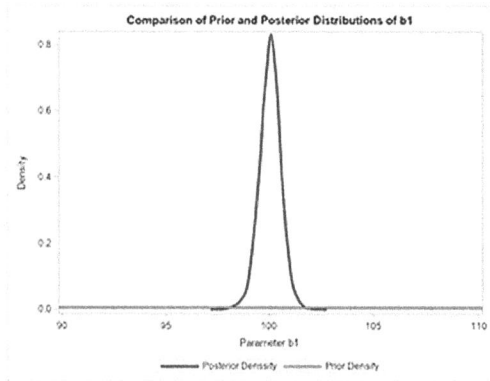

(a)

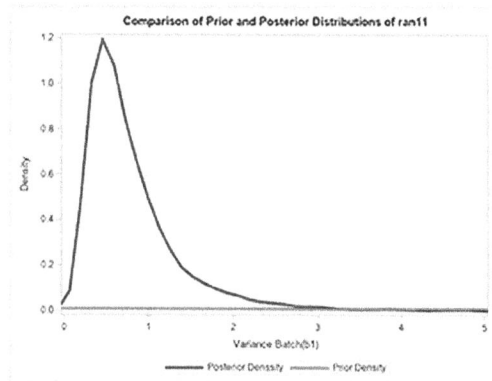

(b)

APPENDIX 7: SAS PROC IML CODE FOR SURROGATE PREDICTIONS

TABLE 16

SAS PROC IML Code	Comment
proc iml;	**Begin code**
use c2a ; read all var _NUM_ into B0 [colname=VNamesB]; close c2a ;	Read in Coefficient Matrix
use g1 ; read all var _NUM_ into Sg [colname=VNamesG] ; print VNamesG ; close g1;	Read in Covariance Matrix Σ_λ
g11 = sg[{**1 2 3**}, {**1 2 3**}] ; g12 = sg[{**1 2 3**}, {**4**}] ; g21 = sg[{**4**}, {**1 2 3**}] ; g22 = sg[{**4**}, {**4**}] ;	Create submatrices of Σ_λ
parname = { "b1", "b2", "b3"}; /* headings for rows */ Coef = { "b1", "b2", "b3" }; /* headings for columns */	Define Column Names
b1 = t(b0[{**1 2 3**},]) ; * dim 3 x r goes to r x 3 ; b2 = t(b0[**4**,]) ; * dim 1 x r goes to r x 1;	Define Coefficient submatrices
cols = {**3 4 5 6 7 8 9 10**} ;	Column locations for model terms
use a2 ; read all var _NUM_ into x0[colname=VNamesX];	Read in data (Table 4)
z0 = j(nrow(x0),**3**) ; z1 = j(**1,8**) ;/* ENTER NUMBER OF MODEL TERMS inc INTERCEPT */ nrx = j(nrow(x0),**1**) ; condb = g12*inv(g22) ;	Define dimensions for matrix and vectors needed later Regression coefficient vector

SAS PROC IML Code	Comment

do i = **1** to nrow(x0);
nr = x0[i,**2**] ; /* define nir column */
z1 = x0[i,cols] ;
m0 = t(z1*b1);
nrx[i,**1**] = z1*b2 ;
 	
z0[i, **1:3**] = t(m0 + condb*(nr − nrx[i,**1**])) ;
end;
	Cycle through by tablet and calculate surrogate prediction z0

w0 = x0 ‖ nrx ‖ z0 ; /* concatenate three matrices */ /* print w0 ; */	Create final dataset
xname = vnamesX ‖ {"NRX" "b1_sur" "b2_sur" "b3_sur"} ; /* print xname ; */	Name columns
create FitPar from w0[colname = xname]; append from w0 ; close fitpar ;	Write surrogate predictions out to SAS dataset

QUIT ;

APPENDIX 8: CONGRUENCE PLOTS OF EMPIRICAL WEIBULL PARAMETERS WITH SURROGATE MODEL PREDICTED WEIBULL PARAMETERS AT RUN AVERAGE LEVEL

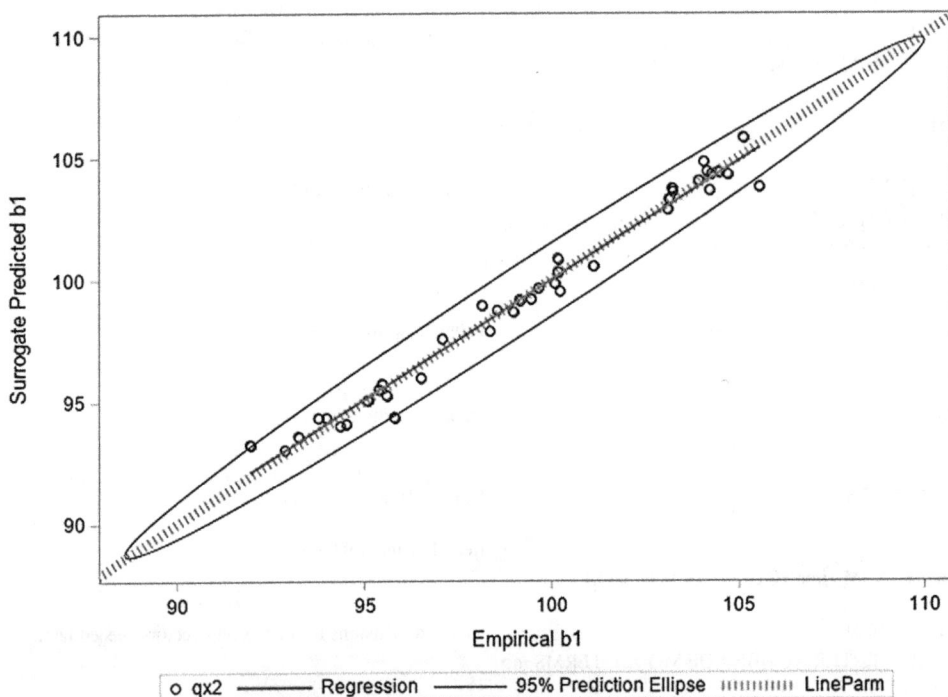

FIGURE A1   Congruence Plot of Surrogate b1 vs Empirical b1.

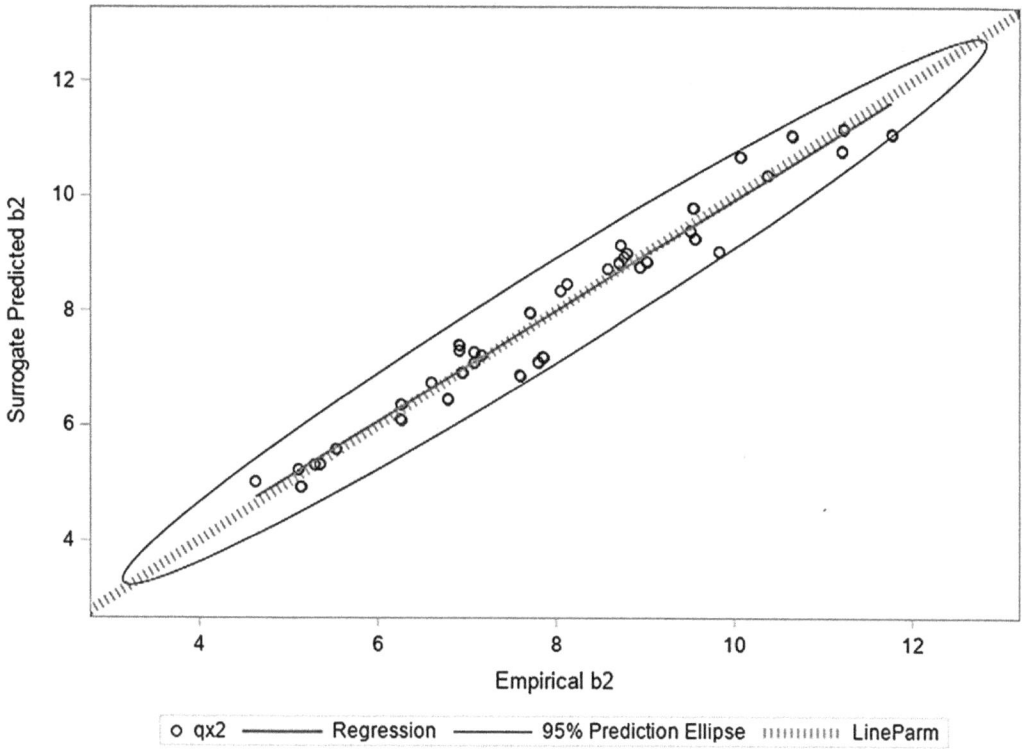

FIGURE A2 Congruence Plot of Surrogate b2 vs Empirical b2.

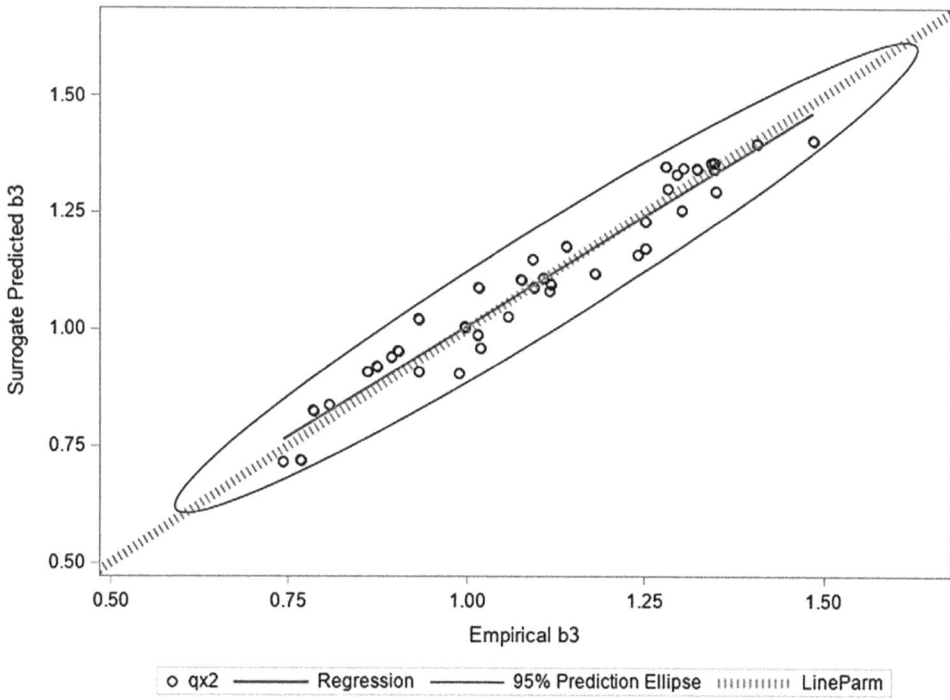

FIGURE A3 Congruence Plot of Surrogate b3 vs Empirical b.

APPENDIX 9: PLOT OF EMPIRICAL PROFILES WITH SURROGATE MODEL PREDICTED PROFILES OF RUN AVERAGES AT THE 3 LEVELS OF FACTOR 4 BY EXPERIMENTAL RUN

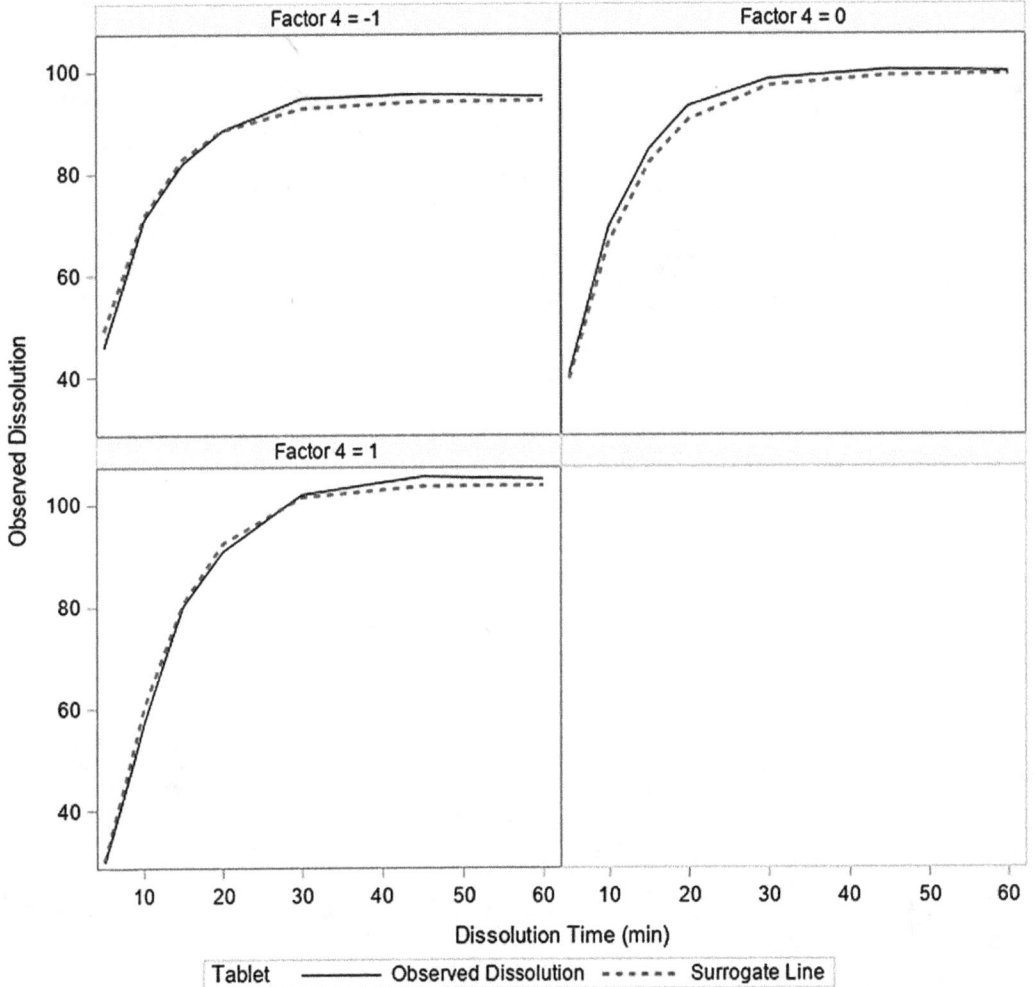

FIGURE A4   Comparison of empirical with surrogate predicted average profiles Experimental Run 1.

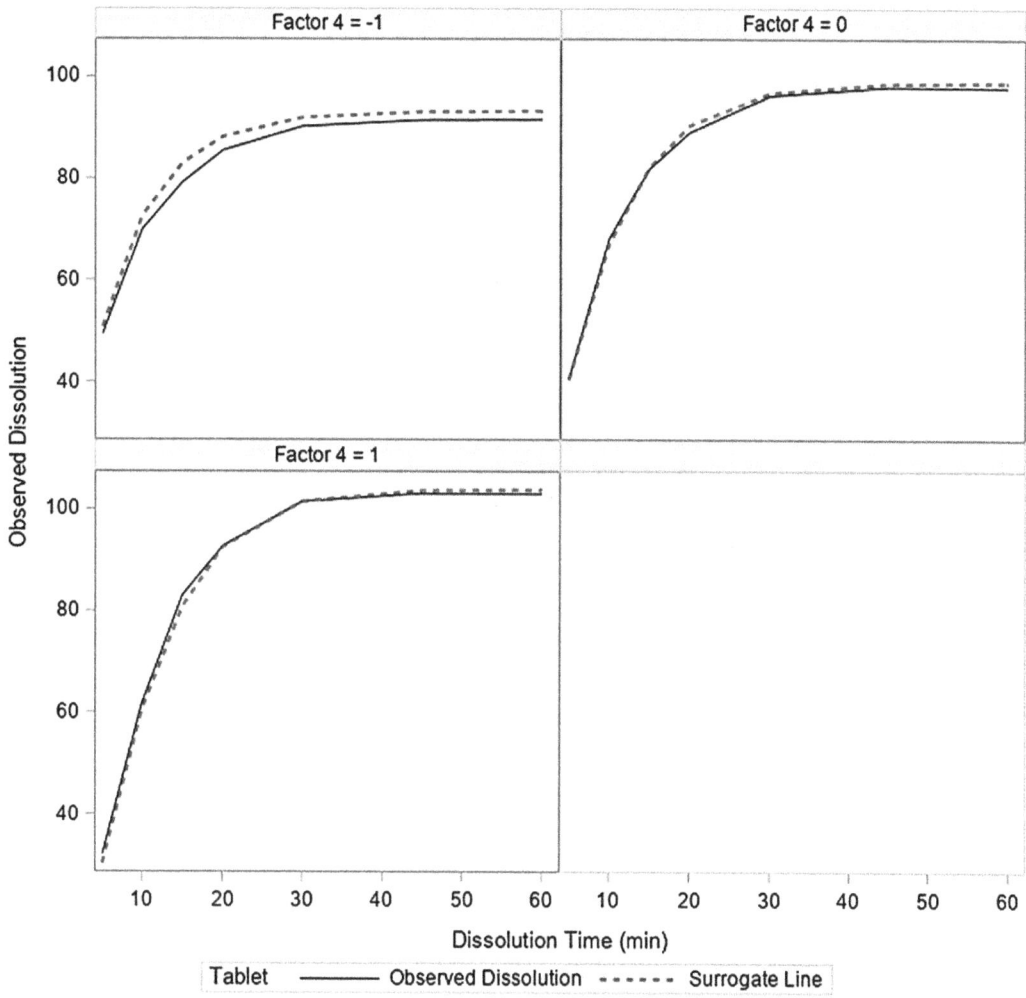

FIGURE A5 Comparison of empirical with surrogate predicted average profiles Experimental Run 2.

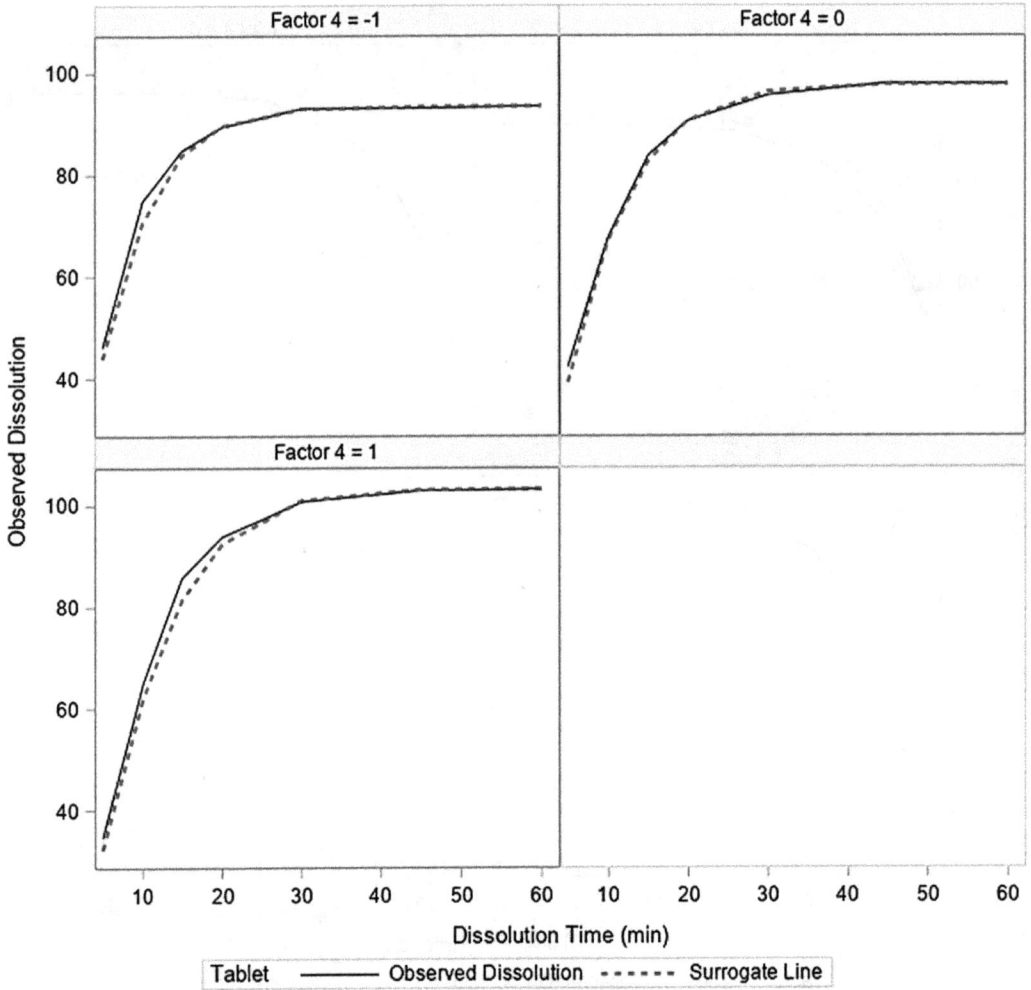

FIGURE A6 Comparison of empirical with surrogate predicted average profiles Experimental Run 3.

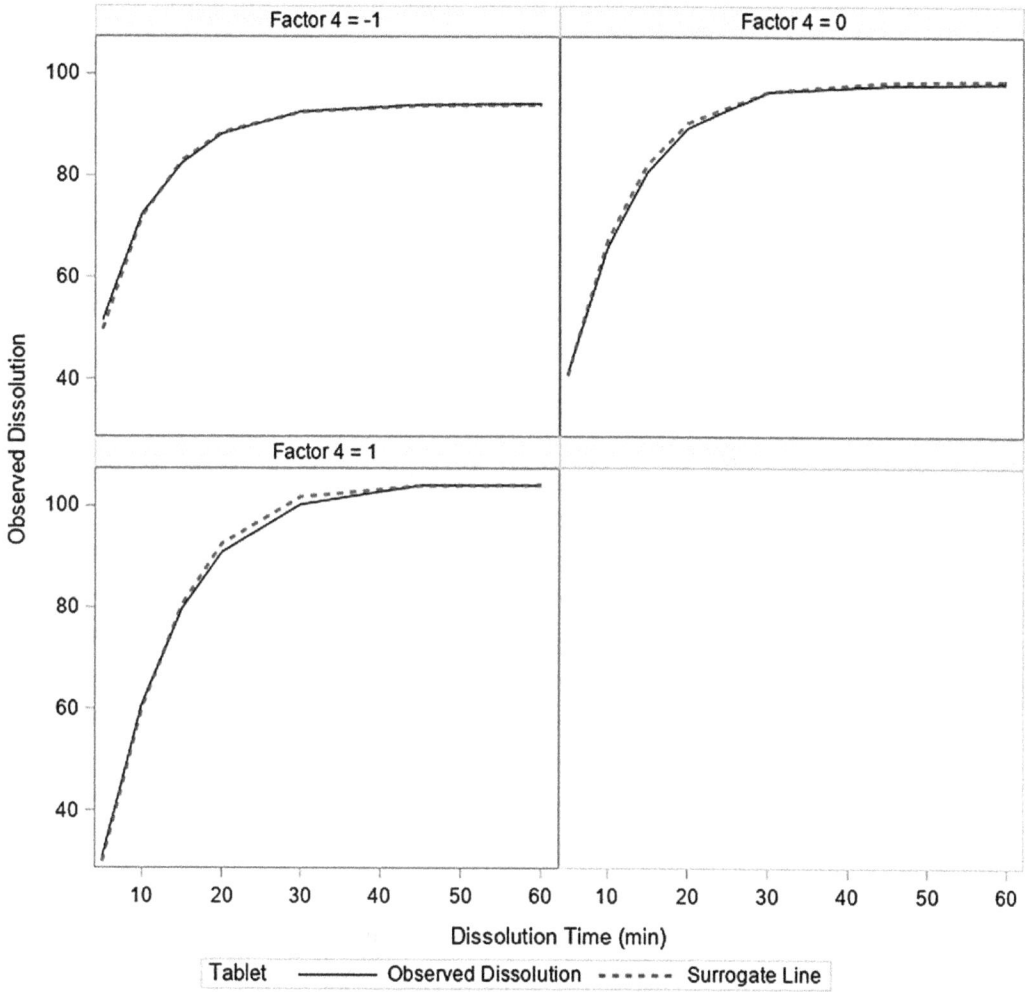

FIGURE A7 Comparison of empirical with surrogate predicted average profiles Experimental Run 4.

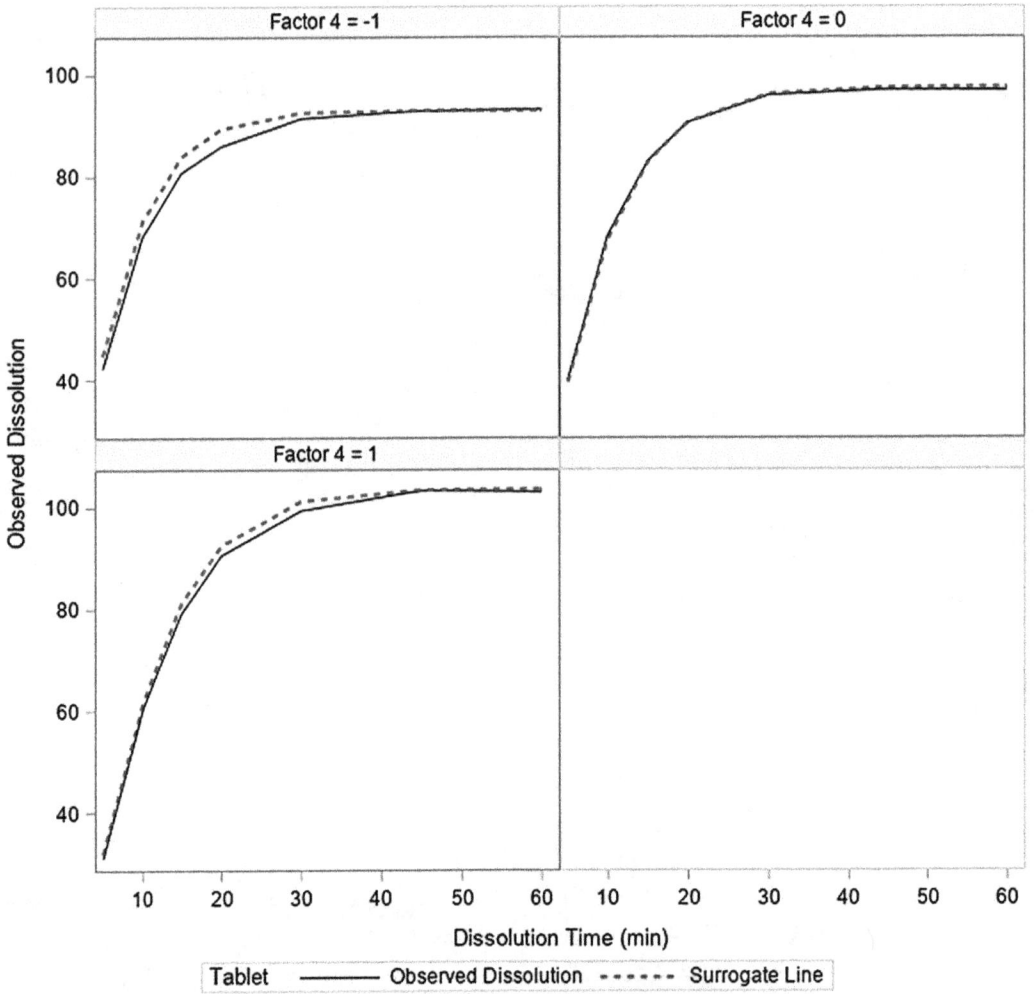

FIGURE A8   Comparison of empirical with surrogate predicted average profiles Experimental Run 5.

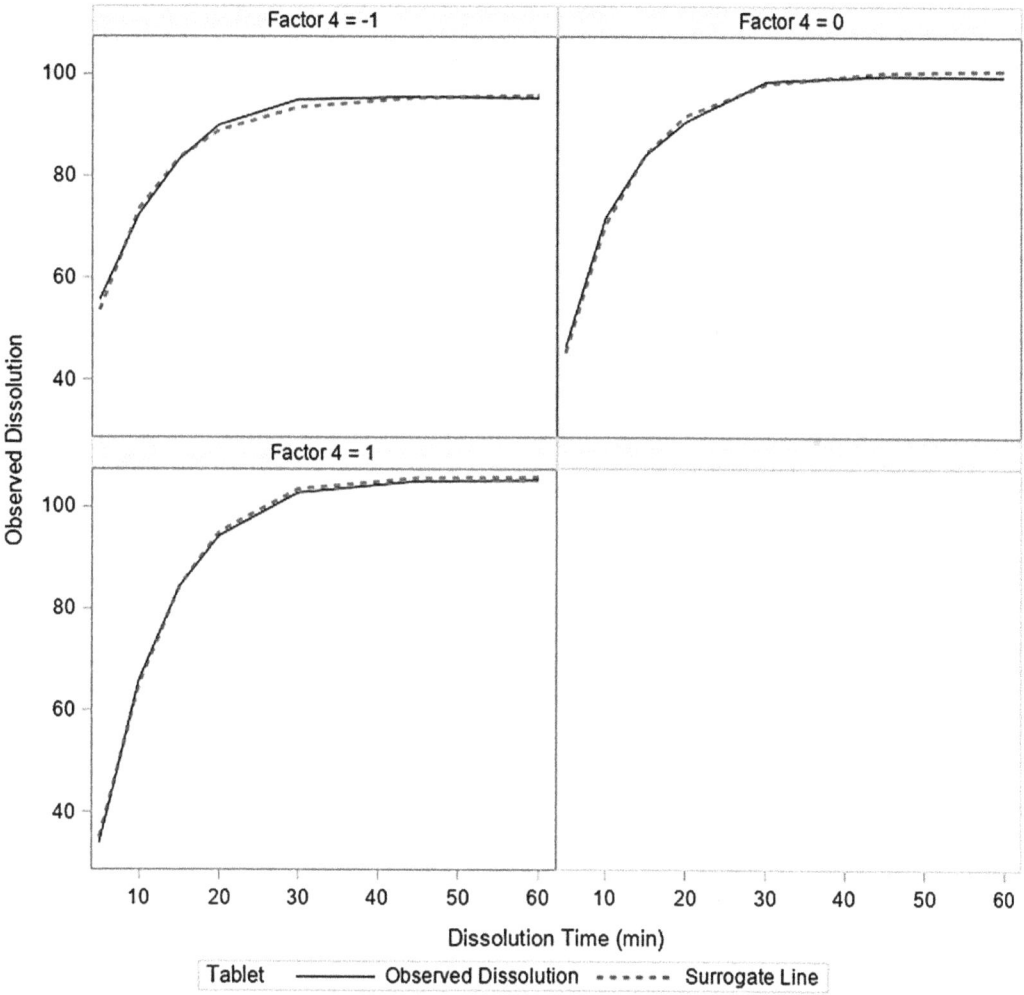

FIGURE A9   Comparison of empirical with surrogate predicted average profiles Experimental Run 6.

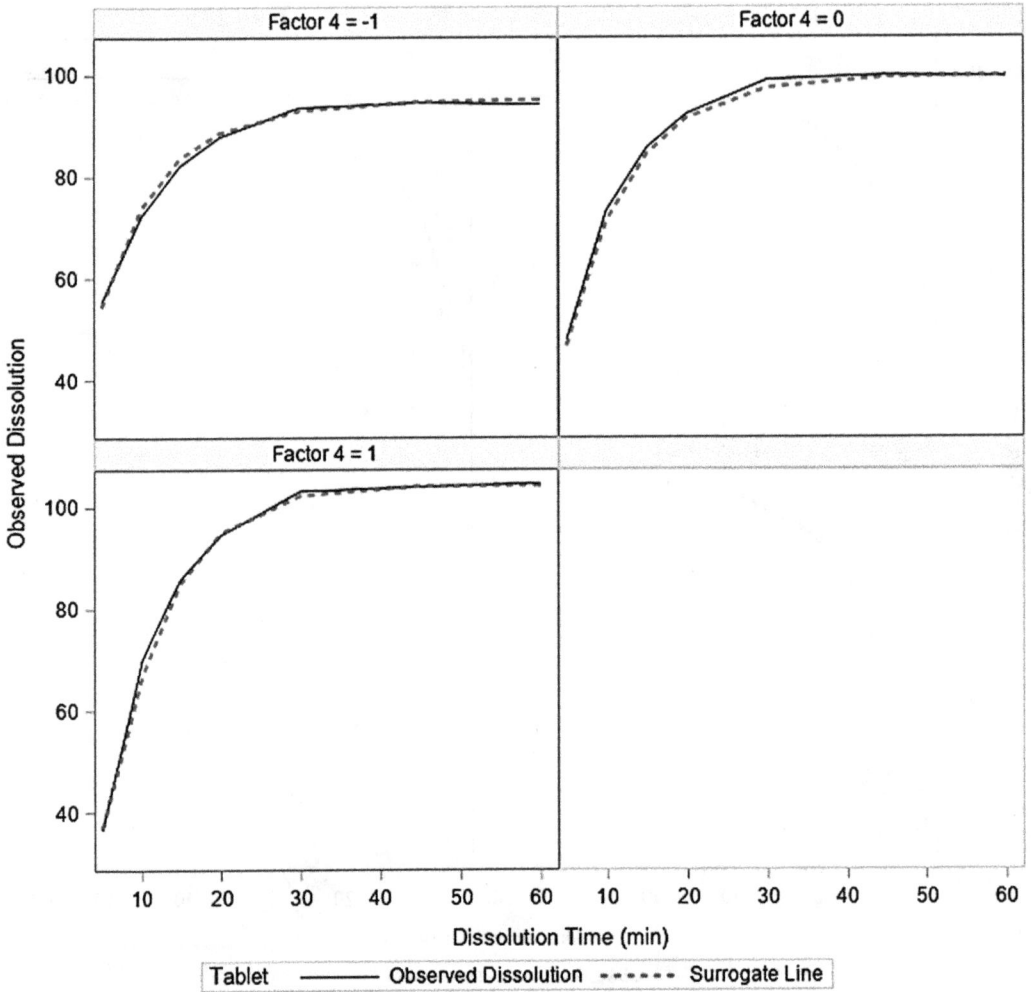

FIGURE A10 Comparison of empirical with surrogate predicted average profiles Experimental Run 7.

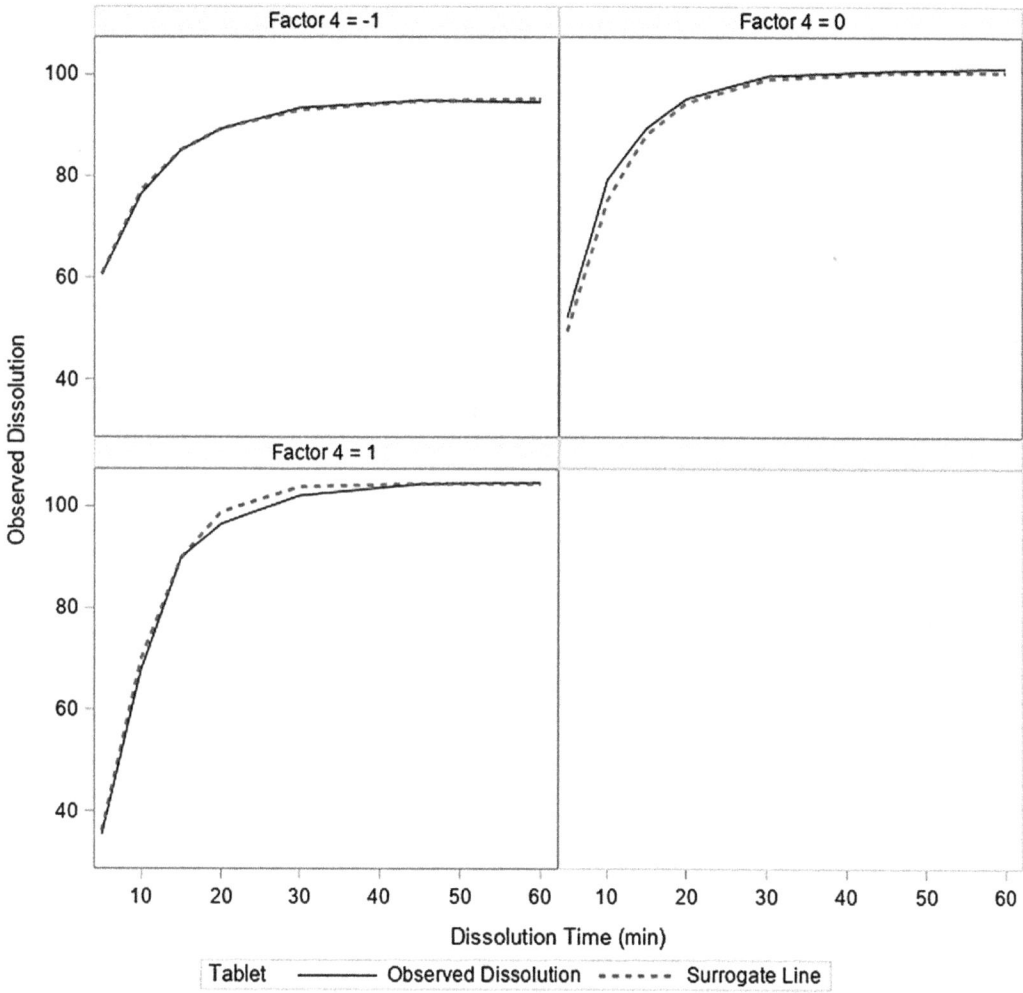

FIGURE A11 Comparison of empirical with surrogate predicted average profiles Experimental Run 8.

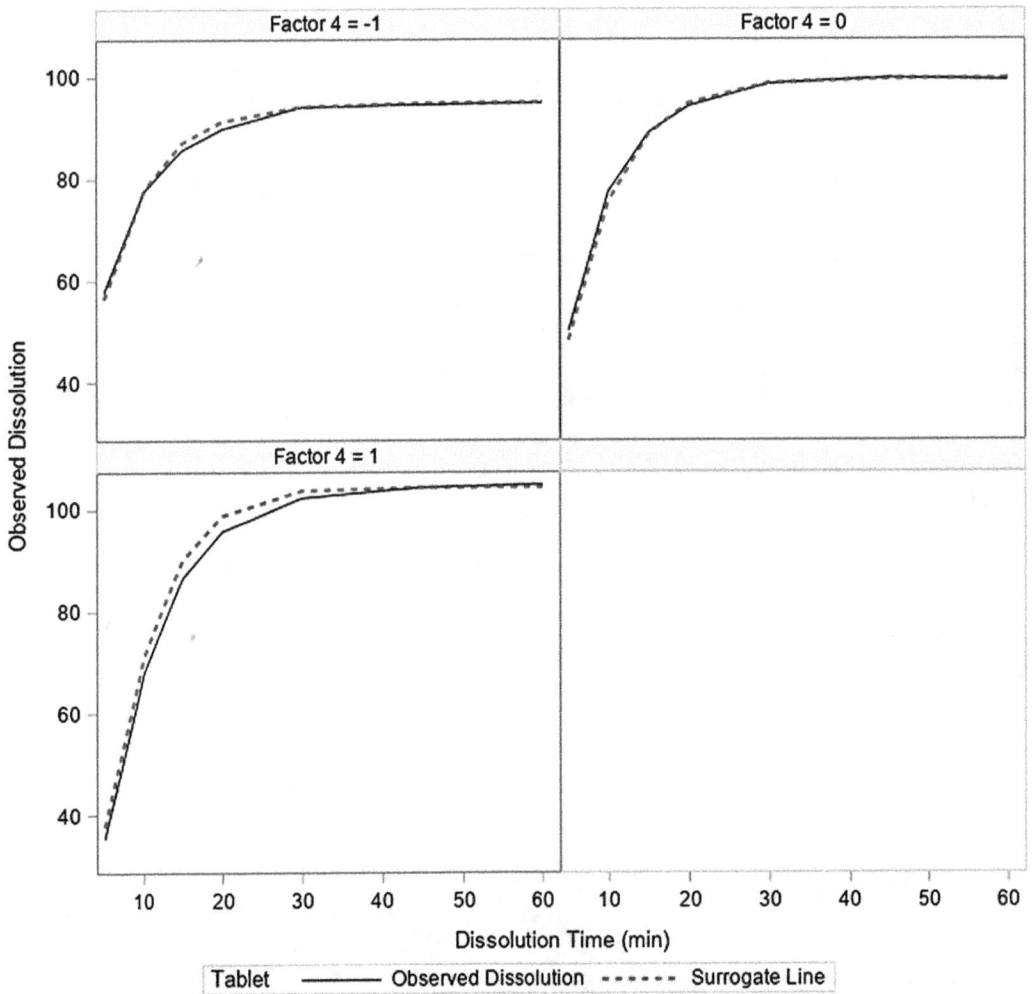

FIGURE A12   Comparison of empirical with surrogate predicted average profiles Experimental Run 9.

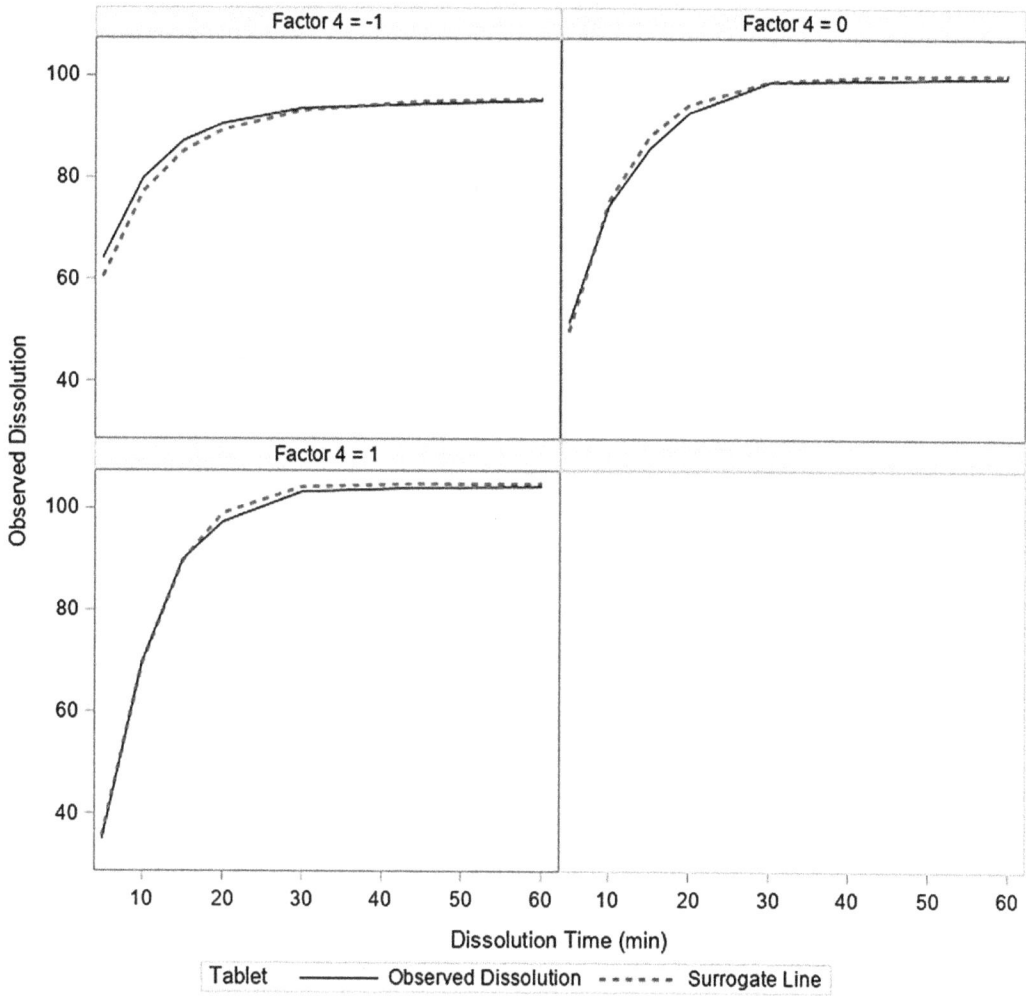

FIGURE A13 Comparison of empirical with surrogate predicted average profiles Experimental Run 10.

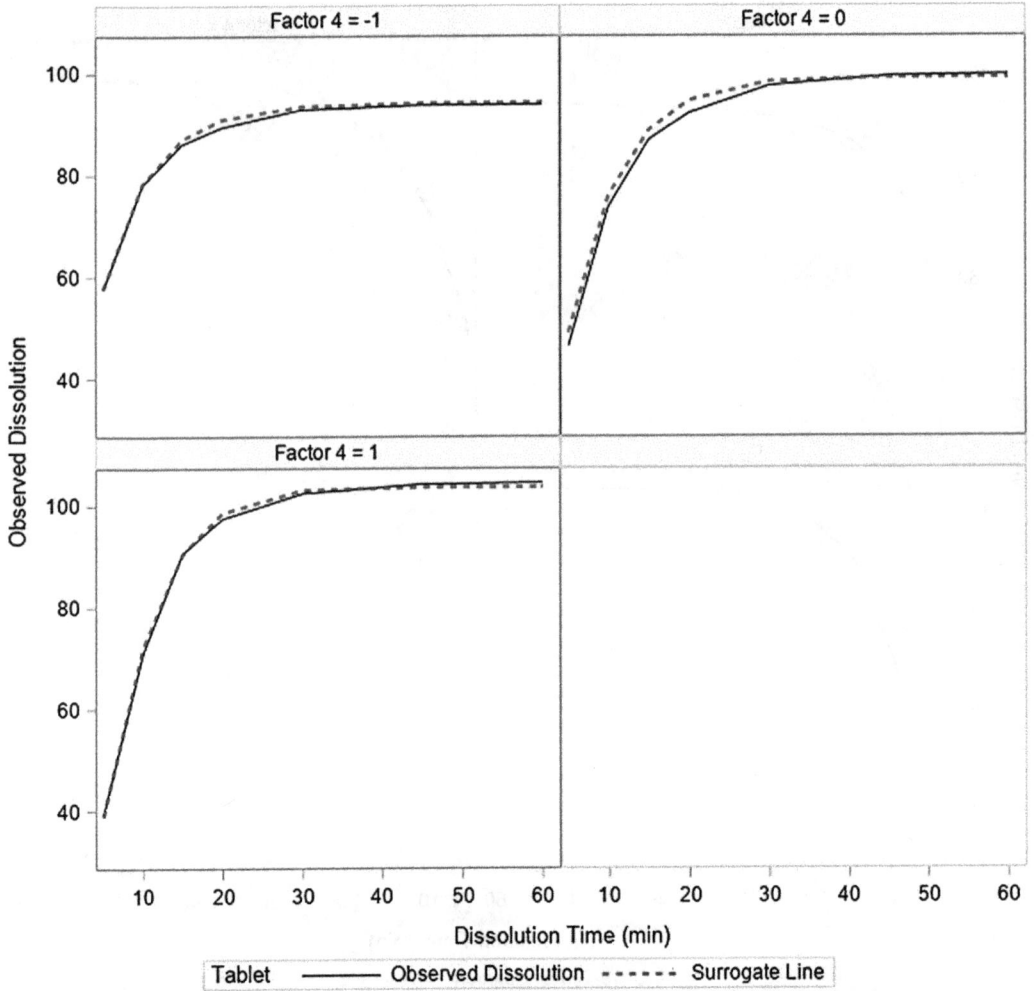

FIGURE A14 Comparison of empirical with surrogate predicted average profiles Experimental Run 11.

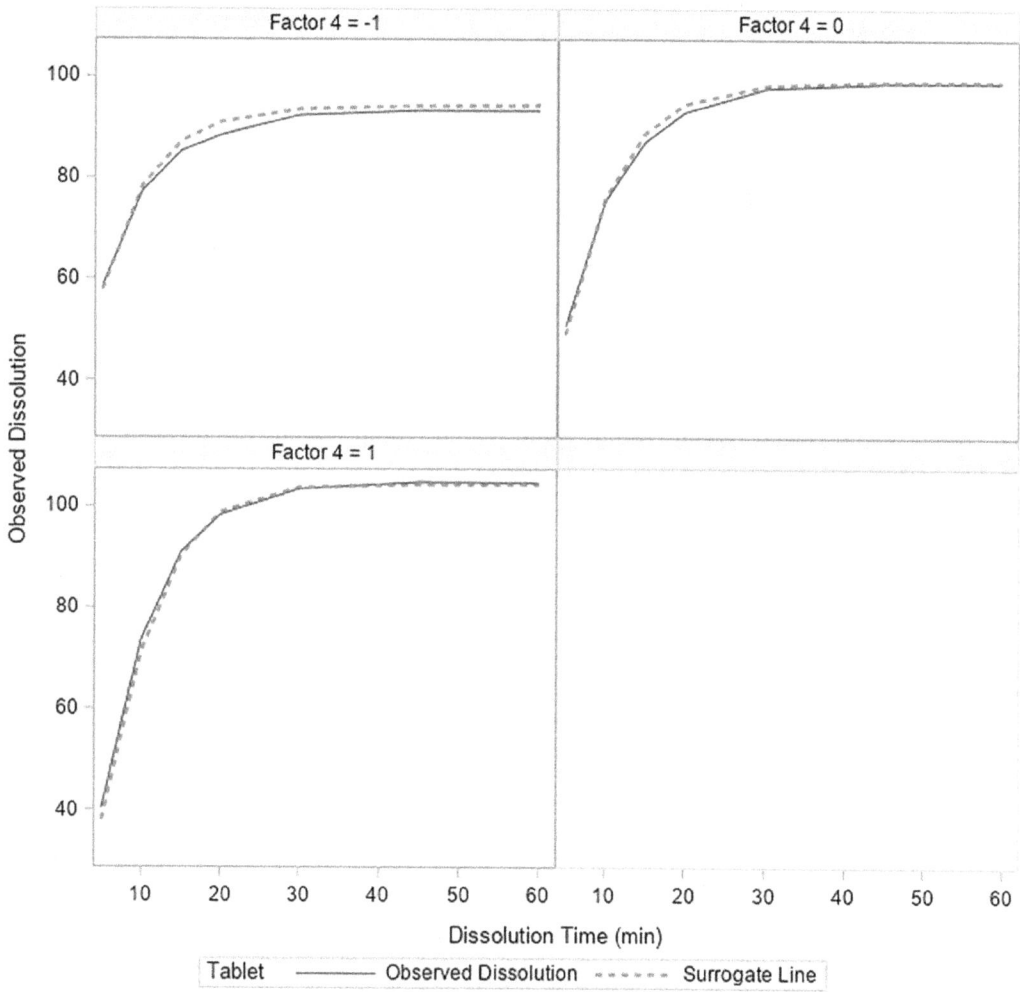

FIGURE A15 Comparison of empirical with surrogate predicted average profiles Experimental Run 12.

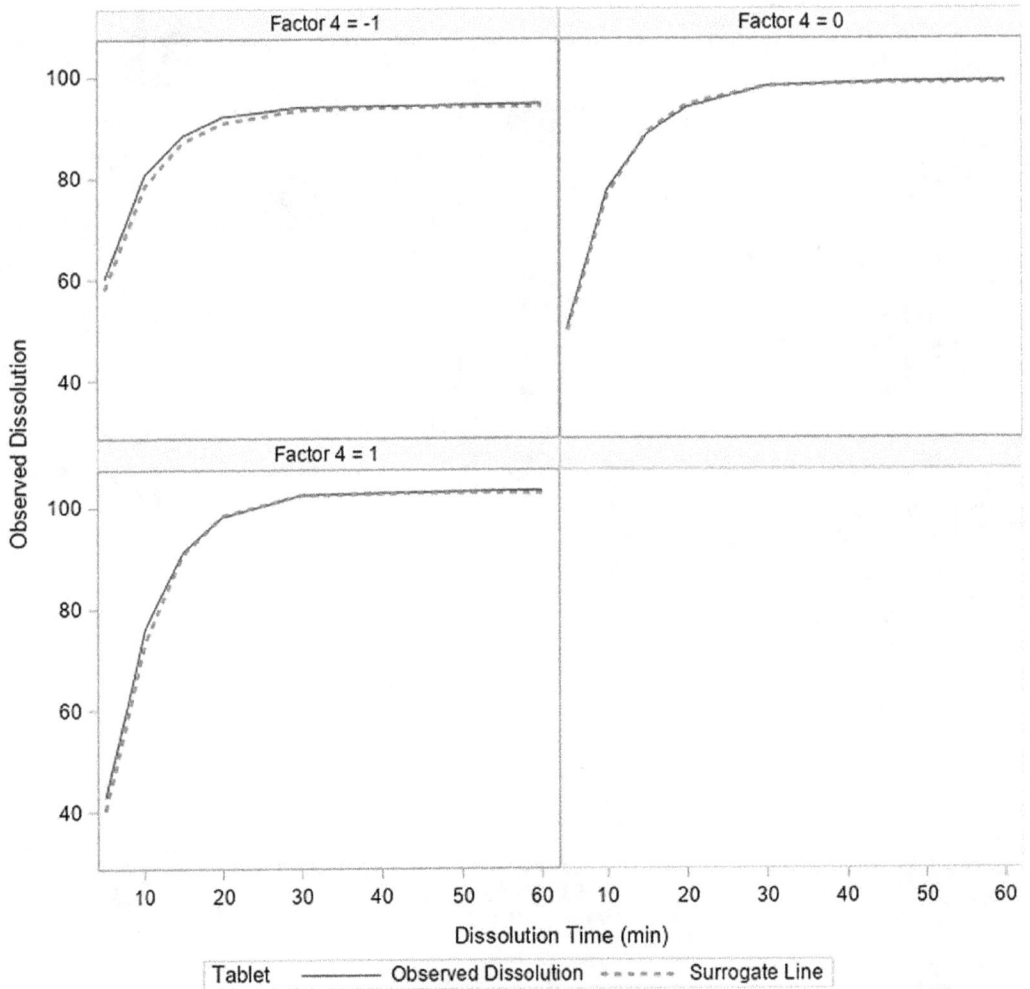

FIGURE A16 Comparison of empirical with surrogate predicted average profiles Experimental Run 13.

APPENDIX 10: SAS MACRO SIM 1

TABLE A17

```
%macro SIM1(n1, n2, n0) ;

%do i= &n1 %to &n2 ;

data line0 ; set post2 ;
if _N_ = &i ;
keep b1 b2 b3 nir b10 b20 b30 NIR0 res11 res21 res22 res31 res32 res33 res41 res42 res43 res44 ;
run ;

DATA LINE1 ; SET LINE0 ;
  rename b10 = b1 b20 = b2 b30 = b3 nir0 = nir ;
  keep b10 b20 b30 NIR0 ;
RUN ;

data r11 ; set line0 ;
b1 = res11/&n0 ; b2 = res21/&n0 ; b3 = res31/&n0 ;
  NIR = res41/&n0 ; output ;
b1 = res21/&n0 ; b2 = res22/&n0 ; b3 = res32/&n0 ;
  NIR = res42/&n0 ; output ;
b1 = res31/&n0 ; b2 = res32/&n0 ; b3 = res33/&n0 ;
  NIR = res43/&n0 ; output ;
b1 = res41/&n0 ; b2 = res42/&n0 ; b3 = res43/&n0 ;
  NIR = res44/&n0 ; output ;
keep b1 b2 b3 NIR ;
run ;

* Generate random measured tablet ;

proc iml;

use line1 ; * mean row vector ;
  read all var _NUM_ into Mean [colname= Mname];
  close line1 ;

use r11 ; * covariance matrix ;
  read all var _NUM_ into rv1 ;
  close r11 ;

call randseed(1043721);
X = RandNormal(1, Mean, rv1);

create line7 from X[colname = Mname];
  append from x ;
  close line7 ;
  quit ;

data line7 ; set line7 ; /* this is the measured values of b0 b1 b2 NIR from n0 tablets*/
  k = &i ; /* Get a measured Q30, get a surrogate Q30 compare to true */
  run ;
```

```
data line7a ; set line7 ;
  rename b1 = mb1 b2=mb2 b3=mb3 NIR=mNIR ; /* measured batch mean */
  run;

data line8 ;
  retain k b1 b2 b3 NIR mb1 mb2 mb3 mNIR sb1 sb2 sb3 ;
  merge line1 line7a ;
  sb1 = 100.059 + 0.3667134 * (mNIR – 99.0050) ;
  sb2 = 8.04726 + 0.1359137 * (mNIR – 99.0050) ;
  sb3 = 0.99245 + 0.0061006 * (mNIR – 99.0050) ;
  run;

data line9 ; set line8 ;
  d20t = b1*(1-exp(-(20/b2)**b3));/* true batch mean */ ;
  d30t = b1*(1-exp(-(30/b2)**b3));
  d20m = mb1*(1-exp(-(20/mb2)**mb3));/* measured batch mean */ ;
  d30m = mb1*(1-exp(-(30/mb2)**mb3));
  d20s = sb1*(1-exp(-(20/sb2)**sb3));/* surrogate prediction */ ;
  d30s = sb1*(1-exp(-(30/sb2)**sb3));
  diffs_t20 = d20s – d20t ;
  diffs_t30 = d30s – d30t ;
  diffs_m20 = d20s – d20m ;
  diffs_m30 = d30s – d30m ;
  run;

data sim0 ; set sim0 line9 ;
  run;

%end ;

%mend SIM1 ;
```

REFERENCES

1. Hermans A, Abend AM, Kesisoglou F, Flanagan T, Cohen MJ, Diaz DA, Mao Y, Zhang L, Webster GK, Lin Y, Hahn DA, Coutant CA, Grady H 2017. Approaches for establishing clinically relevant dissolution specifications for immediate release solid oral dosage forms. *AAPS J 19*(6):1537–1549.
2. Nicolaides E, Symillides M, Dressman JB, Reppas C 2001. Biorelevant dissolution testing to predict the plasma profile of lipophilic drugs after oral administration. *Pharm Res 18*(3):380–388.
3. Zaborenko N, Shi Z, Corredor CC, Smith-Goettler BM, Zhang L, Hermans A, Neu CM, Alam MA, Cohen MJ, Lu X, Xiong L, Zacour BM 2019. First-principles and empirical approaches to predicting in vitro dissolution for pharmaceutical formulation and process development and for product release testing. *AAPS J 21*(3):32.
4. FDA. 2017. *Waiver of in vivo Bioavailability and Bioequivalence Studies for Immediate-Release Solid Oral Dosage Forms Based on a Biopharmaceutics Classification System*. Services USDoHaH, ed.
5. ICH. 1999. Specifications: Test procedures and acceptance criteria for new drug substances and new drug products: Chemical substances: Q6a. In: *International Conference on Harmonisation of Technical Requirements for Registration of Pharmaceuticals for Human Use*, ed.
6. USFDA. 2017. *Waiver of In Vivo Bioavailability and Bioequivalence Studies for Immediate-Release Solid Oral Dosage Forms Based on a Biopharmaceutics Classification System*. In: Services USDoHaH, ed.
7. USP. 2019. *Chemometrics*. <1039>, ed.
8. USP. 2008. *Validation of Compendial Methods*. <1225>, ed.
9. Chen Y, McCall TW, Baichwal AR, Meyer MC 1999. The application of an artificial neural network and pharmacokinetic simulations in the design of controlled-release dosage forms. *J Control Release 59*(1):33–41.

10. Darwish MK 2013. Application of quality by design principles to study the effect of coprocessed materials in the preparation of mirtazapine orodispersible tablets. *Int J Drug Delivery* 5(3):309–322.

11. El-Harras SA 2005. Optimization and characterization of meclizine hydrochloride fast dissolving tablets. *Farmatsiya (Sofia, Bulgaria)* 52(1–2):142–146.

12. Fan CX, Liang WQ 2006. Using artificial neural network (ANN) to quantitatively predict allopurinol release from HPMC sustained release tablets. *Xibei Yaoxue Zazhi* 21(5):214–219.

13. Fan CX, Liang WQ, Chen ZX, Yu ZL 2007. An artificial neural network to predict water soluble drug release from HPMC sustained release tablets. *Zhongguo Xiandai Yingyong Yaoxue* 24(1):9–12.

14. Leane MM, Cumming I, Corrigan OI 2003. The use of artificial neural networks for the selection of the most appropriate formulation and processing variables in order to predict the in vitro dissolution of sustained release minitablets. *AAPS PharmSciTech* 4(2):E26.

15. Madgulkar A, Kadam S, Pokharkar V 2008. Studies on formulation development of mucoadhesive sustained release itraconazole tablet using response surface methodology. *AAPS PharmSciTech* 9(3):998–1005.

16. Sammour OA, Hammad MA, Megrab NA, Zidan AS 2006. Formulation and optimization of mouth dissolve tablets containing rofecoxib solid dispersion. *AAPS PharmSciTech* 7(2):E55.

17. Zaghloul A, Khattab I, Nada A, Al-Saidan S 2008. Preparation, characterization and optimization of probucol self-emulsified drug delivery system to enhance solubility and dissolution. *Pharmazie* 63(9):654–660.

18. FDA. 2004. Guidance for Industry: PAA — T Framework for Innovative Pharmaceutical Development, Manufacturing, and Quality Assurance. ed., http://www.fda.gov/downloads/Drugs/GuidanceCompliance RegulatoryInformation/Guidances/ucm070305.pdf.

19. Buice RG, Pinkston P, Lodder RA 1994. Optimization of acoustic-resonance spectrometry for analysis of intact tablets and prediction of dissolution rate. *Applied Spec* 48(4):517–524.

20. Donoso M, Ghaly ES 2004. Prediction of drug dissolution from tablets using near-infrared diffuse reflectance spectroscopy as a nondestructive method. *Pharm Dev Technol* 9(3):247–263.

21. Donoso M, Ghaly ES 2005. Prediction of tablets disintegration times using near-infrared diffuse reflectance spectroscopy as a nondestructive method. *Pharm Dev Technol* 10(2):211–217.

22. Drennen JK, Lodder RA 1991. Qualitative analysis using near-infrared spectroscopy. A comparison of discriminant methods in dissolution testing. *Spectroscopy* 6(8):34–39.

23. Freitas MP, Sabadin A, Silva LM, Giannotti FM, do Couto DA, Tonhi E, Medeiros RS, Coco GL, Russo VF, Martins JA 2005. Prediction of drug dissolution profiles from tablets using NIR diffuse reflectance spectroscopy: a rapid and nondestructive method. *J Pharm Biomed Anal* 39(1–2):17–21.

24. Gendre C, Boiret M, Genty M, Chaminade P, Pean JM 2011. Real-time predictions of drug release and end point detection of a coating operation by in-line near infrared measurements. *Int J Pharm* 421(2):237–243.

25. Hernandez E, Pawar P, Keyvan G, Wang Y, Velez N, Callegari G, Cuitino A, Michniak-Kohn B, Muzzio FJ, Romanach RJ 2016. Prediction of dissolution profiles by non-destructive near infrared spectroscopy in tablets subjected to different levels of strain. *J Pharm Biomed Anal* 117:568–576.

26. Hiroyuki A, Makoto O 2012. Effects of lubricant-mixing time on prolongation of dissolution time and its prediction by measuring near infrared spectra from tablets *Drug Dev Ind Pharm* 38(4):412–419.

27. Ho L, Muller R, Gordon KC, Kleinebudde P, Pepper M, Rades T, Shen Y, Taday PF, Zeitler JA 2008. Applications of terahertz pulsed imaging to sustained-release tablet film coating quality assessment and dissolution performance. *J Control Release* 127(1):79–87.

28. Ho L, Muller R, Romer M, Gordon KC, Heinamaki J, Kleinebudde P, Pepper M, Rades T, Shen YC, Strachan CJ, Taday PF, Zeitler JA 2007. Analysis of sustained-release tablet film coats using terahertz pulsed imaging. *J Control Release* 119(3):253–261.

29. Otsuka M, Tanabe H, Osaki K, Otsuka K, Ozaki Y 2007. Chemoinformetrical evaluation of dissolution property of indomethacin tablets by near-infrared spectroscopy. *J Pharm Sci* 96(4):788–801.

30. Pawar P, Wang Y, Keyvan G, Callegari G, Cuitino A, Muzzio F 2016. Enabling real time release testing by NIR prediction of dissolution of tablets made by continuous direct compression (CDC). *Int J Pharm* 512(1):96–107.

31. Tabasi SH, Moolchandani V, Fahmy R, Hoag SW 2009. Sustained release dosage forms dissolution behavior prediction: a study of matrix tablets using NIR spectroscopy. *Int J Pharm* 382(1–2):1–6.

32. Tatavarti AS, Fahmy R, Wu H, Hussain AS, Marnane W, Bensley D, Hollenbeck G, Hoag SW 2005. Assessment of NIR spectroscopy for nondestructive analysis of physical and chemical attributes of sulfamethazine bolus dosage forms. *AAPS PharmSciTech* 6(1):E91–99.

33. Wu HQ, Lyon RC, Khan M, Voytilla RJ, Drennen JK 2015. Integration of near-infrared spectroscopy and mechanistic modeling for predicting film-coating and dissolution of modified release tablets. *Ind Eng Chem Res 54*(22):6012–6023.

34. Yamada H, Terada K, Suryanarayanan R 2010. Non-destructive determination of the coating film thickness by X-ray powder diffractometry and correlation with the dissolution behavior of film-coated tablets. *J Pharm Biomed Anal 51*(4):952–957.

35. Zannikos PN, Li WI, Drennen JK, Lodder RA 1991. Spectrophotometric prediction of the dissolution rate of carbamazepine tablets. *Pharm Res 8*(8):974–978.

36. Galata DL, Farkas A, Konyves Z, Meszaros LA, Szabo E, Csontos I, Palos A, Marosi G, Nagy ZK, Nagy B 2019. Fast, spectroscopy-based prediction of in vitro dissolution profile of extended release tablets using artificial neural networks. *Pharmaceutics 11*(8).

37. Galata DL, Konyves Z, Nagy B, Novak M, Meszaros LA, Szabo E, Farkas A, Marosi G, Nagy ZK 2021. Real-time release testing of dissolution based on surrogate models developed by machine learning algorithms using NIR spectra, compression force and particle size distribution as input data. *Int J Pharm 597*:120338.

38. Nagy B, Petra D, Galata DL, Demuth B, Borbas E, Marosi G, Nagy ZK, Farkas A 2019. Application of artificial neural networks for Process Analytical Technology-based dissolution testing. *Int J Pharm 567*:118464.

39. Q14 I. 2021. Analytical Procedure Development and Revision of Q2(R1) Analytical Validation. ed.

40. Lin LI (1989). A concordance correlation coefficient to evaluate reproducibility. *Biometrics 45*(1):255–268.

41. USFDA. 1997. *Guidance for Industry – Dissolution Testing of Immediate Release Solid Oral Dosage Forms*. In: Services USDoHaH, ed.

42. USFDA. 2012. *Q8, Q9, & Q10 Questions and Answers -- Appendix: Q&As from Training Sessions (Q8, Q9, & Q10 Points to Consider)*. In: Services USDoHaH, ed.

43. Altan S et al. 2022. Survey and recommendations on the use of P-values driving decisions in nonclinical pharmaceutical applications. Accepted for publication, Statistics in Biopharmaceutical Research.

44. Box GEP, Hunter JS, Hunter WG 2005. *Statistics for Experimenters: Design, Innovation, and Discovery*, 2nd Edition. Wiley, New York. ISBN: 978-0-471-71813-0

45. Box GEP, Meyer RD 1986. An analysis for unreplicated fractional factorials. *Technometrics 28*:11–18.

46. Box GEP, Meyer RD 1993. Finding the active factor in fractionated screening experiments. *Journal of Quality Technology 25*: 94–105.

47. Cochran WG, Cox GM 1992. *Experimental Designs*, 2nd Edition. Wiley, New York. ISBN: 978-0-471-54567-5

48. Dokoumetzidis A, Papadopoulou V, Macheras P 2006. Analysis of dissolution data using modified versions of noyes–whitney equation and the weibull function. *Pharm Res 23*:256–261.

49. Gelman A, Carlin JB, Stern HS, Dunson DB, Vehtari A, Rubin DB 2013. *Bayesian Data Analysis*, 3rd Edition. Chapman and Hall/CRC, New York. https://doi.org/10.1201/b16018

50. Graybill FA (1976). *Theory and Application of the Linear Model*. Wadsworth Publishing Company, Belmont, CA, 94002

51. John JA, Quenoille MH 1977. *Experiments: Design and Analysis*. 2nd Edition. Macmillan Publishing Co. Inc., New York

52. Jones B, Nachtsheim CJ 2011. A class of three-level designs for definitive screening in the presence of second-order effects. *J Qual Technol 43*(1):https://doi.org/10.1080/00224065.2011.11917841

53. Kadane JB, Lazar NA 2004. Methods and criteria for model selection. *J Am Stat Assoc 99*(465). https://doi.org/10.1198/016214504000000269

54. Lenth RV 1989. Quick and easy analysis of unreplicated factorials. *Technometrics 31*: 469–473.

55. Portet S 2019. A primer on model selection using the Akaike Information Criterion. *Infect Dis Model 2020*(5):111–128.

56. Lin LI 1989. A concordance correlation coefficient to evaluate reproducibility. *Biometrics 45*:255–268.

57. Lin L 2000. A note on the concordance correlation coefficient. *Biometrics 56*:324–325.

58. The output/code/data analysis for this chapter was generated using SAS/STAT® 15.1, SAS/IML® 15.1 and SAS® software, Version 9.4 (M6) of the SAS System for Windows 10, SAS Institute Inc., Cary, NC.

Part II

Design and Control

Continuous Manufacturing of Large Molecule Drug Substances and Products

8

Continuous Manufacturing of Biologics Drug Products: Challenges of Implementing Innovation in cGMP

Erinc Sahin
Global Product Development & Supply, Bristol Myers Squibb, New Brunswick, NJ, USA

James Angelo, Jay West and Xuankuo Xu
Global Product Development & Supply, Bristol Myers Squibb, Devens, MA, USA

CONTENTS

8.1 Preface

Adoption of continuous manufacturing (CM) has strong motivators such as "shorter processing times, smaller equipment footprint, enhanced development approaches such as use of quality by design (QbD) principles, process analytical technologies (PAT) and models, real time quality monitoring, flexible scale-up/scale-out/scale-down in response to changes in supply/demand" as well as "reduced drug product (DP) quality issues, lower manufacturing costs, and improved availability of quality medicines to patients"[1]. Despite these strong value propositions (that are presented as improvements over batch processes), adoption of CM has been slow in the biopharmaceutical industry.

DOI: 10.1201/9781003149835-10

This chapter will discuss some of the advances in CM of biologics (therapeutic proteins) that moved the needle, especially for some of the drug substance (DS) manufacturing processes (i.e. process intensification); however, the industry could not necessarily achieve the holy grail of *end-to-end, DS-to-DP integrated manufacturing with embedded PAT and automated feedback/feedforward controls, concluded with real-time release.* Authors will attempt to identify the contributors of the "activation energy" that prevents a faster adoption; by doing so, hopefully helping the industry recognize and address them more directly and efficiently. As a result, the authors owe the reader the following disclaimer: the tone of this chapter may be more philosophical than technical in its nature. We encourage the reader to refer to the well-written, detailed, and widely applicable CM guidance documents [1, 2] for a deep dive into technical content.

8.2 Introduction

Manufacturing of biologics DPs has a relatively short history (since recombinant insulin in 1982), in comparison to the long legacy of oral solid dosage form manufacturing. As a result, the early years of biologics DP manufacturing had a regulatory philosophy – both by developers/manufacturers of these products and the regulatory bodies – which was initially under the influence of "fear of the unknown". The mantra "in biologics, process is the product" (i.e. any change in the process can change the product) dominated the first two to three decades of regulatory interactions. Situation-specific data (e.g. comparison of complete analytical panels from the exact same process run at two different sites) were expected and generated. However, there was a growing appetite for leveraging a deeper understanding of molecular liabilities as well as targeted and intentional study of the impact of formulation and process changes on quality attributes, as evidenced by encouragements toward filing with quality by design (QbD) principles [3]. In these novice times, guided by the discomfort that *any* quality attribute may turn out to be a critical quality attribute (CQA), and therefore *any* process parameter (PP) may be a critical process parameter (CPP), the industry (rightfully at the time) over-flagged the risks. Some of these early "risks" were found to be remote, or low impact as the accumulated knowledge in the field grew bigger and stronger: the regulatory mantra evolved from the mystical and fearful "process is the product" to deterministic and pragmatic "identify your liabilities and use risk-balanced approach". Unfortunately, by the time the mantra had changed, biopharmaceutical companies had built their platform processes, established their raw material supply chains and quality controls, wrote their SOPs, achieved duly valued familiarity with these SOPs in their cGMP facilities, and enjoyed regulatory, launch, and commercial success through these elements. Once the adaptation of traditional (e.g. small molecule oral solid dosage forms) drug-making paradigms to biologics manufacturing brought success, making changes – especially within cGMP operations – became non-trivial. Proposed changes – including but not limited to CM – were measured with traditional short-sighted valuation metrics such as "return on investment (ROI)" that assigned financial value to individual/ step changes but failed to appropriately value "the cost of doing nothing" in competitive, technology-driven fields, as well as how a change would enable the next ones, thereby triggering "a chain reaction of innovation" (e.g. incorporation of real-time analytics [RTA] is an enabler of multiple additional advances such as continuous quality monitoring; automated feedback/feedforward process control; real-time release testing [RTRT], etc.). Additionally, implementation of new technologies/approaches (rightfully) propagate from development (non-GMP) to clinical manufacturing (small-scale GMP) to commercial manufacturing (large-scale GMP), the latter using the former as a trial run in this chain of collaborators. The use of ROI as a valuation metric poses a significant problem at the development-to-clinical manufacturing interface since it is harder to make a case for a process change when the financial impact is minimal (sometimes even negative) at these small scales. As a result, the development-to-clinical manufacturing interface is frequently a "valley of death" for innovative manufacturing technologies [4].

It should be noted that in the early days described above, manufacturing via conservative/familiar approaches resulted in a heavy bias toward building batch processes that used fixed volume vessels and discrete batches of DPs. After all, putting all ingredients in a single vessel and mixing/homogenizing while there is no material flow in or out of the vessel was the oldest and most familiar way to manufacture any mixture, giving an unmatched sense of control. In this conservative environment, narrow ranges of

PPSs and their impacts on quality attributes were studied, validated, and implemented for cGMP manufacturing. Any changes to these target parameters were not acceptable; therefore, the use of RTA (PAT) for catching such changes within a cGMP process and re-centering the process was out of scope (i.e. if re-centering was needed, lack of process control would be assumed).

Additionally, the familiarity with batch process offered an easily conceivable way to document, process, and sequester DP unit doses. This one-to-one correspondence between "mixing vessel used in manufacturing" and "unit doses that came out of that vessel" dominated the lot definition, and is frequently used as an argument against continuous manufacturing (CM) even though regulatory guidance documents [1, 2] offered clear lot/batch definitions applicable to CM.

8.3 CM in Manufacturing of Biologics Drug Substance

Even though the industry had some success in the implementation of elements of CM in biologics DS manufacturing, these were mostly incremental cases of "process intensification" rather than complete CM implementation. One such example of process intensification is to integrate elements of CM into individual unit operations to increase their efficiency and specific productivity, thus providing a stepping stone to full-scale integration. Hybrid approaches to the CM process that utilize a mixture of batch and continuous unit operation may alleviate and mitigate this concern [5]. As the inherent structure of the process remains unchanged, many producers of biologics decide on this approach as a first pass to CM, as the barrier for entry is much lower.

For biologics DS, the implementation of CM may be categorized into either upstream (i.e. cell culture) or downstream (i.e. purification) operations. Often, the concept of CM in DS manufacturing is centered around perfusion applications [6, 7] that blend the transfer of product between the upstream and downstream areas by affording near continuous harvest and processing of cell culture supernatant. While perfusion operations for upstream cell culture have been explored extensively, lending more to a true CM approach, alternating tangential flow filtration (ATF) perfusion in the n-1 bioreactor (i.e. the penultimate bioreactor) has also been shown to maximize cellular productivity while minimizing cell culture duration [8, 9] This would mean that batch definition would no longer be an issue, as a continuous output from the production bioreactor is not a factor and it intensifies the overall production capability using elements of CM. In certain instances, however, perfusion of the production bioreactor would be preferable due to the ability of the product in intermediate process pools [10].

As biologics titers continue to increase [11] there is an increased need to streamline drug substance (DS) purification operations to maintain processing cadences and reduce bottlenecks. In addition, there has also been a drive to reduce costs of goods in both raw materials (chromatography resins, membrane filters, etc.) and buffer/solvent consumption for downstream processing steps to improve manufacturing efficiency and productivity.

Technologies that have been evolving in the downstream purification space include single-pass tangential flow filtration for product concentration and diafiltration [12, 13], multicolumn capture chromatography [14–16], continuous viral inactivation [17–20] and viral filtration [21], and pool-less or straight-though processing [22]. While all these technologies act to provide process compression through the optimization of parameters such as loading or throughput, there remains the need for PAT tools to be developed in tandem to allow for full integration from one unit operation to the next to take effect. A more sophisticated process control strategy is needed to adjust operational parameters and keep product quality constant during long-term CM operations [23]. A detailed compilation of biologics unit operations, associated CM/intensification approaches, and CM-enabling technologies are reviewed by Chopda et al.

Many outfits have employed a hybrid approach to continuous downstream processing to prepare for this eventuality of more sophisticated systems integration. By optimizing and reducing process bottlenecks within individual operational steps, the specific productivities of these operations may be matched with each other to provide a more efficient transition of product from step to step. However, the bottlenecks outside of the operational parameter space (e.g. system setup and takedown, cleaning/sanitization-in-place, etc.) will always remain within this strategy, as true process compression cannot be achieved without both technological intensifications as well as activity (i.e. labor) scheduling intensifications.

The barriers for CM in the DS space are synonymous with what had been described previously: not enough ROI for incremental changes and benefits in terms of reduction of the COGs or speed to complete a batch. While individual unit operations may be intensified (e.g. ATF perfusion in the n-1 bioreactor, multicolumn capture, and polishing chromatography), the process – inclusive of the activity scheduling and day-to-day operations – must be viewed holistically, and independent of the parameter space defined by the process description/in-process controls, in order to make judgments on the strengths of adopting a CM approach. Heuristics (ease of operation, manufacturability, intensity of operational activities, etc.) must be considered as well, which cannot be captured or boiled down to singular metrics that preclude the adoption and implementation of new technologies into cGMP spaces.

8.4 CM in Manufacturing of Biologics Drug Product

The primary driver of quality considerations is patient safety. Therefore, as sequential cGMP manufacturing unit operations get closer to the final DP that the patient will receive, any changes to time-tested/familiar manufacturing processes tend to face a higher level of resistance and scrutiny by manufacturing and quality organizations. This well-meaning conservatism presents greater activation energy for DP (in comparison to DS) against embracing innovation, for this discussion – CM implementation.

Some DP manufacturing processes have innate advantages that favor CM. For example, manufacturing self-assembling modalities (e.g. lipid nanoparticles, liposomes [24, 25], and protein-coated microparticles [26]) in batch mode may result in a process that has different ratios of free (available to react/interact) ingredients in the mixing tank at the beginning vs. the end of the process, potentially having an impact on the distributions of certain attributes of the self-assembled particles. In contrast, a continuous process may ensure constant ratios of self-assembling components throughout the process. As a result, depending on the specific nature of the self-assembly in question, CM may enable tighter distributions of quality attributes, which may be desirable or even necessary depending on the safety and efficacy profiles of the DP.

It should be noted that in cases where CM has the potential for a positive impact on quality attributes, strong conservatism/resistance is not expected. Development (improvement bias) and manufacturing (consistency bias) organizations will unite around the same common goal: doing what's best for the patient.

There are cultural enablers of bringing innovation to DP manufacturing: development and manufacturing organizations should accept their biases (improvement and consistency, respectively) and acknowledge that both biases are coming from the same place: making safer, efficacious, and accessible DPs… *for the patients.*

8.5 Enablers and Challenges of CM (Innovation) Implementation in Biologics Drug Products

For the sake of fidelity to the context of this book, the following discussions are written from the perspective of CM. However, many are equally applicable to any form of innovative changes offered to cGMP operations.

8.5.1 Project Timeline vs. Innovation Timeline

In the fields of science and engineering, most innovation is inspired by problems and risks: efforts to mitigate risks or solve problems give birth to new technologies and approaches. However, solving a problem through developing a new technology – or even scouting, internalizing, and implementing an existing technology – typically does not fit the timeline of the portfolio project (asset in clinical development) that had the problem. As a result, the problem is usually addressed by a combination of alternate (but not necessarily ideal) approaches with precedent; thereby, removing the pressing and immediate need for the new technology. This "need/obsolescence cycle" is detrimental to the momentum of innovative technology development and the team's ability to deliver the long-term goal. *Therefore, even though the initial motivation for innovation is typically a project need, the innovation project (e.g. development of CM process and its implementation in cGMP) should be seen as a future portfolio enabler and managed in a way that is decoupled from the needs of any one portfolio project.*

If CM development efforts yield successful results on a portfolio project that is manufactured via batch mode, the chemistry-manufacturing-controls (CMC) team will be facing a decision on when to pivot the existing (batch) process to CM. Typically, by the time CMC team is ready to discuss a process switch through governances, clinical studies have precious data available using DP manufactured by batch processes. The cost and uncertainties surrounding pre-clinical and clinical bridging activities present steep activation energy. At this point, most CMC teams are influenced into switching the process into CM as part of life cycle management (LCM).

Executing a batch-to-CM switch in LCM is easier said than done. After the launch of the product, CM is not only "swimming against the current of" comparability and bridging studies, but a batch-to-CM switch would also trigger the preparation of a very stringent comparability package, as well as significant updates and amendments on a successful past filing. ICH-Q12 [27] provides guidance on how to manage post-approval CMC changes efficiently; however, typically there is limited appetite (from the company) for making substantial changes on a successfully filed product unless there is a strong incentive. Availability of more biosimilars on the market may be one such incentive, which is a recently increasing pressure as compared to generic small molecule APIs, and will drive the prices far lower in the coming decades, forcing innovator companies to find more cost-efficient ways to develop and manufacture biologics.

Extension of exclusivity for the product via process patent comes to mind as an incentive for the batch-to-CM switch. However, due to sensitivities around "evergreening" [28], improvement (not matching) of existing quality attributes is necessary to argue extended protection through a process patent: a batch-to-CM switch purely for business drivers (e.g. smaller footprint, lower cost, faster process, etc.) may not be enough to justify the extension of intellectual property protection for a DP. However, if CM offers an advantage to the patient through improved quality attributes (e.g. tighter distribution, lower impurity) in addition to the business drivers, a process patent has a higher chance of securing an extension to the existing exclusivity.

8.5.2 Dedication to Developing and Implementing CM

8.5.2.1 Organizational Factors

In most pharmaceutical development organizations, scientists and engineers spend most of their time advancing portfolio projects, as the successful launch of these assets is directly tied to the future sustainability of the company. This model results in only part-time attention to innovation projects that are longer-term and indirect enablers of business sustainability. One potential strategy to achieve faster development and adoption of CM (and other innovative approaches) may be tied to the organization's commitment to creating well-resourced groups that are focused on longer-term modernization, independent of shorter-term portfolio support [29]. A risk should be noted here: these dedicated and focused groups need to be hierarchically and operationally well-integrated into both development and manufacturing organizations, and the generation of unintentional silos should be actively avoided.

Such dedicated development teams (non-GMP) tasked with the modernization of manufacturing will benefit from mirroring the capabilities and equipment of clinical supply manufacturing (cGMP) facilities. By doing so, gradual modernization of the manufacturing process (i.e. stepwise implementation of RTA, building feedback controls, automation, and RTRT) can be studied while designing disruption-minimized implementation plans (shorter times needed for line closures and re-validations) in cGMP environment.

8.5.2.2 Cultural Factors

Implementation of changes in the cGMP environment (i.e. manufacturing) through the knowledge generated in non-GMP space (i.e. development) is – rightfully, and by design – a high resistance task. The organizational biases (without negative connotation) described before – improvement bias and consistency bias – collectively ensure modernized approaches without compromising quality. The organizations that realize the following about these biases will have a paramount cultural and operational advantage: improvement and consistency biases (i) exist by design, (ii) are meant to complement each other, and (iii) are not opposing forces (they both point to the benefit of the patients). Embracing the intentional presence of these biases will improve the quality of the partnership and mitigate (avoidable) resistance to the implementation of new approaches such as CM and its prerequisites (e.g. RTA, use of models).

Especially in cases the partnership philosophy described above is not fully embraced, operationalizing CM and its prerequisites will be scrutinized using traditional metrics of worthiness. The most commonly misused example of such metrics is ROI or "break even" analysis, which has the potential to be weaponized in advocating for inaction. Classical ROI analysis is inappropriate for evaluating innovation and modernization (e.g. CM and its prerequisites) and alternative valuation analysis approaches have to be used [30, 31]. Moving away from classical ROI analysis will result in a more accurate valuation of innovative and disruptive efforts as well as acceptance of short-term-neutral (or short-term-negative) incremental changes that are enablers of multiple long-term-positive modernizations that are stepwise improvements upon previously implemented innovation. For example, the implementation of a strong RTA presence in manufacturing lines would enable automation of workflows through feedback/feedforward controls that leverage data from existing RTA capabilities. Therefore, earlier modernization efforts on manufacturing operations will decrease the "activation energy" and time needed to implement connected future modernizations. This realization, combined with alternate valuation approaches (maybe a variant of ROI analysis that takes "the cost of doing nothing" as the correct baseline reference) has the potential to change the industry's stance toward the implementation of innovation in cGMP operations (Figure 8.1).

One example of such incremental changes is the tests in the release panel of biologics DPs: it is easy (but wrong) to advocate against the investments/costs of implementing RTA for real-time release (RTR), given that some of the tests (i.e. sterility) currently require longer durations; therefore, RTR is not achievable as long as a rate-limiting test is present in the release panel. However, a more appropriate approach is to resolutely build RTRT capabilities to achieve partial RTR, and be "only one test away from real-time release" [32]. The current industry goal is not "true" same-day RTR, but a faster and consistent release of the DP. At present, the release of DS or DP may require over a month but any approach that would shorten release timelines will be a welcome improvement, allowing faster supply to patients, and likely facilitating better inventory management.

Incorporation of RTA is a prerequisite of RTR, and it will require embracing changes in traditional and deeply established ways of working. For example, something as fundamental as establishing system suitability and use of reference standards will need alternative strategies when the analytical method is modified for in-line RTA (e.g. the feasibility of using reference standards in an analytical instrument that is plumbed into a closed-system aseptic operation, or use of optical filters, etc.). Additionally, CM implementation requires a change in the traditional mindset of "generation of circumstance-specific data" toward "the use of predictive models that receive input from RTA and describe a wide but realistic design space" and will require appropriate validation and documentation of high-impact models used in manufacturing [33].

In addition to the inadequacy of ROI for valuation of innovation (e.g. CM), another common mistake is the failure to include the process heuristics of manufacturability (i.e. ease of manufacturing): intensity of on-the-floor activities is poorly considered to counterbalance the economic advantages/disadvantages of CM. In a culture where these heuristics are not fully appreciated and formed into hard metrics, their importance is undercounted when comparing more advanced ways of processing vs. the status quo.

Modern drug development paradigm is shifting away from "catering to unmet patient need" more toward "product differentiation via satisfying needs *and wants* of the patient". With that substantial shift in target product profiles, all traditional approaches within the pharmaceutical industry need to be reconsidered. Other "consumer's choice" sectors such as food, automotive, electronics, and software industries had to be fast adopters of manufacturing modernization since product characteristics are heavily

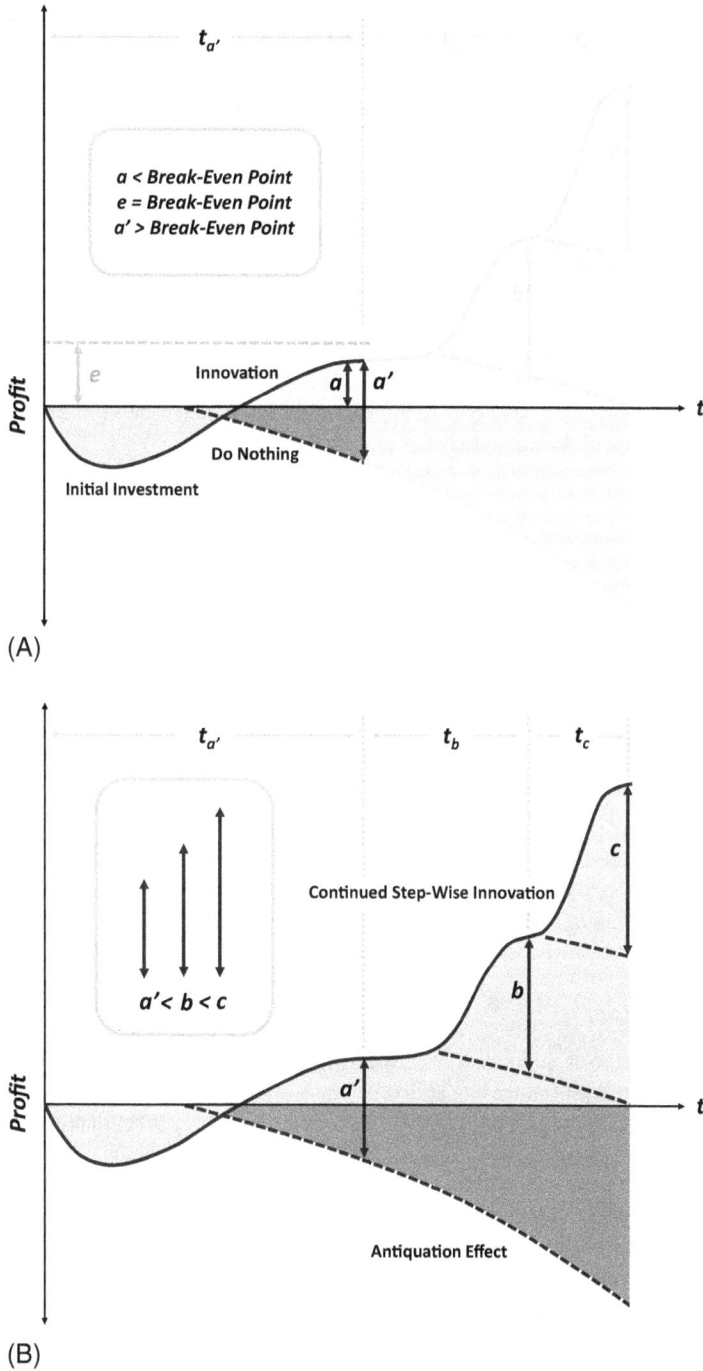

FIGURE 8.1 (A) When the cost of doing nothing is not considered, the value added by innovation (*a*), seems to be less than the break-even value (*e*), resulting in an apparent negative ROI, based on classical ROI analysis. If the correct frame of reference – "Do Nothing" curve – is used, the value added by innovation (*a'*) is greater than the break-even point (*e*), making it a worthy investment. (B) In many cases, earlier steps of modernization are enablers of subsequent steps, leading to shorter development times and steeper differences in realized value once the initial activation energy is overcome. If subsequent innovation is not pursued, the Antiquation Effect is still in play, albeit offset by the value generated by prior innovation.

influenced/designed by ever-evolving user preferences ("wants" rather than "needs"), and the lack of innovation quickly and harshly penalizes complacent company while elevating competition. As an extension, cross-pollination of pharmaceutical industry management with executives from these "innovate-or-die" industries may facilitate the transition of traditional pharmaceutical (manufacturing) practices into modern approaches such as heavier use of RTA, automation, and CM.

Another cultural element is buried within the corporate strategic priorities which are drawn by the vision of the leaders of involved organizations (process development, manufacturing, IT/automation, business operations, finance, etc.). Developing a CM process or implementing a batch-to-CM switch requires careful operational and financial considerations which would be approved by cross-functional alignment across (the leaders of) multiple departments. Unfortunately, innovation efforts impactful enough to require such high-ranking endorsement may be at the mercy of leaders with sustained motivation in advocating for substantial cGMP changes and executing toward the long-term future of the industry. For many leaders, staying the course and not deviating from convention may be in their best interest, especially for those who have had a long career in the industry, and this is not in support of the multidecade strategies that CM require to become the norm.

8.5.2.3 Geographical Factors

The biopharmaceutical industry is at the beginning of its CM journey. There are success stories, but they are mostly a subset of DS manufacturing unit operations, and can be categorized as process intensification rather than end-to-end integrated CM. We are far from the "holy grail": end-to-end, DS-to-DP, "from host cell to product in device" version of CM. Even if the industry overcomes all technical challenges of CM, we should acknowledge that current biopharmaceutical companies are not built with an end-to-end CM vision. In most cases, DS and DP operations are in different campuses, often in different states. Companies that are truly committed to achieving a supply model that feeds from on-demand end-to-end CM may need to consolidate their DS and DP operations within the same campus.

Similarly, the current popular use of a combination of internal and external (contract) manufacturing capabilities for DS and DP manufacturing creates not only an inter-facility, but also an inter-company separation. For a seamless end-to-end CM vision to realize, the advantages of end-to-end CM will need to grossly surpass the advantages of (semi-)externalized manufacturing model.

8.5.2.4 Financial Factors

Biopharmaceutical manufacturing facilities are operating with equipment, isolation, and control systems, and their corresponding infrastructure that collectively cost hundreds of millions of dollars. Larger scale commercial operations (as opposed to typically smaller scale clinical manufacturing) further increase the cost of the equipment in the facility. As a result, "economics of change" at the development-to-clinical manufacturing interface is not readily translatable to commercial manufacturing, which is one of the strongest reasons for making changes in clinical manufacturing before moving onto commercial facilities. Significant facility modifications (e.g. equipment purchasing and validations, etc.) and major interruptions to existing manufacturing schedules are required for a commercial facility to be ready for the implementation of innovative manufacturing technologies.

Additionally, the parts and servicing of existing manufacturing equipment are supported by vendors that have decades of experience in batch-mode manufacturing equipment. As a result, switching site capabilities from batch processes to CM has a steep financial burden as well as notable long-term maintenance and support risks. Once again, companies are faced with a costly and risky transition to CM, which would only realize if the promised changes in product quality, supply chain management, long-term operational costs, and other metrics have a significant advantage over current ways of working. That said, it should be restated that these risk-reward considerations should take into account that there is a heavy cost to doing nothing in innovative sectors [30].

8.5.3 Scale Optimization and Agility

CM has advantages over batch processes in scale-up and scale-out from clinical into commercial operations. The presence of scale-dependent physical phenomena (e.g. mixing, interfacial stresses) present more challenging cases for batch processes, while CM scale-up may simply mean demonstrating consistent product quality over a longer duration of use of CM equipment without fouling of channels and surfaces [1]. This simplicity is applicable to individual unit operations; however, the scale of material flow between consecutive unit operations requires more careful considerations in the case of CM.

8.5.3.1 Scale Compatibility between Unit Operations

A simplified representation of end-to-end biologics manufacturing can be described with the following sequence of unit operations: Thaw of frozen culture → expansion → growth/production → harvest → combination of viral inactivation and chromatographic separations (affinity, ion exchange, hydrophilic interaction, and mixed mode) and filtrations → buffer exchange and concentration via ultrafiltration/ diafiltration (UF/DF) → dilution/formulation/compounding → sterile filtration → fill → lyophilization (when applicable) → device assembly (when applicable) → secondary packaging → shipping/storage.

Material handoffs between some unit operations listed above are well-suited for CM execution (e.g. filtration → fill); however, others have material loading limitations for optimal outcomes (e.g. chromatographic separation) while others require large volume reductions between consecutive unit operations (e.g. capture, in-line concentration, etc.), or typically done via cyclic exposure of recirculated bulk (batch) within the same equipment (e.g. batch mode UF/DF), therefore they do not present the ideal circumstances for an end-to-end CM process. These misalignments between the scales of consecutive unit operations resulted in fragmented successes (i.e. process intensification) as opposed to achieving an end-to-end CM process. Optimization and adjustment of scales of consecutive unit operations as well as switching to CM-enabling technologies (e.g. single-pass UF/DF) are required to graduate from intensified processes to true CM operations.

The aforementioned geographic separations at the interface of DS and DP operations (e.g. UF/DF → dilution/ formulation/compounding) are additional derailers of the industry's ability to achieve end-to-end CM of biologics products. Collectively, the industry's inability to build demand-optimized true CM processes creates an expensive and risky need to manage inventory and expiry, as well as store and ship (temperature-controlled) large quantities of sensitive material.

8.5.3.2 Real-time Response to Patient Demand

A strong enabler of on-demand (or inventory-minimized) end-to-end CM would be the ability to accurately gauge demand and provide quick supply. The current evolution of industry toward personalized medicine modalities (e.g. CAR-T therapies) is a notable force toward building on-demand supply capabilities. These capabilities require electronic systems and predictive models that reliably communicate or project the patient demand, thereby informing fast-responding manufacturing schedules at the correct scales. In effect, the scale optimization described before would originate from the patient demand if we have integrated electronic systems that connect the patient or clinicians to manufacturing operations.

COVID-triggered global supply chain issues in 2020–2021 reminded the world about the fragile connectivity of our supply network. From toilet paper to computer chips, hard-to-predict interconnectivities created bottlenecks that are only obvious in hindsight. Given the rude awakening on the fragility of our supply chains, as well as the importance of quality and consistency in raw materials as a prerequisite of CM, the industry is expected to be hesitant and pessimistic about a switch to on-demand manufacturing (especially in cases where it is optional). Keeping DP inventory – albeit having its own risks – is an established risk mitigation strategy against unpredictable and rather stochastic disruptions in the raw material supply chain. Therefore, it is safe to assume "inventory" mode of supply will not easily surrender its place to on-demand supply, and CM efforts may be negatively impacted by their association with the on-demand supply model.

Considering the high cost of personalized medicine and on-demand CM, the reliability of demand information/projections is extremely important for sustainability of the commercial product, unless an inventory-based (backup) supply model is available. A reliable global information network that collects and projects patient demand is an enabler (if not a prerequisite) of on-demand supply that can be fed by CM. Additionally, the time between demand trigger and supply availability will define the success of this new paradigm (CM and on-demand supply).

8.5.4 Systems Integration: Software and Hardware

The complexity in modern manufacturing requires increased use of PAT, automation, and feedback/feed-forward controls within and between unit operations. CM necessitates seamless integration of sequential unit operations. Additionally, the importance of raw material (input material) quality and consistency and studying the impact of input material quality attributes on the process and final product are clear regulatory expectations [1, 2]. Collectively, these requirements point to a need for heavy systems integration, both at hardware and software levels, sometimes between companies. Commitment (sometimes across companies) to develop these manufacturing and integration technologies and to implement them in cGMP environments present steep financial implications, and therefore require exceptional motivation toward innovation and modernization.

8.5.4.1 Integration Between Raw Material Vendor and DP Manufacturer

Considering the importance of raw material quality and consistency in CM, healthy communication and a strong partnership between raw material suppliers and DP manufacturers are necessary. The future of CM will greatly benefit from inter-company-integrated electronic environments that offer easy access to key information about raw materials such as batch records, analytical data, investigation/deviation reports, and change management documents. Similarly, an ideal business partnership (within the context of CM regulatory expectations) would extend to currently unavailable services such as: (i) maintaining material libraries for different lot numbers of raw materials (facilitation of validation efforts by easy access to multiple lots, especially useful in case of low demand/supply raw materials), (ii) building impurity libraries (ability to spike typical raw material impurities to achieve worst-case levels within a design space), and (iii) providing stronger development packages in support of a regulatory filing for the product that would use their raw material as an ingredient. It should be noted that the authors are encouraged to see their recent requests for such partnerships/services are well-received and resulting in commitments from some raw material vendors.

8.5.4.2 Integration between Equipment that Serve Sequential Unit Operations

As previously described, biopharmaceutical manufacturing involves more than a dozen sequential unit operations. Each of these unit operations requires specialized equipment that is designed and serviced by its vendor. Unfortunately (and surprisingly), it is relatively uncommon for the same vendor to cater to the needs of more than one unit operation. As a result, the hardware and software platforms built for these equipment are not *designed* to be compatible and parts of a continuum; instead, custom integrations have to be designed and built (e.g. communication between instrument A and B being established by exporting ASCII format data from A and importing into B). These "forced integrations" are particularly suboptimal in the cGMP environment since the custom hardware and software will need to be qualified, validated, networked, owned (as the responsibility of a support team), maintained, and updated (aligned with operating system upgrades) according to cGMP requirements including but not limited to 21 CFR Part 11, outside of the vendor-performed servicing of the custom-integrated manufacturing equipment. Manufacturing groups prefer to avoid such custom integration hardware/software since the associated workload described above will likely create pockets of expertise that will be person-dependent (in contrast to the availability of a larger number of service technicians from an instrument vendor), which is a threat to the non-negotiable sustainability of a manufacturing operation. Considering the suboptimality of "forced integrations", there is a need for (i) companies that would handle the integration projects in cGMP environments and their continued servicing and (ii) existing instrument vendors to collaborate or consolidate toward satisfying the instrument integration needs of consecutive unit operations.

The lack of inherent/by-design integration capabilities (rather than "hooks" that can be used to enable a "forced integration") stems from the strength of the batch process tradition. The current expert pool in most instrument vendors does not yet subscribe to the vision of CM: their instrument (hardware and software) designs cater to each unit operation as a separate entity with clean borders and limited scope. However, there are also emerging technologies that are aligned with a CM-enabled future: in-/online concentration and volumetric flow measurements enabling real-time yield and mass balance calculations, data analytics for advanced control of CQAs, bioprocessing modeling and simulations, single-pass UF/DF, in-line conditioning and buffer formulation, continuous lyophilization technology, continuous spray freeze-drying of proteins, filling lines fitted with automated visual inspection, container closure integrity testing with accept/reject/sequester routing options, rapid bioburden and sterility testing, and similar CM-enabling technologies knock on the doors of a modernized future for biologics DP manufacturing…if we choose to let them in.

ACKNOWLEDGEMENTS

Authors thank Gary McGeorge and Dilbir Bindra for discussions on "process changes and exclusivity extension through secondary patents"; George Currier, Mark Howansky, Alpa Bhattacharyya, and Robert Forest for discussions on "valuation approaches for implementation of innovation"; and George Currier for creating the figure that visually highlights the shortcomings of classical ROI approach in evaluating innovation efforts such as CM.

REFERENCES

1. (CDER) FaDA-CfDEaR: *Quality Considerations for Continuous Manufacturing – Guidance for Industry.* Edited by FDA.
2. (ICH) ICfH: Q13 – Continuous Manufacturing of Drug Substances and Drug Products. In *Q13.* Edited by ICH.
3. Yu LX, Amidon G, Khan MA, Hoag SW, Polli J, Raju GK, Woodcock J: Understanding pharmaceutical quality by design. *The AAPS Journal* 2014, **16**:771–783.
4. National Academies of Sciences Engineering, Medicine, Division on Earth, Life S, Board on Chemical S, Technology: Book Section: Continuous Manufacturing for the Modernization of Pharmaceutical Production: Proceedings of a Workshop. In *Continuous Manufacturing for the Modernization of Pharmaceutical Production: Proceedings of a Workshop.* Edited by: National Academies Press (US), Copyright 2019 by the National Academy of Sciences. All rights reserved.; 2019.
5. Konstantinov KB, Cooney CL: White paper on continuous bioprocessing May 20-21 2014 continuous manufacturing symposium. *Journal of Pharmaceutical Sciences* 2015, **104**:813–820.
6. Voisard D, Meuwly F, Ruffieux PA, Baer G, Kadouri A: Potential of cell retention techniques for large-scale high-density perfusion culture of suspended mammalian cells. *Biotechnology and Bioengineering* 2003, **82**:751–765.
7. Chotteau V, Zhang Y, Clincke M-F: Very High Cell Density in Perfusion of CHO Cells by ATF, TFF, Wave Bioreactor, and/or CellTank Technologies – Impact of Cell Density and Applications. In *Continuous Processing in Pharmaceutical Manufacturing.* Edited by; 2014:339–356.
8. Woodgate JM: Chapter 37 – Perfusion N-1 Culture—Opportunities for Process Intensification. In *Biopharmaceutical Processing.* Edited by Jagschies G, Lindskog E, Łącki K, Galliher P: Elsevier; 2018:755–768.
9. Xu J, Rehmann MS, Xu M, Zheng S, Hill C, He Q, Borys MC, Li ZJ: Development of an intensified fed-batch production platform with doubled titers using N-1 perfusion seed for cell culture manufacturing. *Bioresources and Bioprocessing* 2020, **7**:17.
10. Warikoo V, Godawat R, Brower K, Jain S, Cummings D, Simons E, Johnson T, Walther J, Yu M, Wright B, et al.: Integrated continuous production of recombinant therapeutic proteins. *Biotechnology and Bioengineering* 2012, **109**:3018–3029.

11. Rader RAL, Eric S: 30 years of upstream productivity improvements. *Bioprocess International* 2015, **13**:10–14.

12. Arunkumar A, Singh N, Peck M, Borys MC, Li ZJ: Investigation of single-pass tangential flow filtration (SPTFF) as an inline concentration step for cell culture harvest. *Journal of Membrane Science* 2017, **524**:20–32.

13. Rucker-Pezzini J, Arnold L, Hill-Byrne K, Sharp T, Avazhanskiy M, Forespring C: Single pass diafiltration integrated into a fully continuous mAb purification process. *Biotechnology and Bioengineering* 2018, **115**:1949–1957.

14. Godawat R, Brower K, Jain S, Konstantinov K, Riske F, Warikoo V: Periodic counter-current chromatography – Design and operational considerations for integrated and continuous purification of proteins. *Biotechnology Journal* 2012, **7**:1496–1508.

15. Angarita M, Müller-Späth T, Baur D, Lievrouw R, Lissens G, Morbidelli M: Twin-column CaptureSMB: A novel cyclic process for protein A affinity chromatography. *Journal of Chromatography A* 2015, **1389**:85–95.

16. Angelo Jea: Scale-up of twin-column periodic counter-current chromatography for MAb purification. *Bioprocess International* 2018, **16**:28–37.

17. Klutz S, Lobedann M, Bramsiepe C, Schembecker G: Continuous viral inactivation at low pH value in antibody manufacturing. *Chemical Engineering and Processing: Process Intensification* 2016, **102**:88–101.

18. Parker SA, Amarikwa L, Vehar K, Orozco R, Godfrey S, Coffman J, Shamlou P, Bardliving CL: Design of a novel continuous flow reactor for low pH viral inactivation. *Biotechnology and Bioengineering* 2018, **115**:606–616.

19. Gillespie C, Holstein M, Mullin L, Cotoni K, Tuccelli R, Caulmare J, Greenhalgh P: Continuous in-line virus inactivation for next generation bioprocessing. *Biotechnology Journal* 2019, **14**:1700718.

20. Martins DL, Sencar J, Hammerschmidt N, Tille B, Kinderman J, Kreil TR, Jungbauer A: Continuous solvent/detergent virus inactivation using a packed-bed reactor. *Biotechnology Journal* 2019, **14**:1800646.

21. David L, Niklas J, Budde B, Lobedann M, Schembecker G: Continuous viral filtration for the production of monoclonal antibodies. *Chemical Engineering Research and Design* 2019, **152**:336–347.

22. Zhang J, Conley L, Pieracci J, Ghose S: Pool-less processing to streamline downstream purification of monoclonal antibodies. *Engineering in Life Sciences* 2017, **17**:117–124.

23. Helgers H, Schmidt A, Lohmann LJ, Vetter FL, Juckers A, Jensch C, Mouellef M, Zobel-Roos S, Strube J: Towards autonomous operation by advanced process control—Process analytical technology for continuous biologics antibody manufacturing. *Processes* 2021, **9**:172. https://doi.org/10.1002/jctb.6765

24. Pace JR, Jog R, Burgess DJ, Hadden MK: Formulation and evaluation of itraconazole liposomes for Hedgehog pathway inhibition. *Journal of Liposome Research* 2020, **30**:305–311.

25. Worsham RD, Thomas V, Farid SS: Potential of continuous manufacturing for liposomal drug products. *Biotechnology Journal* 2019, **14**:e1700740.

26. König C, Bechtold-Peters K, Baum V, Schultz-Fademrecht T, Bassarab S, Steffens KJ: Development of a pilot-scale manufacturing process for protein-coated microcrystals (PCMC): Mixing and precipitation – Part I. *European Journal of Pharmaceutics and Biopharmaceutics* 2012, **80**:490–498.

27. (ICH) ICfH: Q12 – Implementation Considerations for FDA-Regulated Products – Guidance for Industry. In *Q12*. Edited by ICH.

28. Gurgula O: Strategic Patenting by Pharmaceutical Companies – Should Competition Law Intervene? *IIC; International Review of Industrial Property and Copyright Law*; 2020:1–24.

29. Nepveux K, Sherlock JP, Futran M, Thien M, Krumme M: How development and manufacturing will need to be structured--heads of development/manufacturing. May 20-21, 2014 Continuous Manufacturing Symposium. *Journal of Pharmaceutical Sciences* 2015, **104**:850–864.

30. Vayghan J: Transformation ROI versus the High Cost of Doing Nothing: Why Inaction is Unaffordable. In *Forbes*. Edited by; 2017.

31. Christensen CM, Kaufman SP, Shih WC: *Innovation Killers: How Financial Tools Destroy Your Capacity to Do New Things*: Harvard Business Review Press; 2010.

32. CHMP E: Guideline on Real Time Release Testing (formerly Guideline on Parametric Release). In *EMA/CHMP/QWP/811210/2009-Rev1*. Edited by (CHMP) EMA-CfMPfHU; 2012.

33. (ICH) ICfH: Guidance for Industry – Q8, Q9, & Q10 – Questions and Answers. In *Q8, Q9, Q10 – Questions and Answers*. Edited by ICH; 2012.

9

Modernizing Manufacturing of Parenteral Products: From Batch to Continuous Lyophilization

Roberto Pisano, Merve B. Adali, and Lorenzo Stratta
Politecnico di Torino, Torino, Italy

CONTENTS

DOI: 10.1201/9781003149835-11

9.1 Introduction

The concept of continuous manufacturing has widely been implemented in many applications and industrial fields. In a continuous process, the raw materials endure a series of interconnected unit operations, including physical and chemical transformations, to achieve a continuous flow of the final product. A continuous production plant can operate 24 hours a day, 7 days a week, for several years without any interruptions. The dead times typical of batch production and its intrinsic batch-to-batch variability reduce drastically, improving both the process economy and the final product quality. Among the others, steel production, oil refining, natural gas processing, and paper and chemicals production have been converted into continuous processes starting from the late 1700s. However, even today, the pharmaceutical industry strongly relies on batch production. Due to the incredibly strict regulations applying to the implementation of new technologies, the pharmaceutical industry preferred to stick to well-established batch technologies, hampering the development of new continuous strategies. In order to improve pharmaceutical production flexibility and product quality, the U.S. Food and Drug Administration (FDA) has heavily sponsored the application of continuous manufacturing. Public declarations have been made on the compatibility of continuous manufacturing with the current regulatory guidelines, and numerous funds granted to projects aimed at the development of innovative continuous technologies (Gottlieb, 2021). The Office of Pharmaceutical Quality, a subsection of the Centre for Drug Evaluation and Research (CDER), created on purpose the Emerging Technology Program (ETP). Industries applying to the program can work directly with the Emerging Technology Team (ETT) to "discuss, identify, and resolve potential technical and regulatory issues related to the development and implementation of a novel technology before filing a regulatory submission" (FDA, 2021).

In addition, the ongoing COVID pandemic has highlighted how important this topic is, and how fast we should respond to future threats by being prepared.

In this scenario, the pharmaceutical industry is also facing a profound renovation, shifting from conventional, chemically synthesized drugs to biopharmaceuticals. The global biopharmaceutical market has grown considerably in the last few years and is expected to expand remarkably in the near future. The global sales of biopharmaceuticals resulted in a total of US\$ 228 billion in 2016 (Moorkens et al. 2017), US\$ 325 billion in 2020, and are estimated to be valued at US\$ 497 billion in 2026 (Mordor Intelligence, 2021). Many benefits have been pushed toward this turnover, as their few side effects and targeted action, the easy engineering of new drugs, and the potential to treat diseases long considered untreatable. However, these kinds of drug products often fall into the category of active compounds that require freeze-drying as a downstream operation.

Freeze-drying is a dehydration technique often used to remove solvents from the active components that are unstable in solutions for long periods and degrade when exposed to the high temperatures typical of conventional drying. It is composed of three main steps; freezing, primary drying, and secondary drying. First, the solution is frozen and cooled to a temperature close to −50 °C. Then, during primary drying, the pressure inside the freeze-dryer is reduced to several Pascals below the ice-vapor equilibrium point using a vacuum pump and a condenser working at temperatures close to −80 °C, thus promoting the separation of the ice via sublimation. The required latent heat is supplied by the temperature-controlled shelves of the freeze-dryer. Once all the ice is sublimated, the temperature of the shelves is further increased to promote the desorption of the remaining water from the porous matrix. The freeze-drying process usually constitutes the bottleneck of the entire production chain of a biopharmaceutical product and, compared to other downstream operations, it does not have commercial technological solutions that allow it to be run continuously.

The next sections will highlight the importance of continuous manufacturing in freeze-drying and its advantages compared to batch production. Then, a brief historical background on the applications of continuous freeze-drying will be provided, and lastly, a description of the most up-to-date technological solutions will be presented to the reader.

9.2 Pros and Cons of Batch Lyophilization

There are several reasons why the pharmaceutical industry, and in particular freeze-drying, is still so profoundly attached to batch production. Firstly, the technology is well established, and the personnel trained to use it. In a field as strictly regulated as the pharmaceutical industry, the development of a new technology requires huge investments in the design, the validation of the equipment, and the training of the personnel. Moreover, the actual productivity already fulfils the world demand and, therefore, the return of the investments is not always guaranteed in short times. Lastly, even for new production plants, it is more convenient to stick to the old, reliable batch apparatus as conventional freeze-dryers are extremely easy to design. However, there are several reasons that push toward the development of continuous freeze-dryers.

9.2.1 Time Consumption

Freeze-drying is a tremendously time-consuming process. The duration of a freeze-drying cycle can range from tens of hours to a few days or even weeks. In addition, there are numerous other unavoidable activities that add dead times to the total duration. Among those, the most relevant are:

- Filling and loading and unloading of the vials in the freeze-dryer
- Cleaning-in-place (CIP) and sterilization-in-place (SIP)
- Filter integrity tests
- Leak tests of the unit
- Condenser defrosting

For productions of hundreds of thousands of vials, even with completely automatic filling and loading machines, the time required to fill and load all the vials into the freeze dryer could take several hours.

Moreover, apart from filling, which could be performed in parallel between consequent cycles, the other operations must be done in series. Therefore, they correspond to operational times contributing directly to the total processing time, thus reducing the productivity and profitability of the cycles.

9.2.2 Scale-Up Issues

Batch lyophilization, *as is*, reacts incredibly slowly to the introduction of new products on the market. Every time a product is scaled up to the production line, a new validation campaign is required. The laboratory equipment can be useful for preliminary studies to obtain the basic process information, but the scale-up remains quite troublesome. Heat and mass transfer characteristics can change significantly between laboratory scale freeze-dryers operating with a few hundreds of vials to the industrial scale apparatuses containing hundreds of thousands of vials. Even small variations in the product temperature caused by the different conditions at the two scales can lead to the loss of entire batches. It is evident that precise knowledge of the machines and extensive and time-consuming experimental campaigns are needed in order to bring a new product to the production line. The application of the Quality by Design (QbD) approaches could mitigate the risks, and mathematical modeling has proven to be a great tool in reducing experimental times (Fissore et al. 2011, 2015; Pisano et al. 2011, 2013). However, this approach is still not self-sufficient, as it requires a certain number of experiments in order to obtain the mathematical model parameters.

9.2.3 Impossible Quality Assurance

Another main disadvantage of batch lyophilization is the impossibility to operate in-line Quality Assurance, as most of the vials are not available for inspections during the cycle. Probes like thermocouples or the wireless Tempris® are invasive to the product, and monitored vials will then be discarded.

Non-invasive methods like thermal imaging are currently too space-consuming and infrared (IR)-cameras can monitor only edge vials that behave differently from the rest of the batch. Moreover, in conventional freeze-dryers, the vials are tightly packed and only a small portion of the product, that is, the top of the cake, is free to be inspected. In addition, if the vials are pre-stoppered before loading, as usually happens, the product is completely out of sight of the IR lens. Other methods can indirectly and non-invasively estimate the product temperature but can hardly be referred to the state of individual vials (Fissore et al., 2018; Pisano et al., 2016).

9.2.4 Unpredictable Freezing

Due to the stochastic behavior of nucleation, the freezing step induces great vial-to-vial variability. It is widely known that the number and dimension of the ice crystals in the frozen product are directly related to the nucleation temperature of the solution (Nakagawa et al. 2007; Arsiccio et al. 2017; Colucci et al. 2020). Then, as the cake dries, the remaining pores assume the same structure and morphology as the sublimated ice crystals. Therefore, the product resistance to mass transport during primary drying sensibly depends on the freezing step. Higher nucleation temperatures produce larger pores, which offer lower resistances to the vapor transport, reducing the drying time and the maximum temperature reached by the product. The nucleation temperature, when triggered spontaneously during a predefined cooling ramp of the shelf, can vary several degrees from vial to vial, which could potentially correspond to differences in drying time of several hours among vials of the same batch (Capozzi and Pisano, 2018). To mitigate this phenomenon, various solutions have been proposed to control the nucleation temperature. Vacuum-induced surface freezing (VISF) (Oddone et al. 2016, 2020; Arsiccio et al. 2018; Pisano et al. 2019a), high-pressure shift freezing, depressurization technique, ice-fog technique (Patel et al. 2009), electric field-induced nucleation (Petersen et al. 2006), and ultrasound-assisted nucleation, among the others, are the most advanced. Some of them require hardware modifications of the conventional freeze-dryer, while others can easily be performed with state-of-the-art apparatus such as the VISF. However, even those techniques cannot guarantee uniform nucleation temperatures among the whole batch of vials when applied to large-scale batch freeze-dryers. Geometrical asymmetries in the chamber, pressure gradients, difficulties in reaching all the vials, and lags in the propagation of nucleators are unsolved challenges.

9.2.5 Vial-to-Vial Heterogeneity during Drying

Unexpected heat transfer variations within the batch can occur also during primary and secondary drying. Changes of a few degrees in product temperature can potentially induce the collapse of the cake and consequent loss of the product. Moreover, even if the temperature in each vial remains below the critical values, heterogeneity in heat transfer can result in unavoidable variations in the cake appearance, residual moisture content, and drug activity that are unacceptable in Quality Assurance. It has been demonstrated that small variations in the geometry of the vials have a huge impact on the amount of heat transferred from the shelves to the vials (Pikal et al. 1984). Moreover, vials in different positions on the shelves are subjected to the so-called *edge-vials effect* (Rambhatla and Pikal 2003; Pikal et al. 2016). In a freeze-dryer, the walls of the chamber are not temperature-controlled and, therefore, tend to reach higher temperatures compared to the rest of the system. The vials positioned at the edge of the batch receive a considerable amount of additional energy, by means of thermal radiation from the chamber walls, compared to the central vials. To mitigate this effect and avoid product collapse in the external vials, the recipe must be defined in such a way that the central vials dry under conservative conditions, that is, lower-than-optimal shelf temperatures and pressures, prolonging the drying times.

9.3 Continuous Freeze-Drying as a Solution to the Batch Freeze-Drying Problems

The application of continuous manufacturing to the freeze-drying industry represents an opportunity to solve most of the problems that batch lyophilization is currently facing, as detailed in the following sections.

9.3.1 Time Consumption

Continuous manufacturing consists of a series of uninterrupted unit operations. In continuous equipment, the reduction of the dead times is remarkable as most of the batch freeze-drying bottleneck operations can be executed in parallel to the process itself. Filling, loading, and unloading of the vials are performed continuously alongside the other process steps. Filter integrity tests and the condenser defrosting are performed by switching between duplicates working in parallel without stopping production. Finally, operations such as CIP or SIP can be performed sporadically as the machine is less exposed to external contaminations.

As the dead times represent a remarkable fraction of the total duration, their elimination reduces drastically the total processing time, with benefits in terms of productivity, economical profit, reactivity to changes in production, etc.

9.3.2 Scale-Up and Process Conditions Uniformity

The scale-up of batch freeze-drying cycles is particularly complicated for one main reason: it is difficult to replicate the same product's thermal history among different freeze-driers under constant processing conditions. However, a continuous apparatus works on single units, or small groups of units, of the product and guarantees the same processing conditions for each. A scale difference does not necessarily translate into modifications of heat- and mass-transfer characteristics. A laboratory-scale freeze-dryer would thus be able to precisely replicate the industrial conditions.

Moreover, in a continuous freeze-dryer, it would be possible to quickly test many different process conditions on small groups of units. The experimental campaign duration would therefore reduce tremendously.

Finally, due to the continuous single-unit approach, it would be trivial to implement the induced-nucleation techniques, such as VISF, ice-fog, high-pressure shift freezing, depressurization, etc. Nucleation could be triggered in each vial individually and not simultaneously in a batch of hundreds of thousands of units, thus allowing uniform conditions throughout the whole batch.

9.3.3 Quality Assurance and Process Analytical Technologies (PATs)

In a continuous freeze dryer, the vials are not packed in large batches and are therefore free to be inspected by non-invasive methods, most of which have already been developed and extensively studied in literature. With IR-imaging, it is possible to obtain the whole temperature distribution of the product during freezing (Harguindeguy et al. 2021) and drying (Van Bockstal et al. 2018; Lietta et al. 2019; Harguindeguy and Fissore 2021). Subsequently, suitable mathematical models can infer the internal solid structure of the cake, allowing in-line optimization of the process conditions for each vial (Nakagawa and Hottot 2012; Arsiccio et al. 2017, 2019; Colucci et al. 2020).

On the other hand, near-IR imaging has already been demonstrated to be a powerful, non-invasive tool for providing information on the cake residual moisture (Jones et al. 1993; Derksen et al. 1998; Zheng et al. 2008; Clavaud et al. 2016; Brouckaert et al. 2018; Bobba et al. 2021). The in-line knowledge of the residual moisture of each vial is crucial to determine the end of primary and secondary drying, therefore speeding up the process by eliminating useless dead times. Moreover, as it consists of a non-invasive procedure, it represents a valuable Quality Assurance alternative to the old, product-destructive Karl-Fisher titration that is the standard procedure for residual moisture inference.

9.3.4 Economic Impact

Freeze-drying is a time- and energy-consuming process and has often been considered an expensive procedure for a small fraction of high-added-value products. However, a recent economic evaluation of a freeze-drying cycle has demonstrated that the operative costs (OC) are not prohibitive (Stratta et al. 2020). In an industrial-scale freeze-dryer, working for seven days per week without production interruptions, the OC account for only 15% of the total costs (TC), while the capital costs (CC) cover the remaining 85%.

Continuous manufacturing would impact significantly on the CC. Comparing two apparatuses with similar footprints and initial investments, a continuous freeze-dryer would have a higher production rate than a batch freeze-dryer. As already mentioned, continuous manufacturing eliminates the dead times, thus decreasing the total process time and increasing productivity. With higher productivity, the CC can be divided into a larger number of doses, thus reducing the CC per dose, or per batch, which represents the major contribution to the actual freeze-drying costs.

9.3.5 Delocalization and Stockpiles

Among the other advantages of continuous freeze-drying already presented, there are at least two more that are worth mentioning.

In a world where the majority of pharmaceutical companies delocalize their production plants in order to exploit the low-cost labor and shady regulations of foreign countries, continuous freeze-drying relies on advanced technology and trained personnel, contributing to the economy of the end-users' countries.

Finally, by having the ability to respond promptly to sudden changes in demand, the risk of stock-outs can be eliminated, and stockpiles can be drastically reduced (Pisano 2020).

9.4 The History of Continuous Lyophilization

Although continuous freeze-drying has not yet been fully implemented in the pharmaceutical industry, the concept of a continuous freeze-dryer dates back more than 70 years. The first proposal focused on food rather than drugs and consisted of the lyophilization of bulk products, mostly beverages. In 1947, Sluder et al. designed a pilot plant for the continuous lyophilization of juice (Sluder et al. 1947), in 1969, Oetjen et al. (Rey 2016) proposed a continuous freeze-dryer designed for milk products, and in the 1970s, the Atlas company built the Conrad freeze-dryer (Rey 2016), a fully continuous line for the lyophilization of instant coffee, which was also compatible with milk, vegetable, fish, and meat. Since then, many different strategies were applied to continuous freeze-drying but a few of them have even been implemented in the industry. However, only the food sector has benefited from those innovations since the regulations regarding product sterility and handling safety are less stringent compared to the pharmaceutical industry.

Continuous lyophilization of pharmaceuticals can be divided into two main categories: freeze-drying of unit doses and freeze-drying of bulk products. In the following sections, the most promising technologies, belonging to the two aforementioned categories, will be described in detail.

9.5 Freeze-Drying of Unit Doses

9.5.1 Continuous Freeze-Drying of Unit Doses Based on the Concept of Spin/Shell Freezing and Vacuum Drying

The application of the concept of spin- or shell-freezing as a first step to the continuous lyophilization of active compounds in vials dates back to 1957 when Becker proposed the first prototype of a continuous freeze dryer of unit doses (Becker 1957). Each vial is inserted into a guide capsule, which then rotates quickly under vacuum conditions. The rotation induces the liquid to stick to the lateral walls of the vial forming a thin layer while the vacuum promotes the evaporation of the solvent removing the latent heat that freezes the rest of the solution. Once the vials are completely frozen, the capsule releases them into the drying chamber and returns back to host a new vial. The vials are then moved by gravity in the drying chamber, which is a long, inclined, and heated conduit under vacuum.

In 1965, Broadwin presented a new version designed to treat highly sensitive enzymes and living cells (Broadwin 1965). The containers are inserted into a centrifuge that provides the rotation needed to spread the liquid over the bottle walls. A vacuum is then applied in order to evaporate some of the liquid and, at the same time, cool the solution until the temperature drops below $-15\ °C$. When this temperature is reached, the centrifuge stops to avoid damaging the cells and heat is applied by conduction to evaporate the remaining liquid solvent. Finally, the product completes the dehydration at −50 °C in the same chamber or in a different apparatus.

Both these concepts had, however, their flaws. The design by Becker was particularly traumatic for the vials and the risks of spillage of the solution or ruptures of the frozen products were high. On the other hand, the vacuum freezing proposed in the Broadwin design could impair the product structure due to bubbling and boiling of the solution. Many other approaches involving the concept of spin-freezing have been proposed over the years trying to solve the above problems. However, even though particularly detailed and elaborated, as the one proposed by Oughton (2001), none of them was ever developed. Recently, RheaVita proposed a new plant design to make spin freeze-drying a doable solution to support continuous manufacturing.

9.5.2 IR-Assisted Drying of Previously Spin-Frozen Samples

The design is based on the spin-freezing concept, previously developed by Becker, Broadwin, and Oughton (Figure 9.1). The vials rotate at about 2500 rpm along their vertical axis during freezing and the liquid freezes on the walls of the container forming a thin shell. A stream of cold inert gas provides the required refrigeration for its solidification.

Due to the area of the lateral walls being greater than the vial cross section, the thickness of the liquid layer decreases. Both freezing and drying complete faster as the resistance to the heat and mass transport in the product is lower. It was estimated that the primary drying duration could be reduced by more than 93% and 88% for amorphous and crystalline excipients, respectively, compared to batch freeze-drying (Leys et al. 2020). However, careful consideration of a few aspects is necessary as, for example, a certain number of proteins tend to be sensitive to an augmented air- or glass-to-liquid surface. Lammens et al. (2018) found that, in general, proteins are not strongly affected by the shear stresses generated inside the solution during the spinning step of spin-freezing. However, viruses or bacteria have a greater sedimentation velocity compared to proteins and it is crucial to respect a maximum freezing time in order to avoid intra-product inhomogeneity due to sedimentation. Moreover, Vanbillemont et al. (2020), demonstrated that, for the human intravenous immune globulin (IVIG), with an accurate choice of solution formulation, it is possible to obtain similar residual protein activities in spin-freeze-dried and conventional-freeze-dried samples. However, each formulation must be product-specific as different proteins can react differently to the spin- and spin-freezing-induced stresses.

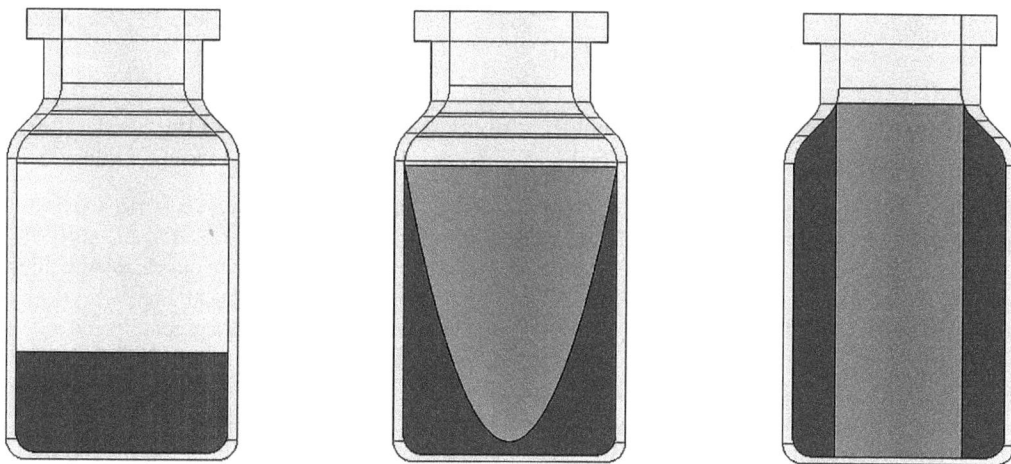

FIGURE 9.1 Concept of the Spin-Freezing. Each vial is rotated along its vertical axis. The centrifugal force acting on the solution inside the vial spread the solution over the vial wall. After the rotational speed reaches a certain value, a thin, uniform layer forms inside the vial, which can then be frozen and dried.

During drying, each vial is rotated at about 5–12 rpm and the required heat is supplied by an individual IR-heater along the whole surface of the vial. The product temperature can precisely be controlled with a feedback controller that adjusts the corresponding IR-radiator temperature in order to maximize the efficiency while restraining the product from surpassing its collapse temperature. The residual moisture level, on the other hand, depends on the radiator power and the vial residence time inside the drying module.

9.5.3 Suspended-Vials Concept

The vials enter in a series of specialized channels in which all the process steps are carried out. A schematic representation of the prototype design can be seen in Figure 9.2.

Firstly, the vials are cooled to the desired nucleation temperature by means of a stream of cold nitrogen and passed through a load-lock to enter the nucleation chamber. Here VISF is applied; the pressure lowers to about 1–2 mbar and the vacuum produces isenthalpic evaporation of the solvent, which cools the solution close to the top surface of the liquid and hence triggers ice nucleation which, then, extends to the entire volume of the solution. This technique has proven beneficial for the whole process (Oddone et al. 2014, 2016, 2017, 2020; Arsiccio et al. 2018). First, as nucleation is induced at the same temperature in all the vials, the variability in the pore size distribution typical of spontaneous nucleation reduces drastically. Then, due to the nucleation temperature being several degrees higher than the spontaneous one, the average pore diameter is larger, which reduces the mass transport cake resistance and, therefore, the drying time.

After nucleation, the vials proceed to move into the actual freezing channel, where a cold stream of nitrogen completes the solidification process and cools the products to the target temperatures of about −50°C. To control the cooling rate, it is possible to act on two main variables, the temperature of the cold gas stream and its flow rate.

Once the vials are completely frozen, they pass through another load-lock to enter the drying section. Radiating fins supply the required heat to each vial, and the power supplied to the vials can be controlled by modifying the fin's temperature.

Once the solvent is sublimated completely and the moisture levels are within the desired ranges, the vials move to the backfilling chamber and are stoppered automatically. The entire process is carried out continuously without the need for any manual intervention.

The machine fills the vials with the solution and suspends them over a moving track as shown schematically in Figure 9.3. The aim of the suspension is to avoid any contact with the freeze-dryer surfaces. The small manufacturing imperfections of the vial's bottom no longer affect the suspended vial heat transfer, which is, therefore, more uniform from vial to vial. Moreover, as heat is transferred only by means of thermal radiation, the pressure inside the chamber can be reduced as desired to maximize the sublimation driving force without inhibiting the heat transfer.

9.5.4 Freeze-Drying of Unconventional Containers – Zydis®, Example of the Semi-Continuous Lyophilization of Orally Disintegrating Tablets (ODT) from Catalent

Dysphagia (difficulty in swallowing) is a widespread condition that affects geriatric, paediatric, and institutionalized patients, and people who suffer from nausea and vomiting. Orally disintegrating tablets (ODT) offer an easy and comfortable drug administration route to all those patients who are unable, or unwilling, to swallow their medication (Rao et al. 2008; Dey and Maiti 2010; Ghosh et al. 2011). Freeze-drying has been intensively applied in the production of ODTs as the dried products solubilize readily and with a particularly low amount of saliva. Even though no fully continuous apparatus involving freeze-drying has been implemented, Catalent developed the Zydis® technology, which consists of a semi-continuous process involving freeze-drying for the production of ODTs, as shown in Figure 9.4.

The process can be divided into four main stages: preparation of the solution, filling and freezing of the tablets, vacuum drying, and sealing.

As mentioned, the process is almost completely continuous and the only step still remaining batch is drying, which is performed in conventional industrial freeze dryers. The active ingredient is formulated into a solution, which is then injected into a continuous pre-formed sheet of blisters. The blisters are then

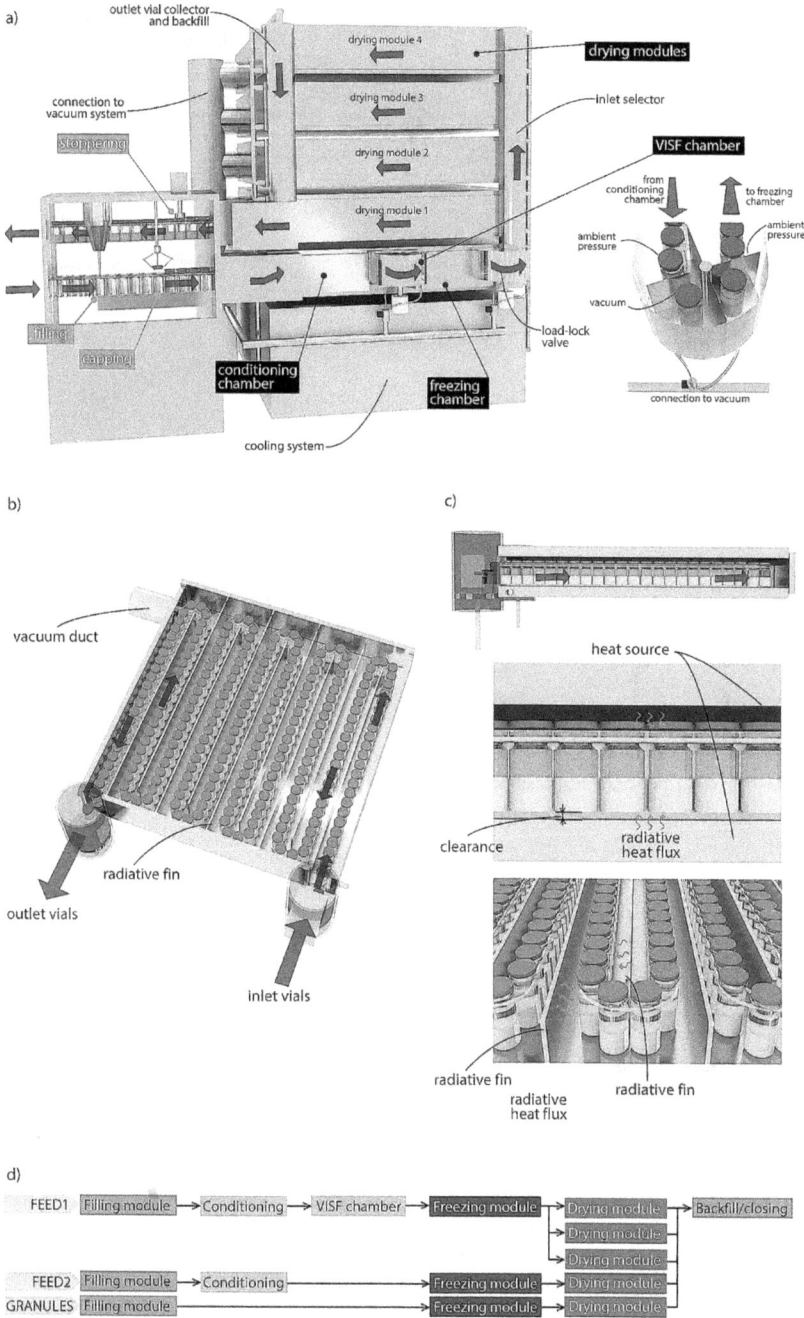

FIGURE 9.2 Design of the continuous freeze-dryer proposed by the group from Polito and MIT in 2015. (Reprinted with permission from Capozzi et al. 2019.)

cut and frozen in the freezing channel, where liquid nitrogen serves as refrigerating medium. The frozen blisters are transported into a large-scale freeze-dryer where drying is carried out under vacuum. After completing this step, the blisters return to a continuous roller for the heat sealing and are divided into primary packings.

Even though the drying step of this process remains batch, this is the tangible proof that continuous manufacturing has the potential to be implemented in the pharmaceutical industry, even if only partially.

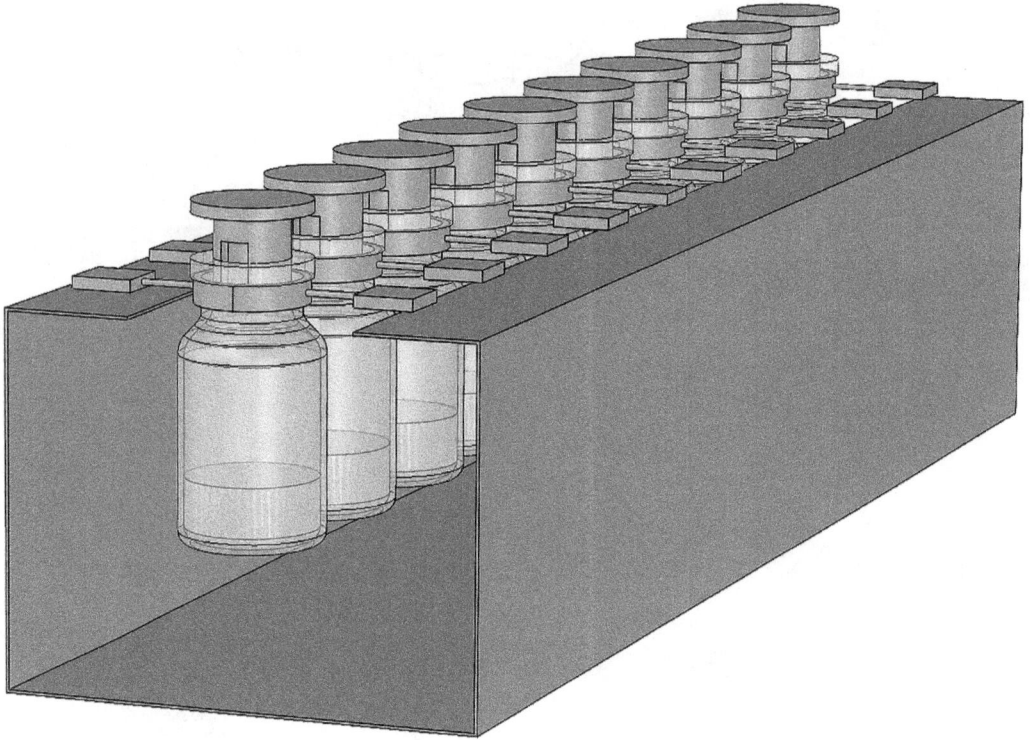

FIGURE 9.3   Concept of suspended vials. Each vial is treated singularly and is not in contact with the freeze-dryer.

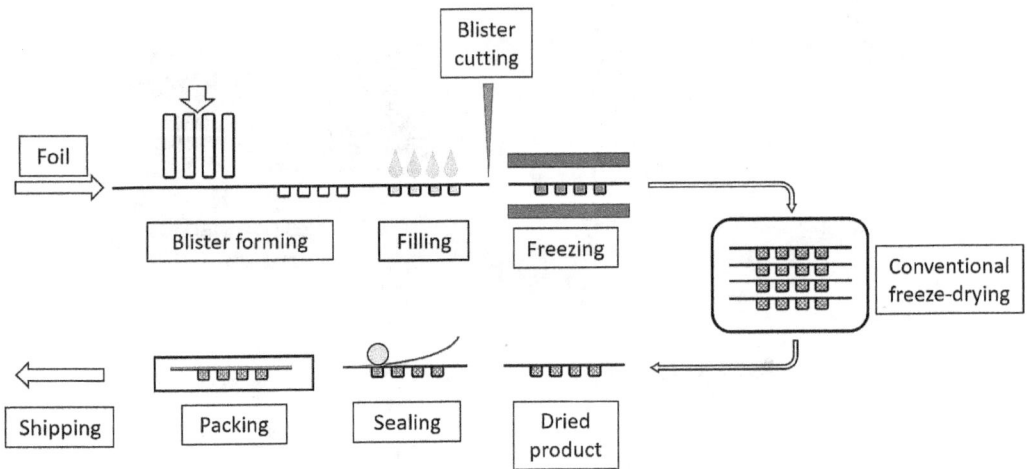

FIGURE 9.4   Schematic description of the Zydis technology.

9.6 Freeze-Drying of Bulk Products

Freeze-drying of pharmaceuticals – whether liquids or suspensions – to ensure good manufacturing practices (GMP) and sterility requirements of the final dried product is commonly performed in glass vials, but, in certain circumstances, bulk freeze-drying is employed to handle larger volumes of liquid (Walters et al. 2014; Luy and Stamato 2020). As an alternative to conventional batch freeze-drying in vials/trays, newer and more advanced techniques such as spray drying, supercritical fluid technology, and more recently spray freeze-drying (SFD) are constantly being developed because of their capacity to produce particles with physical and chemical properties appropriate for pharmaceutical applications (Walters et al. 2014; Emami et al. 2018b). Spray-drying technique is now an established and well-understood process for a wide range of products, but it is potentially dangerous for pharmaceuticals due to thermal stress. While the utility of supercritical fluid technology using compressed fluids (mostly supercritical carbon dioxide) as solvent and anti-solvent has already been demonstrated, the main disadvantage of this technique is the lack of a supercritical liquid extraction method suitable for different matrix types and the low solubility of most organic solids in supercritical carbon dioxide (Rogers et al. 2001; Bin et al. 2020). In contrast, a variety of products can be processed by SFD, including heat-sensitive compounds and organic solutions. SFD may provide fast processing time for bulk material with large-scale production in line with the FDA regulations and a significant cost reduction. Unfortunately, little is known about tailoring the properties of particles using SFD (Sonner et al. 2002; Maltesen and van de Weert 2008). It is worth noting that the main argument in the present contribution is the process and equipment design of SFD for continuous production. Combining continuous processes with GMP standards (FDA 2019) for the highest quality and safety is, of course, a crucial issue in pharmaceutical manufacturing.

9.6.1 Spray Freeze-Drying Overview

The SFD technique, which involves producing a flowable micronized powder from a solution or suspension, has received a great deal of attention in pharmaceutical research over the last 60 years. The first known article in the literature describing this technique for proteins and peptides dates back to the late 1940s (Benson and Ellis 1948). Although the application of SFD was first demonstrated by Meryman in the late 1950s (Meryman 1959); its active research in the pharmaceutical industries only began in the early 1990s to prepare amorphous forms of poorly water-soluble drugs (Mumenthaler and Leuenberger 1991; Dugas and Williams III 2016), and was followed by many patents issued over the subsequent years (Maa and Nguyen 2001; Williams et al. 2002; Maa et al. 2003; Wang and Finlay 2008). Conventional methods of processing biopharmaceuticals into powders, such as mechanical milling and precipitation, most likely result in protein degradation, loss of stability, and lack of sterility (Shoyele and Cawthorne 2006; Wu et al. 2011; Sinha et al. 2013). SFD is unique in its ability to produce pharmaceutical powders with proper sphericity, small particle size, and high porosity without altering their natural conformation (Schiffter 2007; Wanning et al. 2015). As a result, the small particle size and high surface area promote greatly improved wettability, dispersibility, and solubility of formulated drugs (Hu et al. 2002; Bi et al. 2008; Kondo et al. 2009; Ishwarya et al. 2017). This technique consists of a low-temperature drying process and is therefore widely used for the production of pharmaceutical products, such as proteins (Carrasquillo et al. 2001; Yu et al. 2006; Lo et al. 2021), antibodies (Emami et al. 2018a, 2019; Daneshmand et al. 2019), vaccines (Amorij et al. 2007; Saluja et al. 2010; Tonnis et al. 2014), dry powder aerosols (Sweeney et al. 2005; Kho and Hadinoto 2011; Braig et al. 2019), and nanoparticles (Cheow et al. 2011) to improve their stability and ease of administration. Examples of SFD application in pharmaceutical products reported in the literature are given in Table 9.1. These advantages make SFD the preferred process for continuous manufacturing of bulk active ingredients in the pharmaceutical industry.

Fundamentally, SFD is divided into three basic steps: atomization, spray freezing, and freeze-drying. To manufacture an SFD process, a spray solution of drug products, and sometimes additional pharmaceutical excipients, is atomized in a freezing chamber using an atomizer. The atomized droplets are instantly frozen into microparticles by contact with a cryogenic medium. The frozen solvent in the particles is then sublimated at low temperature and pressure, leaving behind dried porous particles (Maa et al. 2004; Costantino et al. 2000). The final particle size and properties depend on the selected operating conditions such as atomizer type, spray freezing process, and drying temperature (Ishwarya et al. 2015; Vishali et al. 2019). Atomization, the breaking up of a liquid bulk solution into fine droplets, predominantly controls the particle size of the resulting powder (Cal and Sollohub 2010). The selection of an atomizer is a critical choice for the SFD design and is made based on the feedstock properties, the desired particle characteristics, and the atomizer capacity (Walters et al. 2014; Vishali et al. 2019). Four different types of atomizers are used for most SFD applications: hydraulic (pressure) atomizers, pneumatic (multifluid) atomizers, ultrasonic atomizers, and monodisperse droplet-stream generations.

TABLE 9.1

Some of the Published Studies on Spray Freeze-Drying Application in Pharmaceutical Research

Name of API	Polymer/Excipient Used	Specific Aim	Reference
Salbutamol sulfate	Excipient free	Dry powder inhaler	(Mueannoom et al. 2012)
	Alginate	Pulmonary delivery	(López-Iglesias et al. 2019)
	Glycine	Dry powder inhaler	(Ogienko et al. 2017)
Insulin	Trehalose dihydrate, dextran, mannitol	Needle-free injection	(Schiffter et al. 2010)
Azithromycin	Polyvinyl alcohol	Drug solubility	(Adeli 2017)
Voriconazole	Mannitol	Pulmonary delivery	(Liao et al. 2019)
Naproxen	Lactose	Drug solubility	(Braig et al. 2019)
Adalimumab	Trehalose, leucine, phenylalanine, glycine, arginine	Pulmonary delivery	(Emami et al. 2019)
Clarithromycin	Mannitol, sucrose	Pulmonary delivery	(Ye et al. 2017)
Kanamycin	Excipient free	Pulmonary delivery	(Her et al. 2010)
Hepatitis B vaccine	Dextran, trehalose, inulin	Drug stability	(Tonnis et al. 2014)
Albuterol sulfate	Polyethylene glycol	Drug delivery	(Barron et al. 2003)
SHetA2	Trehalose	Oral administration	(Ibrahim et al. 2019)
Small interfering RNA	Mannitol	Pulmonary delivery	(Liang et al. 2018)
Naked plasmid DNA	Polyethylenimine, hyaluronic acid	Pulmonary gene therapy	(Ito et al. 2019)
Ciclosporin A	Mannitol	Dry powder inhaler	(Niwa et al. 2012)
Salmon calcitonin	Trehalose, hydroxyl propyl-β-cyclodextrin, maltose	Pulmonary delivery	(Poursina et al. 2016)
Sildenafil citrate	Poly (lactic-co-glycolic acid)	Pulmonary arterial hypertension	(Shahin et al. 2021)
Rizatriptan Benzoate	Leucine, phenylalanine, mannitol, trehalose	Dry powder inhaler	(Faghihi et al. 2021)
Human IgG	Trehalose, hydroxypropyl-β-cyclodextrin	Aerosolization efficiency	(Milani et al. 2020)
Bromelain	Maltodextrin, chitosan	Pulmonary delivery	(Lavanya et al. 2020)
Bovine serum albumin	Hydroxypropyl-β-cyclodextrin	Dry powder inhaler	(Lo et al. 2021)

The most common atomizers used in SFD studies are hydraulic and two-fluid atomizers. The disadvantage of hydraulic atomizers is that they are not suitable for atomizing high-viscosity liquids and can be easily clogged (Cal and Sollohub 2010). Two-fluid atomizers generally produce coarser, free-flowing powders with respect to hydraulic atomizers, but they are expensive to operate due to the high cost of compressed air used during the atomization of the liquid feed (Cal and Sollohub 2010). In recent years, new nozzles have been developed for spraying uniformly sized droplets to achieve more uniform drying times, such as ultrasonic atomizers and monodisperse droplet-stream generators (Ishwarya et al. 2015). Ultrasonic nozzles atomize the feed liquid by vibrating longitudinally at a high frequency via piezoelectric transducers (Ramisetty et al. 2013), whereas monodisperse droplet-stream generators rely on Rayleigh disintegration of the liquid by applying a regular constant vibration to a laminar liquid jet (Süverkrüp et al. 2013). An alternative approach to using monodisperse nozzles is ink-jet printing systems. These systems are classified by the two main operational modes used to generate the droplets: "continuous" (CIJ) and "drop on demand" (DOD) techniques. CIJ methods involve spraying a continuous stream of liquid, while DOD ejects the liquid only when a drop is needed (Castrejón-Pita et al. 2013). The generation of small droplets of equal size would be an ideal atomization process for the production of pharmaceutical powders, for which the use of ink-jet printers has recently been under extensive investigation. In practice, the method still needs to be improved, but it has the potential to be integrated into continuous operation to control the spray characteristics and maximize the uniformity of the final product.

Once the atomized droplets enter the freezing chamber, where the droplets come in contact with a cryogenic medium, rapid freezing of the droplets occurs. The SFD is classified based on the physical state of the cryogen, typically a cold gas stream or liquid nitrogen, used for the freezing action as shown in

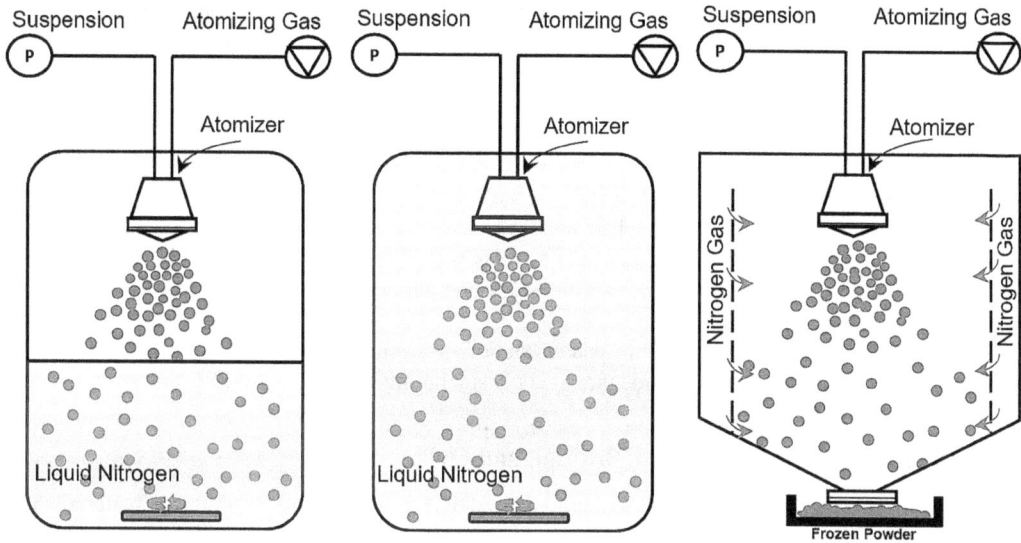

FIGURE 9.5 Schematic of the various spray freezing configuration. Spray freezing into vapor over liquid (left), Spray freezing into liquid (middle), Spray freezing into vapor (right). (Reprinted with permission from Adali et al. 2020.)

Figure 9.5. Spray freezing into liquid (SFL) was presented by the University of Texas in a patent dated 2001 (Hu et al. 2002) and commercialized by Dow Chemical Company, recently by Enavail LLC (Dugas and Williams III 2016). In this technique, a feed liquid is sprayed through an insulated nozzle which is placed directly into a cryogenic liquid (Costantino et al. 2000), such as compressed fluid carbon dioxide, helium, propane, ethane, nitrogen, or argon. However, as mentioned earlier, the most common cryogen used is liquid nitrogen, which is relatively inexpensive, safe, and accepted for use in certain medical applications (Surasarang and Williams III 2016). During the SFL process, it is recommended to stir the cryogenic liquid with an impeller to prevent the aggregation of frozen particles. The frozen material is then collected to remove the solvent by sublimation. The advantage of the SFL is the fast-freezing rates combined with the intense atomization resulting from the liquid–liquid impingement between the pressurized feed solution coming out of the nozzle and the cryogenic liquid (Hu et al. 2003; Rogers et al. 2003). Some studies have proven that the fast-freezing rates achieved due to intense atomization can promote amorphous glass formation, high surface area, enhanced dissolution, and minimized phase separation of solutes (Hu et al. 2004; Rogers et al. 2003). A major issue of this method is nozzle clogging due to ice formation. Generally, the nozzle used for SFL is composed of an insulating material, like a capillary made of polyether–ether ketone (PEEK) characterized by very low thermal conduction. Occasionally, the liquid solution may be sprayed into a cryogenic fluid via a heated nozzle. However, this solution can strengthen the Leidenfrost effect, which causes an insulating layer around the droplets and leads to low thermal conductivity, lowering the freezing rate (Engstrom et al. 2007).

In the configuration of spray freezing into vapor (SFV), frozen microspheres are produced by spraying bulk liquid into a chamber containing a cold vapor (acting as a cryogenic medium). Mumenthaler and Leuenberger proposed a process in which the sprayed droplets are frozen into the stream of cold air and then dried in an integrated fluidized bed at atmospheric pressure (Mumenthaler and Leuenberger 1991). However, the need for huge amounts of cold dry gas to be circulated in the bed is a disadvantage of the system. In addition, the use of counter-current flow is also a disadvantage that affects collection efficiency and particle elutriation. As a possible solution to the latter drawback, cooled nitrogen gas was fed from lateral porous walls into the chamber to create a co-current flow process for delivering the frozen particles to the exit filter, where they dry at atmospheric pressure (Wang et al. 2006).

Spray freezing into vapor over liquid (SFV/L) is the most applied method, especially in the field of pharmaceutical research. The feed solution is sprayed through an atomizer placed at a distance above a boiling cryogenic medium, where the atomized droplets begin to solidify as they fall from the vapor phase and freeze completely when they encounter the cryogenic liquid. Finally, the suspended frozen particles are collected by sieving or by letting the cryogen evaporate, followed by sublimation to obtain a dry powder (Chow et al. 2007).

Following spray freezing, the product is freeze-dried by direct sublimation of the ice at low temperature under reduced pressure. The high surface area-to-mass ratio achieved in the atomization process can potentially improve heat transfer and associated mass transfer during lyophilization of bulk drugs compared to conventional freeze-drying in vials (Vishali et al. 2019). Freeze-drying can also vary according to the respective pressure ranges, such as atmospheric or sub-atmospheric pressure SFD. The use of a fluidized bed with the integration of the SFD process was likewise applied either under atmospheric or sub-atmospheric conditions (Wang et al. 2006; Leuenberger et al. 2006; Anandharamakrishnan et al. 2010; Vishali et al. 2019).

The next section will present some of the patents and/or new concepts developed over the years working on bulk materials and granules to provide practical considerations for successful SFD industrialization.

9.6.2 Patented Concepts by Arsem, Bruttini, and Oyler

Arsem (1986) registered a patent for continuous freeze-drying that operates a slurry of material to be freeze-dried under pressure. In this method, the slurry is continuously flowing along a vertical tower including a freezing section and a drying chamber. The slurry is loaded into a refrigerated tank having cooling plates with numerous vertical holes or pores. These holes open into a vacuum vertical tower having heated walls, and the ice in the frozen slurry sublimates, thanks to the radiant heat from the walls as it falls to the bottom of the tower. Even though the freezing and the drying chambers are connected, vacuum conditions can be maintained in the drying chamber, thanks to the incredible pressure drop developed in the frozen slurry flowing in the connection pores. However, without atomization of the material, the final dried product is not uniform in size and morphologically uncontrolled, thus, it requires additional size reduction processing (Arsem 1986).

Bruttini (1993) suggested a nebulizing system to spray the product to be frozen onto the surface of a cylindrical shaft, from which the frozen product is removed by scraping. The frozen material is then collected and distributed onto a series of revolving planes to be dried. The heat required for sublimation is provided by heating elements consisting of radiating plate or lamp elements placed between the revolving planes. Finally, the freeze-dried product is passed through a dimensional selector and loaded into a removable container. Bruttini claimed that the system enables continuous control of the powdery granule size without subjecting the final product to a heavy mechanical action that would alter the morphological structure of the product (Bruttini 1993).

Another patented system, which can be considered as a combination of Arsem and Bruttini systems, has been proposed by Oyler (1993). In the method, liquid substances are sprayed into a freezing vessel containing a cold gas, usually air, at ambient pressure. The frozen particles settle at the bottom of the vessel and are then transferred into a vertical drying tower by a rotary valve. The drying tower is equipped with a vacuum lock, ice condensers, and a heat source on the walls. While the particles fall through the vacuum tower, the heat emitted from the tower walls causes the ice in the particles to sublimate. The resulting sublimated vapor is removed from the tower by low-temperature condensation, while the final dried particles are collected at the bottom and transferred to a container via a vacuum lock (Oyler 1993).

9.6.3 LyoMotion System by Meridion

The LyoMotion freeze-drying system developed by Meridion Technologies is known as the first industrial-scale unit tested as a batch technology. And the concept of an integrated spray freezing chamber (SprayCon) connected to the cylindrical rotating drum (LyoMotion) in a full line was introduced by Meridion Technologies to manufacture the SFD process. A liquid feed is first split into droplets, which are in the range of 300–600 μm in diameter, by laminar jet disintegration via a nozzle placed on top of a double-walled cylindrical chamber cooled with gas (−110°C) (Meridion Technologies 2021). The droplets are frozen as they pass through the chamber and are continuously discharged into the pre-chilled drum of the rotary dryer, where dynamic bulk lyophilization takes place by constant gentle mixing under vacuum. The required sublimation energy is supplied by radiating sources and temperature-controlled surfaces. The dried particles are then transported as bulk powder to a container that can be connected to a sterile isolator for powder filling. One of the main problems with the LyoMotion system is that the lyophilized product cannot be continuously separated from the SprayCon chamber, thus requiring a subsequent intervention. The use of multibatch rotary dryers can be an alternative solution for the separation of dried powders, making this technology highly suitable for continuous processing (Adali et al. 2020; Luy and Stamato 2020).

9.6.4 Stirred Freeze-Drying by Hosokawa Micron

Hosokawa Micron proposed the Vrieco-Nauta conical dryer, a universal batch dryer called Active Freeze Dryer which, in principle, could allow continuous freeze-drying at low temperatures and pressures (Hosokawa Micron 2021). The raw material is frozen using a freezing medium and then, is fed into the drying chamber, which consists of a conical body with a mixing screw attached to a rotating arm. The thermal energy required for drying is supplied to the product through a jacketed wall heated by steam or hot water/oil. Thanks to continuous mixing, the Vriesco-Nauta vacuum dryer ensures rapid heat distribution to the product. Moreover, continuous mixing eliminates the additional post-processing steps required to obtain a powder after freeze-drying. When the sublimated vapor is removed, the product temperature begins to rise until it is equal to the jacket temperature. The dried particles are then transported to the filter alongside the dryer, offering ease of discharge with a low amount of residue (Bullich 2015; Adali et al. 2020).

9.6.5 Fine-Spray Freeze-Drying by ULVAC

The fully packaged process system for sterile production including powder filling and capping was introduced by ULVAC Technologies, namely fine-spray freeze-drying technology (Micropowderdry™ System). In the system, liquid droplets are gradually dispersed from the liquid column to the vacuum chamber through a special nozzle, and droplets self-freezing occurs thanks to the vapor flash-off cooling the droplets while falling in the vacuum chamber. Therefore, the self-freezing and frozen particle formation take place almost instantly in the vacuum chamber. The frozen particles are then collected on the heated belt in the chamber to obtain a dried powder. The main problem of the system is that the relatively thick layer of the frozen particle can impair the heat transfer to the center of the frozen layer. By combining 150L/Batch capacity mass production equipment and powder filling system, a completely closed design for sterile formulation has been established. ULVAC Technologies and Azbil Telstar Technologies have a cooperation agreement to further develop the fine-spray freeze-drying technology as a continuous process, but the system is still under development (Bullich 2015; Adali et al. 2020).

9.6.6 Rey's Concept

Another heated conveyor system was proposed by Rey in 2010. There is no atomization process in this system, however, liquid droplets are obtained by regularly dropping the liquid in a counter-current cold air stream. The frozen particles placed on the heated conveyor subsequently pass through a vacuum lock system and are continuously loaded into the dryer. A controlled infrared-, or microwave-heating system mounted on top of the drying chamber provides the energy required for sublimation. Following the drying process, the dried powders are transferred to the filling section, where pre-sterilized vials are continuously filled and then capped (Rey 2010; Pisano et al. 2019b).

9.6.7 LYnfinity by IMA

The IMA Group has recently proposed a new continuous aseptic SFD concept, shown in Figure 9.6, that can be considered an improvement of Rey's concept. In this system, the liquid is continuously sprayed into a cryogenically cooled freezing tower via a special nozzle operated at a specific frequency. The precise atomization control allows for uniform droplet size and, thus, consistent drying times. The resultant

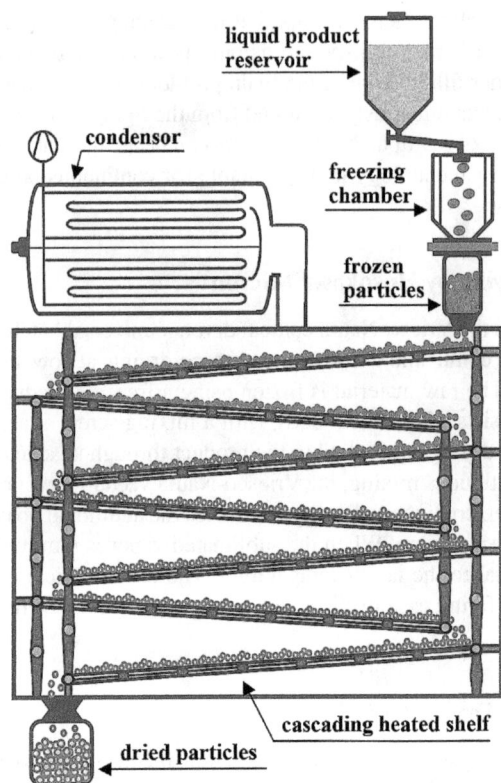

FIGURE 9.6   Schematic design of LYnfinity, continuous aseptic spray freeze-drying, proposed by IMA Group.

frozen particles are continuously settled on heated and cascading vibratory shelves in the drying module. Finally, the dried powder is discharged into a container, ensuring high levels of sterility (Adali et al. 2020; IMA Group 2021).

9.7 Conclusion

The present contribution is a comprehensive description of freeze-drying concepts proposed over the years, which can be applied to the continuous production of pharmaceutical products. While significant progress has been made in the development of new approaches to continuous manufacturing, efforts to implement the technique in a GMP environment are still necessary. Continuous freeze-dryers for either unit doses or bulk materials can replace batch processes in the production of pharmaceutical products only if they guarantee sterility and product quality requirements. The application of the new technologies described above may help the pharmaceutical industry in the development of continuous manufacturing. Some hurdles to the application of continuous manufacturing remain, such as costs for the replacement of existing equipment and for the training of operators, but those drawbacks are largely overcome by the benefits of continuous manufacturing, including better quality control, increased productivity, and smaller footprints.

REFERENCES

Adali, Merve B., Antonello A. Barresi, Gianluca Boccardo, and Roberto Pisano. 2020. "Spray freeze-drying as a solution to continuous manufacturing of pharmaceutical products in bulk." *Processes 8* (6). https://doi.org/10.3390/PR8060709.

Adeli, Ehsan. 2017. "The use of spray freeze drying for dissolution and oral bioavailability improvement of Azithromycin." *Powder Technology 319*: 323–331. https://doi.org/10.1016/j.powtec.2017.06.043.

Amorij, J.P., V. Saluja, A.H. Petersen, W.L.J. Hinrichs, A. Huckriede, and H.W. Frijlink. 2007. "Pulmonary delivery of an inulin-stabilized influenza subunit vaccine prepared by spray-freeze drying induces systemic, mucosal humoral as well as cell-mediated immune responses in BALB/c mice." *Vaccine 25* (52): 8707–8717. https://doi.org/10.1016/j.vaccine.2007.10.035.

Anandharamakrishnan, Chinnaswamy, Chris D. Rielly, and Andrew G.F. Stapley. 2010. "Spray-freeze-drying of whey proteins at sub-atmospheric pressures." *Dairy Science and Technology 90*: 321–334. https://doi.org/10.1051/dst/2010013.

Arsem, Harold B. 1986. "Continuous freeze drying." US Patent US 4590684, May 1986.

Arsiccio, A., A. C. Sparavigna, R. Pisano, and A. A. Barresi. 2019. "Measuring and predicting pore size distribution of freeze-dried solutions." *Drying Technology 37* (4): 435–47. https://doi.org/10.1080/07373937.2018.1430042.

Arsiccio, Andrea, Antonello A. Barresi, and Roberto Pisano. 2017. "Prediction of Ice crystal size distribution after freezing of pharmaceutical solutions." *Crystal Growth & Design 17* (9): 4573–81. https://doi.org/10.1021/acs.cgd.7b00319.

Arsiccio, Andrea, Antonello A. Barresi, Thomas De Beer, Irene Oddone, Pieter Jan Van Bockstal, and Roberto Pisano. 2018. "Vacuum induced surface freezing as an effective method for improved inter- and intra-vial product homogeneity." *European Journal of Pharmaceutics and Biopharmaceutics 128* (March): 210–19. https://doi.org/10.1016/j.ejpb.2018.04.002.

Barron, Melisa K., Timothy J. Young, Keith P. Johnston, and Robert O. Williams. 2003. "Investigation of processing parameters of spray freezing into liquid to prepare polyethylene glycol polymeric particles for drug delivery." *AAPS PharmSciTech 4*: 1–13. https://doi.org/10.1208/pt040212.

Becker, W. 1957. Gefriertrocknungsverfahren. DE 967120 C, issued 1957.

Benson, Sidney W., and David A. Ellis. 1948. "Surface areas of proteins. I. Surface areas and heats of absorption." *Journal of the American Chemical Society 70*: 3563–3569. https://doi.org/10.1021/ja01191a007.

Bi, Ru, Wei Shao, Qun Wang, and Na Zhang. 2008. "Spray-freeze-dried dry powder inhalation of insulin-loaded liposomes for enhanced pulmonary delivery." *Journal of Drug Targeting 16*: 639–648. https://doi.org/10.1080/10611860802201134.

Bin, Liew K., Ashok K. Janakiraman, Fashli S. A. Razak, A. B. M. Helal Uddin, Md Zaidul I. Sarker, Long C. Ming, Bey H. Goh. 2020. "Supercritical Fluid Technology and Its Pharmaceutical Applications: A Revisit with Two Decades of Progress." *Indian Journal of Pharmaceutical Education and Research 54* (2): 1–11. https://doi.org/10.5530/ijper.54.2s.56.

Bobba, Serena, Nunzio Zinfollino, and Davide Fissore. 2021. "Application of near-infrared spectroscopy to statistical control in freeze-drying processes." *European Journal of Pharmaceutics and Biopharmaceutics 168* (August): 26–37. https://doi.org/10.1016/j.ejpb.2021.08.009.

Bockstal, Pieter-Jan Van, Jos Corver, Laurens De Meyer, Chris Vervaet, and Thomas De Beer. 2018. "Thermal imaging as a noncontact inline process analytical tool for product temperature monitoring during continuous freeze-drying of unit doses." *Analytical Chemistry 90* (22): 13591–99. https://doi.org/10.1021/acs.analchem.8b03788.

Braig, Veronika, Christoph Konnerth, Wolfgang Peukert, and Geoffrey Lee. 2019. "Can spray freeze-drying improve the re-dispersion of crystalline nanoparticles of pure naproxen?" *International Journal of Pharmaceutics 564*: 293–298. https://doi.org/10.1016/j.ijpharm.2019.04.061.

Broadwin, Samuel M. 1965. Centrifugal freeze drying apparatus, issued 1965. US3203108A.

Brouckaert, Davinia, Laurens De Meyer, Brecht Vanbillemont, Pieter-Jan Van Bockstal, Joris Lammens, Séverine Mortier, Jos Corver, Chris Vervaet, Ingmar Nopens, and Thomas De Beer. 2018. "Potential of near-infrared chemical imaging as process analytical technology tool for continuous freeze-drying." *Analytical Chemistry 90* (7): 4354–62. https://doi.org/10.1021/acs.analchem.7b03647.

Bruttini, Roberto. 1993. Continuous freeze drying apparatus. issued 1993. US Patent US 5269077.

Bullich, R. 2015. Telstar industry session: Continuous freeze drying. In *Proceedings of the Innovation Forum in Pharmaceutical Process Professional, Pharmaprocess Forum*, Barcelona, Spain, 27–28 October 2015.

Cal, Krzysztof, and Krzysztof Sollohub. 2010. "Spray drying technique. I: Hardware and process parameters." *Journal of Pharmaceutical Sciences 102*: 1165–1172. https://doi.org/10.1002/jps.

Capozzi, Luigi C., Bernhardt L. Trout, and Roberto Pisano. 2019. "From batch to continuous: Freeze-drying of suspended vials for pharmaceuticals in unit-doses." *Industrial & Engineering Chemistry Research 58* (4): 1635–49. https://doi.org/10.1021/acs.iecr.8b02886.

Capozzi, Luigi C., Pisano, Roberto. 2018. "Looking inside the 'black box': Freezing engineering to ensure the quality of freeze-dried biopharmaceuticals." *European Journal of Pharmaceutics and Biopharmaceutics 129*: 58–65.

Carrasquillo, Karen G., Ann M. Stanley, Juan C. Aponte-Carro, Patricia De Jésus, Henry R. Costantino, Carlos J. Bosques, and Kai Griebenow. 2001. "Non-aqueous encapsulation of excipient-stabilized spray-freeze dried BSA into poly(factide-co-glycolide) microspheres results in release of native protein." *Journal of Controlled Release 76*: 199–208. https://doi.org/10.1016/S0168-3659(01)00430-8.

Castrejón-Pita, J. R., W. R.S. Baxter, J. Morgan, S. Temple, G. D. Martin, and I. M. Hutchings. 2013. "Future, opportunities and challenges of inkjet technologies." *Atomization and Sprays 23*: 571–595. https://doi.org/10.1615/AtomizSpr.2013007653.

Cheow, Wean Sin, Mabel Li Ling Ng, Katherine Kho, and Kunn Hadinoto. 2011. "Spray-freeze-drying production of thermally sensitive polymeric nanoparticle aggregates for inhaled drug delivery: Effect of freeze-drying adjuvants." *International Journal of Pharmaceutics 404*, 289–300. https://doi.org/10.1016/j.ijpharm.2010.11.021.

Chow, Albert H.L., Henry H.Y. Tong, Pratibhash Chattopadhyay, and Boris Y. Shekunov. 2007. "Particle engineering for pulmonary drug delivery." *Pharmaceutical Research 24*: 411–437. https://doi.org/10.1007/s11095-006-9174-3.

Clavaud, Matthieu, Yves Roggo, Klara Dégardin, Pierre-Yves Sacré, Philippe Hubert, and Eric Ziemons. 2016. "Moisture content determination in an antibody-drug conjugate freeze-dried medicine by near-infrared spectroscopy: A case study for release testing." *Journal of Pharmaceutical and Biomedical Analysis 131*: 380–90. https://doi.org/10.1016/j.jpba.2016.09.014.

Colucci, Domenico, Davide Fissore, Antonello A. Barresi, and Richard D. Braatz. 2020. "A new mathematical model for monitoring the temporal evolution of the ice crystal size distribution during freezing in pharmaceutical solutions." *European Journal of Pharmaceutics and Biopharmaceutics 148* (January): 148–59. https://doi.org/10.1016/j.ejpb.2020.01.004.

Costantino, Henry R., Laleh Firouzabadian, Ken Hogeland, Chichih Wu, Chris Beganski, Karen G. Carrasquillo, Melissa Córdova, Kai Griebenow, Stephen E. Zale, and Mark A. Tracy. 2000. "Protein spray-freeze drying. Effect of atomization conditions on particle size and stability." *Pharmaceutical Research 17*: 1374–1383. https://doi.org/10.1023/A:1007570030368.

Daneshmand, Behnaz, Homa Faghihi, Maryam Amini Pouya, Shabnam Aghababaie, Majid Darabi, and Alireza Vatanara. 2019. "Application of disaccharides alone and in combination, for the improvement of stability and particle properties of spray-freeze dried IgG." *Pharmaceutical Development and Technology 24*: 439–447. https://doi.org/10.1080/10837450.2018.1507039.

Derksen, Marco W.J., Piet J.M. Van De Oetelaar, and Frans A. Maris. 1998. "The use of near-infrared spectroscopy in the efficient prediction of a specification for the residual moisture content of a freeze-dried product." *Journal of Pharmaceutical and Biomedical Analysis 17* (3): 473–80. https://doi.org/10.1016/S0731-7085(97)00216-1.

Dey, Paramita, and Sabyasachi Maiti. 2010. "Orodispersible tablets: A new trend in drug delivery." *Journal of Natural Science, Biology and Medicine 1* (1): 2. https://doi.org/10.4103/0976-9668.71663.

Dugas, Helene L., and Robert O. Williams III. 2016. "Nanotechnology for Pulmonary and Nasal Drug Delivery". In *Nanotechnology and Drug Delivery*, edited by Jose L. Arias, 102–145. Boca Raton: CRC Press.

Emami, Fakhrossadat, Alireza Vatanara, Abdolhosein Rouholamini Najafabadi, Yejin Kim, Eun Ji Park, Soroush Sardari, and Dong Hee Na. 2018a. "Effect of amino acids on the stability of spray freeze-dried immunoglobulin G in sugar-based matrices." *European Journal of Pharmaceutical Sciences 119*: 39–48. https://doi.org/10.1016/j.ejps.2018.04.013.

Emami, Fakhrossadat, Alireza Vatanara, Eun Ji Park, and Dong Hee Na. 2018b. "Drying technologies for the stability and bioavailability of biopharmaceuticals." *Pharmaceutics 10*: 1–22. https://doi.org/10.3390/pharmaceutics10030131.

Emami, Fakhrossadat, Alireza Vatanara, Faezeh Vakhshiteh, Yejin Kim, Tae Wan Kim, and Dong Hee Na. 2019. "Amino acid-based stable adalimumab formulation in spray freeze-dried microparticles for pulmonary delivery." *Journal of Drug Delivery Science and Technology 54*:101–249. https://doi.org/10.1016/j.jddst.2019.101249.

Engstrom, Josh D., Dale T. Simpson, Edwina S. Lai, Robert O. Williams, and Keith P. Johnston. 2007. "Morphology of protein particles produced by spray freezing of concentrated solutions." *European Journal of Pharmaceutics and Biopharmaceutics 65*: 149–162. https://doi.org/10.1016/j.ejpb.2006.08.005.

FDA. 2021. "About the emerging technology program." Accessed November 17, 2021. https://www.fda.gov/about-fda/center-drug-evaluation-and-research-cder/emerging-technology-program.

Fissore, Davide, Roberto Pisano, and Antonello A. Barresi. 2011. "Advanced approach to build the design space for the primary drying of a pharmaceutical freeze-drying process." *Journal of Pharmaceutical Sciences 100*: 4922–33. https://doi.org/10.1002/jps.22668.

Fissore, Davide, Roberto Pisano, and Antonello A. Barresi. 2015. "Using Mathematical Modeling and Prior Knowledge for QbD in Freeze-Drying Processes." In *AAPS Advances in the Pharmaceutical Sciences Series, 18*:565–93. https://doi.org/10.1007/978-1-4939-2316-8_23.

Fissore, Davide, Pisano, Roberto, Barresi, Antonello A. 2018. "Process analytical technology for monitoring pharmaceuticals freeze-drying. A comprehensive review." *Drying Technology 36* (15): 1839–1865.

Ghosh, Tanmoy, Amitava Ghosh, and Devi Prasad. 2011. "A review on new generation orodispersible tablets and its future prospective." *International Journal of Pharmacy and Pharmaceutical Sciences 3* (1): 1–7.

Gottlieb, Scott. 2021. "FDA statement on FDA's modern approach to advanced pharmaceutical manufacturing." Accessed November 17, 2021. https://www.fda.gov/news-events/press-announcements/fda-statement-fdas-modern-approach-advanced-pharmaceutical-manufacturing.

Harguindeguy, Maitê, and Davide Fissore. 2021. "Temperature/end point monitoring and modelling of a batch freeze-drying process using an infrared camera." *European Journal of Pharmaceutics and Biopharmaceutics 158*: 113–22. https://doi.org/10.1016/j.ejpb.2020.10.023.

Harguindeguy, Maitê, Lorenzo Stratta, Davide Fissore, and Roberto Pisano. 2021. "Investigation of the freezing phenomenon in vials using an infrared camera." *Pharmaceutics 13*: 1664. https://doi.org/10.3390/pharmaceutics13101664.

Her, Jae Young, Chi Sung Song, Seung Ju Lee, and Kwang Geun Lee. 2010. "Preparation of kanamycin powder by an optimized spray freeze-drying method." *Powder Technology 199*: 159–164. https://doi.org/10.1016/j.powtec.2009.12.018.

Hosokawa Micron. 2021. "Active freeze dryer." Accessed November 5, 2021. https://www.hosokawa-micron-bv.com/technologies/industrial-dryers/batch-drying-technologies/active-freeze-dryer.html.

Hu, J., T. L. Rogers, J. Brown, T. Young, K. P. Johnston, and R. O. Williams. 2002. "Improvement of dissolution rates of poorly water soluble APIs using novel spray freezing into liquid technology." *Pharmaceutical Research 19*: 1278–1284. https://doi.org/10.1023/A:1020390422785.

Hu, Jiahui, Keith P. Johnston, and Robert O. Williams. 2003. "Spray freezing into liquid (SFL) particle engineering technology to enhance dissolution of poorly water soluble drugs: Organic solvent versus organic/aqueous co-solvent systems." *European Journal of Pharmaceutical Sciences 20*: 295–303. https://doi.org/10.1016/S0928-0987(03)00203-3.

Hu, Jiahui, Keith P. Johnston, and Robert O. Williams. 2004. "Rapid dissolving high potency danazol powders produced by spray freezing into liquid process." *International Journal of Pharmaceutics 271*: 145–154. https://doi.org/10.1016/j.ijpharm.2003.11.003.

Ibrahim, Mariam, Manolya Kukut Hatipoglu, and Lucila Garcia-Contreras. 2019. "Cryogenic fabrication of dry powders to enhance the solubility of a promising anticancer drug, SHetA2, for oral administration." *AAPS PharmSciTech 20*:1–10. https://doi.org/10.1208/s12249-018-1204-z.

IMA Group. 2021. "LYnfinity: Continuous Aseptic Spray-Freeze-Drying." Accessed November 10, 2021. https://ima.it/pharma/machine/lynfinity/.

Ishwarya, S. Padma, Chinnaswamy Anandharamakrishnan, and Andrew G.F. Stapley.. 2015. "Spray-freeze-drying: A novel process for the drying of foods and bioproducts." *Trends in Food Science and Technology Technol. 41*: 161–181. https://doi.org/10.1016/j.tifs.2014.10.008.

Ishwarya, S. Padma, Chinnaswamy Anandharamakrishnan, and Andrew G.F. Stapley. 2017. "Spray Freeze Drying". In *Handbook of Drying for Dairy Products*, edited by C. Anandharamakrishnan, 123–148. Chichester: Wiley-Blackwell.

Ito, Takaaki, Tomoyuki Okuda, Yoshimasa Takashima, and Hirokazu Okamoto. 2019. "Naked pDNA inhalation powder composed of hyaluronic acid exhibits high gene expression in the lungs." *Molecular Pharmaceutics 16*: 489–497. https://doi.org/10.1021/acs.molpharmaceut.8b00502.

Jones, J. A., I. R. Last, B. F. MacDonald, and K. A. Prebble. 1993. "Development and transferability of near-infrared methods for determination of moisture in a freeze-dried injection product." *Journal of Pharmaceutical and Biomedical Analysis 11* (11–12): 1227–31. https://doi.org/10.1016/0731-7085(93)80108-D.

Faghihi, Homa, Majid Darabi, Maryam Mirmoeini, and Alireza Vatanara. 2021. "Formulation and evaluation of inhalable microparticles of rizatriptan benzoate processed by spray freeze-drying." *Journal of Drug Delivery Science and Technology 62*: 102356. https://doi.org/10.1016/j.jddst.2021.102356.

Kho, Katherine, and Kunn Hadinoto. 2011. "Optimizing aerosolization efficiency of dry-powder aggregates of thermally-sensitive polymeric nanoparticles produced by spray-freeze-drying." *Powder Technology 214*: 169–176. https://doi.org/10.1016/j.powtec.2011.08.010.

Kondo, Masahiro, Toshiyuki Niwa, Hirokazu Okamoto, and Kazumi Danjo. 2009. "Particle characterization of poorly water-soluble drugs using a spray freeze drying technique." *Chemical and Pharmaceutical Bulletin 57*: 657–662. https://doi.org/10.1248/cpb.57.657.

Lammens, Joris, Séverine Thérèse F.C. Mortier, Laurens De Meyer, Brecht Vanbillemont, Pieter-Jan Van Bockstal, Simon Van Herck, Jos Corver, et al. 2018. "The relevance of shear, sedimentation and diffusion during spin freezing, as potential first step of a continuous freeze-drying process for unit doses." *International Journal of Pharmaceutics 539* (1–2): 1–10. https://doi.org/10.1016/j.ijpharm.2018.01.009.

Lavanya, M.N., R. Preethi, J.A. Moses, and C. Anandharamakrishnan. 2020. "Production of bromelain aerosols using spray-freeze-drying technique for pulmonary supplementation." *Drying Technology 39*: 358–370. https://doi.org/10.1080/07373937.2020.1832514.

Leuenberger, Hans, Matthias Plitzko, and Maxim Puchkov. 2006. "Spray freeze drying in a fluidized bed at normal and low pressure." *Drying Technology 24*: 711–719. https://doi.org/10.1080/07373930600684932.

Leys, L., B. Vanbillemont, P.J. Van Bockstal, J. Lammens, G. Nuytten, J. Corver, C. Vervaet, and T. De Beer. 2020. "A primary drying model-based comparison of conventional batch freeze-drying to continuous spin-freeze-drying for unit doses." *European Journal of Pharmaceutics and Biopharmaceutics 157*: 97–107. https://doi.org/10.1016/j.ejpb.2020.09.009.

Liang, Wanling, Alan Y.L. Chan, Michael Y.T. Chow, Fiona F.K. Lo, Yingshan Qiu, Philip C.L. Kwok, and Jenny K.W. Lam. 2018. "Spray freeze drying of small nucleic acids as inhaled powder for pulmonary delivery." *Asian Journal of Pharmaceutical Sciences 13*: 163–172. https://doi.org/10.1016/j.ajps.2017.10.002.

Liao, Qiuying, Long Yip, Michael Y.T. Chow, Shing Fung Chow, Hak Kim Chan, Philip C.L. Kwok, and Jenny K.W. Lam. 2019. "Porous and highly dispersible voriconazole dry powders produced by spray freeze drying for pulmonary delivery with efficient lung deposition." *International Journal of Pharmaceutics 560*: 144–154. https://doi.org/10.1016/j.ijpharm.2019.01.057.

Lietta, Elena, Domenico Colucci, Giovanni Distefano, and Davide Fissore. 2019. "On the use of infrared thermography for monitoring a vial freeze-drying process." *Journal of Pharmaceutical Sciences 108* (1): 391–98. https://doi.org/10.1016/j.xphs.2018.07.025.

Lo, Jason C.K., Harry W. Pan, and J. K.W. Lam. 2021. "Inhalable protein powder prepared by spray-freeze-drying using hydroxypropyl- β -cyclodextrin as excipient." *Pharmaceutics 13*: 615. https://doi.org/10.3390/pharmaceutics13050615.

López-Iglesias, Clara, Alba M. Casielles, Ayça Altay, Ruggero Bettini, Carmen Alvarez-Lorenzo, and Carlos A. García-González. 2019. "From the printer to the lungs: Inkjet-*printed* aerogel particles for pulmonary delivery." *Chemical Engineering Journal 357*: 559–566. https://doi.org/10.1016/j.cej.2018.09.159.

Luy, Bernhard, and Howard Stamato. 2020. "Part III Next Generation Drying *Technologies*". In *Drying Technologies for Biotechnology and Pharmaceutical Applications*, edited by Satoshi Ohtake, Ken-ichi Izutsu, and David Lechuga-Ballesteros, 217–237. Germany:Wiley-VCH.

Maa, Y.F., M. Ameri, C. Shu, L.G. Payne, and D. Chen. 2004. "Influenza vaccine powder formulation development: Spray-freeze-drying and stability evaluation." *Journal of Pharmaceutical Sciences 93*: 1912–1923.

Maa, Yuh-Fun, and Phuong-Anh Nguyen. 2001. Method of spray freeze drying proteins for *pharmaceutical* administration, issued 2001. US Patent 6284282.

Maa, Yuh-Fun, Steven J. Prestreski, and Terry L. Burkoth. 2003. Spray freeze dried compositions, issued 2003. US Patent 20030202978A1.

Maltesen, Morten Jonas, and Marco van de Weert. 2008. "Drying methods for protein pharmaceuticals." *Drug Discovery Today: Technologies 5*: 81–88. https://doi.org/10.1016/j.ddtec.2008.11.001.

Meridion Technologies. 2021. "Freeze drying of microspheres by spray freezing and dynamic bulk freeze drying." Accessed November 1, 2021. http://meridiontechnologies.de/en/technologien.php#spray

Meryman, H.T. 1959. "Sublimation freeze-drying without vacuum." *Science 130*: 628–629. https://doi.org/10.1126/science.130.3376.628.

Milani, Shahriar, Homa Faghihi, Abdolhosein R. Najafabadi, Mohsen Amini, Hamed Montazeri, and Alireza Vatanara. 2020. "Hydroxypropyl beta cyclodextrin: A water-replacement agent or a surfactant upon spray freeze-drying of IgG with enhanced stability and aerosolization." *Drug Development and Industrial Pharmacy 46*: 403–411. https://doi.org/10.1080/03639045.2020.1724131.

Moorkens, Evelien, Nicolas Meuwissen, Isabelle Huys, Paul Declerck, Arnold G. Vulto, and Steven Simoens. 2017. "The market of biopharmaceutical medicines: A snapshot of a diverse industrial landscape." *Frontiers in Pharmacology 8*. https://doi.org/10.3389/fphar.2017.00314.

Mordor Intelligence. 2021. "Biopharmaceuticals market – growth, trends, covid-19 impact, and forecasts (2021–2026)." Accessed November 16, 2021. https://www.mordorintelligence.com/industry-reports/global-biopharmaceuticals-market-industry.

Mueannoom, Wunlapa, Amon Srisongphan, Kevin M.G. Taylor, Stephan Hauschild, and Simon Gaisford. 2012. "Thermal ink-jet spray freeze-drying for preparation of excipient-free salbutamol sulphate for inhalation." *European Journal of Pharmaceutics and Biopharmaceutics 80*: 149–155. https://doi.org/10.1016/j.ejpb.2011.09.016.

Mumenthaler, M., and H. Leuenberger. 1991. "Atmospheric spray-freeze drying: A suitable alternative in freeze-drying technology." *International Journal of Pharmaceutics 72*: 97–110. https://doi.org/10.1016/0378-5173(91)90047-R.

Nakagawa, K., and Aurelie Hottot. 2012. "Modeling of freezing step during freeze-drying of drugs in vials." *AIChE Journal 59* (4): 215–28. https://doi.org/10.1002/aic.

Nakagawa, Kyuya, Aurélie Hottot, Séverine Vessot, and Julien Andrieu. 2007. "Modeling of freezing step during freeze-drying of drugs in vials." *AIChE Journal 53* (5): 1362–72. https://doi.org/10.1002/aic.11147.

Niwa, Toshiyuki, Daisuke Mizutani, and Kazumi Danjo. 2012. "Spray freeze-dried porous microparticles of a poorly water-soluble drug for respiratory delivery." *Chemical and Pharmaceutical Bulletin 60*: 870–876. https://doi.org/10.1248/cpb.c12-00208.

Oddone, Irene, Andrea Arsiccio, Chinwe Duru, Kiran Malik, Jackie Ferguson, Roberto Pisano, and Paul Matejtschuk. 2020. "Vacuum-induced surface freezing for the freeze-drying of the human growth hormone: How does nucleation control affect protein stability?" *Journal of Pharmaceutical Sciences 109* (1): 254–63. https://doi.org/10.1016/j.xphs.2019.04.014.

Oddone, Irene, Antonello A. Barresi, and Roberto Pisano. 2017. "Influence of controlled ice nucleation on the freeze-drying of pharmaceutical products: The secondary drying step." *International Journal of Pharmaceutics 524* (1–2): 134–40. https://doi.org/10.1016/j.ijpharm.2017.03.077.

Oddone, Irene, Pieter-Jan Van Bockstal, Thomas De Beer, and Roberto Pisano. 2016. "Impact of vacuum-induced surface freezing on inter- and intra-vial heterogeneity." *European Journal of Pharmaceutics and Biopharmaceutics 103*: 167–78. https://doi.org/10.1016/j.ejpb.2016.04.002.

Oddone, Irene, Roberto Pisano, Robert Bullich, and Paul Stewart. 2014. "Vacuum-induced nucleation as a method for freeze-drying cycle optimization." *Industrial & Engineering Chemistry Research 53* (47): 18236–44. https://doi.org/10.1021/ie502420f.

Ogienko, A.G., E.G. Bogdanova, N.A. Trofimov, S.A. Myz, A.A. Ogienko, B.A. Kolesov, A.S. Yunoshev, et al. 2017. "Large porous particles for respiratory drug delivery. Glycine-based formulations." *European Journal of Pharmaceutical Sciences 110*: 148–156. https://doi.org/10.1016/j.ejps.2017.05.007.

Oughton, Dominic Micheal. 2001. Freeze-drying process and apparatus. EP 0 812 411 B1, issued 2001.

Oyler, James R. Jr. 1993. Systems and methods for the deliquification of liquid-containing substances by flash sublimation, issued 1993. US Patent US 5230162.

Patel, Sajal M., Chandan Bhugra, and Michael J. Pikal. 2009. "Reduced pressure ice fog technique for controlled ice nucleation during freeze-drying." *AAPS PharmSciTech 10* (4): 1406–11. https://doi.org/10.1208/s12249-009-9338-7.

Petersen, Ansgar, Guenter Rau, and Birgit Glasmacher. 2006. "Reduction of primary freeze-drying time by electric field induced ice nucleus formation." *Heat and Mass Transfer/Waerme- Und Stoffuebertragung 42* (10): 929–38. https://doi.org/10.1007/s00231-006-0153-3.

Pikal, M.J., M.L. Roy, and Saroj Shah. 1984. "Mass and heat transfer in vial freeze-drying of pharmaceuticals: role of the vial." *Journal of Pharmaceutical Sciences 73* (9): 1224–37. https://doi.org/10.1002/jps.2600730910.

Pikal, Michael J., Robin Bogner, Vamsi Mudhivarthi, Puneet Sharma, and Pooja Sane. 2016. "Freeze-drying process development and scale-up: scale-up of edge vial versus center vial heat transfer coefficients, K V." *Journal of Pharmaceutical Sciences 105* (11): 3333–43. https://doi.org/10.1016/j.xphs.2016.07.027.

Pisano, Roberto, Andrea Arsiccio, Kyuya Nakagawa, and Antonello A. Barresi. 2019a. "Tuning, measurement and prediction of the impact of freezing on product morphology: A step toward improved design of freeze-drying cycles." *Drying Technology 37* (5): 579–99. https://doi.org/10.1080/07373937.2018.1528451.

Pisano, Roberto, Andrea Arsiccio, Luigi C. Capozzi, and Bernhardt L. Trout. 2019b. "Achieving continuous manufacturing in lyophilization: Technologies and approaches." *European Journal of Pharmaceutics and Biopharmaceutics 142*: 265–279. https://doi.org/10.1016/j.ejpb.2019.06.027.

Pisano, Roberto, Davide Fissore, and Antonello A. 2011. "Heat Transfer in Freeze-Drying Apparatus." In *Developments in Heat Transfer*. InTech. https://doi.org/10.5772/23799.

Pisano, Roberto, Davide Fissore, Antonello A. Barresi, Philippe Brayard, Pierre Chouvenc, and Bertrand Woinet. 2013. "Quality by design: Optimization of a freeze-drying cycle via design space in case of heterogeneous drying behavior and influence of the freezing protocol." *Pharmaceutical Development and Technology 18* (1): 280–95. https://doi.org/10.3109/10837450.2012.734512.

Pisano, Roberto, Fissore, Davide, Barresi, Antonello A. 2016. "noninvasive monitoring of a freeze-drying process for tert-butanol/water cosolvent-based formulations." *Industrial and Engineering Chemistry Research 55* (19): 5670–5680.

Pisano, Roberto. 2020. "Continuous manufacturing of lyophilized products: Why and how to make it happen." *American Pharmaceutical Review*. 2020. https://www.americanpharmaceuticalreview.com/Featured-Articles/563771-Continuous-Manufacturing-of-Lyophilized-Products-Why-and-How-to-Make-it-Happen/.

Poursina, Narges, Alireza Vatanara, Mohammad R. Rouini, Kambiz Gilani, and Abdolhossein Rouholamini Najafabadi. 2016. "The effect of excipients on the stability and aerosol performance of salmon calcitonin dry powder inhalers prepared via the spray freeze drying process." *Acta Pharmaceutica 66*: 207–218. https://doi.org/10.1515/acph-2016-0012.

Rambhatla, Shailaja, and Michael J. Pikal. 2003. "Heat and mass transfer scale-up issues during freeze-drying, I: Atypical radiation and the edge vial effect." *AAPS PharmSciTech 4* (2): 22–31. https://doi.org/10.1208/pt040214.

Ramisetty, Kiran A., Aniruddha B. Pandit, and Parag R. Gogate. 2013. "Investigations into ultrasound induced atomization." *Ultrasonics Sonochemistry 20*: 254–264. https://doi.org/10.1016/j.ultsonch.2012.05.001.

Rao, YamsaniMadhusudan, Suresh Bandari, RajendarKumar Mittapalli, and Ramesh Gannu. 2008. "Orodispersible tablets: An overview." *Asian Journal of Pharmaceutics 2* (1): 2. https://doi.org/10.4103/0973-8398.41557.

Rey, Louis. 2010. "Glimpses into the Realm of Freeze-Drying: Classical Issues and New Ventures." In *Freeze-Drying/Lyophilization of Pharmaceutical and Biological Products*: 3rd Edition.

Rogers, True L., Keith P. Johnston, and Robert O. Williams. 2001. "Solution-based particle formation of pharmaceutical powders by supercritical or compressed fluid CO2 and cryogenic spray-freezing technologies." *Drug Development and Industrial Pharmacy 27* (10): 1003–1015. https://doi.org/10.1081/DDC-100108363

Rogers, True L., Andrew C. Nelsen, Marazban Sarkari, Timothy J. Young, Keith P. Johnston, and Robert O. Williams. 2003. "Enhanced aqueous dissolution of a poorly water soluble drug by novel particle engineering technology: Spray-freezing into liquid with atmospheric freeze-drying." *Pharmaceutical Research 20*: 485–493. https://doi.org/10.1023/A:1022628826404.

Saluja, V., J.P. Amorij, J.C. Kapteyn, A.H. de Boer, H.W. Frijlink, and W.L.J. Hinrichs. 2010. "A comparison between spray drying and spray freeze drying to produce an influenza subunit vaccine powder for inhalation." *Journal of Controlled Release 144*: 127–133. https://doi.org/10.1016/j.jconrel.2010.02.025.

Schiffter, Heiko A. 2007. "Spray-freeze-drying in the manufacture of pharmaceuticals." *European Pharmaceutical Review 12*: 67–71.

Schiffter, Heiko, Jamie Condliffe, and Sebastian Vonhoff. 2010. "Spray-freeze-drying of nanosuspensions: The manufacture of insulin particles for needle-free ballistic powder delivery." *Journal of the Royal Society Interface 7*: 483–500. https://doi.org/10.1098/rsif.2010.0114.focus.

Shahin, Hend, Bhavani P. Vinjamuri, Azza A. Mahmoud, Suzan M. Mansour, Mahavir B. Chougule, and Lipika Chablani. 2021. "Formulation and optimization of sildenafil citrate-loaded PLGA large porous microparticles using spray freeze-drying technique: A factorial design and in-vivo pharmacokinetic study." *International Journal of Pharmaceutics 597*: 120320. https://doi.org/10.1016/j.ijpharm.2021.120320.

Shoyele, Sunday A., and Simon Cawthorne. 2006. "Particle engineering techniques for inhaled biopharmaceuticals." *Advanced Drug Delivery Reviews 58*: 1009–1029. https://doi.org/10.1016/j.addr.2006.07.010.

Sinha, Biswadip, Rainer H. Müller, and Jan P. Möschwitzer. 2013. "Bottom-up approaches for preparing drug nanocrystals: Formulations and factors affecting particle size." *International Journal of Pharmaceutics 453*: 126–141. https://doi.org/10.1016/j.ijpharm.2013.01.019.

Sluder J.C., Olsen R.W., Kenyon E.M. 1947. "Methods for production of dry powdered orange juice." *Food Technology 1*: 85–94.

Sonner, Christine, Yuh Fun Maa, and Geoffrey Lee. 2002. "Spray-freeze-drying for protein powder preparation: Particle characterization and a case study with trypsinogen stability." *Journal of Pharmaceutical Sciences 91*: 2122–2139. https://doi.org/10.1002/jps.10204.

Stratta, Lorenzo, Luigi C. Capozzi, Simone Franzino, and Roberto Pisano. 2020. "Economic analysis of a freeze-drying cycle." *Processes 8* (11): 1399. https://doi.org/10.3390/pr8111399.

Surasarang, S. Hengsawas, and R.O. Williams III. 2016. "Pharmaceutical Cryogenic Technologies." In *Formulating Poorly Water Soluble Drugs*, edited by Robert O. Williams III, Alan B. Watts, and Dave A. Miller, 527–607. Switzerland: Springer.

Süverkrüp, Richard, Sören N. Eggerstedt, Katja Gruner, Matthias Kuschel, Martin Sommerfeld, and Alf Lamprecht. 2013. "Collisions in fast droplet streams for the production of spherolyophilisates." *European Journal of Pharmaceutical Sciences 49*: 535–541. https://doi.org/10.1016/j.ejps.2013.05.010.

Sweeney, Lyle G., Zhaolin Wang, Raimar Loebenberg, Jonathan P. Wong, Carlos F. Lange, and Warren H. Finlay. 2005. "Spray-freeze-dried liposomal ciprofloxacin powder for inhaled aerosol drug delivery." *International Journal of Pharmaceutics 305*: 180–185. https://doi.org/10.1016/j.ijpharm.2005.09.010.

Tonnis, W.F., J.P. Amorij, M.A. Vreeman, H.W. Frijlink, G.F. Kersten, and W.L.J. Hinrichs. 2014. "Improved storage stability and immunogenicity of hepatitis B vaccine after spray-freeze drying in presence of sugars." *European Journal of Pharmaceutical Sciences 55*: 36–45. https://doi.org/10.1016/j.ejps.2014.01.005.

U.S. Food and Drug Administration (FDA). 2019. Quality Considerations for Continuous Manufacturing. In *Guidance for Industry*. Accessed November 5, 2021. https://www.fda.gov/regulatory-information/search-fda-guidance-documents/quality-considerations-continuous-manufacturing.

Vanbillemont, Brecht, John F. Carpenter, Christine Probst, and Thomas De Beer. 2020. "The impact of formulation composition and process settings of traditional batch versus continuous freeze-drying on protein aggregation." *Journal of Pharmaceutical Sciences 109* (11): 3308–18. https://doi.org/10.1016/j.xphs.2020.07.023.

Vishali, D.A., J. Monisha, S.K. Sivakamasundari, J.A. Moses, and C. Anandharamakrishnan. 2019. "Spray freeze drying: Emerging applications in drug delivery." *Journal of Controlled Release 300*: 93–101. https://doi.org/10.1016/j.jconrel.2019.02.044.

Walters, Robert H., Bakul Bhatnagar, Serguei Tchessalov, Ken I. Izutsu, Kouhei Tsumoto, and Satoshi Ohtake. 2014. "Next generation drying technologies for pharmaceutical applications." *Journal of Pharmaceutical Sciences 103*: 2673–2695. https://doi.org/10.1002/jps.23998.

Wang, Z.L., W.H. Finlay, M.S. Peppler, and L.G. Sweeney. 2006. "Powder formation by atmospheric spray freeze drying." *Powder Technology 170*: 45–52 https://doi.org/10.1016/j.powtec.2006.08.019

Wang, Zhaolin, and Warren H. Finlay. 2008. "Powder formation by atmospheric spray-freeze drying." US Patent 8322046 B2, 4 December 2012.

Wanning, Stefan, Richard Süverkrüp, and Alf Lamprecht. 2015. "Pharmaceutical spray freeze drying." *International Journal of Pharmaceutics 488*: 136–153. https://doi.org/10.1016/j.ijpharm.2015.04.053.

Williams, R., K. Johnston, T. Young, T. Rogers, M. Barron, Z. Yu, and J. Hu. 2002. "Process for production of nanoparticles and microparticles by spray freezing into liquid." US Patent 6862890 B2, 8 March 2005.

Wu, Libo, Jian Zhang, and Wiwik Watanabe. 2011. "Physical and chemical stability of drug nanoparticles." *Advanced Drug Delivery Reviews 63*: 456–469. https://doi.org/10.1016/j.addr.2011.02.001.

Ye, Tiantian, Jiaqi Yu, Qiuhua Luo, Shujun Wang, and Hak Kim Chan. 2017. "Inhalable clarithromycin liposomal dry powders using ultrasonic spray freeze drying." *Powder Technology 305*: 63–70. https://doi.org/10.1016/j.powtec.2016.09.053.

Yu, Zhongshui, Keith P. Johnston, and Robert O. Williams. 2006. "Spray freezing into liquid versus spray-freeze drying: Influence of atomization on protein aggregation and biological activity." *European Journal of Pharmaceutical Sciences. 27*: 9–18. https://doi.org/10.1016/j.ejps.2005.08.010.

Zheng, Yiwu, Xuxin Lai, Susanne Wrang Bruun, Henrik Ipsen, Jørgen Nedergaard Larsen, Henning Løwenstein, Ib Søndergaard, and Susanne Jacobsen. 2008. "Determination of moisture content of lyophilized allergen vaccines by nir spectroscopy." *Journal of Pharmaceutical and Biomedical Analysis 46* (3): 592–96. https://doi.org/10.1016/j.jpba.2007.11.011.

Part III

Process Analytical Technologies

10

Near-infrared Spectroscopy as Process Analytical Technology in Continuous Solid Dosage Form Manufacturing

Michiel Peeters, Thomas De Beer, and Ashish Kumar
Ghent University, Ghent, Belgium

CONTENTS

10.1 Introduction

It took until the late 1980s before there was a clear interest in near-infrared spectroscopy (NIRS) for pharmaceutical applications. There was a sharp increase in attention for NIRS after the introduction of the process analytical technology (PAT) guidance from the FDA, as reflected by the increasing number of publications utilizing NIRS from the mid-2000s onward. Now, NIRS is one of the most commonly used PAT process analyzers in the pharmaceutical industry (Burns and Ciurczak 2008; Markl et al. 2020; Zhong et al. 2020; FDA 2004) (Figure 10.1).

Several advantages make NIRS very attractive as an alternative to traditional analytical techniques for process monitoring applications. NIR spectra can give information about a great number of process variables simultaneously. Furthermore, different phases of the pharmaceutical manufacturing process may be monitored in real-time because measurements of complex matrices are performed without the need for sample preparation and optical fiber probes enable measurements of samples directly in the process stream (De Beer et al. 2011; Jamrógiewicz 2012; OZAKI 2012).

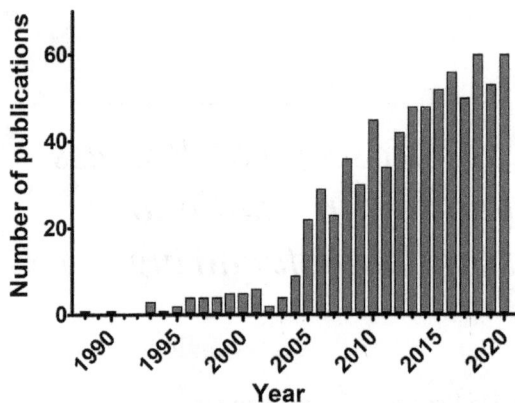

FIGURE 10.1 Number of pharmaceutical publications utilizing NIR spectroscopy. (Source: https://www.webof knowledge.com.)

10.2 Theory

10.2.1 NIR Fundamentals

Infrared spectroscopy studies the vibration properties of a sample. The most intense molecular vibrations are located in the mid-infrared range from 400 to 4000 cm^{-1} (2500–25000 nm). The near-infrared region covers the range before the mid-infrared and extends up to the visible region from 4000 to 12500 cm^{-1} (800–2500 nm). It contains absorption bands corresponding to overtone or combination vibrations with much lower intensity than the fundamental molecular vibrations (Siesler et al. 2006; Burns and Ciurczak 2008).

The basic physical principle of infrared spectroscopy can be described by the harmonic and anharmonic oscillator models. The harmonic oscillator is represented as a diatomic molecule with vibrating masses m$_1$ and m$_2$ in Figure 10.2.

The potential energy of the diatomic molecule, V, can be calculated by:

$$V = \frac{1}{2} \times k \times (r - r_e)^2 = \frac{1}{2} \times k \times x^2 \tag{10.1}$$

where r is the internuclear distance, r_e is the equilibrium bond length, k is the force constant of the bond, and $x = r - r_e$ is the displacement coordinate. The harmonic potential function is parabolic in shape and symmetrical about r_e, as seen in Figure 10.3.

The harmonic oscillator model leads to the vibrational frequency v_0:

$$v_0 = \frac{1}{2\pi} \sqrt{\frac{k}{m}} \tag{10.2}$$

where m is the reduced mass, such that:

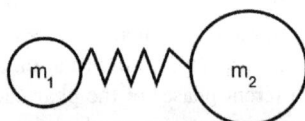

FIGURE 10.2 The harmonic oscillator, represented as a diatomic molecule with vibrating masses m$_1$ and m$_2$.

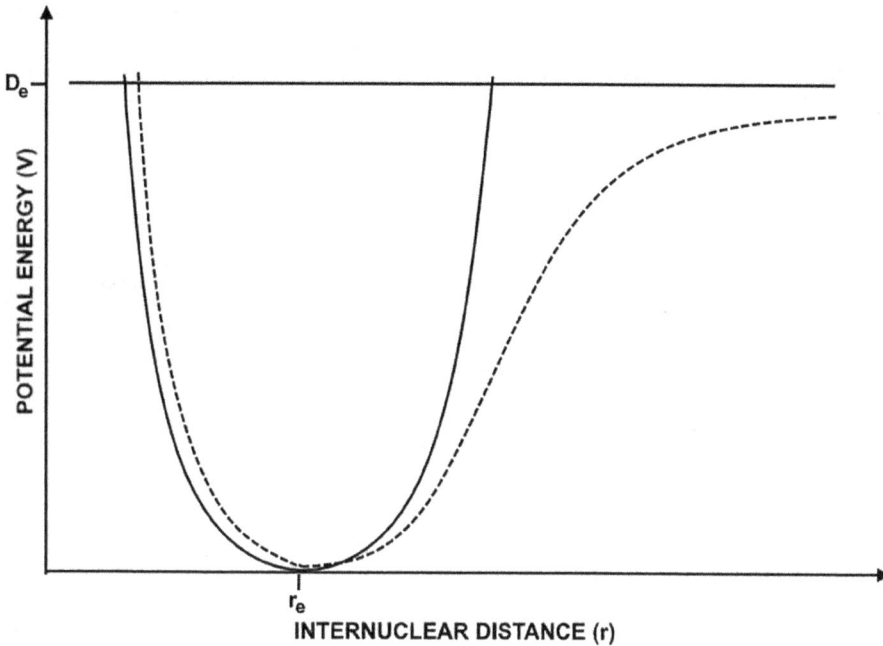

FIGURE 10.3 The harmonic (solid black line) and anharmonic (dotted black line) potential function showing the potential energy (V) in function of the internuclear distance (r). The dissociation energy (D_e) is indicated in the figure.

$$m = \frac{m_1 m_2}{m_1 + m_2} \qquad (10.3)$$

The Schrodinger equation shows that the vibrational energy E_{vib} can only have certain discrete values that are given by:

$$E_{vib} = h v_0 \left(n + \frac{1}{2} \right) \qquad (10.4)$$

where h is Planck's constant, v_0 is the vibrational frequency defined above, and n is the vibrational quantum number that can only have integer values 0, 1, 2, 3... The energy levels are expressed in wavenumber units (cm^{-1}) by G_{vib}:

$$G_{vib} = \frac{E_{vib}}{hc} = \bar{v}_0 \left(n + \frac{1}{2} \right) \qquad (10.5)$$

Where c is the speed of light and $\bar{v}_0$ the wavenumber of the vibrational transition.

Only heteronuclear diatomic molecules will interact with infrared radiation and exhibit vibrational energy level transitions. For the harmonic oscillator, the gap between the different vibrational energy levels is identical. Transitions are only allowed between neighboring energy levels and not across more than one energy level. From the Boltzmann distribution, most molecules at room temperature populate the ground level $n = 0$, and consequently, the so-called fundamental transitions between n = 0 and $n = 1$ dominate the vibrational absorption spectrum. These fundamental transitions give rise to absorption bands generally located in the min-infrared range. The harmonic oscillator model needs to be modified to explain the vibrational spectroscopic transitions responsible for the absorption bands in the near-infrared region. The harmonic oscillator model is no longer valid at larger amplitudes of vibration and shorter wavelengths because of the repulsive forces acting between the vibrating atoms and the possibility of dissociation when the internuclear distance is strongly extended (Watts and Hussain 2005; Burns and Ciurczak 2008; Siesler et al. 2006). An anharmonicity constant χ is introduced in the expression of the allowed energy levels G_n of the anharmonic oscillator model:

$$G_n = \frac{E_n}{hc} = \bar{v}_0 \left(n + \frac{1}{2} \right) - \chi \bar{v}_0 \left(n + \frac{1}{2} \right)^2 \tag{10.6}$$

The vibrational energy levels are not equally spaced as it was in the simple harmonic case, and overtone transitions such as $n = 0$ to $n = 2, 3, 4\ldots$ are allowed. The potential energy of the anharmonic oscillator model is represented by an asymmetric potential energy function in Figure 10.3 and expressed by the empirical Morse equation:

$$V = D_e (1 - e^{-bx})^2 \tag{10.7}$$

Where b is a constant, x is the difference between the internuclear distance and the equilibrium bond distance, and De is the dissociation energy measured from the equilibrium position, which is the minimum of the curve in Figure 10.3.

The intensity of the overtones depends on the anharmonicity constant of the chemical bonds (Burns and Ciurczak 2008). As seen in Table 10.1, functional groups containing a hydrogen atom such as C-H have a high anharmonicity constant, and hence dominate the overtone spectra. Polar carbonyl stretching bands which strongly absorb in the mean-infrared region have a low anharmonicity constant and their higher overtones are found to be very low in intensity.

Besides overtones, combinations of different fundamental vibrational transitions are responsible for the spectral absorption bands in the near-infrared region. These overtone and combination vibrations have much lower intensity than the fundamental vibrational transitions and their overlap decreases the specificity of NIR spectroscopy. Therefore, NIR spectroscopy was neglected for a long time by spectroscopists. However, the intensity and frequency of the C-H absorption bands are strongly influenced by near neighbors in the molecular structure, increasing the information content in NIR spectra and improving the specificity of NIRS. Furthermore, the weak absorptivity of most samples in NIRS can be positively exploited. Physically thick samples can be measured without sample dilution, being especially beneficial for PAT applications requiring direct measurement of the sample. Another benefit of the low intensity of the overtone and combination vibrations is the high penetration depth of the sampling beam in diffuse reflectance NIR measurements of powders. Relatively large volumes of material can be measured, avoiding problems of sample non-homogeneity and surface contamination (Burns and Ciurczak 2008; Watts and Hussain 2005).

10.2.2 Mainstream and Emerging Analyzer Technologies for Process Analytical Technology Applications

A NIRS system generally consists of a light source, an optical configuration for wavelength separation, a sample holder, and a detector. The tungsten-halogen lamp is the standard NIR source, being an

TABLE 10.1

Anharmonicity Constants χ for Selected Chemical Bonds

Anharmonicity Constants χ for Selected Chemical Bonds	
–CH	1.9×10^{-2}
–CD	1.5×10^{-2}
–CF	4×10^{-3}
–CCl	6×10^{-3}
–C=O	6.5×10^{-3}

inexpensive broadband light source with a long lifetime. When LEDs will become able to emit higher power in the lower energy region (1600–2500 nm) and will become less expensive in the future, their use as a NIR radiation source will probably increase. A continuous radiation source based on an arrangement of LEDs or specially constructed LEDs may replace the standard tungsten-halogen lamp in the newer NIRS. They could improve the SNR and robustness of these systems because they are fast responding and easily modulated (Pasquini 2018). Semi-conductor and thermal detectors are the two basic types of photodetectors for NIRS. Semi-conductor detectors are divided into photoconductive and photodiode detectors. Lead sulfide (PbS) and lead selenide (PbSe) are photoconductive materials used in the earliest detectors. Because of their limitations in linearity, speed, and sensitivity, they have largely been replaced by indium gallium arsenide (InGaAs) photodiode detectors (Bhakeev 2010). Thermal detectors are commonly used in Fourier-transform NIR (FT-NIR) instruments. The deuterated triglycine sulfate (DTGS) detector is a low-cost, wideband thermal NIR detector well suited for use in FT-NIR instruments. It contains a ferroelectric DTGS crystal in which the molecules are naturally aligned with a permanent electric dipole. The amount of charge stored at the crystal surface changes upon changes in the temperature of the DTGS crystal when infrared radiation hits the detector surface. The current that subsequently flows across a load resistor generates a signal voltage (Burns and Ciurczak 2008). The requirements of a NIRS PAT system mainly depend on whether it is used for at-line, online, or in-line measurements. The speed of systems used for at-line measurements is generally less important, but they should be more flexible in terms of the capacity to be used for a diversity of measurement tasks. The online and in-line instruments are selected based on their sensitivity, robustness, and speed. They should be robust toward environmental variations because they are often exposed to vibrations, temperature, and humidity fluctuations. Also, frequent maintenance is often difficult due to access and scheduling restrictions. The speed of in-line sensors is important because they are typically used to measure flowing materials. The materials in motion might be wet, sticky, or abrasive, and therefore, a robust design of the sampling system is critical. The spectrometer window should be made of a hard material and can have an automated cleaning mechanism. Sometimes, probes are heated slightly above the process temperature to reduce the risk of probe fouling (Harry G. Brittain, 2006).

The mainstream NIR analyzer technologies used for PAT applications in the pharmaceutical field are the scanning grating monochromator, the polychromator photodiode array (PDA) analyzer, the acousto-optical tunable filter (AOTF) instruments, and the FT-NIR analyzers (Bhakeev 2010). Their most important quality features are listed in Table 10.2. The scanning grating monochromator is the most conventional NIR analyzer and uses a concave holographic grating and an exit slit for wavelength separation and selection. This analyzer needs to make a direct compromise between spectroscopic resolution and signal-to-noise ratio (SNR). The slits need to be sufficiently wide to achieve an appropriate level of SNR. In order to achieve adequate resolution, the slits need to be sufficiently narrow. Another disadvantage of this type of analyzer is the issue of reproducible wavelength scanning and accurate wavelength registration related to the mechanical rotation of the grating. In the PDA analyzer, the exit slit from the scanning grating monochromator is replaced by a linear array of photodiodes, each recording a specific wavelength in the spectrum. Therefore, these instruments show better SNR and faster data acquisition times. The AOTF analyzer uses an optically anisotropic crystal lattice connected to a piezotransducer for wavelength selection. A radio frequency driver causes a high-frequency vibration of the transducer and hence the AOTF crystal is subjected to an acoustic wave. An incident NIR beam is scattered by the acoustic wave and only a very narrow band of wavelengths is directed to the sample. The key operational advantage of an AOTF analyzer is the very rapid wavelength selection and extremely rapid scanning. The most important practical issues are those of temperature control of the anisotropic crystal and insufficient wavelength accuracy (Bhakeev 2010). The FT-NIR analyzers use the principle of interferometry, where the interference between two beams with an optical path difference creates an interferogram. The interferometer of the FT-NIR analyzer consists of a beamsplitter and two mutually perpendicular plane mirrors, one of which moves along its axis. The beamsplitter partially reflects the incoming NIR light onto the fixed mirror and transmits the remaining to the moving mirror. The two reflected beams with an optical path difference are recombined at the beamsplitter and directed to the sample and finally to the detector. The recombination of the two beams creates the interferogram (Burns and Ciurczak 2008). The main advantages of the FT-NIR analyzers are: (i) the multiplex advantage; all wavelengths are measured

TABLE 10.2

Important Quality Features of the Mainstream and Emerging Analyzer Technologies for Process Analytical Technology Applications

	Mainstream				Emerging			
	Scanning Grating Monochromator	PDA	AOTF	FT-NIR	MEMS FT-NIR	Hadamard Device	Fabry-Perot Interferometer	LVF
Measurement speed (scans/s)	Fast – up to 50	Very fast – 200	Fast – 100	Average – 5	Very fast – 400	Average – 3	Average – 10	Average – 2–4
Width spectral range (nm)	Average, 900–1700, 1100–2100, 1400–2400	Average, 900–1700, 1100–2100, 1400–2400	Average, 900–1800, 1000–2000, 1200–2400	Very broad, 700–20000	Broad, 800–2300	Broad, 900–2400	Average, 1100–1850, 1750–2150, 1550–1950	Average, 950–1650, 1150–2150 (extended)
Signal-to-noise ratio	Average	Good	Good	Very good (>10000:1)	Good (3000:1)	Good (6000:1)	Very good (10000:1)	Very good (25000:1)
Reproducibility	Poor, needs mathematical treatment	Poor, needs mathematical treatment	Poor	Very good	Good	Poor, needs mathematical treatment	Good	NA
Stability (wavelength repeatability)	Limited	Limited	Limited	Very good	Good	Good	Limited	NA
Straylight effects	Sensitive	Sensitive	Sensitive	Insensitive	Insensitive	Insensitive	Insensitive	NA
Optical resolution (nm)	Average – good (5–20)	Average – good (5–20)	Average – good (3–10)	Good -Excellent (1–8)	Average (10)	Average (10–20)	Good (5)	Average (15–20)
Robust to vibrations	Very	Very	Good	Medium	Very	Very	Good	Very
Size	Compact	Compact	Compact	Compact	Very compact	Very compact	Very compact	Very compact
Temperature sensitivity	Little effect	Little effect	Sensitive	Sensitive	NA	Little effect	Insensitive	Insensitive

Polychromator photodiode array (PDA), Acousto-optical tunable filter (AOTF), Fourier transform near-infrared (FT-NIR), Micro-electro-mechanical systems (MEMS), Linear variable filter (LVF); NA = no information available. (Information obtained from Alcalà et al. 2013; Bhakeev 2010; Pasquini 2018).

simultaneously, allowing to have a fast measurement speed and high SNR; (ii) throughput advantage; there are no exit slits or other wavelength selecting devices, allowing to have a short measurement time and high SNR; (iii) cones advantage or wavelength repeatability; the FT-NIR uses a HeNe laser acting as an internal reference for each scan and hence it has high long-term stability and wavelength precision; (iv) immune to straylight effects; and (v) high optical resolution. These advantages have made FT-NIR analyzers very attractive for NIR applications. The high optical resolution, high SNR, wavelength accuracy, and lack of straylight effects are essential for the development and maintainability over time of near-infrared chemometric calibration models (Burns and Ciurczak 2008; Bhakeev 2010). The other mainstream NIR analyzers (i.e., scanning grating monochromator, PDA analyzer, and AOTF devices) all depend on some form of wavelength selection, and therefore spectral repeatability and reproducibility can become an issue (Bhakeev 2010).

Most of the emerging analyzer technologies are using micro-electro-mechanical systems (MEMS) technology to produce miniaturized NIRS systems. MEMS methods enable the manufacturing of microscaled and integrated devices using various techniques from the semi-conductor industry for chip manufacturing. These devices are typically small, light (about 100g), operate wirelessly, and have built-in batteries. Most recent miniaturized NIRS systems are using one of these four different technologies: (i) MEMS FT-NIR, (ii) Hadamard masks, (iii) Fabry-Perot interferometers, and (iv) linearly variable interference filters (LVFs) (Be et al. 2020; Pasquini 2018; Bhakeev 2010). The first technology was employed by the company Si-Ware Systems to make a micro-interferometer for an FT-NIR spectrophotometer. The Hadamard devices are multiplex devices that observe more than one wavelength at a time using masks. The light from the NIR source passes through a sample and is dispersed by a grating. Then, the mask selects only a part of the wavelengths and passes that light onto a single element detector. The spectrum is then obtained through an inverse Hadamard transform. Either digital micromirror devices (DMD) or MEMS chips can be used as a Hadamard mask. A DMD is used in digital light projector devices. The DMD is a matrix of micromirrors whose surface angle is controlled by a voltage applied individually to each mirror and hence wavelengths can be focused and collected on the single element detector. The NanoNIR from Texas Instruments is an example of a NIRS using a DMD. A MEMS chip is used in the MicroPhasir instrument from ThermoFisherScientific. Fabry-Perot interferometers use a wavelength filter consisting of two mirrors, facing each other and separated by a distance d. By changing the electrical potential applied to the filter, the distance d and hence the wavelengths that are transmitted can be adapted. The Fabry-Perot interferometers are typically very compact fast-scanning and mechanically robust devices. It is used in the NIRONE 2.0 device from Spectral Engines. LVFs are the fourth main technology used to produce miniaturized NIRS systems. LVF are optical wavelength filters using a coating of varying thickness across their surface. Therefore, the transmitted wavelength varies linearly across the filters. It results in low cost, very compact, low power consumption, and high spectral resolution NIRS devices. The MicroNIR from Viavi Solutions is an example of a miniature device using LVF. It only weighs 100g, it uses an array of 124 InGaAs sensors, and two small tungsten filament radiation sources. It is a rugged device, tolerant to vibrations, and can be wirelessly operated. An acceptable SNR can be achieved by using an integration time in the range of a few tens of milliseconds per scan. Although the effective optical resolution is lower compared to the typical FT-NIR devices (i.e., between 15 and 20 nm), it is sufficient for several pharmaceutical analytical applications (Alcalà et al. 2013). Every year, new developments in miniaturized NIRS systems are introduced. A recent example is the nano-FTIR NIR spectrometer from SouthNest Technology. Whereas the first MEMS spectrometers had limitations with respect to optical throughput, the nano-FTIR uses a MEMS Michelson interferometer with a large mirror in order to increase the light output and optical throughput. Another advantage of this device is that it has a high spectral resolution of 6 nm at 1600 nm, it has a broad working spectral region (800–2600 nm), a high SNR, and rapid scanning, while being very compact and having a low weight (Be et al. 2020). Although these emerging NIRS could offer significant operational advantages in terms of robustness, reproducibility, and ease of mounting in hard-to-reach and hazardous process environments, they still need to prove their performance in terms of sensitivity, spectral working range, spectral resolution, and long-term stability compared to the traditionally used NIRS (Be et al. 2020; Bhakeev 2010). Another disadvantage of these miniaturized NIRS is the poor representativeness of the measurement because the spot size of these instruments is usually very small. The NanoNIR from Texas instruments for example has a probing area of only 0.05 mm² compared to almost 20 mm² for the SentroPAT FO diode array NIRS from Sentronic. The miniaturized NIRS still need to prove their adequate performance through performing comprehensive validation studies in well-equipped laboratories (Be et al. 2020).

10.3 NIRS as a PAT Tool for Process Monitoring and Control in Solid Dosage Form Manufacturing

Many PAT tools used in the pharmaceutical industry are based on NIR spectroscopy since it allows the rapid chemical and physical characterization of in-process and final materials during the production process without sample preparation (Laske et al. 2017). Chemical quality attributes such as content uniformity, homogeneity, and residual moisture content can be measured by at-line, online, and in-line NIR applications. Also, physical properties such as ribbon density during roller compaction processes and tablet hardness, disintegration time, and dissolution can be predicted. The use of NIRS as a process analyzer to monitor and control solid dosage form manufacturing has been extensively described by several authors (Razuc et al. 2019; Reich 2005; Roggo et al. 2007; OZAKI 2012; De Beer et al. 2011). The critical quality attributes (CQAs) measured using NIRS for the typical unit operations in solid dosage manufacturing, and the measurement location are listed in Table 10.3.

10.3.1 Quantitative Chemometric Model Development

A NIR spectrum is a result of overtone absorbances and combinations of different fundamental vibrational transitions (see Section 10.2.1). In addition, a NIR spectrum is influenced by the physical conditions of both the sample and the instrument (e.g., sample particle size and shape, instrument geometry). The resulting NIR spectrum is therefore a combination of several chemical and physical effects, making it difficult to interpret using univariate methods. This is the reason why multivariate data analytical methods are necessary to derive specific and useful information from NIR spectra (Phatak 2004). Chemometrics apply multivariate, empirical modeling methods to chemical data (Martens and Naes 1989). The development of chemometrics for analytical chemistry was largely driven by the increasing popularity and use of NIRS for a wide range of industrial applications through the 1980s and 1990s (Bhakeev 2010). Quantitative chemometric models are needed to predict certain properties of interest from the collected NIR spectra. Five important steps can be distinguished when developing a quantitative chemometric model and these will be discussed in this section: (i) collection of the calibration dataset (DoE based), (ii) pre-processing step, (iii) application of a chemometric modeling technique, (iv) outlier detection and remediation, and (v) validation of the developed chemometric model. The first step uses a DoE experimental design to specify an efficient and effective set of calibration samples, which should be representative of the commercial production process. DoE tools are generally considered to be some of the most important tools in the development of calibration models for PAT (Hunter and Hunter 1978). The first step in experimental design is to identify suitable design variables that may affect the spectral response (i.e., concentrations of sample constituents, physical properties, and process variables), which may lead to an incorrect assessment of quality and/or "false positives". These variables should be identified using a risk assessment (EMA 2014). The next step is to specify the number of target levels. In PAT, one often needs to determine more than two target levels for one or more of the design variables, so that any non-linear relationships between these design variables and the analyzer response can be sufficiently modeled (Bhakeev 2010). Then, the value ranges of the different design variables must be specified, being a "balancing act" for PAT applications. The ranges should cover the values expected to occur during the real-time operation of the PAT analyzer. At the same time, however, one must avoid using ranges that are too wide, as this might result in a decrease in model accuracy and precision due to local non-linearities. Finally, an experimental design type must be selected. These different design types vary in the total number of experiments that are required and the ability to characterize various interaction effects between design variables. Before collecting any NIR spectra, the presentation of the sample to the device should

TABLE 10.3

Overview of the Critical Quality Attributes (CQAs) Analyzed by NIRS for the Typical Unit Operations in Oral Solid Dosage Form Manufacturing

Unit Operation	Measurement Location	CQA	Reference
Blending	In-line in blender	Blend uniformity (blending end-point)	(El-Hagrasy et al. 2001; Li et al. 2007; Sulub et al. 2009; Singh et al. 2015)
	In-line in transfer line from blender to tablet press	Density	
	In-line above the tablet press in the buffer hopper	Blend uniformity	(Palmer et al. 2020)
	In-line in tablet press feed frame	Blend uniformity	(De Leersnyder et al. 2018)
Wet granulation (Twin-screw/ high-shear/ Fluid-bed)	At-line	Granule potency	(Blanco and Alcalá 2006)
	Online through glass window of the fluid-bed	Moisture content	(Alcalà et al. 2010; Findlay et al. 2005)
	Online through glass window of the fluid-bed	Granule size distribution	(Alcalà et al. 2010; Findlay et al. 2005)
	Online through glass window of the fluid-bed	Bulk density	(Alcalà et al. 2010)
	At-line	API polymorphic form	(Li et al. 2005)
Roller compaction	In-line (directly downstream of roller compactor)	Ribbon density	(Austin et al. 2013; Gupta et al. 2005)
	In-line (directly downstream of roller compactor)	Granule content uniformity	
	In-line (directly downstream of roller compactor)	Granule moisture content	(Gupta et al. 2005; Austin et al. 2013)
Hot melt extrusion	In-line (on the die of the extruder)	API content and content uniformity	(Vo et al. 2020)
	In-line (transmission probe on the die of the extruder, reflectance probe in the first mixing zone of the extruder)	Solid state properties	(Islam et al. 2015)
Tableting	At-line	Dissolution	(Freitas et al. 2005; Hernandez et al. 2016; Otsuka et al. 2007; Pawar et al. 2016; Smetiško and Miljanić 2017)
	At-line	Disintegration time	(Pestieau et al. 2014; Tomuta et al. 2013, 2014)
	Online (conveyor belt), online (on the tablet press), at-line	API content and content uniformity	(Boiret and Chauchard 2017; Casian et al. 2017; Colón et al. 2017; Goodwin et al. 2018; Järvinen et al. 2013; Kandpal et al. 2017; Pestieau et al. 2014; Tomuta et al. 2013, 2014; Vargas et al. 2018)
	On-line (conveyor belt), at-line	Hardness/tensile strength	(Boiret and Chauchard 2017; Casian et al. 2017; Kandpal et al. 2017; Pestieau et al. 2014; Tomuta et al. 2014)
	At-line	Friability	(Pestieau et al. 2014)
Coating	At-line and in-line	Film thickness	(Andersson et al. 1999, Andersson et al. 2000, Möltgen et al. 2012, Marković et al. 2014)
	In-line	Moisture content	(Möltgen et al. 2012)
	In-line	Residual solvent(s)	(Marković et al. 2014)
	In-line	Dissolution	(Gendre et al. 2011a)
	In-line	Curing progression	(Gendre et al. 2012)
	At-line	Active ingredient content	(Avalle et al. 2014)
	In-line	Pellet size distribution	(Marković et al. 2014)
	In-line	Acidic resistance	(Marković et al. 2014)

Note: The measurement location and literature references are added to the table.

be optimized and validated. Examples of variables that should be considered for in-line NIR methods include the probe location, the effective sample size, and the risk of probe fouling. After collecting the NIR spectra, preprocessing of the data is important because often a large part of the analyzer response is irrelevant to predicting the properties of interest (i.e., baseline variations and multiplicative effects). Nevertheless, care should be taken when performing any pre-treatment to avoid loss of essential information, for example, when only using a partial spectral NIR range. The three most common preprocessing techniques in PAT applications are offsetting (i.e., mean centering and baseline correction), sample-wise scaling (i.e., multiplicative signal correction and standard normal variate), and filtering (i.e., Savitsky-Golay derivatives) (Rinnan et al. 2009). Usually, a combination of different preprocessing techniques is applied to spectral data. Multiplicative variations between spectra originate from uncontrolled differences in sample path length, caused by changes in sample physical properties, sample presentation, and variations in spectrometer optics. They cannot be removed by offsetting or Savitsky-Golay derivatives but SNV can correct for these undesired effects by normalizing the single spectra (i.e., resulting in single spectra having intensities with a mean of 0 and a standard deviation of 1). In the following step, a chemometric modeling technique is applied to the preprocessed data. These quantitative modeling methods can be divided into direct (e.g., classical least squares) and inverse (e.g., multiple linear regression, partial least squares regression[PLS]) linear regression techniques, and learning methods (e.g., neural networks, support vector machines) (Brown and Obremski 2006; Marbach 2005; Haaland and Melgaard 2000; Blanco et al. 2000; Fearn 1983). The learning methods use non-linear transform functions allowing the efficient modeling of non-linear and complex data structures. Outlier detection and remediation is one of the most important steps in chemometric model development because the outlier's extremeness can give them a disproportionally high influence in the construction of the calibration model. One can run into three different types of outliers: (i) an x-sample outlier, based on the sample's spectrum, (ii) an x-variable outlier, based on its behavior relative to the other x-variables, and (iii) a y-sample outlier, based on its property value. Part of the x-sample and y-sample outliers can be removed by simply plotting the data. More subtle outliers can be detected using modeling methods such as PCA and PLS. PCA can be used to detect x-sample and x-variable outliers by looking at the Hotelling T^2 statistic and the Q residuals. PLS can be effective for removing y-sample outliers. The final step in chemometric model construction is the validation of the developed model. The validation method uses either an independently collected dataset (i.e., external validation) or the calibration dataset itself (i.e., cross-validation) to assess the model. While cross-validation is used to optimize the model by determining the optimal model complexity, external validation is used to evaluate the model's performance for new samples. The use of such an external data set is a minimum requirement for the validation of chemometric NIR models. Several cross-validation methods are described in literature (Bro et al. 2008), all of them returning the root-mean-square error of cross-validation (RMSECV) to quantify the chemometric model's performance. The method using an independent dataset simulates the case where the models are applied to future samples and returns the root-mean-square error of prediction (RMSEP). It is important that the independent dataset is sufficiently representative of future samples, otherwise, the validation results can be misleading. Before the quantitative NIR model can be applied to a new sample spectrum, the spectral quality should be tested to determine whether the characteristics of the sample fall within the range of variation for which the model was calibrated and validated. Statistical tests such as Hotelling T^2 or Q residuals are typically performed for this purpose.

10.3.2 Blending

Blending is a critical process step in the production process of many solid dosage forms because the homogeneity of the final drug product depends on the degree of mixing of their constituents. In-line NIR has frequently been used to assess the powder blend uniformity during blending (Wu et al. 2009; Li et al. 2007; El-Hagrasy et al. 2001; Sulub et al. 2009). Bulk density is another important physical property of a powder blend during a tableting process because it can have an effect on the final tablet weight and hardness. In a publication from Singh et al. (2015), the blend bulk density was measured by a NIRS installed inside the chute between the continuous blender and tablet press. The NIRS could monitor changes in blend density because of changes in excipient particle size or changes in blend composition.

A feed-forward controller was developed where variations in the measured powder bulk density (input) could be compensated by changing the fill depth (output), and therefore, allowing to control of the tablet weight and hardness in real-time. NIRS has also been used for blend potency monitoring inside the feed frame of a tablet press. In a recent study by De Leersnyder et al. (2018), a NIR probe (SentroPAT FO) was implemented into the feed frame of a rotary tablet press to monitor physical mixtures of sodium saccharin with two different target concentrations: 5 and 20% (w/w). When collecting spectra during tableting with the original paddle wheel, disturbances caused by the passing paddle wheel fingers could be clearly noticed in the raw spectra. Therefore, the NIRS interface was optimized by comparing the variation in absorbance at one wavelength (i.e., 1300 nm), not influenced by API concentration fluctuations, between measurements performed using paddle wheels with and without notches in the paddle wheel fingers. Cutting notches reduced the variation in absorbance at 1300 nm and positively influenced the spectral quality of the NIR data acquired in the feed frame.

Furthermore, the influence of paddle speed, notch dimensions, and the probe distance-to-finger on the quality of the NIR spectra was studied by calculating the standard deviation between the measured absorbance at four different wavelengths during one experimental run. The first wavelength was not influenced by concentration fluctuations (i.e., 1300 nm), two wavelengths were lactose-selective (i.e., 1530 and 1586 nm), and one wavelength was selective for sodium saccharin (i.e., 1664 nm). The paddle speed did not have an effect on the spectral quality. Cutting notches of 3 mm deep and 30 mm wide resulted in a lower standard deviation at the four wavelengths compared to paddle wheels having notches of 2 mm deep and 16 mm wide because the larger notches created a more stable powder bed underneath the probe. The standard deviation between the absorption values increased with increasing probe distance-to-finger. Increasing the distance between the probe and the paddle wheel finger increased the variability in sample presentation caused by powder wave behavior inside the feed frame. A probe distance-to-finger of 1 mm or 2 mm was found to be appropriate for the NIRS measurements in this study. Finally, two PLS models and two ratio models were built for each sodium saccharin target concentration, and their predictive performance was calculated using accuracy profiles. The effect of notch dimensions, paddle speed, and tableting speed on the predictive performance of the models was evaluated. Cutting notches inside the paddle wheel fingers and increasing the paddle wheel speed improved the model performance by avoiding disturbances in the NIR spectra and improving the flow behavior inside the feed frame, respectively. The turret speed did not have an effect on the predictive performance. Overall, the PLS-based models had better predictive performance than the ratio models, which could be explained by the fact that for the development of the PLS models, the wavelengths are reduced to PLS components, excluding possible noise in the spectral data.

10.3.3 Granulation

A granulation step often follows powder blending in the manufacturing of solid dosage forms. It is often necessary for later tablet compression or capsule filling. Granulates are produced by either wet granulation (i.e., twin-screw granulation, high-shear granulation, and fluid bed granulation) or dry granulation (i.e., roller compaction). The granule moisture content is an important quality attribute during wet granulation as it describes the granule growth kinetics and is important for later processing. NIRS allows monitoring the granule moisture content in real-time and much faster than the classical measurement methods such as infrared dryers. NIRS has also been used during wet granulation to monitor the granule size distribution, density, potency, and solid state (Jørgensen et al. 2004; Li et al. 2005; Blanco and Alcalá 2006; Alcalá et al. 2010; Findlay et al. 2005).

Austin et al. (2013) developed two PLS models to monitor ribbon envelope density and granule moisture content using NIRS during a roller compaction process. A Turbido OFS-12S-120H NIR probe was placed directly downstream of the roller compactor. No spectral pre-treatment was used for the envelope density model because the largest observable change in the spectra of different density ribbons was a shift in their baselines. A PLS model with two principal components and a root mean squared error (RMSE) of 0.073g/mL was obtained. A three-factor PLS model using the spectral range between 1440 and 1630 nm was constructed for moisture content monitoring. An RMSE of 0.115% was obtained using "leave one out" cross-validation. Gupta et al. (2005) demonstrated the use of in-line NIRS as a rapid and non-destructive method for real-time determination of ribbon density, content uniformity, and moisture content of roller-compacted material. Their NIRS method was able to respond in real-time to environmental and process conditions (i.e., roll speed and relative humidity) and predict the effect of such changes on key ribbon attributes.

10.3.4 Hot Melt Extrusion

NIRS is the most widely applied PAT tool in hot melt extrusion (HME) processes, where it is used to determine the drug concentration, the API solid-state, and drug–polymer interactions. NIRS is generally implemented using a heated probe inserted into the extruder die. The melt is measured through a sapphire window and typically using diffuse reflectance or transmission for opaque and transparent melts, respectively (Saerens et al. 2012; Kelly et al. 2015; Islam et al. 2015). Reflectance NIRS contains a large amount of noise in the spectra when a transparent formulation is monitored. However, Vo et al. (Vo et al. 2020) were able to measure the ketoprofen concentration of a transparent melt in a holt melt extrusion-spheronization process using diffuse reflectance NIRS measurements. They positioned a custom stainless steel reflector opposite to and distanced 2 mm from the NIR probe to enhance the intensity of the collected signal. As the drug content was measured every 20 seconds and the residence time of the formulation in the extruder barrel was approximately 10 minutes, the FT-NIR system could be used for feedback control of the drug content. Islam et al. (2015) implemented an in-line reflectance NIR probe in the first mixing zone of the barrel and a transmission NIR probe in the extruder die during HME. As the processed formulations were not fully melted in the first mixing zone near the feeder, spectra could be collected using the reflectance NIR probe. The extrudates were converted to a transparent melt along the mixing zones and spectra could be collected using the transmission probe placed at the extruder die. A die orifice with a 1 mm slit size was used to obtain a sufficiently thin and transparent sheet for NIR transmission measurements at the extruder die. Using both probes allowed monitoring the transformation of the API (indomethacin), in the presence of polymers (Soluplus and Kollidon VA64), from a crystalline phase to an amorphous phase. The in-line collected NIR spectra showed peak shifts, indicating molecular interactions between the drug and polymer. The shift was smaller for the reflectance probe in the first mixing zone (5243 cm^{-1}), where indomethacin is still crystalline, compared to the peak shift in the spectra collected by the transmission probe in the third mixing zone (5251 cm^{-1}), where indomethacin was molecularly dispersed within the polymer matrix. The peaks were larger and the shifts were more intense in the transmission spectra with increasing indomethacin concentration because of the formation of stronger, and more drug–polymer intermolecular interactions.

10.3.5 Tableting

NIRS allows the fast and non-destructive measurement of both physical and chemical tablet properties. NIR analytical methods have been developed to measure the API content, excipient concentration, content uniformity, hardness, friability, tensile strength, disintegration time, and dissolution rate of tablets (Goodwin et al. 2018; Vargas et al. 2018; Kandpal et al. 2017; Casian et al. 2017; Tomuta et al. 2013; Pestieau et al. 2014; Pawar et al. 2016; Otsuka et al. 2007; Smetiško and Miljanić 2017; Hernandez et al. 2016; Zaborenko et al. 2019; Järvinen et al. 2013; Boiret and Chauchard 2017; Colón et al. 2017). At-line NIRS has been used to predict the dissolution behavior of tablets by several researchers (Freitas et al. 2005; Otsuka et al. 2007; Smetiško and Miljanić 2017; Hernandez et al. 2016; Pawar et al. 2016). Otsuka et al. (2007) compared a diffuse reflectance and a transmittance NIRS method to predict the dissolution properties of tablets. Principal component regression models were established to predict the time required for 75% dissolution (T75) and mean dissolution time (MDT) based on the NIR spectra of tablets. The standard errors of cross-validation for T75 and MDT of the transmittance method were smaller than those obtained with the diffuse reflectance method because with the former, the whole tablet was measured instead of only a limited part of the tablet surface. The loading vectors of the first and second principal components used to construct the regression models were shown to have a strong linear relationship with the internal pore structure of the tablets, a physical property known to affect the water penetration rate and dissolution of a tablet. In the transmittance method, the intensity of the transmitted light increased with decreasing internal pore volume because of the larger solid/solid boundary surface area. More light will transmit through the denser tablets, and air/solid boundary surfaces will reflect less light in low porosity tablets. Conversely, in the diffuse reflectance method, the intensity of diffused reflectance spectra decreased with decreasing internal pore volume because light can penetrate more deeply into the tightly packed tablet and is then absorbed between the matrices. Pestieau et al. (2014) developed and validated at-line NIRS methods for tablet CU, tablet hardness, disintegration time, and friability. Tablets were produced on an eccentric tablet press at three different compaction pressures (25, 45, and 65 kg/cm^2) and contained three different API dosages (80, 100, and 120% of the target dosage). An FT-NIR spectrometer analyzed tablets in transmission mode. PLS models were built for CU, tablet hardness, and disintegration time. The PLS models for CU and tablet hardness were successfully validated using accuracy profiles. The robustness and accuracy of the disintegration PLS model were indicated by an RMSECV and an RMSEP of 1.67s and 4.18s, respectively. A qualitative method for friability based on multivariate pattern recognition (K-nearest neighbors) was developed and was able to classify tablets on two levels (tablets that failed and passed the friability reference test). The non-destructive, offline NIRS methods allowed for replacing the time-consuming pharmacopoeia reference methods, offering significant advantages in batch release time. It was shown that offline NIRS could be an interesting technique to support real-time release. Measurements on the final tablets are usually performed at-line (i.e., tablets are first sampled and then analyzed away from the process stream), but there are a few examples of applications where tablets are measured immediately on the tablet press (i.e., online and in-line measurements) (Karande et al. 2010; Boiret and Chauchard 2017; Järvinen et al. 2013). Transmission spectra are preferred over reflection spectra for offline NIRS as they permit the interaction of the NIR radiation with a larger part of the tablet, which is especially advantageous for measuring the API concentration in low drug content formulations. For real-time measurements of tablets being ejected from a tablet press, diffuse reflectance spectra are collected because transmission measurements are not possible (Karande et al. 2010; Boiret and Chauchard 2017; Järvinen et al. 2013). Järvinen et al. (2013) developed an in-line NIRS method for the 100% inspection of the drug content of tablets during a continuous tableting process. A VisioNIR LS instrument (Uhlmann VisioTec GmbH, Laupheim, Germany) was used to acquire spectra of each individual tablet on the rotary tablet press at a tableting speed between 25000 and 125000 tablets/h. The constructed PLS model using 20 to 30% (w/w) API content calibration tablet samples yielded an R-square and RMSEC value of 0.943 and 0.75% (w/w), respectively. The predictability of the PLS model was demonstrated by an RMSEP of 1.37% (w/w), obtained during a test run. Boiret and Chauchard (2017) used NIRS to collect spectral and spatial information from tablets being loaded onto a conveyor belt. The NIR probe contained three different classes of fibers collecting spectra at a speed of 2500 tablets/h. The first class of fibers evaluated the tablet surface level, the signal received from the second class of fibers provided subsurface information, and the third set of fibers provided information on the physical tablet properties (density, hardness, particle size, and shape). The NIRS allowed measuring the API content and its distribution within each analyzed tablet.

10.3.6 Coating

Pan and fluid-bed coaters are the two most common types of coating systems. During pan coating, a large rotating perforated pan mixes the tablets while they are sprayed with an atomized solution and dried with hot air. Fluidized-bed coating utilizes a Wurster column and an atomized spray from the center bottom to coat the fluidized tablets or pellets, which are subsequently dried by heated air. The coating thickness can be critical in coating applications, as it can influence both the release profile in the case of a functional coating and the potency in the case of active coating. NIRS can be used for at-line and in-line monitoring of coating thickness and detection of polymorphic changes (Tabasi et al. 2008; Kirsch and Drennen 1996; Andersson et al. 1999, 2000; Pérez-Ramos et al. 2005; Römer et al. 2008; Kamada et al. 2009; Lee et al. 2010; Korasa and Vrečer 2018). Andersson et al. (1999) used an at-line NIRS system to measure the amount of tablet coating on individual tablets. NIR absorbance appeared to be very sensitive to the coating thickness at specific wavelengths (i.e., at 1450–1650 and 1900–2250 nm). A PLS model was obtained correlating the spectra to the total amount of tablet coating suspension added and the total time the tablets spent in the coater after starting the spraying. As the Y matrix did not contain any reference coating thickness measurements, the model could not estimate the coating thickness directly. Andersson et al. (2000) developed an in-line NIRS method to measure the coating thickness and its variation during a fluidized bed pellet coating process. An NIR probe was mounted through a side port of the fluidized bed reactor and the probe tip was located close to the middle of the pellet bed during fluidization. A sample collector that was emptied by compressed air was used inside the vessel to ensure representative sampling. A programmable logical controller (PLC) was used to control the cycle time of one sampling sequence. The cycle time was set between 54 and 66 seconds to keep the amount of coating applied constant between each acquisition of a spectrum. The Y variable (coating thickness) in the calibrated PLS model was calculated using a theoretical growth model where the coating thickness is calculated in function of pellet dimensions and coater process settings. The calibrated PLS model showed a good fit and predictability, yielding an $R^2 = 0.97$ and an RMSEP = 2.2 µm. Several studies demonstrated the potential of NIRS for the determination of several other critical tablet characteristics during film coating processes such as moisture content, drug release, API content, residual solvent content, curing progression, pellet size distribution, and acidic resistance (Möltgen et al. 2012; Gendre et al. 2013; Gendre et al. 2011b; Gendre et al. 2012; Avalle et al. 2014; Marković et al. 2014; Korasa et al. 2016; Pomerantsev et al. 2011; Tabasi et al. 2008). An important advantage of NIRS is that it can be used to measure several pellet and tablet characteristics simultaneously. Möltgen et al. (2012) mounted an FT-NIRS inside an industrial-scale pan coater to monitor the coating growth and tablet moisture content. The tablets were coated with a thin hydroxypropyl methylcellulose (HPMC) film. The intense NIR band region between 5800 cm^{-1} and 5500 cm^{-1}, characteristic of HPMC, and the water bands situated at 6835 cm^{-1} and at 5190 cm^{-1}, allowed to monitor coating growth and tablet moisture content simultaneously. Marković et al. (2014) demonstrated that NIRS can be used to monitor multiple pellet characteristics at the same time during a film coating operation. They used a two-window retractable version of the GEA Lighthouse Probe™ (GEA Pharma Systems NV, Belgium), installed through a port approximately 15 cm above the inlet air distributor plate of a fluid bed coater (Huettlin HDGC 400). PLS models were calibrated predicting pellet size sieve fraction, residual solvent content, coating film thickness, and the enteric performance. Gendre et al. (2011a) demonstrated the use of in-line NIRS to predict the drug release from sustained release coated tablets during a pan coating process. Tablets were coated with an ethylcellulose-based functional coating to obtain a controlled release dosage form over 16 hours. NIR spectra were collected by an NIR probe positioned at the front of the coater drum, parallel to the spray to prevent clogging of the probe tip. Three PLS models were calibrated predicting percentages of the released drug at 4, 8, and 12 hours, respectively. The predictive performance of the PLS models was demonstrated by comparing the predicted values with dissolution reference measurements for three independent coating experiments. The percentages of drug release at 4, 8, and 12 hours were accurately predicted from the in-line NIR measurements. The mean difference between the predicted and reference values (i.e., residuals) was around 1%. The in-line NIR measurements also allowed for predicting the coating end point. For two batches, samples corresponding to the predicted end point were collected and analyzed using the reference dissolution method. All predicted values were close to the reference measurements and within the selected dissolution specifications.

10.4 Implementation of an In-Line NIR Spectrometer Inside the Tablet Press for Blend Uniformity and Tablet Content Uniformity Monitoring

Emergence of continuous manufacturing as a preferred mode of solid dosage manufacturing has increased the importance of control and monitoring of blend composition. Continuous blending is a critical step during tableting to ensure active content uniformity in the end product. While RTD-based transfer functions can keep track of blend composition using mass flow feed rate, there exists a clear gap in monitoring special causes events leading to blend and tablet composition variation. In-line monitoring of blend potency and blend uniformity inside the tablet press can therefore be performed to replace traditional content uniformity release testing on the final tablets. In-line NIRS has been used for blend potency monitoring inside the tablet press at three different locations: (i) the buffer hopper above the tablet press (ii) the feed chute, and (iii) the feed frame (Vargas et al. 2017; Sierra-Vega et al. 2019; Palmer et al. 2020;

Vargas et al. 2018; De Leersnyder et al. 2018). The advantage of measuring inside the buffer hopper or the feed chute is that the powder blend can be removed from the process before reaching the feed frame if it does not meet the specifications. Palmer et al. (2020) installed a GEA lighthouse probe in the buffer hopper above the tablet press to measure the blend saccharin concentration. In-line NIR measurements can be influenced by changes in environmental conditions (i.e., temperature, relative humidity) or build-up of material on the sensor window, hence negatively affecting the concentration predictions. Therefore, the GEA lighthouse probe uses three stages of operation (measurement, window wash, and calibration) to make sure the probe is always clean and regularly calibrated. A PLS model with an RMSEP of 0.483% (w/w) was constructed. Larger variations in the measured sodium saccharin concentration were observed when tablets having the lowest concentration (i.e., 5% (w/w) and 10% (w/w) were produced. This could be related to the feeder struggling to maintain its set point at very small mass flow rates. Vargas et al. (2017) demonstrated the importance of the measurement position inside the feed chute. They developed a NIRS method for real-time measurements of the API concentration in blends from a continuous manufacturing process. An interface was used where NIR spectrometers collected spectra at three different positions inside the feed chute between the blender and the tablet press. Considerable differences in results precision and accuracy were observed between the three NIR measurement locations. NIR measurements at the position closest to the blender outlet yielded the results with the lowest precision and accuracy because the blend exerted greater pressure on the material in front of the NIR spectrometer at this location (Vargas et al. 2017). The feed frame might be a better location because here, additional blend mixing and segregation can occur before the powder blend is compressed into tablets. Measuring inside the feed frame allows immediate diversion of tablets that are not within specifications. Sierra-Vega et al. (2019) were the first to compare blend uniformity in the chute and within the feed frame, along with the content uniformity of the produced tablets. They concluded that the feed frame is preferred over the chute to monitor blend potency because of the lower blend heterogeneity inside the feed frame and because of the reduced sampling error, resulting in better correspondence with the drug concentration in the actual tablets. The sampling error of the feed frame measurements was lower because the effective sample size (i.e., the amount of material scanned to obtain one spectrum) was considerably larger. The effective sample size depends on the diameter of the NIR beam, the penetration depth, the density of the material, the velocity at which the powder blend passes underneath the probe, and the time needed to acquire one NIR spectrum (i.e., the acquisition time). It should be comparable to one unit dose for blend uniformity monitoring according to the FDA guideline "Development and Submission of Near Infrared Analytical Procedures" (FDA 2015). However, it is difficult to calculate the effective sample size because the penetration depth, the density of the material being measured, and the velocity at which the powder blend passes underneath the probe are difficult to obtain. Semi-empirical and empirical approaches are used to determine the effective sample size in NIR spectroscopy. Berntsson et al. (1998) have developed a method to determine the effective sample size where NIR spectra were recorded from powder layers of controlled thickness placed on a strongly absorbing polyamide plate. The effective sample size was found by looking at the powder layer thickness at which the absorption significantly increased (Berntsson et al. 1998, 1999). Nevertheless, their method was developed using measurements of static powder samples while the powder blend flows underneath the NIR probe during in-line or online NIR measurements. For the calculation of the effective sample size of in-line or online NIR measurements, the material movement underneath the probe should be considered (Dalvi et al. 2019). In several recent publications on NIR feed frame monitoring, either the sample size was not considered, or it was calculated using several assumptions for sample area, penetration depth, and blend bulk density inside the feed frame (De Leersnyder et al. 2019; Wahl et al. 2014; Dalvi et al. 2019; De Leersnyder et al. 2018). The effective sample size of an in-line NIR measurement inside the feed chute of a tablet press will be considerably lower compared to the effective sample size of an in-line NIR measurement inside the feed frame when identical spectroscopic settings (i.e., acquisition time) are used. Because of the rotating paddle wheels, the amount of powder that is scanned during one measurement is much higher inside the feed frame compared to one measurement inside the feed chute, where the powder moves much slower in front of the NIR probe. Vargas et al. (2018) calculated the sample mass analyzed by one NIR spectrum collected inside the feed chute of a tablet press. It was estimated to be approximately 37 mg, being considerably lower than the tablet weight (around 1000 mg). Taking into account the acquisition time (i.e., 1.46 seconds) used to obtain an effective sample size of 37 mg, and the time needed by the system to create and save the file on the computer (i.e., 3.54 seconds), it would take 43 seconds ((1.46/37) × 1000 + 3.54 seconds) to obtain one in-line measurement with an effective sample size of 1000 mg. Because of the long measurement time needed to obtain one spectrum having a sufficiently large sample size, and the additional segregation and mixing that can occur inside the feed frame, the latter is the preferred location for in-line NIRS blend potency monitoring. The NIR probe is usually positioned at the top of the feed frame and as close as possible to the die filling station, measuring the powder blend right before being compressed into tablets. De Leersnyder et al. (2019) conducted a study using pulse-response experiments to compare the in-line NIR measurements inside the freed frame with the produced tablets. The study demonstrated that the in-line measured concentration was not fully representative of the produced tablets and this could be attributed to the position of the probe at the top of the feed frame. There was a difference in time and concentration between the in-line response and the produced tablets. Since the penetration depth of NIR is limited, only the upper powder layer inside the feed frame was measured while the dies are filled with powder from the bottom layer inside the feed frame. The existence of different powder layers inside the feed frame was demonstrated by implementing the NIR probe at the bottom of the feed frame. In-line measurements at this location were clearly more representative of the concentration in the final tablets. However, there were issues of probe fouling using this set-up. Because of gravity, the probability of probe fouling is higher when the NIR probe is positioned below instead of on top of the feed frame. The risk of probe fouling would further increase when cohesive and poorly flowing formulations are tableted. Therefore, it was suggested that if probe fouling cannot be avoided, in-line measurements at the top of the feed frame in combination with a model linking the in-line measurements to the actual tablets could be used for real-time tablet content uniformity monitoring and real-time release. The tablet content uniformity can also be determined using NIRS at the compression stage. The quantification of the API content and its uniformity in tablets has been performed at-line, online, and in-line (Chavez et al. 2015; Goodwin et al. 2018; Järvinen et al. 2013; Karande et al. 2010; Pauli et al. 2019). Chavez et al. (2015) developed an at-line NIRS method in transmission mode for the determination of the active content of non-coated pharmaceutical tablets. Tablets were analyzed with a multipurpose analyzer FT-NIR spectrometer (MPA, Bruker Optics, Ettlingen, Germany). The accuracy of the method was proven using accuracy profiles applied to an external validation dataset. The 95% β-expectation tolerance limits were included within the acceptance limits, set at 10%, over the whole investigated concentration range (i.e., between 70–130% (w/w) of the target). Finally, the NIRS model was transferred from the benchtop FT-NIR spectrometer to an online process analyzer (Tandem spectrometer, Bruker, Germany). The Tandem spectrometer was placed just next to the tablet press and automatically sampled tablets during the tableting process to analyze them online. The model used to predict the API concentration from the collected spectra was the same for both equipment. Although the spectroscopic measurement parameters (i.e., number of scans for averaging, resolution, wavelength range, and integration time) were identical, a bias of 1.75% (w/w) between the predictions of the two spectrometers was observed. This could be explained by the sample holders having a difference in terms of size and shape of the measuring window. A difference in the power of the NIR sources could be another possible reason for the observed bias. They proposed to improve the model by adding new spectra collected with the online equipment or by using a transfer algorithm. Goodwin et al. (2018) developed a comprehensive control strategy for the tablet content and content uniformity for a compression unit operation that included: (i) compaction force weight control acting on each tablet made, (ii) periodic IPC measurements for mean and individual tablet weight, and (iii) at-line tablet content monitoring using a Tandem spectrometer (Bruker, Germany). Although the control strategy exceeded the compendial quality standard for uniformity of dosage units, there were limitations in terms of sample size because approximately 12 minutes were required to complete all tests (i.e., tablet weight, thickness, hardness, and tablet content by NIR) and there was no automated sampling plan to enable online analysis. Tablets had to be sampled and transferred to the spectrometer manually. Consequently, the tablet content of only five tablets was measured every 30 minutes while the nominal compression speed of the tablet press was 3000 tablets per minute. Changes in starting material properties, environmental conditions (i.e., temperature, humidity, vibrations), and process parameters over the course of production could cause variations in powder blend content uniformity and hence in tablet API content. These fluctuations might go undetected when analyzing only a limited number of tablets. This could be overcome by implementing the NIR probe directly in the tablet press, measuring every individual tablet (Järvinen et al. 2013; Karande et al. 2010; Pauli et al. 2019). Karande et al. (2010) positioned a NIR probe just adjacent to the tablet ejection area to measure the API content at a speed of 100 tablets/minute. These measurements were compared with offline NIR- and UV analysis on 30 sampled tablets for each time period of 30 minutes. While the off-line NIR- and UV analysis showed that the complete batch met the USP criteria for content uniformity, the in-line NIR measurements revealed a deviation in content uniformity in the second half of the tableting process. The researchers believed that powder blend segregation occurred during the tableting process due to the considerable differences in powder physical characteristics (i.e., size and density) and the hopper geometry. Denser particles (API-coated lactose particles) moved more rapidly downward and the less dense MCC particles trailed behind at the upper part of the powder bed. This led to a severely skewed distribution of the in-line collected content uniformity data, with a significant part of tablets crossing the USP criteria for tablet content in the second part of the tableting process. The offline NIR- and UV analysis on a smaller number of tablets could not identify the content uniformity problems. Other researchers have successfully used NIRS for tablet content uniformity monitoring in processes operating at higher tableting speeds (Järvinen et al. 2013; Pauli et al. 2019). Järvinen et al. (2013) used the VisioNIR to measure the content of each tablet at the exit of a continuous direct compression line at a speed of up to 125000 tablets/hour. A PLS model was constructed to predict the drug content in acetaminophen tablets having a target concentration of 25% (w/w). An RMSEP value of 1.37% (w/w) was obtained for the independent test run and demonstrated the reliability of API content predictions. In-line NIRS at the exit of the tablet press could allow ejecting single tablets that do not meet their predefined quality characteristics and could enable feedback control loops to take action as soon as a drift in API content occurs. Recently, the VisioNIR was used to demonstrate the uniformity of dosage units according to Ph.Eur. 10.5, *chapter 2.10.47 – Demonstration of uniformity of dosage units using large sample sizes* (Pauli et al. 2019). The API content of tablets at the exit of the continuous twin-screw wet granulation tableting line was measured at a speed of up to 70000 tablets/hour. The average predicted API content of 4500 tablets was 98.29% of the target concentration, with a standard deviation = 2.11%. This resulted in an acceptance value of 5.07, being far below the allowed limit of 15. Furthermore, no individual dosage units fell outside the defined API content range of 74–123% of the target concentration.

10.5 NIR as PAT for Advanced Process Control of Oral Solid Dosage Form Manufacturing

The FDA encourages the adoption of Quality by design (QbD) principles in drug product development, manufacturing, and regulation (ICH 2009). QbD is a systematic approach to development and emphasizes process and product understanding and control based on sound scientific knowledge and quality risk management. QbD consists of different elements: (i) a quality target product profile (QTPP) identifying the CQAs of the drug product, (ii) product design including the identification of critical material attributes (CMAs), (iii) process design including the identification of the critical process parameters (CPPs), (iv) a control strategy, and (v) process capability analysis and continuous improvement (Yu et al. 2014). The control strategy is a planned set of controls ensuring process performance, product safety, and efficacy. It requires to detection, monitoring, and controlling of any sources of process and material variations which impact the CQAs of the drug product. However, it is difficult to have a full scientific understanding of all aspects that affect the drug product quality, and hence the typical control strategy applied in the pharmaceutical industry relies on extensive end-product testing and tightly controlled material attributes and process parameters (i.e., level 3 control strategy). Improvements in sensor technology over the last decade have led to the development of industrially robust and reliable process analyzers that can be used for PAT applications, allowing to monitor a wide range of physical and chemical material characteristics during manufacturing (Laske et al. 2017). Process analyzers are used in an advanced process control strategy (i.e., level 1 control strategy) to measure and control the CQAs of in-process and final products. In a level 1 control strategy, process parameters are automatically adjusted to assure that CQAs consistently meet the established acceptance criteria, enabling RTR (Lee et al. 2015; Yu et al. 2014). NIRS is frequently used as a process analyzer in oral solid dosage form manufacturing because it can monitor a wide range of physical and chemical material properties, as shown in Table 10.3. A few examples are described in literature where NIRS is used for the advanced process control of pharmaceutical manufacturing processes (Singh et al. 2014; Huang and Lauri 2017; Zhao et al. 2019; Burggraeve et al. 2012; Markl et al. 2013; Nicolaï et al. 2018; Singh et al. 2015). The conventional control strategy of fluid bed granulation processes consists of monitoring process parameters (e.g., inlet air humidity, volume, process air flow). The progress of the drying process is determined by the granule bed temperature and outlet air temperature combined with the drying time. The fluid bed granulation endpoint is reached when a pre-defined exhaust air temperature is obtained (Parikh et al. 1997). However, direct product quality attribute measurements (e.g., granule size distribution, residual moisture content, and bulk density) should also be considered because these intermediate product properties directly influence the subsequent post-granulation process steps (i.e., tableting) and the product stability during storage. In-line diffuse reflectance FT-NIR measurements were used by Burggraeve et al. (2012) in the development of a feed-forward process control method for a top-spray fluid bed granulation process. In-line collected granulation information during the process spraying phase was used to determine the optimum drying temperature of the consecutive drying phase. The feed-forward control method consisted of (i) PLS models to predict the end product granule bulk and tapped density from the process and product information and (ii) individual DoE regression models to derive the drying temperature needed to reach the desired end product granule bulk and tapped density, respectively. If the density predicted by the PLS model did not meet the predefined quality requirements, the DoE models could be used to predict the required drying temperature to steer the granulation process toward the desired density. The X-matrix of the PLS models consisted of the process (i.e., inlet air temperature, binder addition rate, and drying temperature) and product (i.e., granule size distribution and moisture content) information. The granule size distribution and moisture content were collected in-line by means of spatial filter velocimetry (SFV) and NIR, respectively. Different PLS models were constructed and compared, varying the product information included in the X-matrix. A first model was constructed with the X-matrix consisting of the three process variables settings and the particle size distribution determined at the end of the spraying period. Adding moisture content and particle size distribution data collected during the final minutes of the spraying period improved the models' predictability. Adding granule information collected during the complete spraying phase did not contribute to better predictability. The Y-matrix consisted of the granule bulk and tapped densities. The DoE models were constructed using data collected during a 2-level full factorial design with the response (i.e., Y-variable) being the bulk or tapped density and the X-variables being the process variables (i.e., inlet air temperature, binder addition rate, and drying temperature). The feed-forward process control method was tested during the granulation of several test batches. A first granulation run was performed using an inlet air temperature of 30 °C, a binder addition rate of 12 g/minute, and a drying temperature of 50 °C. The end product granule bulk density was predicted by the PLS models to be 0.52 g/mL using the SFV and NIR data collected during the final minutes of the spraying period. Subsequently, the drying temperature was increased to 67 °C, using the bulk density DoE model, to obtain the desired granule bulk density of 0.48 g/mL. The obtained granule bulk density for this and two additional batches was consistent with the desired granule bulk density of 0.48 g/mL. The case study demonstrated that in-line NIRS and SFV measurements can be used to steer the granulation process to obtain granules with the desired density. An advanced process control solution to monitor and control the granule moisture content during a continuous twin-screw wet granulation process was developed by Nicolaï et al. (2018). A SentroPAT FO photodiode array NIR spectrometer with a SentroProbe DR LS fibre optic probe (Sentronic GmbH, Dresden, Germany) was mounted at the exit of a ConsiGma™-25 production line using a custom-made process-instrument interface to measure the granule moisture content. A rotating plastic paddle wheel was installed on the interface to ensure a continuous granule stream at the probe tip, making the presentation of the sample independent of the powder feed flow rate, and reducing probe fouling because of sticky wet granules. Window fouling was further reduced by heating the probe tip to 30 °C. Outlying spectra caused by the rotating paddle wheel were removed by a linear support vector machine. To develop a solution to monitor and control the granule moisture content, first, a PLS regression model was constructed for the prediction of the granule moisture content from NIR spectra. A PLS model was obtained composed of both calibration and validation data sets having an RMSEP = 0.32% (w/w). Then, a linear time-invariant discrete transfer function was constructed to describe the relationship between the predicted granule moisture content and granulator liquid pump speed, which is needed in the process control loop to actively adjust the pump speed upon changes in predicted granule moisture content. The transfer function was derived using process excitation experiments where the liquid flow rate switched between 20 g/minute and 40 g/minute. Multiple repetitions of both slow (i.e., 12 seconds between two consecutive signals) and fast (i.e., 5 seconds between each consecutive signal) excitation experiments were performed. Subsequently, all excitation data from both slow and fast experiments were combined to construct an autoregressive moving-average with external inputs (ARMAX) model, describing the dynamic relationship between the predicted granule moisture content and pump speed. The ARMAX model was then used to develop both a classical proportional-integral (PI) and a model predictive control design. Finally, the process control designs were validated by performing setpoint tracking and disturbance rejection experiments. The former evaluates how well the controller copes with changes in granule moisture content setpoint whereas for the latter the ability of the controller to maintain the desired granule moisture content upon disturbances introduced into the system is assessed. The results from the setpoint tracking experiments clearly indicated that the simple PI control design is sufficient and that there is no real advantage to using a more complex model predictive controller. Currently, the PI control design is the standard in continuous control because of its acceptable performance and simplicity (Astrom and Hägglund 1995; Visioli 2006). During the disturbance rejection experiments, the powder mass flow rate was deliberately changed to mimic a disturbance in feed factor which could occur when running low on volume or variability in material properties. The model predictive controller was able to actively manipulate the pump speed during the entire experiment to match the setpoint granule moisture content. The relative standard deviation of the controlled granule moisture content was 3.32% and the RMSE between the measured and setpoint granule moisture content was 0.25% (w/w), indicating satisfactory controller performance. The researchers demonstrated that it is possible to monitor and actively control the granule moisture content during a continuous twin-screw wet granulation process using in-line NIRS and either PI or model predictive control. They also encountered several challenges with respect to the NIR spectra data collection and implementation of the control design. Despite the use of a custom-made process-instrument interface to control the wet granule flow in front of the probe window and a heated probe to reduce window fouling, a thin layer of powdered material built up on the sapphire window over time, resulting in a small measurement drift during the setpoint tracking experiments. It was suggested to use a mathematical drift correction post measurement or to further improve the process-instrument interface to avoid measurement errors. The computational performance boundaries of the NIR instrument and the PAT data management software were reached because of the fast dynamics of the twin-screw wet granulator. The NIR instrument and PAT data management software were not implemented on an operating system which serves real-time applications that process data without delays, resulting in a sampling rate that varied and hence reducing the quality of the ARMAX model fit. This observation should be tackled by instrument and software suppliers to facilitate the use of advanced process control in a commercial continuous production environment.

10.6 Chemometric Model Maintenance

After the chemometric model development, it should be periodically validated against the standard quality control results. Chemometric model maintenance activities are performed to preventively and periodically verify the model performance after it has been approved for regular use in a quality-controlled setup. The model maintenance can include steps for accuracy monitoring, method update, and revalidation of the updated model. The most obvious way to determine when a model requires maintenance is by checking the sample property predictions versus the quality control reference method. In the absence of external validation samples, it is possible to use the multivariate model diagnostics based on the orthogonal difference between a sample and the modeled data, that is, the model residual known as Q and how far a sample is from the center of the data set i.e., a leverage measured by Hotelling T^2 statistic. When monitoring the accuracy, periodic tests are performed to check the measurement accuracy, and if the results meet the acceptance criteria, NIR method maintenance is complete. However, when results do not meet the acceptance criteria, the next steps of method maintenance are performed, such as an update of the NIR calibration model might be required due to a sample characteristic for which the model was not robust. When this condition is arising due to the addition of any previously unseen variations (such as particle size distribution changed or the process drifted to a new steady-state), making the qualified model biased, the model update should be performed by including measurements from samples with this new characteristic in the expanded calibration dataset. In another case, while the samples are the same, the measurement system might have changed due to changes in the measurement hardware (new light source, clouding of optics, and wavelength registration shift). Thus, a calibration transfer is required. There are two types of calibration transfer methods: standard-based methods such as direct standardization and piece direct standardization, and standard-free methods such as the dynamic orthogonal projections, domain adaption techniques such as transfer component analysis, and domain-invariant PLS regression, and parameter-free calibration enhancement framework. In the standard-based calibration transfer methods, assuming that the differences in the signals are due to the intrinsic differences in the instruments, the same standard sample is measured on both instruments to model instrumental differences and/or compensate for them. However, the measurement of standard samples on both instruments is often not possible for reasons such as when the instrument is either inaccessible or damaged. In such a situation, standard-free calibration transfer to support model sharing across different instruments is preferred. A detailed review of various methods applied when adopting both of these approaches has been presented by Workman (2017). In this way, an updated NIR test method is obtained post maintenance which is robust to the new variations. The updated NIR calibration model should be revalidated using additional independent measurements.

10.7 Outlook

NIRS has proven its value in the monitoring and control of different formulation and process parameters during solid dosage form manufacturing. However, there are many areas in which new developments are taking place, which will further enable this technology platform. Different chemometric modeling techniques are used to extract useful information from NIRS measurements (see Section 10.3.1). PLS is by far the most applied chemometric model in PAT applications. Nevertheless, PLS regression has some disadvantages. For example, when regressing spectral data containing a large number of variables (i.e., wavelengths) compared to the number of observations (i.e., calibration samples), multicollinearity can result in less statistically robust models. Deep learning in spectral data modeling is an emerging field that is expected to effectively address this challenge. Both supervised as well as unsupervised feature extraction and learning approach for spectral data is possible using a deep learning approach.

Beside data modeling, ground-breaking developments are taking place in the area of nano-photonics, translating into the on-chip miniature spectrometer. These developments in NIR analyzer technology will likely translate into further miniaturization and performance improvements of the NIR sensors in the near future. However, new developments further diversify the available NIR spectrometer technologies. It is already a challenge that spectra collected using one NIR cannot be replaced by a second NIR instrument, due to the instrumental response differences between instruments. Not only development in the area of calibration transfers is sufficient, but a serious industry-wide effort is also needed to drive the standardization of NIR technology is needed.

Extensive development is also taking place in the other sensing technologies. Thus, while NIRS technology is maturing, a further step is to combine, that is, fuse the outputs of multiple instrumental sources by exploiting the synergies of different spectroscopic techniques. This allows an increase in the information obtained from the measurements and can therefore be very beneficial in the field of pharmaceutical manufacturing.

REFERENCES

Alcalà, Manel, Marcelo Blanco, Manel Bautista, and Josep M. González. 2010. "On-Line Monitoring of a Granulation Process by NIR Spectroscopy." *Journal of Pharmaceutical Sciences* 99 (1): 336–45. https:// doi.org/10.1002/jps.21818.

Alcalà, Manel, Marcelo Blanco, Daniel Moyano, Neville W. Broad, Nada O'Brien, Don Friedrich, Frank Pfeifer, and Heinz W. Siesler. 2013. "Qualitative and Quantitative Pharmaceutical Analysis with a Novel Hand-Held Miniature near Infrared Spectrometer." *Journal of Near Infrared Spectroscopy 21* (6): 445–57. https://doi.org/10.1255/jnirs.1084.

Andersson, M., M. Josefson, F. W. Langkilde, and K. G. Wahlund. 1999. "Monitoring of a Film Coating Process for Tablets Using near Infrared Reflectance Spectrometry." *Journal of Pharmaceutical and Biomedical Analysis 20* (1–2): 27–37. https://doi.org/10.1016/S0731-7085(98)00237-4.

Andersson, Martin, Staffan Folestad, Johan Gottfries, Mats O. Johansson, Mats Joseffson, and Karl Gustav Wahlund. 2000. "Quantitative Analysis of Film Coating in a Fluidized Bed Process by In-Line NIR Spectrometry and Multivariate Batch Calibration." *Analytical Chemistry 72* (9): 2099–2108. https://doi.org/10.1021/ac990256r.

Astrom, K. J., and T. Hägglund. 1995. *PID Controllers: Theory, Design, and Tuning.* 2nd Edition. North Carolina: International Society of Automation. https://www.academia.edu/27771107/PID_Controllers_2nd_Edition_Åström_Karl_J_Hägglund_Tore_.

Austin, John, Anshu Gupta, Ryan McDonnell, Gintaras V. Reklaitis, and Michael T. Harris. 2013. "The Use of Near-Infrared and Microwave Resonance Sensing to Monitor a Continuous Roller Compaction Process." *Journal of Pharmaceutical Sciences 102* (6): 1895–1904. https://doi.org/10.1002/jps.23536.

Avalle, P., M. J. Pollitt, K. Bradley, B. Cooper, G. Pearce, A. Djemai, and S. Fitzpatrick. 2014. "Development of Process Analytical Technology (PAT) Methods for Controlled Release Pellet Coating." *European Journal of Pharmaceutics and Biopharmaceutics 87* (2): 244–51. https://doi.org/10.1016/j.ejpb.2014.01.008.

Be, Krzysztof B., Justyna Grabska, Heinz W. Siesler, and Christian W. Huck. 2020. "Handheld Near-Infrared Spectrometers: Where Are We Heading?" *NIR News 31* (3–4): 28–35. https://doi.org/10.1177/0960336020916815.

Berntsson, O., T. Burger, S. Folestad, L. G. Danielsson, J. Kuhn, and J. Fricke. 1999. "Effective Sample Size in Diffuse Reflectance Near-IR Spectrometry." *Analytical Chemistry 71* (3): 617–23. https://doi.org/10.1021/ac980652u.

Berntsson, O., L. G. Danielsson, and S. Folestad. 1998. "Estimation of Effective Sample Size When Analysing Powders with Diffuse Reflectance Near-Infrared Spectrometry." *Analytica Chimica Acta 364* (1–3): 243–51. https://doi.org/10.1016/S0003-2670(98)00196-2.

Bhakeev, Katherine A. 2010. Process Analytical Technology. Edited by Katherine A. Bakeev. *Process Analytical Technology.* 2nd Edition. Wiley. https://doi.org/10.1016/b978-0-08-102824-7.00007-5.

Blanco, M., and M. Alcalá. 2006. "Simultaneous Quantitation of Five Active Principles in a Pharmaceutical Preparation: Development and Validation of a near Infrared Spectroscopic Method." *European Journal of Pharmaceutical Sciences 27* (2–3): 280–86. https://doi.org/10.1016/j.ejps.2005.10.008.

Blanco, M., J. Coello, H. Iturriaga, S. Maspoch, and J. Pagès. 2000. "NIR Calibration in Non-Linear Systems: Different PLS Approaches and Artificial Neural Networks." *Chemometrics and Intelligent Laboratory Systems 50* (1): 75–82. https://doi.org/10.1016/S0169-7439(99)00048-10.

Boiret, Mathieu, and Fabien Chauchard. 2017. "Use of Near-Infrared Spectroscopy and Multipoint Measurements for Quality Control of Pharmaceutical Drug Products." *Analytical and Bioanalytical Chemistry 409* (3): 683–91. https://doi.org/10.1007/s00216-016-9756-10.

Bro, R., K. Kjeldahl, A. K. Smilde, and H. A. Kiers. 2008. "Cross-Validation of Component Models: A Critical Look at Current Methods." *Analytical and Bioanalytical Chemistry 390* (5): 1241–51. https://doi.org/10.1007/S00216-007-1790-1.

Brown, C. W., and R. J. Obremski. 2006. "Multicomponent Quantitative Analysis." *Applied Spectroscopy Reviews 20* (3–4): 373–418. https://doi.org/10.1080/05704928408060424.

Burggraeve, Anneleen, Ana F. T. Silva, Tom Van Den Kerkhof, Mario Hellings, Chris Vervaet, Jean Paul Remon, Yvan Vander Heyden, and Thomas De Beer. 2012. "Development of a Fluid Bed Granulation Process Control Strategy Based on Real-Time Process and Product Measurements." *Talanta 100* (October): 293–302. https://doi.org/10.1016/j.talanta.2012.07.054.

Burns, Donald A., and Emil W. Ciurczak. 2008. *Handbook of Near-Infrared Analysis.* Edited by Donald A. Burns and Emil W. Ciurczak. 3rd Edition. Boca Raton, FL: CRC Press. https://doi.org/10.1021/ja015320c.

Casian, Tibor, Andra Reznek, Andreea Loredana Vonica-Gligor, Jeroen Van Renterghem, Thomas De Beer, and Ioan Tomuţă. 2017. "Development, Validation and Comparison of near Infrared and Raman Spectroscopic Methods for Fast Characterization of Tablets with Amlodipine and Valsartan." *Talanta 167* (May): 333–43. https://doi.org/10.1016/j.talanta.2017.01.092.

Chavez, Pierre François, Pierre Yves Sacré, Charlotte De Bleye, Lauranne Netchacovitch, Jérôme Mantanus, Henri Motte, Martin Schubert, Philippe Hubert, and Eric Ziemons. 2015. "Active Content Determination of Pharmaceutical Tablets Using near Infrared Spectroscopy as Process Analytical Technology Tool." *Talanta 144* (November): 1352–510. https://doi.org/10.1016/j.talanta.2015.08.018.

Colón, Yleana M., Jenny Vargas, Eric Sánchez, Gilfredo Navarro, and Rodolfo J. Romañach. 2017. "Assessment of Robustness for a Near-Infrared Concentration Model for Real-Time Release Testing in a Continuous Manufacturing Process." *Journal of Pharmaceutical Innovation 12* (1): 14–25. https://doi.org/10.1007/s12247-016-9265-6.

Dalvi, Himmat, Alyssa Langlet, Marie Josee Colbert, Antoine Cournoyer, Jean Maxime Guay, Nicolas Abatzoglou, and Ryan Gosselin. 2019. "In-Line Monitoring of Ibuprofen during and after Tablet Compression Using near-Infrared Spectroscopy." *Talanta 195* (April): 87–96. https://doi.org/10.1016/j.talanta.2018.11.034.

De Beer, T., A. Burggraeve, M. Fonteyne, L. Saerens, J. P. Remon, and C. Vervaet. 2011. "Near Infrared and Raman Spectroscopy for the In-Process Monitoring of Pharmaceutical Production Processes." *International Journal of Pharmaceutics*. https://doi.org/10.1016/j.ijpharm.2010.12.012.

De Leersnyder, Fien, Elisabeth Peeters, Hasna Djalabi, Valérie Vanhoorne, Bernd Van Snick, Ke Hong, Stephen Hammond, et al. 2018. "Development and Validation of an In-Line NIR Spectroscopic Method for Continuous Blend Potency Determination in the Feed Frame of a Tablet Press." *Journal of Pharmaceutical and Biomedical Analysis 151* (March): 274–83. https://doi.org/10.1016/J.JPBA.2018.01.032.

De Leersnyder, Fien, Valérie Vanhoorne, Ashish Kumar, Chris Vervaet, and Thomas De Beer. 2019. "Evaluation of an In-Line NIR Spectroscopic Method for the Determination of the Residence Time in a Tablet Press." *International Journal of Pharmaceutics 565* (June): 358–66. https://doi.org/10.1016/j.ijpharm.20110.05.006.

El-Hagrasy, Arwa S., Hannah R. Morris, Frank D'Amico, Robert A. Lodder, and James K. Drennen. 2001. "Near-Infrared Spectroscopy and Imaging for the Monitoring of Powder Blend Homogeneity." *Journal of Pharmaceutical Sciences 90* (9): 1298–1307. https://doi.org/10.1002/jps.1082.

EMA. 2014. *Guideline on the Use of Near Infrared Spectroscopy (NIRS) by the Pharmaceutical Industry and the Data Requirements for New Submissions and Variations.* European Medicine Agency. Vol. *44*.

FDA. 2004. *Guidance for Industry PAT – A Framework for Innovative Pharmaceutical Development, Manufacturing, and Quality Assurance.* http://www.fda.gov/cvm/guidance/published.html.

FDA. 2015. *FDA. Guidance for Industry, Development and Submission of Near Infrared Analytical Procedures Guidance for Industry.* U.S. Department of Health and Human Services Food and Drug Administration: Silver Spring, MD.

Fearn, T. 1983. "Misuse of Ridge REGRESSION in the Calibration of a Near infrared Reflectance Instrument." *Applied Statistics 32* (1): 73–710. https://doi.org/10.2307/2348045.

Findlay, W. Paul, Garnet R. Peck, and Kenneth R. Morris. 2005. "Determination of Fluidized Bed Granulation End Point Using Near-Infrared Spectroscopy and Phenomenological Analysis." *Journal of Pharmaceutical Sciences 94* (3): 604–12. https://doi.org/10.1002/jps.20276.

Freitas, Matheus P., Andréia Sabadin, Leandro M. Silva, Fábio M. Giannotti, Débora A. Do Couto, Edivan Tonhi, Renato S. Medeiros, Gislaine L. Coco, Valter F. T. Russo, and José A. Martins. 2005. "Prediction of Drug Dissolution Profiles from Tablets Using NIR Diffuse Reflectance Spectroscopy: A Rapid and Nondestructive Method." *Journal of Pharmaceutical and Biomedical Analysis 39* (1–2): 17–21. https://doi.org/10.1016/j.jpba.2005.03.023.

Gendre, Claire, Mathieu Boiret, Muriel Genty, Pierre Chaminade, and Jean Manuel Pean. 2011a. "Real-Time Predictions of Drug Release and End Point Detection of a Coating Operation by in-Line near Infrared Measurements." *International Journal of Pharmaceutics 421* (2): 237–43. https://doi.org/10.1016/j.ijpharm.2011.010.036.

Gendre, Claire, Muriel Genty, Mathieu Boiret, Marc Julien, Loïc Meunier, Olivier Lecoq, Michel Baron, Pierre Chaminade, and Jean Manuel Péan. 2011b. "Development of a Process Analytical Technology (PAT) for in-Line Monitoring of Film Thickness and Mass of Coating Materials during a Pan Coating Operation." *European Journal of Pharmaceutical Sciences 43* (4): 244–50. https://doi.org/10.1016/j.ejps.2011.04.017.

Gendre, Claire, Muriel Genty, Julio César Da Silva, Ali Tfayli, Mathieu Boiret, Olivier Lecoq, Michel Baron, Pierre Chaminade, and Jean Manuel Péan. 2012. "Comprehensive Study of Dynamic Curing Effect on

Tablet Coating Structure." *European Journal of Pharmaceutics and Biopharmaceutics 81* (3): 657–65. https://doi.org/10.1016/j.ejpb.2012.04.006.

Gendre, Claire, Muriel Genty, Barbara Fayard, Ali Tfayli, Mathieu Boiret, Olivier Lecoq, Michel Baron, Pierre Chaminade, and Jean Manuel Peán. 2013. "Comparative Static Curing versus Dynamic Curing on Tablet Coating Structures." *International Journal of Pharmaceutics 453* (2): 448–53. https://doi.org/10.1016/j.ijpharm.2013.06.008.

Goodwin, Daniel J., Sander van den Ban, Mike Denham, and Ian Barylski. 2018. "Real Time Release Testing of Tablet Content and Content Uniformity." *International Journal of Pharmaceutics 537* (1–2). https://doi.org/10.1016/j.ijpharm.2017.12.011.

Gupta, Abhay, Garnet E. Peck, Ronald W. Miller, and Kenneth R. Morris. 2005. "Real-Time near-Infrared Monitoring of Content Uniformity, Moisture Content, Compact Density, Tensile Strength, and Young's Modulus of Roller Compacted Powder Blends." *Journal of Pharmaceutical Sciences 94* (7): 1589–97. https://doi.org/10.1002/jps.20375.

Haaland, David M., and David K. Melgaard. 2000. "New Prediction-Augmented Classical Least-Squares (PACLS) Methods: Application to Unmodeled Interferents." *Applied Spectroscopy 54* (9): 1303–12. https://doi.org/10.1366/0003702001951228.

Hernandez, Eduardo, Pallavi Pawar, Golshid Keyvan, Yifan Wang, Natasha Velez, Gerardo Callegari, Alberto Cuitino, Bozena Michniak-Kohn, Fernando J. Muzzio, and Rodolfo J. Romañach. 2016. "Prediction of Dissolution Profiles by Non-Destructive near Infrared Spectroscopy in Tablets Subjected to Different Levels of Strain." *Journal of Pharmaceutical and Biomedical Analysis 117* (January): 568–76. https://doi.org/10.1016/j.jpba.2015.10.012.

Huang, Jun, and David Lauri. 2017. *GMP Implementation of Advanced Process Control in Tablet Manufacturing | American Pharmaceutical Review – The Review of American Pharmaceutical Business & Technology.* American Pharmaceutical Review. https://www.americanpharmaceuticalreview.com/Featured-Articles/335415-GMP-Implementation-of-Advanced-Process-Control-in-Tablet-Manufacturing/.

Hunter, W. G., and J. S. Hunter. 1978. *Statistics for Experimenters: An Introduction to Design, Data Analysis and Model Building.* New York: John Wiley & Sons, Ltd.

ICH. 2009. *International Conference On Harmonisation of Technical Requirements for Registration of Pharmaceuticals for Human use Pharmaceutical Development Q8(R2)."*

Islam, Muhammad T., Nikolaos Scoutaris, Mohammed Maniruzzaman, Hiren G. Moradiya, Sheelagh A. Halsey, Michael S. A. Bradley, Babur Z. Chowdhry, Martin J. Snowden, and Dennis Douroumis. 2015. "Implementation of Transmission NIR as a PAT Tool for Monitoring Drug Transformation during HME Processing." *European Journal of Pharmaceutics and Biopharmaceutics 96*: 106–16. https://doi.org/10.1016/j.ejpb.2015.06.021.

Jamrógiewicz, Marzena. 2012. "Application of the Near-Infrared Spectroscopy in the Pharmaceutical Technology." *Journal of Pharmaceutical and Biomedical Analysi.* https://doi.org/10.1016/j.jpba.2012.03.0010.

Järvinen, Kristiina, Wolfgang Hoehe, Maiju Järvinen, Sami Poutiainen, Mikko Juuti, and Sven Borchert. 2013. "In-Line Monitoring of the Drug Content of Powder Mixtures and Tablets by near-Infrared Spectroscopy during the Continuous Direct Compression Tableting Process." *European Journal of Pharmaceutical Sciences 48* (4–5): 680–88. https://doi.org/10.1016/j.ejps.2012.12.032.

Jørgensen, Anna Cecilia, Jukka Rantanen, Pirjo Luukkonen, Sampsa Laine, and Jouko Yliruusi. 2004. "Visualization of a Pharmaceutical Unit Operation: Wet Granulation." *Analytical Chemistry 76* (18): 5331–38. https://doi.org/10.1021/ac049843p.

Kamada, Kenji, Shiho Yoshimura, Masami Murata, Hiroshi Murata, Hiroshi Nagai, Hidetoshi Ushio, and Katsuhide Terada. 2009. "Characterization and Monitoring of Pseudo-Polymorphs in Manufacturing Process by NIR." *International Journal of Pharmaceutics 368* (1–2): 103–8. https://doi.org/10.1016/j.ijpharm.2008.10.010.

Kandpal, Lalit Mohan, Jagdish Tewari, Nishanth Gopinathan, Jessica Stolee, Rick Strong, Pierre Boulas, and Byoung Kwan Cho. 2017. "Quality Assessment of Pharmaceutical Tablet Samples Using Fourier Transform near Infrared Spectroscopy and Multivariate Analysis." *Infrared Physics and Technology 85* (September): 300–306. https://doi.org/10.1016/j.infrared.2017.07.016.

Karande, Atul D., Paul Wan Sia Heng, and Celine Valeria Liew. 2010. "In-Line Quantification of Micronized Drug and Excipients in Tablets by near Infrared (NIR) Spectroscopy: Real Time Monitoring of Tabletting Process." *International Journal of Pharmaceutics 396* (1–2): 63–74. https://doi.org/10.1016/j.ijpharm.2010.06.011.

Kelly, A. L., S. A. Halsey, R. A. Bottom, S. Korde, T. Gough, and A. Paradkar. 2015. "A Novel Transflectance near Infrared Spectroscopy Technique for Monitoring Hot Melt Extrusion." *International Journal of Pharmaceutics 496* (1): 117–23. https://doi.org/10.1016/j.ijpharm.2015.07.025.

Kirsch, John D., and James K. Drennen. 1996. "Near-Infrared Spectroscopic Monitoring of the Film Coating Process." *Pharmaceutical Research.* https://doi.org/10.1023/A:1016039014090.

Korasa, Klemen, Grega Hudovornik, and Franc Vrečer. 2016. "Applicability of Near-Infrared Spectroscopy in the Monitoring of Film Coating and Curing Process of the Prolonged Release Coated Pellets." *European Journal of Pharmaceutical Sciences 93* (October): 484–92. https://doi.org/10.1016/j.ejps.2016.08.038.

Korasa, Klemen, and Franc Vrečer. 2018. "Overview of PAT Process Analysers Applicable in Monitoring of Film Coating Unit Operations for Manufacturing of Solid Oral Dosage Forms." *European Journal of Pharmaceutical Sciences.* https://doi.org/10.1016/j.ejps.2017.10.010.

Laske, Stephan, Amrit Paudel, Otto Scheibelhofer, Stephan Sacher, Theresa Hoermann, Johannes Khinast, Adrian Kelly, et al. 2017. "A Review of PAT Strategies in Secondary Solid Oral Dosage Manufacturing of Small Molecules." *Journal of Pharmaceutical Sciences.* https://doi.org/10.1016/j.xphs.2016.11.011.

Lee, Min Jeong, Cho Rong Park, Ah Young Kim, Byung Soo Kwon, Kyu Ho Bang, Young Sang Cho, Myung Yung Jeong, and Guang Jin Choi. 2010. "Dynamic Calibration for the In-Line NIR Monitoring of Film Thickness of Pharmaceutical Tablets Processed in a Fluid-Bed Coater." *Journal of Pharmaceutical Sciences 99* (1): 325–35. https://doi.org/10.1002/jps.21795.

Lee, Sau L., Thomas F. O'Connor, Xiaochuan Yang, Celia N. Cruz, Sharmista Chatterjee, Rapti D. Madurawe, Christine M. V. Moore, Lawrence X. Yu, and Janet Woodcock. 2015. "Modernizing Pharmaceutical Manufacturing: From Batch to Continuous Production." *Journal of Pharmaceutical Innovation.* https://doi.org/10.1007/s12247-015-9215-8.

Li, Weiyong, Mark C. Johnson, Rick Bruce, Henrik Rasmussen, and Gregory D. Worosila. 2007. "The Effect of Beam Size on Real-Time Determination of Powder Blend Homogeneity by an Online near Infrared Sensor." *Journal of Pharmaceutical and Biomedical Analysis 43* (2): 711–17. https://doi.org/10.1016/j.jpba.2006.07.015.

Li, Weiyong, Gregory D. Worosila, Wayne Wang, and Tracy Mascaro. 2005. "Determination of Polymorph Conversion of an Active Pharmaceutical Ingredient in Wet Granulation Using NIR Calibration Models Generated from the Premix Blends." *Journal of Pharmaceutical Sciences 94* (12): 2800–2806. https://doi.org/10.1002/jps.20501.

Marbach, Ralf. 2005. "A New Method for Multivariate Calibration." *Journal of Near Infrared Spectroscopy 13* (5), 241–54. https://www.osapublishing.org/abstract.cfm?uri=jnirs-13-5-241.

Markl, Daniel, Patrick R. Wahl, José C. Menezes, Daniel M. Koller, Barbara Kavsek, Kjell Francois, Eva Roblegg, and Johannes G. Khinast. 2013. "Supervisory Control System for Monitoring a Pharmaceutical Hot Melt Extrusion Process." *AAPS PharmSciTech 14* (3): 1034–44. https://doi.org/10.1208/s12249-013-9992-7.

Markl, Daniel, Martin Warman, Melanie Dumarey, Eva-Lotta Bergman, Staffan Folestad, Zhenqi Shi, Leo Francis Manley, Daniel J Goodwin, and J Axel Zeitler. 2020. "Review of Real-Time Release Testing of Pharmaceutical Tablets: State-of-the Art, Challenges and Future Perspective." *International Journal of Pharmaceutics,* 119353. https://doi.org/10.1016/j.ijpharm.2020.119353.

Marković, Snežana, Ksenija Poljanec, Janez Kerč, and Matej Horvat. 2014. "In-Line NIR Monitoring of Key Characteristics of Enteric Coated Pellets." *European Journal of Pharmaceutics and Biopharmaceutics 88* (3): 847–55. https://doi.org/10.1016/j.ejpb.2014.10.003.

Martens, H., and Naes, T. 1989. *Multivariate Calibration.* Chichester: John Wiley & Sons, Ltd. https://doi.org/10.1002/CEM.1180040607.

Möltgen, C. V., T. Puchert, J. C. Menezes, D. Lochmann, and G. Reich. 2012. "A Novel In-Line NIR Spectroscopy Application for the Monitoring of Tablet Film Coating in an Industrial Scale Process." *Talanta 92* (April): 26–37. https://doi.org/10.1016/j.talanta.2011.12.034.

Nicolaï, Niels, Fien De Leersnyder, Dana Copot, Michiel Stock, Clara M. Ionescu, Krist V. Gernaey, Ingmar Nopens, and Thomas De Beer. 2018. "Liquid-to-Solid Ratio Control as an Advanced Process Control Solution for Continuous Twin-Screw Wet Granulation." *AIChE Journal 64* (7). https://doi.org/10.1002/aic.16161.

Otsuka, Makoto, Hideaki Tanabe, Kazuo Osaki, Kuniko Otsuka, and Yukihiro Ozaki. 2007. "Chemoinformetrical Evaluation of Dissolution Property of Indomethacin Tablets by Near-Infrared Spectroscopy." *Journal of Pharmaceutical Sciences 96* (4): 788–801. https://doi.org/10.1002/jps.20704.

Ozaki, Yukihiro. 2012. "Near-Infrared Spectroscopy—Its Versatility in Analytical Chemistry." *Analytical Sciences 28* (6): 545–63. https://doi.org/10.2116/analsci.28.545.

Palmer, J., C. J. O'Malley, M. J. Wade, E. B. Martin, T. Page, and G. A. Montague. 2020. "Opportunities for Process Control and Quality Assurance Using Online NIR Analysis to a Continuous Wet Granulation Tableting Line." *Journal of Pharmaceutical Innovation 15* (1): 26–40. https://doi.org/10.1007/s12247-018-9364-7.

Parikh, D. M., J. A. Bonck, and M. Mogavero. 1997. *Handbook of Pharmaceutical Granulation Technology.* Edited by D. M. Parikh. New York: Marcel Dekker, Inc.

Pasquini, Celio. 2018. "Near Infrared Spectroscopy: A Mature Analytical Technique with New Perspectives – A Review." *Analytica Chimica Acta.* https://doi.org/10.1016/j.aca.2018.04.004.

Pauli, Victoria, Yves Roggo, Laurent Pellegatti, Nhat Quang Nguyen Trung, Frantz Elbaz, Simon Ensslin, Peter Kleinebudde, and Markus Krumme. 2019. "Process Analytical Technology for Continuous Manufacturing Tableting Processing: A Case Study." *Journal of Pharmaceutical and Biomedical Analysis 162* (January): 101–11. https://doi.org/10.1016/J.JPBA.2018.010.016.

Pawar, Pallavi, Yifan Wang, Golshid Keyvan, Gerardo Callegari, Alberto Cuitino, and Fernando Muzzio. 2016. "Enabling Real Time Release Testing by NIR Prediction of Dissolution of Tablets Made by Continuous Direct Compression (CDC)." *International Journal of Pharmaceutics 512* (1): 96–107. https://doi.org/10.1016/j.ijpharm.2016.08.033.

Pérez-Ramos, José D., W. Paul Findlay, Garnet Peck, and Kenneth R. Morris. 2005. "Quantitative Analysis of Film Coating in a Pan Coater Based on In-Line Sensor Measurements." *AAPS PharmSciTech 6* (1): E127. https://doi.org/10.1208/pt060120.

Pestieau, Aude, Fabrice Krier, Grégory Thoorens, Anaïs Dupont, Pierre François Chavez, Eric Ziemons, Philippe Hubert, and Brigitte Evrard. 2014. "Towards a Real Time Release Approach for Manufacturing Tablets Using NIR Spectroscopy." *Journal of Pharmaceutical and Biomedical Analysis 98* (September): 60–67. https://doi.org/10.1016/j.jpba.2014.05.002.

Phatak, Aloke. 2004. "A User-Friendly Guide to Multivariate Calibration and Classificationtion, T. Næs, T. Isaksson, T. Fearn, T. Davies: Chichester: NIR Publications." *Chemometrics and Intelligent Laboratory Systems 71* (1): 79–81. https://doi.org/10.1016/J.CHEMOLAB.2003.12.010.

Pomerantsev, Alexey L., Oxana Ye Rodionova, Michael Melichar, Anthony J. Wigmore, and Andrey Bogomolov. 2011. "In-Line Prediction of Drug Release Profiles for PH-Sensitive Coated Pellets." *Analyst 136* (22): 4830–38. https://doi.org/10.1039/c0an01033b.

Razuc, M., A. Grafia, L. Gallo, M. V. Ramírez-Rigo, and R. J. Romañach. 2019. "Near-Infrared Spectroscopic Applications in Pharmaceutical Particle Technology." *Drug Development and Industrial Pharmacy.* https://doi.org/10.1080/03639045.20110.1641510.

Reich, Gabriele. 2005. "Near-Infrared Spectroscopy and Imaging: Basic Principles and Pharmaceutical Applications." *Advanced Drug Delivery Reviews 57* (8): 1109–43. https://doi.org/10.1016/j.addr.2005.01.020.

Rinnan, Åsmund, Frans van den Berg, and Søren Balling Engelsen. 2009. "Review of the Most Common Pre-Processing Techniques for near-Infrared Spectra." *TrAC – Trends in Analytical Chemistry 28* (10): 1201–22. https://doi.org/10.1016/j.trac.20010.07.007.

Roggo, Yves, Pascal Chalus, Lene Maurer, Carmen Lema-Martinez, Aurélie Edmond, and Nadine Jent. 2007. "A Review of near Infrared Spectroscopy and Chemometrics in Pharmaceutical Technologies." *Journal of Pharmaceutical and Biomedical Analysis.* https://doi.org/10.1016/j.jpba.2007.03.023.

Römer, Meike, Jyrki Heinämäki, Clare Strachan, Niklas Sandler, and Jouko Yliruusi. 2008. "Prediction of Tablet Film-Coating Thickness Using a Rotating Plate Coating System and NIR Spectroscopy." *AAPS PharmSciTech 9* (4): 1047–53. https://doi.org/10.1208/s12249-008-9142-10.

Saerens, Lien, Lien Dierickx, Thomas Quinten, Peter Adriaensens, Robert Carleer, Chris Vervaet, Jean Paul Remon, and Thomas De Beer. 2012. "In-Line NIR Spectroscopy for the Understanding of Polymer-Drug Interaction during Pharmaceutical Hot-Melt Extrusion." *European Journal of Pharmaceutics and Biopharmaceutics 81* (1): 230–37. https://doi.org/10.1016/j.ejpb.2012.01.001.

Sierra-Vega, Nobel O., Andrés Román-Ospino, James Scicolone, Fernando J. Muzzio, Rodolfo J. Romañach, and Rafael Méndez. 2019. "Assessment of Blend Uniformity in a Continuous Tablet Manufacturing Process." *International Journal of Pharmaceutics 560* (April): 322–33. https://doi.org/10.1016/j.ijpharm.20110.01.073.

Siesler, H. W., Y. Ozaki, S. Kawate, and H. M. Heise. 2006. Near-Infrared Spectroscopy. Principles, Instruments, Applications. Edited by H. W. Siesler, Y. Ozaki, S. Kawate, and H. M. Heise. *Journal of Physics A: Mathematical and Theoretical.* 3rd ed. Wiley. https://doi.org/10.1088/1751-8113/44/8/085201.

Singh, Ravendra, Andrés D. Román-Ospino, Rodolfo J. Romañach, Marianthi Ierapetritou, and Rohit Ramachandran. 2015. "Real Time Monitoring of Powder Blend Bulk Density for Coupled Feed-Forward/Feed-Back Control of a Continuous Direct Compaction Tablet Manufacturing Process." *International Journal of Pharmaceutics 495* (1): 612–25. https://doi.org/10.1016/j.ijpharm.2015.010.0210.

Singh, Ravendra, Abhishek Sahay, Krizia M. Karry, Fernando Muzzio, Marianthi Ierapetritou, and Rohit Ramachandran. 2014. "Implementation of an Advanced Hybrid MPC-PID Control System Using PAT Tools into a Direct Compaction Continuous Pharmaceutical Tablet Manufacturing Pilot Plant." *International Journal of Pharmaceutics 473* (1–2): 38–54. https://doi.org/10.1016/j.ijpharm.2014.06.045.

Smetiško, Jelena, and Snežana Miljanić. 2017. "Dissolution Assessment of Allopurinol Immediate Release Tablets by near Infrared Spectroscopy." *Journal of Pharmaceutical and Biomedical Analysis 145* (October): 322–30. https://doi.org/10.1016/j.jpba.2017.06.055.

Sulub, Yusuf, Busolo Wabuyele, Paul Gargiulo, James Pazdan, James Cheney, Joseph Berry, Abhay Gupta, Rakhi Shah, Huiquan Wu, and Mansoor Khan. 2009. "Real-Time on-Line Blend Uniformity Monitoring Using near-Infrared Reflectance Spectrometry: A Noninvasive off-Line Calibration Approach." *Journal of Pharmaceutical and Biomedical Analysis 49* (1): 48–54. https://doi.org/10.1016/j.jpba.2008.10.001.

Tabasi, Simin Hassannejad, Raafat Fahmy, Dennis Bensley, Charles O'Brien, and Stephen W. Hoag. 2008. "Quality by Design, Part II: Application of NIR Spectroscopy to Monitor the Coating Process for a Pharmaceutical Sustained Release Product." *Journal of Pharmaceutical Sciences 97* (9): 4052–66. https://doi.org/10.1002/jps.21307.

Tomuta, Ioan, Lucia Rus, Rares Iovanov, and Luca Liviu Rus. 2013. "High-Throughput NIR-Chemometric Methods for Determination of Drug Content and Pharmaceutical Properties of Indapamide Tablets." *Journal of Pharmaceutical and Biomedical Analysis 84* (October): 285–92. https://doi.org/10.1016/j.jpba.2012.12.020.

Vargas, Jenny M., Sarah Nielsen, Vanessa Cárdenas, Anthony Gonzalez, Efrain Y. Aymat, Elvin Almodovar, Gustavo Classe, Yleana Colón, Eric Sanchez, and Rodolfo J. Romañach. 2018. "Process Analytical Technology in Continuous Manufacturing of a Commercial Pharmaceutical Product." *International Journal of Pharmaceutics 538* (1–2): 167–78. https://doi.org/10.1016/j.ijpharm.2018.01.003.

Vargas, Jenny M., Andres D. Roman-Ospino, Eric Sanchez, and Rodolfo J. Romañach. 2017. "Evaluation of Analytical and Sampling Errors in the Prediction of the Active Pharmaceutical Ingredient Concentration in Blends From a Continuous Manufacturing Process." *Journal of Pharmaceutical Innovation 12* (2): 155–67. https://doi.org/10.1007/s12247-017-9273-1.

Visioli, A. 2006. *Practical PID Control. Practical PID Control.* Springer: London. https://doi.org/10.1007/1-84628-586-0.

Vo, Anh Q., Gerd Kutz, Herman He, Sagar Narala, Suresh Bandari, and Michael A. Repka. 2020. "Continuous Manufacturing of Ketoprofen Delayed Release Pellets Using Melt Extrusion Technology: Application of QbD Design Space, Inline Near Infrared, and Inline Pellet Size Analysis." *Journal of Pharmaceutical Sciences 109* (12): 3598–3607. https://doi.org/10.1016/j.xphs.2020.010.007.

Wahl, Patrick R., Georg Fruhmann, Stephan Sacher, Gerhard Straka, Sebastian Sowinski, and Johannes G. Khinast. 2014. "PAT for Tableting: Inline Monitoring of API and Excipients via NIR Spectroscopy." *European Journal of Pharmaceutics and Biopharmaceutics 87* (2): 271–78. https://doi.org/10.1016/J.EJPB.2014.03.021.

Watts, D. Christopher, and Ajaz S. Hussain. 2005. "Process Analytical Technology." In *Handbook of Pharmaceutical Granulation Technology*, 2nd Edition, 545–53. CRC Press. https://doi.org/10.1016/b978-0-08-102824-7.00007-5.

Workman, Jerome J., Jr. 2017. "A Review of Calibration Transfer Practices and Instrument Differences in Spectroscopy." *Applied Spectroscopy 72* (3): 340–65. https://doi.org/10.1177/0003702817736064.

Wu, Huiquan, Mobin Tawakkul, Maury White, and Mansoor A. Khan. 2009. "Quality-by-Design (QbD): An Integrated Multivariate Approach for the Component Quantification in Powder Blends." *International Journal of Pharmaceutics 372* (1–2): 39–48. https://doi.org/10.1016/j.ijpharm.20010.01.002.

Yu, Lawrence X., Gregory Amidon, Mansoor A. Khan, Stephen W. Hoag, James Polli, G. K. Raju, and Janet Woodcock. 2014. "Understanding Pharmaceutical Quality by Design." *The AAPS Journal 16* (4): 771–83. https://doi.org/10.1208/s12248-014-9598-3.

Zaborenko, Nikolay, Zhenqi Shi, Claudia C. Corredor, Brandye M. Smith-Goettler, Limin Zhang, Andre Hermans, Colleen M. Neu, et al. 2019. "First-Principles and Empirical Approaches to Predicting In Vitro Dissolution for Pharmaceutical Formulation and Process Development and for Product Release Testing." *AAPS Journal 21* (3): 1–20. https://doi.org/10.1208/s12248-019-0297-y.

Zhao, Yuxiang, James K. Drennen, Shikhar Mohan, Suyang Wu, and Carl A. Anderson. 2019. "Feedforward and Feedback Control of a Pharmaceutical Coating Process." *AAPS PharmSciTech 20* (4). https://doi.org/10.1208/s12249-019-1348-5.

Zhong, Liang, Lele Gao, Lian Li, and Hengchang Zang. 2020. "Trends-Process Analytical Technology in Solid Oral Dosage Manufacturing." *European Journal of Pharmaceutics and Biopharmaceutics*. https://doi.org/10.1016/j.ejpb.2020.06.008.

11

The Role of Process Analytical Technology (PAT) in Biologics Development

Dhanuka P. Wasalathanthri
Global Process Analytical Science, Bristol-Myers Squibb Company, Devens, MA, United States

Bhumit A. Patel
Analytical Research and Development, Merck & Co., Inc., Kenilworth, NJ, United States

CONTENTS

11.1 Introduction

Traditional offline analytics involves the extraction of samples from process streams and the analysis at an analytical laboratory followed by reporting of results. This process typically takes several hours and/or days to complete. In contrast, process analytical technology (PAT) tools feature platforms where analytics are integrated into the process for real-time and/or near-real-time monitoring of attributes and parameters followed by feedback or feedforward control. In 2004, the U.S. Food and Drug Administration (FDA) introduced the formal definition of PAT as a system for designing, analyzing, and controlling manufacturing through timely measurements (i.e., during processing) of performance and critical quality attributes of raw and in-process materials to ensure consistent final product quality (Wasalathanthri et al. 2020c; FDA 2004). There are three main ways of integrating analytics into processes (Figure 11.1). In in-line mode, analytes are measured within the process stream in real-time. On-line mode features the extraction of a sample out of the process stream in an automated fashion; the sample may or may not be introduced back into the process stream. At-line analysis involves the withdrawal of samples from the process stream to analyze on the process floor, in contrast to conventional offline testing, where samples are typically analyzed remotely in analytical testing labs (Figure 11.1). Hence, PAT platforms feature a variety of analytical techniques such as chromatography, spectroscopy, affinity binding assays, and mass spectrometry in conjunction with automated sampling techniques. Automatic data transfer from the analytical instrument, analysis, and visualization are also integral parts of the framework to enable real-time monitoring

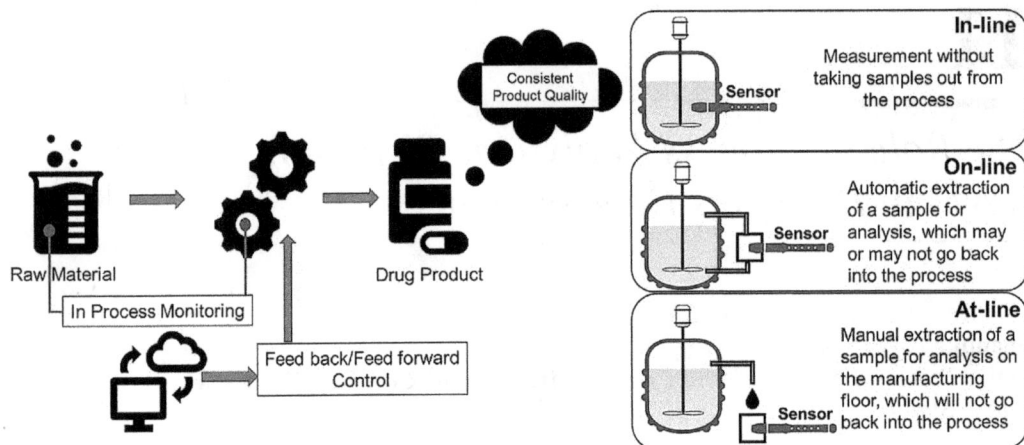

FIGURE 11.1 A schematic representation of the definition of PAT, which describes an analytical system capable of ensuring consistent product quality through monitoring and control of quality attributes and process parameters during the manufacturing process. Standard definitions of in-line, on-line, and at-line integration modes are also highlighted.

of quality attributes and process parameters. As defined by the U.S. FDA guidance, a PAT system not only serves as an analytical technique for monitoring but also controls the process and product quality attributes through feedback or feedforward control loops (Read et al. 2010).

Biologics process development includes the development of upstream and downstream sides of the process followed by formulation development for the final drug product. The functionalities such as cell line development, clone selection, media and feed development, and bioprocess development occur during the upstream process with the goal of generating a product of interest with a defined titer, productivity, and quality (Gronemeyer et al. 2014). The downstream process entails systematic removal of process and product-related impurities to generate a drug substance. Drug substance material is then either lyophilized or buffer exchanged for the final drug product during the formulation development phase (Gronemeyer et al. 2014). Each of these major steps of the process includes multiple unit operations; however, PAT should be deployed at critical control points (CCPs) of the process. A CCP of the bioprocess is defined as a particular unit operation of a production process, after which there is little to no potential for product quality change (Jiang et al. 2017). Typically, critical quality attributes (CQAs) – the physical, chemical, biological, or microbiological properties or characteristics that should be within an appropriate limit, range, or distribution to ensure the desired product quality – are monitored and controlled at the CCPs (ICH Q8(R2), 2009a). Even though the CQAs are dependent upon the type of the molecule and/or the process, some of the common CQAs of antibody therapeutic molecules may include glycosylation, charge variant profiles during cell culture, high molecular weight species, and host cell proteins (HCPs) clearance in the polishing steps. The control of CQAs can be accomplished by controlling critical process parameters (CPPs). CPPs are process parameters whose variability has an impact on critical quality attributes and therefore should be monitored or controlled to ensure the process produces the desired quality (ICH Q8(R2), 2009a). Some of the common process parameters include feed glucose concentration, viable cell density, amino acids, and metabolites such as lactate in the production bioreactor (Figure 11.2). The strategies for systematic development and deployment of PAT tools for biopharmaceutical development are out of the scope of this chapter and are discussed elsewhere (Wasalathanthri et al. 2020c).

11.1.1 Significance of PAT for Biologics Development and Continuous Processes

The regulatory approvals for biologic drugs have nearly doubled from 2009 to 2019 for various therapeutic unmet needs (Mullard 2020). Despite the complexity of the molecules and processes in comparison to small molecular therapeutics, monoclonal antibodies and related products are the fastest-growing modalities of biologics (Beck et al. 2013). Due to these complexities, the number of CQAs of a biotherapeutic

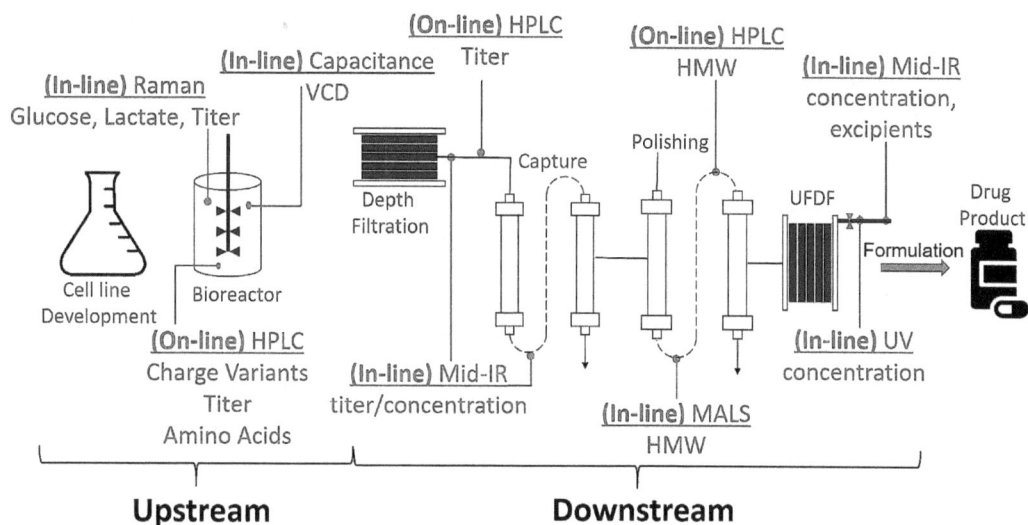

FIGURE 11.2 A schematic representation of some of the common CQAs, CPPs, and CCPs and their corresponding PAT tools.

typically exceeds that of small molecules, and also requires a specialized analytical toolbox to measure some of the critical attributes such as glycosylation, charge variants, and product-related impurities (Beck et al. 2013). Moreover, regulatory agencies encourage the use of quality by design (QbD) approach for biopharmaceutical manufacturing, which is defined as a systematic approach to development that begins with predefined objectives and emphasizes product and process understanding and process control, based on sound science and quality risk management (ICH Q8(R2), 2009a). QbD involves the identification of CPPs and CQAs followed by designing the process with robust control strategies to ensure consistent process performance to achieve the target product profile (Rathore 2009; Rathore and Winkle 2009). Thus, an analytical platform capable of real-time monitoring and control is a necessity for QbD, which is enabled by PAT with the deployment of appropriate analytical tools to measure CPPs and CQAs in real-time. In conjunction with systematic data management infrastructure and advanced data analytical tools, PAT allows holistic process and product understanding, which also plays a vital role in defining an appropriate QbD approach (Herwig et al. 2015; Rathore and Winkle 2009).

Traditional biologics manufacturing is mainly focused on batch process, where the product output from one unit operation is typically collected in a holding tank before moving to the next processing step (Zydney 2015). However, with a rapidly increasing demand for biologic drugs and the constant pressure from biosimilars (Mullard 2020), there is a significant driver for advanced technologies to improve manufacturing efficiency and production cost (Fisher et al. 2019). Thus, cutting-edge technologies focusing on intensified and continuous processes have evolved in recent years (Warikoo et al. 2012; Xu et al. 2020; Coolbaugh et al. 2021). An intensified process can be defined as one with major process improvements (e.g., productivity), which significantly reduce manufacturing costs and facility footprints through the adoption of innovative technologies (Xu et al. 2020). Fully continuous manufacturing platforms focus on end-to-end processes from upstream cell culture to drug products. Even though fully continuous processes are currently non-existent in biologics manufacturing, few noteworthy platforms have been reported with semi-continuous operations (Warikoo et al. 2012; Coolbaugh et al. 2021). Traditional offline analytics where samples are taken out from the process stream, followed by analysis in an analytical laboratory (several hours to days of results turnaround time), fail to meet the agility requirement of intensified or continuous processes, where the availability of real-time analytics is a necessity to maintain the continuous operation from one unit operation to the next (Wasalathanthri et al. 2021). For example, intensified processes of monoclonal antibody products often include multicolumn chromatography (MCC) capture steps (Figure 11.2), where multiple Protein A chromatography columns are run sequentially in a continuous fashion (Xu et al. 2020). In these types of continuous purification steps, adaptive column switching from one to another is required, which cannot be achieved without the use of real-time monitoring of harvest titer or real-time monitoring and control of column loading with the use of appropriate PAT tools (Thakur et al. 2020; Wasalathanthri et al. 2021). Thus, PAT plays a crucial role in enabling continuous and intensified processes for biomanufacturing.

11.1.2 Key Elements of a Typical PAT Platform

The following are a few essential components of any given PAT platform (Wasalathanthri et al. 2020a):

1. Analytical Sensor: To acquire analytical data from the process.
2. Automation: A robotic system for sample extraction, pre-treatment (if required), and analysis – in on-line PAT tools.
3. Data Management and Visualization System: To automatically transfer data from analytical sensors, followed by real-time analysis and visualization on a graphical user interface (GUI).
4. Distribution Control System: For feedback or feedforward control functions.

These components are required for real-time monitoring and control of the process using PAT to ensure consistent product quality. We discuss each of these components and their roles in detail below.

11.1.2.1 Analytical Sensor

An analytical sensor can be defined, in the context of PAT, as the component or technology which integrates with the process sample through in-line, on-line, or at-line modes to acquire data. A variety of analytical technologies serve this purpose. Vibrational spectroscopy techniques such as Raman, Fourier transform mid-infrared (FT-MIR), and Fourier transform near-infrared (FT-NIR) are some of the commonly used in-line analytical sensors (Trunfio et al. 2017; Wasalathanthri et al. 2020d). These techniques acquire vibrational spectra of the analyte of interest (quality attribute or process parameter) in the bioprocess. Separation techniques such as on-line liquid chromatography (on-line LC) such as Waters PATROL© and two-dimensional chromatography systems are also commonly utilized. Analytical technologies are evolving rapidly, with the characteristic of their own capabilities and limitations. For instance, vibrational spectroscopic techniques such as FT-MIR and Raman can generate data within a fraction of a minute time scale; however, they may lack the sensitivity and specificity of chromatographic or mass spectrometric techniques. In contrast, chromatographic techniques are exclusively on-line or at-line PAT techniques where a sample is required to be taken out from the process for analysis and require significantly higher assay time (typically on a minutes-to-hours' time scale). Moreover, it is also important to understand the analytical response time requirement for a given CQA. Some attributes such as the titer, charge variants, and glycan profile of a therapeutic molecule during a typical fed-batch culture process often do not significantly change every several hours or days, thus an on-line chromatographic technology which can monitor these quality attributes once or twice per day is sufficient for real-time understanding during the process. However, the concentration of a therapeutic molecule of interest during the elution step of bind-and-elute unit operation changes on seconds time scale. In such unit operations, a PAT tool such as on-line LC is incapable of providing real-time concentration measurements within the time scale of the bind-and-elute stage, and hence in-line PAT tools with faster response time such as vibrational spectroscopic techniques should be employed.

11.1.2.2 Automation

On-line integration of analytics to the process requires automatic extraction of a sample from the unit operation, hence robotic infrastructure is also important for a typical PAT framework. They could be sampling probes, pretreatment modules, sample distribution systems, fraction collectors, or high throughput autosamplers. Generally, all chromatography-based PAT requires some sort of automation system in place to take a sample from a unit operation for analysis. There are a variety of sample automation techniques available in the market which utilize the flow injection analysis techniques for sample extraction and delivery (Wasalathanthri et al. 2020c). Segflow© systems from Flownamics (Madison, WI, USA), MAST© autosampler from LONZA (Bend, OR, USA) and SIA Analyzers© from FIAlabs (Seattle, WA, USA) are some of the commonly used instruments. They are capable of obtaining cell-free or cell-containing samples from unit operations as necessary. Probes with ceramic microporous membranes are often used in cell-free sampling devices.

11.1.2.3 Data Management and Visualization System

Analytical sensors (Section 11.1.2.1) are capable of acquiring information about the analyte of interest; however, the data are present as a raw spectrum or a chromatogram which may not necessarily provide any value to process scientists until the data are processed and analyzed to convert to a specific CQA or CPP. A data management system of a PAT platform allows automated piping of raw and metadata from the analytical sensors, automated analysis, and storage. GUI interfaces are often a part of these systems where analytical outputs of CQAs and CPPs are displayed on graphs and tables for visualization (Figure 11.3). Therefore, data management and visualization platforms enable real-time monitoring of CQAs and CPPs which is a crucial component of PAT. Several commercially available platforms with 21 CFR Part 11 compatibility are available in the market. SynTQ® from Optimal Industrial Automation, SIPAT® from Siemens, BioPAT SIMCA® from Sartorius, and Unscrambler Process Pulse II® from Camo are some of the most common solutions in the market (Wasalathanthri et al. 2020c). These platforms not only are capable of automated transfer of data from analytical instruments but also provide functions such as data preprocessing, multivariate data analysis (MVDA) analysis, and visualization (Cao et al. 2018). As data are collected throughout the process run in real-time, PAT systems generate larger data sets (Hong et al. 2018), thus a systematic data engineering and repository system is also a necessity (Cao et al. 2018).

11.1.2.4 Distribution Control System

The ability to control CPPs and CQAs to achieve the target product profile is required to ensure consistent quality. A distribution control system (DCS) allows feedback and feedforward control functions to modulate process parameters to maintain consistent product quality within the specifications. Most of

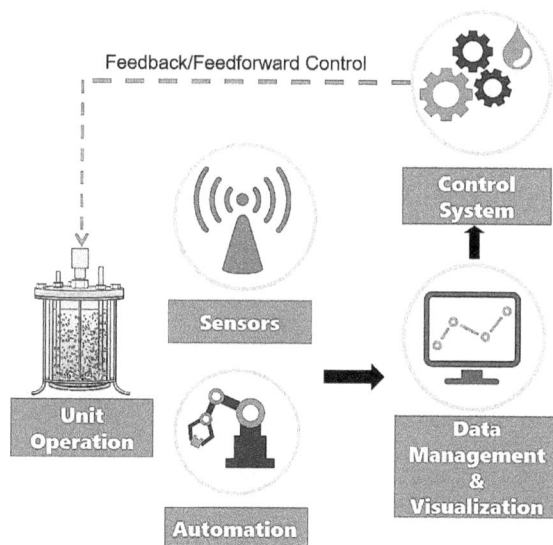

FIGURE 11.3 Main components of a typical PAT framework.

the process control functions can be done manually, and DCS can be used to automate process control through feedback and feedforward closed loops. For example, Berry et al. have demonstrated the modulation product's quality attributes and process performance with the utility of automated control of glucose feed in cell culture using Raman spectroscopy (Berry et al. 2016). The authors have used DeltaV© from Emerson (St. Louis, MO, USA), which is one of the most commonly used platforms in biomanufacturing for process control.

In the subsequent section, we provide a detailed and critical discussion on major types of PAT tools in bioprocess development.

11.2 In-line Vibrational Spectroscopy and MVDA Tools

Raman, FT-MIR, and NIR are well-known vibrational spectroscopic techniques that are used to monitor CPPs and CQAs in bioprocess (Trunfio et al. 2017; Wasalathanthri et al. 2020d). Spectroscopic methods are becoming more and more popular as PAT tools due to their rapid measurement times, non-destructive nature, and ability to monitor multiple different components in a single measurement (Esmonde-White et al. 2017). Unlike wet chemical techniques, they do not require any sample extraction and/or preparation before the measurements and typically come with probes and flow cells that can be integrated into the bioprocess easily. Figure 11.4 demonstrates some of the commonly available spectroscopic analytical sensors that are equipped with probes and flow cells. Some of the FT-MIR probes consist of Silver Halide fiber optic probes with diamond-attenuated total reflection (ATR) sensors at the end to acquire FT-MIR signals which can be integrated into unit operations of bioprocesses (Figure 11.4 (a, c)), while others contain specialized flow cells with built-in ATR sensors (Figure 11.4(e–g)). Modern Raman spectroscopic instruments use high-intensity laser beams of a specific wavenumber to acquire response from the sample due to Raman scattering (Figure 11.4(b)). For most bioprocessing applications, 785-nm wavelength is used to minimize fluorescence interferences. More details about vibrational spectroscopy instruments, theories, and their applications can be found elsewhere (Sathyanarayana 2004).

One of the key advantages of vibrational spectroscopic techniques as PAT in bioprocess is their ability to capture a plethora of information during measurements. For instance, a Raman probe in a bioreactor typically captures a spectrum every 15 minutes and each spectrum contains vibrational spectroscopic information not only on the analyte of interest but also on unique spectral signatures of all the other Raman active components in the bioreactor. Moreover, spectroscopic tools are capable of capturing this

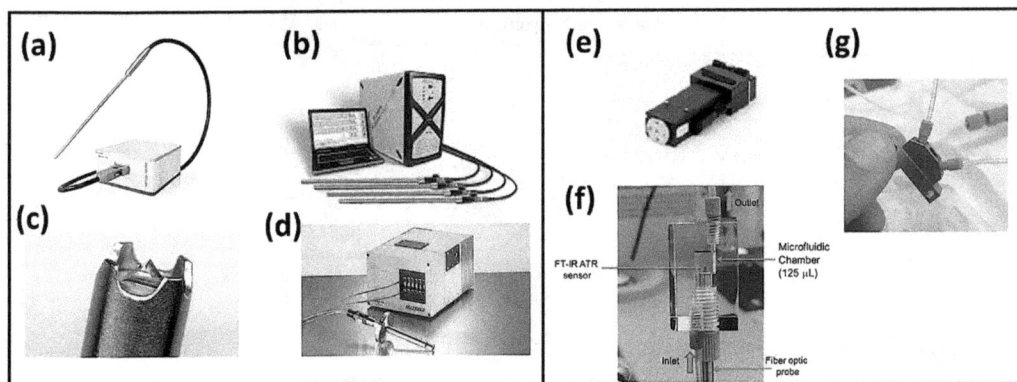

FIGURE 11.4 Some common spectroscopic sensors for bioprocess monitoring: (a) FT-MIR spectrometer with Silver Halide probe and ATR at the tip (ReactIR© Mettler Toledo); (b) Raman spectrometer with the laser-based signal acquisition (Kaiser Raman Rxn2© Kaiser Optical Systems); (c) Diamond ATR tip in an FT-MIR probe (Bruker Optics); (d) FT-NIR spectrometer with a fiber optic probe (MATRIX-F©, Bruker Optics); (e) DS Micro Flow Cell (Mettler Toledo); (f) A custom-made flowcell for FT-MIR applications (Wasalathanthri et al. 2020b); (g) Flowcell for Quantum Cascade Laser based InfraRed spectroscopic measurements (DRS Daylight Solutions).

information throughout the whole bioprocess, which enables one to understand the behavior of the bioprocess upon applying more advanced data interrogation techniques (Trunfio et al. 2017; Li et al. 2013). However, if the interest is in a specific component in the bioprocess, then preprocessing of spectra is required to eliminate any noise, scattering effects, outliers, and other spectral artifacts to "clean" spectral data sets before analysis. Baseline subtraction, smoothing, derivatization, normalization, and multiplicative scatter correction are some of the commonly used preprocessing techniques for vibrational spectra in bioprocess applications. However, which combination and sequence of preprocessing techniques to use are entirely dependent upon the types of spectroscopic data. In bioprocess monitoring applications, typically pre-processed spectral data are subjected to MVDA. Partial least square regression (PLS) modeling is one of the most common quantitative MVDA techniques used in bioprocess applications, which finds a linear regression model by projecting the predicted variables and the observable variables. For example, the PLS model of antibody titer in a bioreactor contains chromatographically measured titer values as observed variables and spectroscopically predicted titer values as predicted variables. Qualitative and classification MVDA models typically involve principal component analysis (PCA) or support-vector machine algorithms for bioprocess applications. A generic workflow of real-time CQA and/or CPP monitoring is depicted in Figure 11.5, where spectra collected from a given unit operation of the bioprocess are channelled automatically to a process monitoring system (PMS) for automatic analysis and visualization of results in GUI. MVDA models must be pre-constructed and loaded into the PMS for automatic processing of spectral data. There is a variety of PMS currently available in the market. SynTQ® from Optimal Industrial Automation, SIPAT® from Siemens, BioPAT SIMCA® from Sartorius, and Unscrambler Process Pulse II® from AspenTech are some of the most common PMS platforms (Wasalathanthri et al. 2021).

Raman spectroscopy has grown in popularity for bioprocess applications since the publication by Abu-Absi et al. describing the use of Raman to monitor multiple upstream process parameters, such as glucose, lactate, and viable cell density, in an in-line fashion (Abu-Absi et al. 2011). The application of FT-MIR or NIR spectroscopy in bioprocess monitoring is not as well-established as Raman, mainly due to the spectral interference from water present in the matri11. However, modern MIR spectrometers are capable of automatically subtracting water absorbance as part of background correction during spectral acquisition, which allows increasing application of infrared PAT technologies, especially for downstream applications in bioprocess (Wasalathanthri et al. 2020b; Thakur et al. 2020). The signal response time of NIR and FT-MIR techniques are comparatively faster than Raman, hence are better suited for downstream applications as CQAs change rapidly during a given unit operation. Some of the

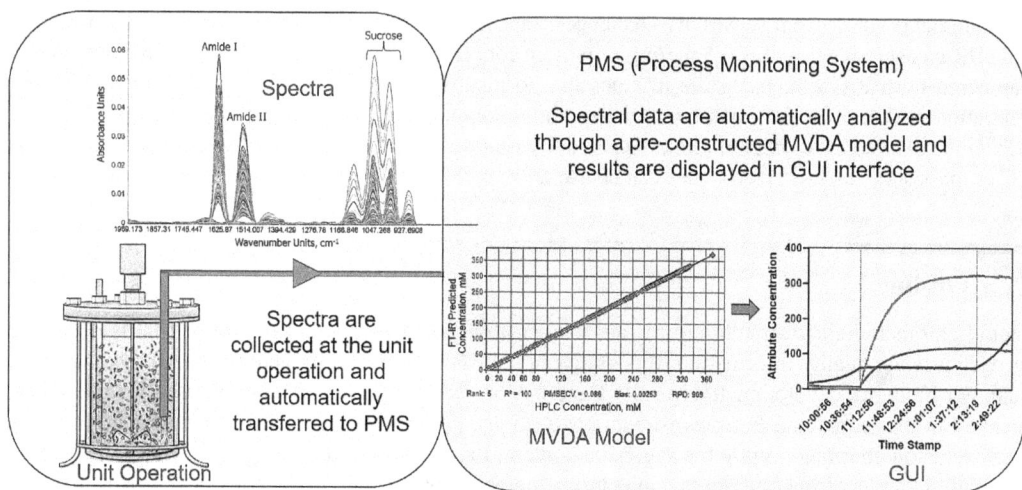

FIGURE 11.5 Typical spectroscopic-based PAT for bioprocess monitoring. A spectroscopic probe or a flow cell is used to acquire spectra from a given unit operation. Vibrational spectra contain unique signatures that correspond to analytes of interest. These spectra are then piped automatically into a PMS platform for analysis and visualization.

TABLE 11.1

Vibrational Spectroscopy and MVDA Technologies for Bioprocess Monitoring

Technique	Mode	Attribute	Reference
Raman	In-line	Glutamine, glutamate, glucose, lactate, ammonia, viable cell density, and osmolality	Webster et al. (2018), Berry et al. (2015), Matthews et al. (2016), Mehdizadeh et al. (2015), Santos et al. (2018)
		Excipients, protein concentration, aggregation, nutrients	Czeterko et al. (2019)
		Antibody concentration	Yilmaz et al. (2020), André et al. (2015)
		Protein titer	Santos et al. (2018)
MIR	At-line	Titer, aggregation, HCP	Capito et al. (2015a)
		Lactate, glutamate, viable cell density, antibody concentration	Capito et al. (2015b)
	In-line	Protein concentration, aggregation, HCP, charge variants	Wasalathanthri et al. (2019)
		protein concentration	Boulet-Audet et al. (2016), Großhans et al. (2018)
		Excipients	Wasalathanthri et al. (2020a)
NIR	At-line	Amino acid, trace metals	Trunfio et al. (2017)
		Cell culture media	Ryder (2018), Rathore et al. (2018)
	On-line	Glucose	Kambayashi et al. (2020)

commonly monitored CQAs and CPPs using vibrational spectroscopic PAT tools are listed in Table 11.1 below. The role of these techniques in biologics development is multifold. As they are capable of providing continuous monitoring of CQA and CPP variations throughout the entire time of the unit operation, it is possible to detect and adjust deviations through feedback control strategies. For example, Berry et al. have demonstrated the use of Raman spectroscopy and MVDA for glucose monitoring followed by process automation to control bolus feeding of glucose (Berry et al. 2016). The use of Raman-enabled automated-glucose feeding into bioreactors eliminates the need for manual measurement and addition of glucose, which in turn saves resources and human errors. Furthermore, spectroscopic PAT techniques allow holistic process understanding as they provide uninterrupted monitoring throughout the process. Despite the widespread utility of spectroscopic MVDA techniques as PAT, there are a few drawbacks worth considering in deploying these tools in biologics process development. Vibrational spectroscopic measurements suffer from sensitivity challenges, especially in complex biologic matrices. For instance, FT-MIR measurements below 0.5 mg/mL of protein concentrations in cell culture media are significantly hampered by matrix effects. While it is possible to identify unique spectral signatures of higher concentration analytes in vibrational spectra, sometimes components with similar vibrational spectroscopic signatures overlap each other leading to specificity issues. In such situations, other PAT such as on-line LC or mass spectrometric techniques can be used.

11.3 On-line LC

Liquid chromatography separation provides the sensitivity, specificity, and resolution that is needed to provide product quality information. It is used routinely as a release assay and to characterize the molecule. For biologics development, typically Protein A or reversed phase methods are used for titer measurement in the bioreactor. For downstream applications, product attributes can be determined by using size exclusion chromatography for aggregate content, ion exchange chromatography for charge variant distribution, and hydrophobic interaction chromatography for oxidation (Haverick et al. 2014). In order to progress offline analytics into PAT-compatible techniques, automation is generally required. There are two main workflows that use liquid chromatography in an on-line manner (on-line LC). One workflow is the use of Waters PATROL® instrument, and the other requires a standard offline LC connected to an

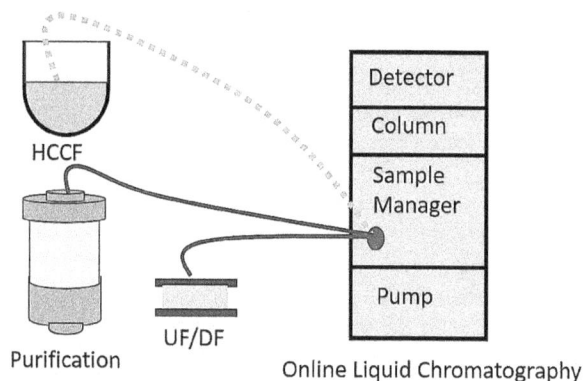

FIGURE 11.6 Representation of an on-line LC connected to an upstream or downstream unit operation.

automated sampling technology. These tools can be connected to upstream and downstream unit operations and can also provide constant analysis of the purification process (Figure 11.6). As continuous processes are typically longer than batch processes, on-line LC is a critical path in ensuring a consistent final product as the unit operations are functioning at the same time (especially for end-to-end continuous).

Figure 11.6 is a demonstration of the on-line LC being integrated with the upstream or downstream unit operation. For upstream processes, the samples must be cell-free in order to perform an analysis. A few examples of attributes that could be evaluated on the harvest cell culture fluid (HCCF) are titer, post translation modifications, and glycan profile. For downstream processes, the on-line LC could be connected to at polishing steps or at ultrafiltration and diafiltration (UF/DF) steps. The attributes that could be measured are aggregates, charge variants, hydrophobic variants (oxidation), post translation modifications and/ or product-related impurities. The detector can be UV, fluorescence, mass spec, and light scattering.

Waters PATROL® UPLC Process Analysis System is designed to provide access to real-time, chromatographic-quality analysis in an automated setting. The PATROL® instrument is ultra-performance liquid chromatography (UPLC) that is similar to an offline LC and has a similar modular design. Two features that allow the PATROL® to be on-line are its portability and Process Sample Manager. As it is on a cart, it can be wheeled next to the process and the Process Sample Manager allows the sample to be drawn in an automated manner from the process stream as well as dilute the sample when necessary. For upstream applications, PATROL® is typically connected to a cell-free sampling probe such as the FISP® probe in Segflow systems. An application of PATROL-Segflow connection is to monitor titer in the HCCF by performing analytical Protein A chromatography (Chemmalil et al. 2021). The combination of the speed of the Protein A assay and automated sampling of on-line LC can replace offline titer measurements and can be fed into the development of an accurate and robust Raman model (Goby et al. 2019).

On-line LC applications can also be connected to all downstream unit operations. Patel et al. showcased an example where the on-line LC unit was connected to an anion exchange purification for multiple weeks as part of monitoring a continuous process (Patel et al. 2017). In addition, the sample can be diluted into the appropriate matrix to allow for proper binding and separation in the analytical chromatography. Customized on-line LC systems have been made with a two-position/six-port valve whereby automated sampling of the product stream can come from a process column, and can then be delivered into a chromatography system for CQA monitoring (Tiwari et al. 2018). On-line LC techniques require automated sampling technologies (AST) for sample extraction from the process and process analyzers for sample preparation and delivery (Pepper 2016; Hofer et al. 2020). Segflow® system (Flownamics) and MAST® (Lonza) are the two most commonly used ASTs. ASTs enable the connection of chromatographic systems and aseptic technologies to bioreactors, surge vessels, and purification column eluents streams (Pepper 2016).

As discussed above, one can perform the same analytical separation/chromatography technique in an on-line fashion by connecting the on-line LC to the downstream unit operations (which contains purified antibody). However, purification is typically required to remove media components including HCPs to obtain quality information from the bioreactor and HCCF. This can be accomplished by placing an AST upstream of two-dimensional LC (2D-LC) (D. R. Stoll and Carr 2017; Chemmalil et al. 2021). By using a Protein A column in the first dimension, one can purify the protein of interest, park the protein of interest in a loop, and deliver it to the second dimension for further analysis. Protein A analytical column followed by SEC, IEX, HIC, and RP are some examples that can be performed (Stoll et al. 2016; Dunn et al. 2020). This ability to detect product quality attributes from the bioreactor in a rapid format is very powerful as the majority of product quality changes happen in the bioreactor. Conventionally, the samples from HCCF are run on an automated liquid handling platform (Bravo®, Tecan®) to purify the antibody and then transferred to an LC for analysis. This procedure may require multiple handoffs which can cause delays and cause sample degradation if the product of interest is unstable in the growth media. 2D-LC can speed these steps up and provide product quality information as fast as 5 minutes (Figure 11.7). The challenges that 2D-LC faced in biologics at the onset of its introduction regarding mobile phase computability and the inability to capture the full peak of interest are alleviated. The active solvent modulation valve allows for proper mixing of the mobile phases before fractions are added to the second-dimension columns to connect two different separations with ease (D. R. Stoll et al. 2017). With the introduction of new technologies in cell culture like the AMBR® system (high throughput automated bioreactor system for process development), the analytics must keep up (Sandner, Pybus, and McCreath 2018). On-line 2D-LC can alleviate these concerns as the sample is purified and analyzed right away. In addition, it may be connected to mass spectrometry for characterization.

Figure 11.7 portrays an AST system working in conjunction with the 2D-LC to provide real-time analysis of an upstream process. The AST system can deliver the upstream samples from the Bioreactor (cell-comprising) or from the HCCF (cell-free) to the 2D-LC. With the 2D-LC, the first dimension can be an analytical Protein A method, separating the monoclonal antibody (mAb) from process-related impurities, in which the purified mAb is then sent to the second dimension for a different quality attribute such as aggregates, charge variants, hydrophobic variants (oxidation), or product-related impurities.

With either of the LC PAT systems described (1D or 2D), data can be measured in real-time in a continuous manner. Time can be minutes, hours, or even days in this illustration depending on the specific application. Quality attributes could be titer, high molecular weight species (aggregates), charge variant, glycan, oxidation, etc. This type of analysis provides the opportunity to monitor the health of the continuous process and detect any quality anomalies.

Figure 11.8 shows hypothetical data that can be measured by either on-line LC or AST + 2D-LC that can be used for process monitoring of the continuous process for days. This type of separation-based PAT may be connected at the unit operation at the point of control or at the end of the process. Regardless of where in the process the PAT is located, measuring quality is key to ensuring a consistent quality product. Of course, if excursion or aberrant data are detected, the material can be diverted and/or the process

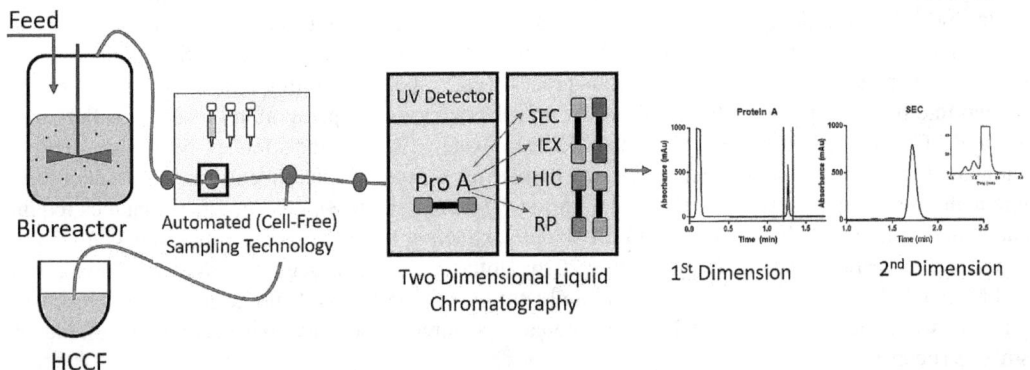

FIGURE 11.7 Representation of an automated sampling technology integrated with a 2D-LC providing different attributes for upstream quality analysis.

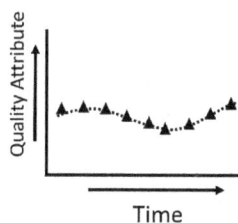

FIGURE 11.8 Hypothetical illustration of data output from on-line LC and/or AST + 2D-LC.

can be corrected. The sampling frequency for on-line LC should be set according to the quality attribute measured and the location that it is connected. For example, in order to monitor aggregates, the on-line LC may be measured after polishing chromatography to assess the clearance of impurities and to serve as a checkpoint to feed forward the material to further downstream unit operations. Of course, these PAT can be used for semi-continuous processes and even discrete steps on the time scale of hours such as monitoring aggregates from a purification column.

11.4 Other Sensors

In addition to vibrational spectroscopic techniques mentioned above, there are other in-line sensors that can be used for various upstream and downstream applications. Some examples of these include capacitance for biomass concentration measurement, UV spectroscopy and refractive index for protein concentration, and multiangle light scattering (MALS) for aggregate content.

Bio-capacitance (dielectric spectroscopy) probes are inserted in the bioreactor to provide real-time measurement of biomass concentration and have been widely used across the biopharmaceutical industry for viable cell density measurement (Moore et al. 2019). The technology applies a periodic alternating electric field to the system and detects the polarization of the cells. Only viable cells with an intact cell membrane can polarize, while dead cells or impurities in the cell media are not detected. The measured capacitance signal can be converted to permittivity for process monitoring or control. However, it is critical to note that as the mammalian cell culture ages and the cell diameter increases, the polarization is different and the signal contribution of each cell increases (S Metze et al. 2020b; Opel et al. 2010). A possible avenue to correct this difference is to calibrate the capacitance with offline techniques such as Trypan Blue Assay-based CEDEX HiRes Cell Counter and Analyzer System® (Roche). Alternatively, multivariate models may be used at stages of cell culture where the permittivity value is unaffected by cell culture age (Metze et al. 2020a).

Another valuable in-line sensor is MALS, which can provide an assessment of aggregation during process development and eventually manufacturing. During purification, the typical workflow for determining high molecular weight species involves time-consuming and laborious steps of fraction collection and offline SEC separation. Most importantly, the analysis (amount of impurity, total protein yield) and pooling decisions are only made after the purification has finished, eliminating the ability to provide feedback control. These decisions are often time-sensitive as the purification conditions involve the protein being susceptible to extreme pH and salt conditions which can degrade the protein. Although MALS is usually used as an analytical detector in conjunction with size exclusion chromatography, it can be used to determine the average molecular weight (M_w) for product characterization through in-line techniques, and therefore has the potential to be an excellent PAT tool. MALS provides a plug-and-play, non-destructive, real-time option to detect M_w. This technology has been demonstrated for flowthrough chromatography steps at a bench scale where the change M_w can be converted to percent high molecular weight species (Patel et al. 2018). Of course, one must have the product and process understanding and know the degradation pathway of the molecule for such an analysis. The connectivity of the MALS to the purification instrument allows for process control decisions to be made, where a predetermined limit/range of M_w can be set. This provides additional quality assurance at the production level. MALS also can be used to screen purification columns and conditions in development as well as load columns more aggressively. Although examples of flowthrough chromatography are cited, proof of concept using MALS for bind-and-elute chromatography would tremendously increase its value. However, for bind-and-elute chromatography, one must take into consideration rapid changes in protein concentration, buffer species, and aggregate levels, which may complicate the MALS analysis. Since the current MALS instrument can accommodate flow rates from (0.1–100 mL/min); a new flow cell/instrument is needed at a larger scale if the analysis were to be performed in a truly in-line fashion. Slipstream approaches can be utilized, but consideration needs to be taken when designing suitable aseptic connections. At the current stage, MALS is one of the few in-line instruments that can provide critical quality attribute information.

Another process requisite is the need to determine accurate, precise, fast, and in-line protein concentration measurements for both fed-batch and continuous processes at various downstream unit operations. In-line variable pathlength UV spectroscopy (in-line VPS) is one such technology that is based on the principles of slope spectroscopy. Briefly, protein concentration is determined by using principles of Beer-Lambert (A= εcl) and the slope of A/l is derived from absorbance measurements made at multiple pathlengths (Huffman et al. 2014). This functionality overcomes the limitation of many UV sensors and broadens the linear range. Moreover, this flexibility can be used for both batch and continuous processes for purification (column loading, pooling) applications as well as UF/DF steps. The current UV-based tools that are integrated on purification skids often saturate, and laborious offline measurements (that are dependent on matrix effects and sample dilution) are used to measure higher concentrations samples from UF/DF. In-line VPS overcomes these challenges and provides a real-time protein concentration that can be used for process control. MVDA can also be performed on UV measurement to provide further insight on product quality attributes like higher molecular weight species by post-acquisition spectral processing and PLS modeling (Brestich et al. 2018).

There are additional devices that can measure protein concentration, although in-line VPS is GMP compatible and has a broad linear range. PendoTech® offers single-use flow cells with different options of hose barb connections and lower UV path length (Fedorenko et al. 2018). Index of refraction (IoR) offers another option to measure concentration as it has been demonstrated for capture chromatography and ultrafiltration downstream steps at low and high concentration ranges (Harris et al. 2021). Although this is a promising option, currently it is limited to the development scale due to flow rate restrictions.

The above-mentioned in-line PAT techniques have a clear advantage as they can be integrated with the process. They are plug and play, require minimal supervision, and manual intervention, and possess fast data acquisition frequencies. However, the specificity and sensitivity of spectroscopic tools suffer compared to their chromatographic counterparts when it comes to measuring product quality attributes.

11.5 Conclusion

In this chapter, we highlighted the role of PAT in biologics development, especially to facilitate intensified initiatives such as integrated and continuous processes. Integrated and continuous processes require rapid analytics to advance from one unit operation to another in a non-stop fashion. Thus, the analytical testing paradigm consisting of PAT was also evolved to meet these demands in development pipelines, and some of these techniques have been progressed into manufacturing suites to ensure consistent product quality. Within the chapter, we discussed some of the basic concepts, common terminologies, and main components of a typical PAT platform. A typical PAT system must contain a sensor, which captures analytical information from the biologics process. Analytical sensors can be spectroscopic, chromatographic, mass spectrometric, or any other analytical technique. Vibrational spectroscopic sensors are generally equipped with probes or flow cells for in-line data acquisition while techniques such as chromatography and/or mass spectrometry require extraction of a sample from the unit operations. Thus, such PAT techniques must be coupled with automated sampling devices. PMS and DCS systems are required for automatic processing of data, result visualization, and feedback control. Vibrational spectroscopic techniques such as Raman, FT-MIR, and NIR in conjunction with MVDA modeling allow real-time monitoring of CQAs and CPPs. Glucose, lactate, glutamate, viable cell density, and protein titer are some of the common attributes and parameters that can be measured by Raman spectroscopy during cell culture processes. Protein and excipient concentrations in downstream unit operations are known to be monitored by FT-MIR and/or NIR PAT tools. However, product- and process-related impurities such as aggregates, HCPs, and protein fragments require more sensitive and specific PAT techniques involving chromatography and mass spectrometry.

PAT relieves the analytical burden, provides a control mechanism, and ensures a consistent quality profile. These benefits propagate the use of PAT from development to clinical to commercial. Well-established technology that has hardware and software compliance should be translatable to commercial manufacturing. However, a thorough evaluation of risk assessment, business value, and technology readiness must be performed prior to the transfer into manufacturing suites for routine applications. PAT Monitoring and Control Team at BioPhorum, an inter-industry coalition of subject matter experts on PAT, recently reported a study on assessing the business and technology value of common PAT tools (Gillespie et al. 2022). This study provides a systematic assessment of the current usage and perceived value of PAT in the biopharma industry today. One common approach to minimize the risk of implementing newer analytical technologies in manufacturing is to use them initially for "information-only" purposes while continuing to rely on existing traditional offline analytics for decision-making. Raman for glucose monitoring and bio-capacitance probes for viable cell density monitoring are some of the common industry examples. The use of PAT tools for "information-only" for a defined period of time will allow the users to gain confidence and ample time for training, and also enable technology optimization for manufacturing needs. At this point, typically it is possible to use it for decision-making purposes while retiring the traditional offline analytical technique.

Regulatory considerations are also important in developing and implementing PAT platforms in manufacturing applications. The use of each of the tools mentioned above will dictate the regulatory strategy that needs to be taken. Most of the PAT is expected to be used as a monitoring tool, where a pre-defined action can be taken if product quality is out of range of experience. Regulatory guidance for method development and validation of general analytical techniques are applicable for PAT platforms. For instance, ICH Q2(R1) guidance on analytical method validation is applicable for PAT tools (ICH Q2(R1), 2005), though there is some specific regulatory guidance such as validation procedures for FT-NIR techniques (EMA 2014). As model-based process monitoring and control platforms of bioprocess are gaining momentum in recent years, it is essential to consider regulatory expectations on such technologies (ICH 2009b). ICH Q8,9,10 Q&A document classifies model-based approaches as low-impact, medium-impact, and high-impact, where low-impact models are information-only models that do not affect the process or the product quality assurance strategy, while high-impact models are the sole control/assurance of product quality. Medium-impact models can affect product quality, but other engineering controls are in place within the process to mitigate any redundancies due to false predictions. One of the key features of all the regulatory guidelines which are available to date is that all clearly emphasize the fact that multivariate models should demonstrate mechanistic, scientific, and statistical understanding with supporting data (ICH 2009b). FDA recommends early engagement with them through an emerging technology team (ETT) before including new technologies such as PAT in regulatory fillings for better alignment, knowledge sharing, and feedback.

REFERENCES

Abu-Absi NR, Kenty BM, Cuellar ME, et al. Real time monitoring of multiple parameters in mammalian cell culture bioreactors using an in-line Raman spectroscopy probe. *Biotechnol Bioeng*. 2011;*108*(5):1215–1221. doi:10.1002/bit.23023.

André S, Cristau L Saint, Gaillard S, Devos O, Calvosa É, Duponchel L. In-line and real-time prediction of recombinant antibody titer by in situ Raman spectroscopy. *Anal Chim Acta*. 2015;*892*:148–152. doi:10.1016/j.aca.2015.08.050.

Beck A, Wagner-Rousset E, Ayoub D, Van Dorsselaer A, Sanglier-Cianférani S. Characterization of therapeutic antibodies and related products. *Anal Chem*. 2013;*85*(2):715–736. doi:10.1021/ac3032355

Berry BN, Dobrowsky TM, Timson RC, Kshirsagar R, Ryll T, Wiltberger K. Quick generation of Raman spectroscopy based in-process glucose control to influence biopharmaceutical protein product quality during mammalian cell culture. *Biotechnol Prog*. 2016;*32*(1):224–234. doi:10.1002/btpr.2205.

Boulet-Audet M, Kazarian SG, Byrne B. In-column ATR-FTIR spectroscopy to monitor affinity chromatography purification of monoclonal antibodies. *Sci Rep.* 2016;*6*(July):1–13. doi:10.1038/srep30526.

Brestich N, Rüdt M, Büchler D, Hubbuch J. Selective protein quantification for preparative chromatography using variable pathlength UV/Vis spectroscopy and partial least squares regression. *Chem Eng Sci.* 2018;*176*:157–164. doi:10.1016/j.ces.2017.10.030

Cao H, Mushnoori S, Higgins B, et al. A systematic framework for data management and integration in a continuous pharmaceutical manufacturing processing line. *Processes.* 2018;*6*(5):1–21. doi:10.3390/pr6050053

Capito F, Skudas R, Kolmar H, Hunzinger C. At-line mid infrared spectroscopy for monitoring downstream processing unit operations. *Process Biochem.* 2015b;*50*(6):997–1005. doi:10.1016/j.procbio.2015.03.005.

Capito F, Zimmer A, Skudas R. Mid-infrared spectroscopy-based analysis of mammalian cell culture Parameters. *Biotechnol Prog.* 2015a;*31*(2):578–584. doi:10.1002/btpr.2026.

Chemmalil L, Wasalathanthri DP, Zhang X, et al. Online monitoring and control of upstream cell culture process using 1D and 2D – LC with SegFlow interface. *Biotechnol Bioeng.* 2021;*118*(9):3593–3603. doi:10.1002/bit.27873.

Coolbaugh MJ, Varner CT, Vetter TA, et al. Pilot-scale demonstration of an end-to-end integrated and continuous biomanufacturing process. *Biotechnol Bioeng.* 2021. doi:10.1002/bit.27670.

Czeterko M, DeBaise A, Pierce W, Conway M, inventors; Regeneron Pharmaceuticals Inc, assignee. In Situ Raman Spectroscopy Systems and Methods for Controlling Process Variables in Cell Cultures. 2019. *United States patent application US 16/160,194.*

Dunn ZD, Desai J, Leme GM, Stoll DR, Douglas D. Rapid two-dimensional Protein-A size exclusion chromatography of monoclonal antibodies for titer and aggregation measurements from harvested cell culture fluid samples. *MAbs.* 2020;*12*(1). doi:10.1080/19420862.2019.1702263

EMA. *Guideline on the Use of Near Infrared Spectroscopy by the Pharmaceutical Industry and the Data Requirements for New Submissions and Variations.* 2014. Retried from https://www.ema.europa.eu/en/use-near-infrared-spectroscopy-nirs-pharmaceutical-industry-data-requirements-new-submissions.

Esmonde-White KA, Cuellar M, Uerpmann C, Lenain B, Lewis IR. Raman spectroscopy as a process analytical technology for pharmaceutical manufacturing and bioprocessing. *Anal Bioanal Chem.* 2017;*409*(3):637–649. doi:10.1007/s00216-016-9824-1.

FDA. *Guidance for Industry PAT – A Framework for Innovative Pharmaceutical Manufacturing and Quality Assurance.* 2004. Retrieved from http://www.fda.gov/cder/OPS/PAT.htm969/.

Fedorenko D, Tan J, Shinkazh O, Annarelli D. In-line turbidity sensors for monitoring process streams in continuous countercurrent tangential chromatography. *Bioprocess Int.* 2018;*16*(10):8–11.

Fisher AC, Kamga MH, Agarabi C, Brorson K, Lee SL, Yoon S. The current scientific and regulatory landscape in advancing integrated continuous biopharmaceutical manufacturing. *Trends Biotechnol.* 2019;*37*(3):253–267. doi:10.1016/j.tibtech.2018.08.008.

Gillespie C, Wasalathanthri DP, Ritz DB, et al. Systematic assessment of process analytical technologies for biologics. *Biotechnol Bioeng.* 2022;*119*:423–434. doi:10.1002/bit.27990.

Goby JD, Khouri JN, Durve A, Zimmerman E, Furuya K. Control of protein a column loading during continuous antibody production: A technology overview of real-time titer measurement methods. *Bioprocess Int.* 2019. https://bioprocessintl.com/analytical/pat/control-of-protein-a-column-loading-during-continuous-antibody-production-real-time-titer-measurement-methods/.

Gronemeyer P, Ditz R, Strube J. Trends in upstream and downstream process development for antibody manufacturing. *Bioengineering.* 2014;*1*:188–212. doi:10.3390/bioengineering1040188.

Großhans S, Rüdt M, Sanden A, et al. In-line Fourier-transform infrared spectroscopy as a versatile process analytical technology for preparative protein chromatography. *J Chromatogr A.* 2018;*1547*:37–44. doi:10.1016/j.chroma.2018.03.005.

Harris SA, Patel BA, Gospodarek A, et al. Determination of protein concentration in downstream biomanufacturing processes by in-line index of refraction. *Biotechnol Prog.* 2021;*37*(5):1–10. doi:10.1002/btpr.3187.

Haverick M, Mengisen S, Shameem M. Separation of mAbs molecular variants by analytical hydrophobic interaction chromatography HPLC: Overview and applications Separation of mAbs molecular variants by analytical hydrophobic interaction chromatography HPLC Overview and applications. *MAbs.* 2014;*0862*. doi:10.4161/mabs.28693.

Herwig C, Garcia-Aponte OF, Golabgir A, Rathore AS. Knowledge management in the QbD paradigm: Manufacturing of biotech therapeutics. *Trends Biotechnol.* 2015;*33*(7):381–387. doi:10.1016/j.tibtech.2015.04.004

Hofer A, Kroll P, Barmettler M, Herwig C. A reliable automated sampling system for on-line and real-time monitoring of CHO cultures. *Processes*. 2020;*8*(6):1–16.

Hong MS, Severson KA, Jiang M, Lu AE, Love JC, Braatz RD. Challenges and opportunities in biopharmaceutical manufacturing control. *Comput Chem Eng*. 2018;*110*:106–114. doi:10.1016/j.compchemeng.2017.12.007.

Huffman S, Soni K, Ferraiolo J. UV-vis based determination of protein concentration. *Bioprocess Int*. 2014;*12*(8):66–73.

ICH. (2005). *Validation of Analytical Procedures: Text and Methodology Q2(R1)*. Retrieved from https://database.ich.org/sites/default/files/Q2_R1__Guideline.pdf.

ICH. (2009a). *Pharmaceutical Development Q8(R2)*. Retrieved from https://database.ich.org/sites/default/files/Q8_R2_Guideline.pdf. Accessed 01 February 2020.

ICH. (2009b). *Quality Implementation Working Group on Q8, Q9 and Q10 Questions & Answers (R2)*. https://database.ich.org/sites/default/files/Q8_Q9_Q10_Q%26As_R4_Points_to_Consider_0.pdf. Accessed 01 February 2020.

Jiang M, Severson KA, Love JC, et al. Opportunities and challenges of real-time release testing in biopharmaceutical manufacturing. *Biotechnol Bioeng*. 2017;*114*(11):2445–2456. doi:10.1002/bit.26383.

Li B, Ray BH, Leister KJ, Ryder AG. Performance monitoring of a mammalian cell based bioprocess using Raman spectroscopy. *Anal Chim Acta*. 2013;*796*:84–91. doi:10.1016/j.aca.2013.07.058.

Matthews TE, Berry BN, Smelko J, Moretto J, Moore B, Wiltberger K. Closed loop control of lactate concentration in mammalian cell culture by Raman spectroscopy leads to improved cell density, viability, and biopharmaceutical protein production. *Biotechnol Bioeng*. 2016;*113*(11):2416–2424. doi:10.1002/bit.26018.

Mehdizadeh H, Lauri D, Karry KM, Moshgbar M, Procopio-Melino R, Drapeau D. Generic Raman-based calibration models enabling real-time monitoring of cell culture bioreactors. *Biotechnol Prog*. 2015;*31*(4):1004–1013. doi:10.1002/btpr.2079.

Metze S, Blioch S, Matuszczyk J, Greller G, Grimm C, Scholz J. Multivariate data analysis of capacitance frequency scanning for online monitoring of viable cell concentrations in small-scale bioreactors. *Anal Bioanal Chem*. 2020b;*412*:2089–2102. 10.1007/s00216-019-02096-3.

Metze S, Greller SRG, Scholz CGJ. Monitoring online biomass with a capacitance sensor during scale – up of industrially relevant CHO cell culture fed – batch processes in single – use bioreactors. *Bioprocess Biosyst Eng*. 2020a;*43*(2):193–205. doi:10.1007/s00449-019-02216-4.

Moore B, Sanford R, Zhang A. Case study: The characterization and implementation of dielectric spectroscopy (biocapacitance) for process control in a commercial GMP CHO manufacturing process. *Biotechnol Prog*. 2019;*35*(3). doi:10.1002/btpr.2782.

Mullard A. 2019 FDA drug approvals. *Nat Rev Drug Discov*. 2020;*19*(2):79–84. doi:10.1038/d41573-020-00001-7.

Opel CF, Li J, Amanullah A. Quantitative modeling of viable cell density, cell size, intracellular conductivity, and membrane capacitance in batch and fed-batch cho processes using dielectric spectroscopy. *Am Inst Chem Eng*. 2010;*92056*:1187–1199. doi:10.1002/btpr.425

Patel BA, Gospodarek A, Larkin M, et al. Multi-angle light scattering as a process analytical technology measuring real-time molecular weight for downstream process control. *MAbs*. 2018;*10*(7):945–950. doi:10.1080/19420862.2018.1505178.

Patel BA, Pinto NDS, Gospodarek A, et al. On-line ion exchange liquid chromatography as a process analytical technology for monoclonal antibody characterization in continuous bioprocessing. *Anal Chem*. 2017;*89*(21):11357–11365. doi:10.1021/acs.analchem.7b02228.

Pepper C. Accelerate cell culture development using the modular automated sampling technology (MASTTM) platform in an integrated bioprocess lab environment. *Eng Conf Int*. 2016:5–10.

Rathore AS. Roadmap for implementation of quality by design (QbD) for biotechnology products. *Trends Biotechnol*. 2009;*27*(9):546–553. doi:10.1016/j.tibtech.2009.06.006.

Rathore AS, Kumar D, Kateja N. Role of raw materials in biopharmaceutical manufacturing: risk analysis and fingerprinting. *Curr Opin Biotechnol*. 2018;*53*:99–105. doi:10.1016/j.copbio.2017.12.022.

Rathore AS, Winkle H. Quality by design for biopharmaceuticals. *Nat Biotechnol*. 2009;*27*(1):26–34.

Read EK, Park JT, Shah RB, Riley BS, Brorson KA, Rathore AS. Process analytical technology (PAT) for biopharmaceutical products: Part I. Concepts and applications. *Biotechnol Bioeng*. 2010;*105*(2):276–284. doi:10.1002/bit.22528.

Ryder AG. Cell culture media analysis using rapid spectroscopic methods. *Curr Opin Chem Eng.* 2018;22:11–17. doi:10.1016/j.coche.2018.08.008.

Sandner V, Pybus LP, McCreath G. Scale-down model development in AMBR systems: An industrial perspective. *Biotechnol J.* 2018:1–31. 10.1002/biot.201700766.

Santos RM, Kessler JM, Salou P, Menezes JC, Peinado A. Monitoring mAb cultivations with in-situ raman spectroscopy: The influence of spectral selectivity on calibration models and industrial use as reliable PAT tool. *Biotechnol Prog.* 2018;34(3):659–670. doi:10.1002/btpr.2635.

Sathyanarayana DN. *Vibrational Spectroscopy—Theory and Applications*, 2nd ed. New Delhi, India: New Age International (P) Limited, 2004.

Stoll D, Danforth J, Zhang K, Beck A. Characterization of therapeutic antibodies and related products by two-dimensional liquid chromatography coupled with UV absorbance and mass spectrometric detection. *J Chromatogr B Anal Technol Biomed Life Sci.* 2016;1032:51–60. doi:10.1016/j.jchromb.2016.05.029.

Stoll DR, Carr PW. Two-dimensional liquid chromatography: A state of the art tutorial. *Anal Chem.* 2017;89(1):519–531. doi:10.1021/acs.analchem.6b03506.

Stoll DR, Shoykhet K, Petersson P, Buckenmaier S. Active solvent modulation: A valve-based approach to improve separation compatibility in two-dimensional liquid chromatography. *Anal Chem.* 2017;89:9260–9267. doi:10.1021/acs.analchem.7b02046.

Thakur G, Hebbi V, Rathore AS. An NIR-based PAT approach for real-time control of loading in Protein A chromatography in continuous manufacturing of monoclonal antibodies. *Biotechnol Bioeng.* 2020;117(3):673–686. doi:10.1002/bit.27236.

Tiwari A, Kateja N, Chanana S, Rathore AS. Use of HPLC as an enabler of process analytical technology in process chromatography. *Anal Chem.* 2018;90(13):7824–7829. doi:10.1021/acs.analchem.8b00897.

Trunfio N, Lee H, Starkey J, Agarabi C, Liu J, Yoon S. Characterization of mammalian cell culture raw materials by combining spectroscopy and chemometrics. *Biotechnol Prog.* 2017;33(4):1127–1138. doi:10.1002/btpr.2480.

Warikoo V, Godawat R, Brower K, et al. Integrated continuous production of recombinant therapeutic proteins. *Biotechnol Bioeng.* 2012;109(12):3018–3029. doi:10.1002/bit.24584

Wasalathanthri DP, Ding J, Li ZJ. Real time process monitoring in biologics development. *Am Pharm Rev.* 2020d;23(April):72–75.

Wasalathanthri DP, Feroz H, Puri N, et al. Real-time monitoring of quality attributes by in-line Fourier transform infrared spectroscopic sensors at ultrafiltration and diafiltration of bioprocess. *Biotechnol Bioeng.* 2020c;117:3766–3774. doi:10.1002/bit.27532.

Wasalathanthri DP, Rehmann MS, Song Y, et al. Technology outlook for real-time quality attribute and process parameter monitoring in biopharmaceutical development—A review. *Biotechnol Bioeng.* 2020a;117:3182–3198. doi:10.1002/bit.27461.

Wasalathanthri DP, Rehmann MS, West JM, Borys MC, Ding J, Li ZJ. Paving the way for real time process monitoring in biomanufacturing. *Am Pharm Rev.* 2020b:1–5. www.americanpharmaceuticalreview.com.

Wasalathanthri DP, Shah R, Ding J, Leone A, Li ZJ. Process analytics 4.0: A paradigm shift in rapid analytics for biologics development. *Biotechnol Prog.* 2021:1–13. doi:10.1002/btpr.3177.

Wasalathanthri DP, Tewari JC, Kang X, Hincapie M, Barrett S. Multivariate spectral analysis and monitoring for biomanufacturing. 2019. *Patent No. US 2019/0272894 A1. United States.*

Webster TA, Hadley BC, Hilliard W, Jaques C, Mason C. Development of generic raman models for a GS-KOTM CHO platform process. *Biotechnol Prog.* 2018;34(3):730–737. doi:10.1002/btpr.2633.

Xu J, Xu X, Huang C, et al. Biomanufacturing evolution from conventional to intensified processes for productivity improvement: A case study. *MAbs.* 2020;12(1). doi:10.1080/19420862.2020.1770669.

Yilmaz D, Mehdizadeh H, Navarro D, Shehzad A, O'Connor M, McCormick P. Application of Raman spectroscopy in monoclonal antibody producing continuous systems for downstream process intensification. *Biotechnol Prog.* 2020;36(3). doi:10.1002/btpr.2947.

Zydney AL. Perspectives on integrated continuous bioprocessing – opportunities and challenges. *Curr Opin Chem Eng.* 2015;10:8–13. doi:10.1016/j.coche.2015.07.005.

12

Moving to Manufacturing: Lessons Learned in a Career in Process Analytical Technology

Rodolfo J. Romañach
University of Puerto Rico, Mayaguez, Puerto Rico

CONTENTS

Introduction – Always Encountering PAT

This is a reflection on a career where process analytical chemistry or process analytical technology (PAT) has always been present. It is an exception to the author's advice to students while writing research papers: "focus on science and leave behind personal experiences". This chapter is the acceptance of a separate advice: "The unexamined life is not worth living". The author hopes that it will be helpful to young scientists starting their careers in the pharmaceutical industry.

The author's first encounter with this exciting field was in graduate studies at the University of Georgia through a seminar by Bruce Kowalski (Callis et al. 1987; Kelly et al. 1989; Pell et al. 2014; Kowalski 1978). Kowalski's seminar brought a clear message that analytical chemistry was not limited to measurements in a chemistry lab, and provided an invitation to open our minds to multivariate data analysis. This seminar strengthened the research group's perspective of industrial applications of process measurements since it was already working on real-time spectroscopic methods (Friedman and De Haseth 1985; Romañach and de Haseth 1988; Robertson et al. 1988). Kowalski's seminar was the beginning of a career in process analytical chemistry where the term "process analytical technology" would later be used to emphasize a systems approach to manufacturing, which was not limited to chemistry (U.S. Department of Health and Human Services, Food & Drug Administration 2004). Hopefully, nobody will be shocked to learn that PAT was not invented by the U.S. Food and Drug Administration (FDA), and it did not start with the PAT guidance (U.S. Department of Health and Human Services, Food & Drug Administration 2004). The ideas in the PAT guidance were developed many years before by Kowalski and other scientists, and became part of an effort to bring innovation into the pharmaceutical manufacturing science.

DOI: 10.1201/9781003149835-15

This reflection requires a special thank you to Ken Morris, who first mentioned that PAT was being discussed in FDA committees and recommended keeping an eye on it, and to Ajaz Hussain for encouraging research in PAT. We invited Ajaz to speak at a session on blend uniformity at a conference in San Juan in 2003. However, as we organized the meeting it became evident that his focus was on PAT, and he did not want to speak about blend uniformity. Ajaz used one minute of his talk to indicate that the blend uniformity guidance which had brought so much discussion and problems was withdrawn a few days before (U.S. Department of Health and Human Services, Food & Drug Administration 2002; Muzzio et al. 1997), and dedicated the remaining 30 minutes to PAT. This was a clear message that it was time to move on to PAT. The author was just starting his research group at the University of Puerto Rico, Mayaguez campus, and focusing on near-infrared (NIR) spectroscopy as a way to reduce the use of liquid chromatography and solvents in content uniformity testing (Ramirez et al. 2001). However, the message from Ajaz was that it was time to monitor pharmaceutical processes, use NIR spectroscopy to monitor processes, and move out of the laboratory.

The author's career started in pharmaceutical manufacturing. Many of the first projects as a recently graduated PhD scientist were related to the lack of robustness of high-performance liquid chromatography (HPLC) methods. In 1987, QC labs were still making a transition from gas chromatography to HPLC; silanol effects and column-to-column variation were barely understood (Köhler and Kirkland 1987; Kirkland et al. 1989). HPLC offered many interesting scientific challenges at this time. The manufacturing site had a very vibrant quality improvement programme which emphasized the importance of estimating the cost of product non-conformance when product quality problems occurred (Covey 2004; Crosby 1980). As the plant examined its processes, it became obvious that the cost of rejecting a lot was much greater than the savings involved in improving a method in the quality control lab. The next step was an invitation to participate in teams that sought to address problems related to production processes.

Looking back, the author can now see that several of his first industrial problems were a clear signal of the need for process knowledge and PAT. The challenges included a product where occasionally 1 out of 12 tablets would fail dissolution. The main thinking was that over-lubrication could be occurring and magnesium stearate could be coating the active pharmaceutical ingredient (API) preventing its release. The homogenization of magnesium stearate and the development of methods to determine its distribution in formulations attracted significant research efforts in later years (Duong et al. 2003; Abe and Otsuka 2012; Green et al. 2005; Zuurman et al. 1999). A second product also developed dissolution problems. This was a high-volume product and the company wanted to reduce its release times. A Quality Improvement team found an opportunity to reduce release times by quickly moving the tablets from the production area to the QC lab. All of a sudden, the product started to fail dissolution, and large portions of tablets would remain intact in the dissolution bath. This was the first encounter with tablet relaxation, a topic to which we returned a few years later (Ropero et al. 2011; Van der Voort Maarschalk et al. 1997). The industrial experience also involved six months at Upjohn headquarters in Kalamazoo in troubleshooting projects with polarized light microscopy (Aldrich and Smith 1999). This short industrial sabbatical was an introduction to the solid state and sparked interest in understanding the interaction among particles in solid oral dosage forms. However, practically all the methods implemented in the quality control laboratories involved the destruction of the tablet structure to make it possible to use HPLC, eliminating all the information related to the physical properties of the materials needed to understand the manufacturing process.

The need to adapt to non-destructive methods of analysis capable of providing information on the chemical composition of formulations and their physical properties is still a hurdle to the implementation of PAT in manufacturing. The adoption of PAT requires an open mind to new methods of analysis. Unfortunately, many analytical chemists are still trained in methods completely focused on the API, considering the physical properties of materials as interferences, and throwing away the information on the physical properties that are needed by process support personnel.

PAT from Development to Manufacturing

PAT is often seen strictly from the product development point of view. The business case for PAT is easy to visualize when the method is needed for approval of a drug product and growth of company sales.

However, PAT projects may also be started by personnel at pharmaceutical manufacturing sites (Vargas et al. 2018; Gray 2016).

Many manufacturing sites are still concerned about observing unexpected variation in processes when PAT measurements are made. Many companies are not aware of the "PAT Safe Harbor" as described in the PAT Guidance (U.S. Department of Health and Human Services, Food & Drug Administration 2004): "When using new measurement tools, such as on-or in-line process analyzers, certain data trends, intrinsic to a currently acceptable process, may be observed. Manufacturers should scientifically evaluate these data to determine how or if such trends affect quality and implementation of PAT tools. FDA does not intend to inspect research data collected on an existing product for the purpose of evaluating the suitability of an experimental process analyzer or other PAT tool. FDA's routine inspection of a firm's manufacturing process that incorporates a PAT tool for research purposes will be based on current regulatory standards (e.g. test results from currently approved or acceptable regulatory methods)." Even though the PAT Guidance was published in 2004, it is not sufficiently known at the manufacturing level. There are still pharmaceutical personnel surprised to learn that PAT research data may be collected while the product is evaluated with the currently approved FDA procedures.

The progress of PAT in manufacturing is also slowed down by projects that were not planned correctly. The author has encountered situations where a NIR or Raman spectrometer was purchased because funds were available at the end of the year, and the operational unit did not want to lose them. The instrument was purchased but without funds for developing or implementing the method, since the salesperson said it was easy to implement. The plan was for the analyst to advance the project in "free time", which never materialized. The author recognizes that these situations are less likely nowadays, but there are still cases where PAT instruments are purchased for a product that was never approved. The reality is that there are millions of dollars invested in PAT equipment that is not used, and too much paperwork and time are needed to donate the instrument to a university. Depreciation is the only deliverable from many PAT instruments.

Lack of communication with subject matter experts within companies or with academic research groups has delayed the progress of PAT. PAT projects were started but ran into difficulties due to lack of expertise, the project stopped and was never re-started. We once visited a manufacturing site where a project to monitor drying within a fluid bed granulator was stopped, since one out of every ten spectra would be noisy with a high baseline. The remaining spectra were excellent, with a high signal-to-noise ratio. Service personnel had come to check the spectrometer twice and could not determine the cause. This visit coincided with a research project that studied the baseline in spectra obtained in real-time (Ropero et al. 2009). The reason for the problem was immediately clear: a paddle (chopper) in the granulator was interrupting the path of light to the NIR spectrometer and causing the high baseline. However, the fundamental problem was the lack of timely communication with subject matter experts.

Several major pharmaceutical companies have now established PAT groups (Guenard and Thurau 2010; Montenegro-Alvarado et al. 2014). These PAT groups include highly specialized personnel with expertise in spectroscopy, chemometrics, and process engineering. The PAT groups participate in conferences such as International Foundation for Process Analytical Chemistry (IFPAC) which serve as a bridge between FDA leaders and industry (Peng et al. 2015). PAT groups play a key role in communicating with the FDA on PAT and in the development and implementation of emerging technologies (O'Connor et al. 2016).

The PAT groups are also a good resource for manufacturing sites to plan successful projects. As companies have gained more experience, they have each developed their own "PAT Tool Box" – a set of successful applications applied in development and manufacturing. However, PAT groups are usually focused on contributing to the approval of new products. The PAT groups need to move to another new product once the method is implemented at the manufacturing site. The successful transition of PAT from development to manufacturing requires dedicated PAT ownership at the manufacturing site. The author has seen too many good projects hampered by the lack of a dedicated process owner. PAT methods require model maintenance which must be performed within the manufacturing facility's quality system. Of course, communication with the original method developers is always important, but it should not require extensive use of their time. A full method transfer where the manufacturing site takes charge is necessary.

The transition of PAT into manufacturing requires that it be implemented within the manufacturing plant's quality system. Quality systems need to transition from the established approach where samples are brought to the quality control laboratory to procedures based on a new paradigm where a process is monitored in real-time (Singh et al. 2014b). Quality systems must consider the effect of process disturbances on the continuous manufacturing system (Taipale-Kovalainen et al. 2019; Vargas et al. 2018; Sánchez-Paternina et al. 2022). Quality systems must describe the control strategy that is now possible through PAT.

Raw Material Identification – An Ideal Starting Point for PAT Projects

The identification of raw materials is a well-developed application and serves as an ideal introductory project to non-destructive analysis and PAT (Miró Vera and Alcalà Bernàrdez 2017). The identification of raw materials and APIs by NIR spectroscopy was described more than 20 years ago (Blanco and Romero 2001). The pioneering work by Marcelo Blanco's group described the development of a spectral library with 125 different raw materials and showed the concept of sub-cascading libraries to discriminate between structurally similar excipients. This spectral library for raw material identification has been expanded and used at Grupo Menarini for over 20 years. The original dispersive NIR spectrometer where the application was developed is no longer in service. A new library was constructed with Fourier transform NIR instruments. A pharmaceutical manufacturing site can now use NIR spectroscopy to determine whether the material received is a specific type of excipient, such as microcrystalline cellulose (MCC). However, it could also be used to identify the type of MCC received. This well-established application is an ideal application for a manufacturing plant to start developing expertise with non-destructive methods of analysis and then move into PAT applications.

A frequent question is whether to use Raman or NIR spectroscopy for the identification of raw materials. Raman spectroscopy has become very popular in recent years through the introduction of various hand-held systems (Matthews et al. 2019; Crocombe 2018; Bakeev 2015). Raman spectra are much easier to interpret than NIR spectra which are characterized by the overlap of overtone and combination bands from the different functional groups. Raman spectroscopy is usually more powerful in discriminating between the different crystal forms of a compound. However, excipients such as MCC and some APIs will exhibit fluorescence adding a low-frequency noise to Raman spectra. Each pharmaceutical company must evaluate the advantages and disadvantages of NIR and Raman spectroscopic approaches.

The Business Case for PAT

A few years ago, after a presentation on PAT, we were asked for advice on how to present the business case for PAT. Industrial scientists need to justify a PAT project through a business case; the most used tool to justify a capital investment (Maes and Van Liedekerke 2006; Kourti and Davis 2012; Fontalvo-Lascano et al. 2020a; Fontalvo-Lascano et al. 2022; BioPhorum 2020). The business case is frequently a highly structured instrument that describes the problem, cost, benefits, possible solutions, and data required to make an investment decision (Stratton 2004; Fontalvo-Lascano et al. 2020b; Romañach 2021). The business case for PAT must be clear before the project is funded.

The requirements for a clear effective business case are very similar to the requirements for presenting a research proposal to the National Science Foundation (NSF) or other funding agency. The approval of a research project also requires a description of the benefits, cost, and risks involved. Therefore, the business case may serve as an instrument for industry–university collaboration. Academic scientists understand the benefits of PAT and the cost of instruments, and can visualize possible delays in developing a new method. Industrial personnel must seek information on the cost structure of their companies and visualize the benefits of PAT in transforming their operations. The cost structure of pharmaceutical manufacturing depends on every single company and varies according to the diversity of their products. PAT projects compete with many other potential investments that company leaders evaluate, just like an NSF proposal. The future advancement of PAT requires greater study of the benefits, costs, and risks associated with each application (Axon et al. 1998; Cogdill et al. 2007). The business case is the starting point of this important evaluation.

PAT and chemometrics will help companies make money (Seasholtz 1999). However, this vision needs to encompass the entire framework for working with the data obtained from a process and extracting information from it. A few years ago, a presentation by Dow scientists indicated a key idea: "where data is working for us, and we are not working for it". This integration of PAT, process data, and relevant information is becoming increasingly important for advanced manufacturing (Huang et al. 2021).

Industry–University Collaboration in PAT

The first request for a "PAT trained scientist" was received over 15 years ago. This and other requests were the basis of an article on this subject (Romañach 2008). Surprisingly, the ideas in that initial article are still fairly accurate. PAT scientists must:

- Obtain and interpret data relevant to the manufacturing process.
- Be interested in the various aspects of pharma manufacturing, data storage and evaluation, and risk management.
- Be able to visualize the interaction between different components in formulations.
- Work with a PAT team to understand FDA guidance, Quality by Design, and ICH guidelines.
- Work with personnel who understand company procedures and practices, and especially with personnel involved in quality control functions who can help implement PAT within the company's quality system.

The main role of universities is in providing the future generation of pharmaceutical scientists that will advance PAT. Research groups at the Universitat Autònoma de Barcelona and Duquesne have provided leaders for the PAT initiative (Blanco et al. 2008, Rosas et al. 2013, Igne et al. 2015, Shi et al. 2012, Càrdenas et al. 2014). The NSF funding of the Engineering Research Center for Structured Organic Particulate Systems (C-SOPS) also led to the training of scientists in continuous manufacturing and PAT at Rutgers, Purdue, NJIT, and our University of Puerto Rico-Mayagüez campus (Hernandez et al. 2016; Román-Ospino et al. 2016; Gupta et al. 2015; Zhang et al. 2014; Jerez-Rozo et al. 2011; Singh et al. 2014a; Pawar et al. 2016; Escotet-Espinoza et al. 2018).

A worldwide academic response to the call for innovation started by the PAT guidance has occurred resulting in advances in material characterization, process measurements, design of experiments and chemometrics, risk management, modeling and simulations, and control strategies (Rantanen and Khinast 2015; Sacher et al. 2022; Thakur et al. 2021; Buckley and Ryder 2017; Bawuah et al. 2021; Durao et al. 2017). The transition toward continuous manufacturing and PAT requires significant training of pharmaceutical personnel (de Matas et al. 2016; Moghtadernejad et al. 2018; Romañach et al. 2014). However, the role of the academic sector has not been limited to human resources. The knowledge obtained in continuous manufacturing at C-SOPS was the basis for industrial processes (Vargas et al. 2017; Vargas et al. 2018), and many current industrial PAT methods have also benefited from previous academic research efforts. The future advancement of PAT into manufacturing will require greater industry–university collaboration. The use of Strategic Doing as a method for collaboration for innovation is highly promising (Morrison et al. 2019).

This is a great opportunity to thank industrial scientists who have encouraged the breaking of the natural academic tendency to highlight good results, emphasizing the results that show good accuracy and precision. This approach might facilitate publication but does not provide the most valuable information for industrial scientists. The description of unexpected results could help the industry save a lot of time and money. Throughout the years, a number of scientists have encouraged the publication of these not-so-good, but valuable unexpected results.

PAT and Company Culture

One of the lessons learned during these years has been that progress in PAT and industry–university collaboration depends to a large degree on company culture. The cultures that limit progress are as follows:

- This is a regulated industry, and nothing can be changed.
- We do not want to open Pandora's box.
- We do not want to be leaders, we will focus on the state of the art. We could be leaders, but then others will catch up. Leading is too much trouble!!
- We do not have expertise in PAT or chemometrics. We need to check with headquarters first. We will let you know later.

PAT is an opportunity to be a leader, and an opportunity to transform a company through manufacturing science and innovation. Just visualize the following scenario: Will an FDA inspector arrive at a manufacturing plant while thinking:

- Will I have to go over the same documentation and quality problems as last time, which required over 2 months of work? or,
- Let's see what's new this time. On my last visit, they showed me a new PAT system, and a thorough understanding of their granulation process. It was quite interesting! They are true PAT and QbD leaders, this is always a nice refreshing visit.

A few years ago, we conducted hundreds of customer interviews through the NSF I-Corps (Innovation Corps) program (Pinzon de la Rosa et al. 2017). The best winning culture that we found was: "We will invest in the right tools and people to bring our products to market first. We do not want to delay new sales because we lack technology or scientific knowledge". PAT is part of the science and technology that can bring products to market first, and then contribute to the manufacturing of a quality product.

Further Analytical Challenges/Implementing in Manufacturing

Many of the PAT methods employ NIR spectroscopy to obtain real-time spectra directly in the production area. Spectra may be obtained for samples in their native state without having to reduce their particle size or dissolve them. The fact that sample preparation is not required makes NIR spectroscopy an excellent analytical method for the study of solids. However, NIR spectra depend on both the chemical composition and physical properties of materials, and the deconvolution of the chemical information and the physical properties is not simple (Razuc et al. 2019; Griffiths and Dahm 2007; Dahm and Dahm 2007; Dahm et al. 2000; Alcala et al. 2009).

NIR spectra are often obtained through diffuse reflection. As the NIR radiation travels through particles, some of it is absorbed, some transmitted, and some diffusely reflected in other directions. Figure 12.1 shows the NIR spectra of sucrose and sucrose ground with a mortar and pestle. The ground sucrose has a much greater surface area and more diffuse radiation reaches the detector. Therefore, the ground sucrose appears to absorb less radiation. The right side of Figure 12.1 shows that baseline differences are eliminated through the second derivative, but spectral differences are still observed. The spectra shown in Figure 12.1 clearly show the ability of NIR spectroscopy to identify materials with different physical properties.

One of the difficulties or challenges in working with NIR spectroscopy is that the exact mass of material that is analyzed is not known. The mass analyzed may only be estimated (Bellamy et al. 2008; Colón et al. 2014; Iyer et al. 2002; Hetrick et al. 2021; Ortega-Zuñiga et al. 2017; Dahm and Dahm 2007). There is always strong interest in analyzing the mass of a single dose. However, the depth of penetration of the radiation is practically impossible to determine in real-time measurements in the feed frame of a tablet

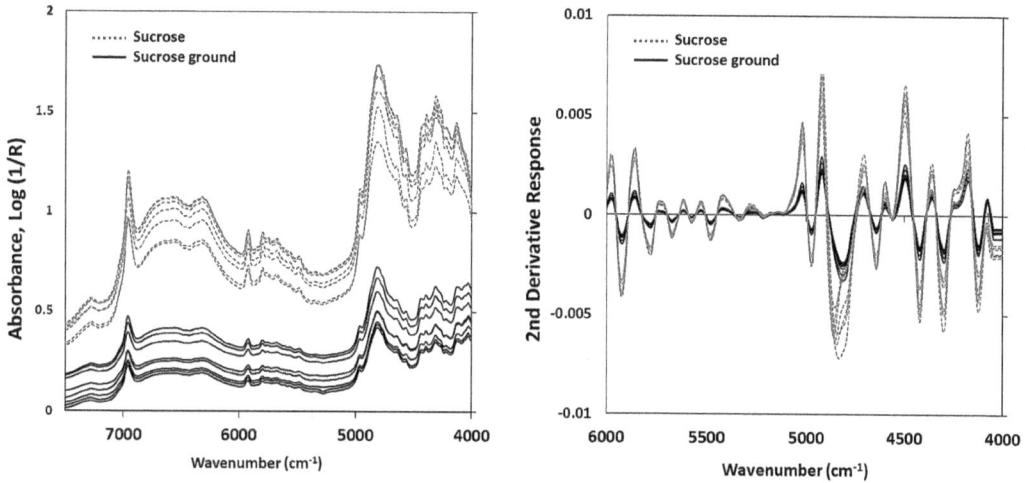

FIGURE 12.1 NIR spectra of sucrose and sucrose ground with mortar and pestle. Differences are observed in the original spectra and after second derivative preprocessing.

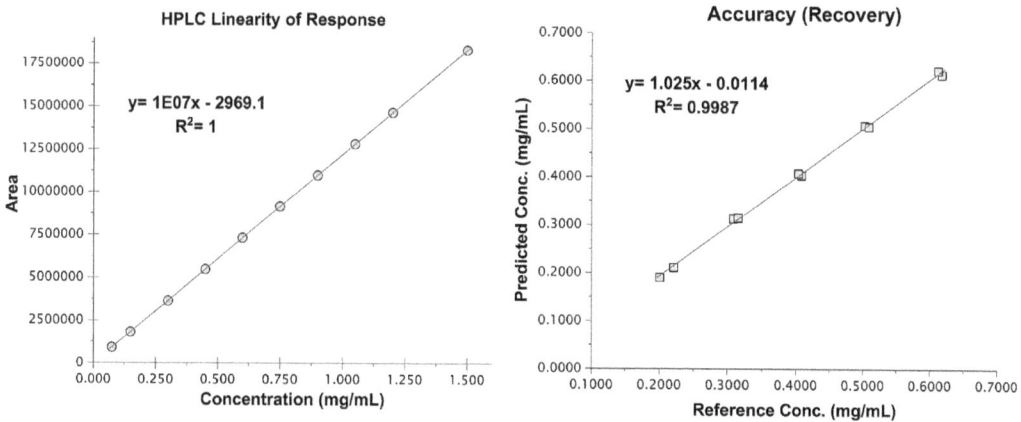

FIGURE 12.2 Two different ways in which linearity may be evaluated. Left – linearity of detector response. Right – linearity of accuracy at the different concentrations.

press and other operations. The depth of penetration also varies according to physical properties such as the bulk density of a powder blend.

The implementation of NIR or Raman spectroscopy is also affected when method validation is approached as a checklist. For example, the checklist may indicate method linearity. In an HPLC method, linearity is conducted with solutions of a single solute in a non-interfering solvent. Linearity is often plotted as the response of the detector response in absorbance units, peak area, or peak height versus concentration as shown in Figure 12.2. However, in the NIR or Raman methods, the pharmaceutical product is measured in its native state. The response of the detector is not plotted when performing linearity in the NIR spectroscopy method. Instead, in a NIR spectroscopic method, linearity is determined by plotting the predicted concentration vs. the expected or reference concentration. The linearity in the NIR method involves all the steps in the determination: spectral acquisition and prediction. The linearity in the HPLC method does not involve all the steps in the determination, it is based on single solute solutions and does not involve extractions from the sample matrix.

The figures of merit (FOM) used in PAT methods for indicating accuracy may be confusing to personnel who are used to reviewing HPLC validations and are often unfamiliar with the root mean square error of prediction (RMSEP). PAT validations do not measure accuracy through the percent API extracted (recovered) from a sample matrix, as shown on the left side of Table 12.1. In PAT methods, the FOM most often used to express accuracy are bias and the RMSEP (Næs et al. 2002; Esbensen and Swarbrick 2018). Bias is the average difference of the residuals obtained after comparing the predicted value, $\hat{y}_i$ and y_i, the expected or reference result for the independent validation samples. Table 12.1 presents on the first columns the FOM which would be used in an HPLC validation and those that would be used in a PAT validation on the right side. All results in this didactic example have been expressed with four significant figures or four decimal places. Accuracy would be expressed as 99.22% recovery in HPLC validations, while the validation of an NIR spectroscopic method would indicate an RMSEP of 6.514×10^{-3} grams, and as a bias of -0.0011 grams in PAT FOM. These two approaches appear initially to be somewhat difficult to compare as recovery is expressed in relative terms and bias on an absolute basis. The two approaches can be compared by calculating the residual in relative terms. Each residual value may be divided by the reference amount and multiplied by 100% as shown in the column labeled residual (%) in Table 12.1. The percent relative bias for the results shown in Table 12.1 is -0.7842 %, and it is now easy to visualize that it refers to the 99.22% recovery.

$$bias = \frac{\sum_{i=1}^{Np} (\hat{y}_i - y_i)}{N_p} \tag{12.1}$$

$$\text{Percent relative bias} = \frac{\sum_{i=1}^{Np} \left(\frac{\hat{y}_i - y_i}{y_i} \times 100 \right)}{N_p} \tag{12.2}$$

The RMSEP is also often used to indicate accuracy in PAT methods. The RMSEP expresses the variability of the difference between the predicted $\hat{y}_i$ and the reference values for the validation samples (Davies and Fearn 2006). A low RMSEP indicates accurate predictions where the results are close to the reference value and have low variability. The predicted values, $\hat{y}_i$, may be corrected by the bias, to define the standard error of performance or prediction (SEP; Næs et al. 2002). This correction is shown in Table 12.1 in the column labeled bias corrected. The RMSEP and SEP are defined as shown below (Næs et al. 2002; Davies and Fearn 2006).

$$RMSEP = \sqrt{\frac{\sum_{i=1}^{Np} (\hat{y}_i - y_i)^2}{N_p}} \tag{12.3}$$

$$SEP = \sqrt{\frac{\sum_{i=1}^{Np} \left(\hat{y}_i - y_i - bias \right)^2}{(N_p - 1)}} \tag{12.4}$$

The definition of the SEP makes it possible to express the RMSEP in terms of two components:

$$RMSEP^2 \approx SEP^2 + Bias^2 \tag{12.5}$$

This relationship is approximate since the bias and the RMSEP are divided by the number of predicted samples, N_p, while the SEP is divided by $N_p - 1$ samples. Table 12.1 shows the calculation of the SEP^2 and $Bias^2$, and their addition to obtain the $RMSEP^2$. When the results obtained are close to each other (low SEP), the bias could be very similar to the RMSEP. However, there are many situations where the contribution of the SEP and bias to the RMSEP are similar. Therefore, it is always a good idea to calculate

TABLE 12.1

Comparison of a Set of Results Using Figures of Merit Typically Used in HPLC and PAT Methods

| | Linearity of Accuracy (Recovery) | | | | PAT (NIR or Raman) Chemometric Model | | | | |
Level	Amount Added (g)	Amount Found (g)	% Recovered	Residual (g)	Residual (g)^2	Bias Corrected (g)	Residual (%)	Ref Value (g)^2
1	0.2208	0.2108	95.5	−0.01000	1.000E−04	7.850E−05	−4.529	0.04875
	0.2003	0.1897	94.7	−0.01060	1.124E−04	8.949E−05	−5.292	0.04012
2	0.3087	0.3127	101.3	0.004000	1.600E−05	2.642E−05	1.296	0.09530
	0.3153	0.3141	99.6	−0.001200	1.440E−06	3.600E−09	−0.3806	0.09941
3	0.4084	0.4035	98.8	−0.004900	2.401E−05	1.414E−05	−1.200	0.1668
	0.4037	0.4078	101.0	0.004100	1.681E−05	2.746E−05	1.016	0.1630
4	0.5024	0.5076	101.0	0.005200	2.704E−05	4.020E−05	1.035	0.2524
	0.5087	0.5051	99.3	−0.003600	1.296E−05	6.052E−06	−0.7077	0.2588
5	0.6178	0.6136	99.3	−0.004200	1.764E−05	9.364E−06	−0.6798	0.3817
	0.6123	0.6221	101.6	0.009800	9.604E−05	1.197E−04	1.601	0.3749
Average recovery			99.22	**Bias** (Average residual) −0.0011	**PRESS** (Sum of residuals^2) 4.243E−04	**RMSEP** 6.514E−03	**% Relative bias** (Average % Residual) −0.7842	**(Sum Ref values)^2** 1.881
Standard deviation recovery			2.387			SEP^2 2.823E−04		
%RSD			2.405		RSEP (%)	bias^2 1.300E−06		
					2.26E−02	RMSEP^2 2.836E−04		

Note: Dotted lines indicate the relationship between the values and the results in the same column. The result has been maintained with four significant figures.

the bias and the RMSEP, and to calculate the SEP. The 99.22% recovery and 2.4% standard deviation in the usual HPLC FOM also indicate that the bias is lower than the variation in the results.

The RMSEP describes the absolute error of the method. However, the relative error is also needed. Consider the case of a 0.51-mg RMSEP when the label claim of a formulation is 1 mg, versus when it is 500 mg. The relative error in the first case is about 50%, and 0.1% in the second case. The relative standard error of prediction (RSEP (%)) may be used (Blanco and Alcalà 2009). The RSEP (%) may be calculated with the data used in Table 12.1; the squared reference values are shown in the last column.

$$RSEP\left(\%\right) = \sqrt{\frac{\sum_{i=1}^{Np}(\hat{y}_i - y_i)^2}{\sum_{i=1}^{Np}(y_i)^2}} \times 100 \tag{12.6}$$

Table 12.1 also shows five different levels of addition of an API to a placebo mixture. The results at the lower concentration level are not as accurate as at the other concentration levels. Inaccuracies at a specific level are hidden when the RMSEP is calculated across all concentration levels. Table 12.1 provides an example where the results are not as accurate at the 0.2-g level. The RMSEP and bias should be calculated for each level.

The repeatability or short-term precision study is one of the simplest tests that may be performed during validation. This test may be performed with six or more consecutive spectra obtained without moving the sample or the NIR probe. The standard deviation is calculated using the predictions for the consecutive spectra. The objective is to estimate the minimum variation that may be obtained from using a NIR or Raman spectroscopic method, by analyzing the same sample through consecutive spectra. Unfortunately, this simple evaluation is missing in a number of publications where PAT methods are described.

Precision may also be estimated through intermediate precision and reproducibility studies (International Conference on Harmonisation of Technical Requirements for Registration of Pharmaceuticals for Human Use 1995). However, the advantage of the repeatability study is that it provides the variation associated with the method. When multiple samples are analyzed from a process, the variation observed is both from the process and the method.

The implementation of PAT methods is also affected by the significant differences in nomenclature observed in the chemometrics scientific literature. One possible solution could be to use the nomenclature of the FDA and EMA guidelines (Food and Drug Administration 2021; European Medicines Agency 2014a, b). When a scientist is not in agreement with a term, it is always possible to indicate that a term was used according to the guidance on the submission of documents to a regulatory agency. Even though significant progress has been made in the development of PAT methods, it is still difficult to indicate possible acceptance requirements for a method in a protocol as required by some quality systems, and to set adequate robustness studies (Colón et al. 2014). We need to continue understanding the sources of errors in NIR spectroscopic methods to achieve this goal.

On several occasions, we have been asked why we do not use HPLC as a reference method throughout the entire development of a calibration model. Many pharmaceutical companies consider HPLC the gold standard, and often use it to determine the reference concentration of every calibration sample. We do not see a reason for this wasteful approach. First, HPLC is also a gravimetric method. All reference concentrations used in HPLC depend on an analytical balance. The HPLC would likely add more errors from the dilutions and extractions in the sample preparation, injection, and detection error. We prefer to develop the method based on blends prepared gravimetrically and challenge it in the same manner. We have only used HPLC when the NIR method was fully developed, and was being implemented at the pharmaceutical company (Vargas et al. 2018).

Sampling Considerations

One of the more rewarding aspects of this career has been meeting a community of scientists who are focused on sampling instead of analysis (Esbensen and Holmes 2017). Their focus on sampling is a strong contrast to analytical chemistry textbooks that dedicate 900 pages to analysis and at the most two pages to sampling. The learning curve in Theory of Sampling (TOS) has been steep, it required opening the mind to new ideas on sampling. The TOS evolved with the great vision of Pierre Gy within the mining and geochemical industries (Gy 2004; Holmes 2004; Esbensen 2020). The initial reading of articles from these fields was a struggle, as one part of the brain tried to pay attention to the inorganic materials described in TOS articles, while the other part thought of MCC and ibuprofen particles. However, the lessons learned include that there are many opportunities to apply the TOS in pharmaceutical manufacturing, and not just in mining (Romañach and Esbensen 2015). The goal of TOS is to perform representative sampling, overcoming the challenges imposed by the unavoidable heterogeneity of materials.

Sampling of pharmaceutical processes involves many more steps than just estimating the sample size analyzed or trying to approximate a unit dose. A guiding theory is needed for sampling, and it is provided by the TOS (Gy 1998; Petersen et al. 2005). The six governing principles and four sampling unit operations have provided the guidance needed for much of our work since 2014 (Esbensen et al. 2016; Esbensen and Romañach 2021; Esbensen et al. 2018).

TOS establishes that all materials are heterogeneous regardless of the scale of scrutiny. This heterogeneity is the source of all sampling errors. TOS has provided a new perspective to NIR spectroscopy. The heterogeneity so prominently discussed in TOS answers many of the early questions on NIR spectroscopy where a scientist would indicate that the technique was not reliable because: "you place the probe on one part of the blend and get a result, and then obtain a different result at a second sample". NIR and Raman spectroscopic results do not depend solely on the analytical method, they depend to a large degree on the heterogeneity of the materials analyzed (Esbensen and Romañach 2021; Esbensen et al. 2018).

TOS has also provided the guidance needed for defining a representative sample. A representative sample is the result of performing a multistage sampling process that complies with the Fundamental Sampling Principle (FSP) ensuring that all sampling units (increments or samples) of the lot have an equal probability of being selected and are not altered in any way, while all sampling units that do not belong to the lot shall have zero probability of being selected (Danish-Standards-Foundation 2013; Esbensen and Romañach 2021; Esbensen 2020). Representative samples only occur when a representative sampling process is performed. Certainly, the use of thief sampling with preselected sample locations completely violates the principles of TOS (Muzzio et al. 1997). The FSP is followed when blend uniformity is determined in the feed frame as all parts of the lot have the same opportunity of being sampled (Sierra-Vega et al. 2019; Sierra-Vega et al. 2021; Hetrick et al. 2017; Li et al. 2018). The FSP was also followed in the development of a new stream sampler for real-time monitoring of powder blends (Romañach and Mendez 2019; Alvarado-Hernández et al. 2020; Sierra-Vega et al. 2020a, b).

Concluding Remarks

The success of PAT projects requires integrating knowledge from the various areas of research described in this chapter. PAT must move from development to manufacturing to reach its full benefits.

The greatest satisfaction has been in seeing former students working with operators and engineers in the implementation of PAT in commercial pharmaceutical manufacturing. This is the mark of success; chemists do not have to be limited to the QC lab. Our graduates are making a difference with real-time measurements in manufacturing processes, contributing to product quality. We have moved to manufacturing!

ACKNOWLEDGMENTS

The Economic Development Administration (01-70-14889) is thanked for the funding that has made the study of PAT business cases possible. The Puerto Rico Science Technology and Research Trust and the National Science Foundation are thanked for funding that has contributed to the development of the stream sampler and bringing the TOS into pharmaceutical manufacturing. Graduate students Nathaly Movilla Meza and José Puche Mercado are thanked for help with the tables and figures. This wonderful career has been possible, thanks to many dedicated students and collaborators.

REFERENCES

Abe, H., and M. Otsuka. 2012. "Effects of lubricant-mixing time on prolongation of dissolution time and its prediction by measuring near infrared spectra from tablets." *Drug Development and Industrial Pharmacy* 38 (4):412–9. 10.3109/03639045.2011.608679.

Alcala, M., J. Ropero, R. Vazquez, and R. J. Romanach. 2009. "Deconvolution of chemical and physical information from intact tablets NIR spectra: Two- and three-way multivariate calibration strategies for drug quantitation." *Journal of Pharmaceutical Sciences* 98 (8):2747–2758. 10.1002/jps.21634.

Aldrich, D. S., and M. A. Smith. 1999. "Pharmaceutical applications of infrared microspectroscopy (Reprinted from Practical Guide to Infrared Microspectroscopy, pg 323–375, 1995)." *Applied Spectroscopy Reviews* 34 (4):275–327. 10.1081/asr-100101218.

Alvarado-Hernández, Barbara B., Nobel O. Sierra-Vega, Pedro Martínez-Cartagena, Manuel Hormaza, Rafael Méndez, and Rodolfo J. Romañach. 2020. "A sampling system for flowing powders based on the theory of sampling." *International Journal of Pharmaceutics* 574:118874. 10.1016/j.ijpharm.2019.118874.

Axon, T. G., R. Brown, S. V. Hammond, S. J. Maris, and F. Ting. 1998. "Focusing near infrared spectroscopy on the business objectives of modern pharmaceutical production." *Journal of Near Infrared Spectroscopy* 6 (A):A13–A19. 10.1255/jnirs.161.

Bakeev, K. A. 2015. "Using handheld Raman spectroscopy to reduce risks in materials used for manufacturing." *Pharmaceutical Engineering* 35 (3):77–79.

Bawuah, P., D. Markl, A. Turner, M. Evans, A. Portieri, D. Farrell, R. Lucas, A. Anderson, D. J. Goodwin, and J. A. Zeitler. 2021. "A fast and non-destructive terahertz dissolution assay for immediate release tablets." *Journal of Pharmaceutical Sciences* 110 (5):2083–2092. 10.1016/j.xphs.2020.11.041.

Bellamy, L. J., A. Nordon, and D. Littlejohn. 2008. "Real-time monitoring of powder mixing in a convective blender using non-invasive reflectance NIR spectrometry." *Analyst* 133 (1):58–64. 10.1039/b713919e.

BioPhorum. 2020. *In-line Monitoring/Real-Time Release Testing in Biopharmaceutical Processes -Prioritization and Cost-Benefit Analysis.*

Blanco, M, and M Alcalà. 2009. "Multivariate Calibration for Quantitative Analysis." In *Infrared Spectroscopy for Food Quality Analysis and Control*, 51–82.

Blanco, M., M. Bautista, and M. Alcala. 2008. "Preparing calibration sets for use in pharmaceutical analysis by NIR spectroscopy." *Journal of Phamaceutical Sciences* 97 (3):1236–45. 10.1002/jps.21105.

Blanco, M., and M. A. Romero. 2001. "Near-infrared libraries in the pharmaceutical industry: a solution for identity confirmation." *Analyst* 126 (12):2212–2217. 10.1039/b105012p.

Buckley, Kevin, and Alan G. Ryder. 2017. "Applications of raman spectroscopy in biopharmaceutical manufacturing: A short review." *Applied Spectroscopy* 71 (6):1085–1116. 10.1177/0003702817703270.

Callis, James B., Deborah L. Illman, and Bruce R. Kowalski. 1987. "Process analytical chemistry." *Analytical Chemistry* 59 (9):624A–637A. 10.1021/ac00136a001.

Càrdenas, V., M. Blanco, and M. Alcalà. 2014. "Strategies for selecting the calibration set in pharmaceutical near infrared spectroscopy analysis. A comparative study." *Journal of Pharmaceutical Innovation* 9 (4):272–281. 10.1007/s12247-014-9192-3.

Cogdill, Robert P., Thomas P. Knight, Carl A. Anderson, and James K. Drennen. 2007. "The financial returns on investments in process analytical technology and lean manufacturing: Benchmarks and case study." *Journal of Pharmaceutical Innovation* 2 (1):38–50. 10.1007/s12247-007-9007-x.

Colón, Y. M., M. A. Florian, D. Acevedo, R. Mendez, and R. J. Romañach. 2014. "Near infrared method development for a continuous manufacturing blending process." *Journal of Pharmaceutical Innovation* 9 (4):291–301. 10.1007/s12247-014-9194-1.

Covey, Stephen R. 2004. *The 7 habits of highly effective people: Powerful lessons in personal change*: Simon and Schuster.

Crocombe, Richard A. 2018. "Portable spectroscopy." *Applied Spectroscopy* 72 (12):1701–1751. 10.1177/0003702818809719.

Crosby, Philip B. 1980. *Quality is Free: The Art of Making Quality Certain*: Signet Book.

Dahm, D. J., Dahm, K. D. 2007. *Interpreting Diffuse Reflectance and Transmittance: A Theoretical Introduction to Absorption Spectroscopy of Scattering Materials.* Chichester, West Sussex: NIR Publications.

Dahm, Donald J., Kevin D. Dahm, and Karl H. Norris. 2000. "Test of the representative layer theory of diffuse reflectance using plane parallel samples." *Journal of Near Infrared Spectroscopy* 8 (3):171–181. 10.1255/jnirs.276.

Danish-Standards-Foundation. 2013. DS 3077(2013). In *Representative Sampling – Horizontal Standard*. Danish Standards Foundation.

Davies, Anthony M. C., and T. Fearn. 2006. "Back to basics: Calibration statistics." *Spectroscopy 18* (2):31–32. 10.1255/sew.2008.a1.

de Matas, Marcel, Thomas De Beer, Staffan Folestad, Jarkko Ketolainen, Hans Lindén, João Almeida Lopes, Wim Oostra, Marco Weimer, Per Öhrngren, and Jukka Rantanen. 2016. "Strategic framework for education and training in Quality by Design (QbD) and process analytical technology (PAT)." *European Journal of Pharmaceutical Sciences 90*:2–7. 10.1016/j.ejps.2016.04.024.

Duong, N. H., P. Arratia, F. Muzzio, A. Lange, J. Timmermans, and S. Reynolds. 2003. "A homogeneity study using NIR spectroscopy: tracking magnesium stearate in Bohle bin-blender." *Drug Development and Industrial Pharmacy 29* (6):679–87. 10.1081/ddc-120021317.

Durao, P., C. Fauteux-Lefebvre, J. M. Guay, N. Abatzoglou, and R. Gosselin. 2017. "Using multiple process analytical technology probes to monitor multivitamin blends in a tableting feed frame." *Talanta 164*:7–15. 10.1016/j.talanta.2016.11.013.

Esbensen, K. E., and B. Swarbrick. 2018. *Multivariate Data Analysis – In practice. An Introduction to Multivariate Analysis, Process Analytical Technology and Quality by Design*. 6th ed. Oslo, Norway: CAMO Software AS.

Esbensen, K. H. 2020. *Introduction to the Theory and Practice of Sampling*. Chichester, UK: IMP Open.

Esbensen, K. H., A. D. Román-Ospino, A. Sanchez, and R. J. Romañach. 2016. "Adequacy and verifiability of pharmaceutical mixtures and dose units by variographic analysis (Theory of Sampling) – A call for a regulatory paradigm shift." *International Journal of Pharmaceutics 499* (1–2):156–174. 10.1016/j.ijpharm.2015.12.038.

Esbensen, Kim H, and Rodolfo J. Romañach. 2021. "A Framework for Representative Sampling for NIR Analysis–Theory of Sampling (TOS)." In *Handbook of Near-Infrared Analysis*, edited by E. W. Ciurczak, B. Igne, Jerry Workman and D. B. Burns. Boca Raton, FL: Taylor & Francis Group.

Esbensen, Kim H., Rodolfo J. Romañach, and Andrés D. Román-Ospino. 2018. "Chapter 4 - Theory of Sampling (TOS): A Necessary and Sufficient Guarantee for Reliable Multivariate Data Analysis in Pharmaceutical Manufacturing " In *Multivariate Analysis in the Pharmaceutical Industry*, edited by Ana Patricia Ferreira, José C. Menezes and Mike Tobyn, 53–91. London, UK: Academic Press.

Esbensen, Kim, and Ralph Holmes. 2017. "International pierre Gy sampling association (IPGSA)." *TOS Forum 7*:4–6.

Escotet-Espinoza, M. Sebastian, Sara Moghtadernejad, James Scicolone, Yifan Wang, Glinka Pereira, Elisabeth Schäfer, Tamas Vigh, Didier Klingeleers, Marianthi Ierapetritou, and Fernando J. Muzzio. 2018. "Using a material property library to find surrogate materials for pharmaceutical process development." *Powder Technology 339*:659–676. doi: 10.1016/j.powtec.2018.08.042.

European Medicines Agency. 2014a. *Addendum to EMA/CHMP/CVMP/QWP/17760/2009 Rev 2: Defining the Scope of an NIRS Procedure. edited by European Medicines Agency*.

European Medicines Agency. 2014b. *Guideline on the Use of Near Infrared Spectroscopy (NIRS) by the Pharmaceutical Industry and the Data Requirements for New Submissions and Variations*.

Fontalvo-Lascano, M. A., B. B. Alvarado-Hernández, C. Conde, E. J. Sánchez, M. I. Méndez-Piñero, R. J. Romañach. 2022. Development and application of a business case model for a stream sampler in the pharmaceutical industry. *The Journal of Pharmaceutical Innovation*. doi: 10.1007/s12247-022-09634-0

Fontalvo-Lascano, M. A., M. I. Méndez-Piñero, and R. J. Romañach. 2020a. "Design and development of a cost model for the implementation of process analytical technology in the pharmaceutical industry." *9th Annual World Conference of the Society for Industrial and Systems Engineering*, September 17–18, 2020.

Fontalvo-Lascano, María A, Mayra I Méndez-Piñero, and Rodolfo J Romañach. 2020b. "Development of a business case model for process analytical technology implementation in the pharmaceutical industry." *Proceedings of the 5th NA International Conference on Industrial Engineering and Operations Management*, Detroit, Michigan, August 10–14, 2020.

Food and Drug Administration. 2021. *Development and Submission of Near Infrared Analytical Procedures Guidance for Industry*. Silver Spring, MD: U.S. Department of Health and Human Services Center for Drug Evaluation and Research (CDER).

Friedman, C. R., and J. A. De Haseth. 1985. "Rapid scanning FT-IR/time resolved spectrometry (TRS) for gas phase systems." *Proceedings of SPIE – The International Society for Optical Engineering*.

Gray, N. 2016. In first, FDA approves Janssen's switch to continuous manufacturing for HIV drug. *BioPharma Dive*. Accessed November 3, 2017.

Green, R. L., M. D. Mowery, J. A. Good, J. P. Higgins, S. M. Arrivo, K. McColough, A. Mateos, and R. A. Reed. 2005. "Comparison of near-infrared and laser-induced breakdown spectroscopy for determination of magnesium stearate in pharmaceutical powders and solid dosage forms." *Applied Spectroscopy 59* (3):340–7. 10.1366/0003702053585354.

Griffiths, P. R., and D. J. Dahm. 2007. "Continuum and Discontinuum Theories of Diffuse Reflection." In *Handbook of Near-Infrared Analysis*, 3rd Edition, edited by E. W. Ciurczak and D.A. Burns, 21–64. CRC Press.

Guenard, Robert, and Gert Thurau. 2010. "Implementation of Process Analytical Technologies." In *Process Analytical Technology*, 17–36. John Wiley & Sons, Ltd.

Gupta, Anshu, John Austin, Sierra Davis, Michael Harris, and Gintaras Reklaitis. 2015. "A novel microwave sensor for real-time online monitoring of roll compacts of pharmaceutical powders online—A comparative case study with NIR." *Journal of Pharmaceutical Sciences 104* (5):1787–1794. 10.1002/jps.24409.

Gy, P. 1998. *Sampling for Analytical Purposes*. 1st ed. New York: Wiley.

Gy, P. 2004. "Sampling of discrete materials – A new introduction to the theory of sampling – I. Qualitative approach." *Chemometrics and Intelligent Laboratory Systems 74* (1):7–24. 10.1016/j.chemolab.2004.05.012.

Hernandez, Eduardo, Pallavi Pawar, Golshid Keyvan, Yifan Wang, Natasha Velez, Gerardo Callegari, Alberto Cuitino, Bozena Michniak-Kohn, Fernando J. Muzzio, and Rodolfo J. Romañach. 2016. "Prediction of dissolution profiles by non-destructive near infrared spectroscopy in tablets subjected to different levels of strain." *Journal of Pharmaceutical and Biomedical Analysis 117*:568–576. 10.1016/j.jpba.2015.10.012.

Hetrick, E. M., Z. Shi, Z. D. Harms, and D. P. Myers. 2021. "Sample mass estimate for the use of near-infrared and raman spectroscopy to monitor content uniformity in a tablet press feed frame of a drug product continuous manufacturing process." *Applied Spectroscopy 75* (2):216–224. 10.1177/0003702820950318.

Hetrick, Evan M., Zhenqi Shi, Lukas E. Barnes, Aaron W. Garrett, Robert G. Rupard, Timothy T. Kramer, Tony M. Cooper, David P. Myers, and Bryan C. Castle. 2017. "Development of near infrared spectroscopy-based process monitoring methodology for pharmaceutical continuous manufacturing using an offline calibration approach." *Analytical Chemistry 89* (17):9175–9183. 10.1021/acs.analchem.7b01907.

Holmes, R. J. 2004. "Correct sampling and measurement - the foundation of accurate metallurgical accounting." *Chemometrics and Intelligent Laboratory Systems 74* (1):71–83. 10.1016/j.chemolab.2004.03.019.

Huang, Jun, Thomas O'Connor, Kaschif Ahmed, Sharmista Chatterjee, Chris Garvin, Krishna Ghosh, Marianthi Ierapetritou, Malcolm Jeffers, David Lauri Pla, Sau L. Lee, David Lovett, Olav Lyngberg, John Mack, Eoin McManus, Saly Romero-Torres, Cenk Undey, Venkat Venkatasubramanian, and Martin Warman. 2021. "AIChE PD2M advanced process control workshop-moving APC forward in the pharmaceutical industry." *Journal of Advanced Manufacturing and Processing 3* (1):e10071. 10.1002/amp2.10071.

Igne, Benoît, Sameer Talwar, Hanzhou Feng, James K. Drennen, and Carl A. Anderson. 2015. "Near-infrared spatially resolved spectroscopy for tablet quality determination." *Journal of Pharmaceutical Sciences 104* (12):4074–4081. 10.1002/jps.24618.

International Conference on Harmonisation of Technical Requirements for Registration of Pharmaceuticals for Human Use. 1995. *ICH Q2 (R1) Validation of analytical procedures: text and methodology, Step 5.* edited by IInternational Conference on Harmonisation.

Iyer, Meenakshy, Hannah Morris, and James Drennen III. 2002. "Solid dosage form analysis by near infrared spectroscopy: comparison of reflectance and transmittance measurements including the determination of effective sample mass." *Journal of Near Infrared Spectroscopy 10* (4):233–245. 10.1255%2Fjnirs.340.

Jerez-Rozo, J. I., A. Zarow, B. Zhou, R. Pinal, Z. Iqbal, and R. J. Romañach. 2011. "Complementary near-infrared and raman chemical imaging of pharmaceutical thin films." *Journal of Pharmaceutical Sciences 100* (11):4888–4895. 10.1002/jps.22653.

Kelly, J. J., C. H. Barlow, T. M. Jinguji, and J. B. Callis. 1989. "Prediction of gasoline octane numbers from near-infrared spectral features in the range 660–1215 nm." *Analytical Chemistry 61* (4):313–320. 10.1021/ac00179a007.

Kirkland, J. J., J. L. Glajch, and R. D. Farlee. 1989. "Synthesis and characterization of highly stable bonded phases for high-performance liquid chromatography column packings." *Analytical Chemistry 61* (1):2–11. 10.1021/ac00176a003.

Köhler, J., and J. J. Kirkland. 1987. "Improved silica-based column packings for high-performance liquid chromatography." *Journal of Chromatography A 385* (C):125–150. 10.1016/S0021-9673(01)94628-X.

Kourti, Theodora, and Bruce Davis. 2012. "The business benefits of quality by design (QbD)." *Pharmaceutical Engineering 32* (4):1–10.

Kowalski, B. R. 1978. "Analytical chemistry: The Journal and the science, the 1970's and beyond." *Analytical Chemistry 50* (14):1309A–1313A. 10.1021/ac50036a718.

Li, Yi, Carl A. Anderson, James K. Drennen, Christian Airiau, and Benoît Igne. 2018. "Method development and validation of an inline process analytical technology method for blend monitoring in the tablet feed frame using raman spectroscopy." *Analytical Chemistry 90* (14):8436–8444. 10.1021/acs.analchem.8b01009.

Maes, Ingrid, and Beatrijs Van Liedekerke. 2006. "The need for a broader perspective if process analytical technology implementation is to be successful in the pharmaceutical sector." *Journal of Pharmaceutical Innovation 1* (1):19–21.

Matthews, T. E., C. Coffman, D. Kolwyck, D. Hill, and J. E. Dickens. 2019. "Enabling robust and rapid raw material identification and release by handheld raman spectroscopy." *PDA Journal of Pharmaceutical Science and Technology 73* (4):356–372. 10.5731/pdajpst.2018.009563.

Miró Vera, Aira Y., and Manel Alcalà Bernàrdez. 2017. "Near-Infrared Spectroscopy in Identification of Pharmaceutical Raw Materials." In *Encyclopedia of Analytical Chemistry*, 1–19.

Moghtadernejad, Sara, M. Sebastian Escotet-Espinoza, Sarang Oka, Ravendra Singh, Zhanjie Liu, Andrés D. Román-Ospino, Tianyi Li, Sonia Razavi, Savitha Panikar, James Scicolone, Gerardo Callegari, Douglas Hausner, and Fernando Muzzio. 2018. "A training on: continuous manufacturing (direct compaction) of solid dose pharmaceutical products." *Journal of Pharmaceutical Innovation 13* (2):155–187. 10.1007/s12247-018-9313-5.

Montenegro-Alvarado, J., B. Diehl, J. M. Guay, S. Hammond, H. Isaac, B. Lyons, C. McSweeney, S. O'Neill, J. S. Simard, and J. Timmermans. 2014. "PAT for packaging: Review of applications for expeditious, non-destructive quality testing." *European Pharmaceutical Review 19* (2):47–52.

Morrison, Edward, Scott Hutcheson, Elizabeth Nilsen, Janyce Fadden, and Nancy Franklyn. 2019. *Strategic Doing: Ten Skills for Agile Leadership*. Wiley.

Muzzio, F. J., P. Robinson, C. Wightman, and D. Brone. 1997. "Sampling practices in powder blending." *International Journal of Pharmaceutics 155* (2):153–178. 10.1016/s0378-5173(97)04865-5.

Næs, T., T. Isaksson, T. Fearn, and T. Davies. 2002. *A User-Friendly Guide to Multivariate Calibration and Classification*. Chichester, UK: NIR Publications.

O'Connor, Thomas F., Lawrence X. Yu, and Sau L. Lee. 2016. "Emerging technology: A key enabler for modernizing pharmaceutical manufacturing and advancing product quality." *International Journal of Pharmaceutics 509* (1–2):492–498. 10.1016/j.ijpharm.2016.05.058.

Ortega-Zuñiga, Carlos, Kerimar Reyes-Maldonado, Rafael Méndez, and Rodolfo J. Romañach. 2017. "Study of near infrared chemometric models with low heterogeneity films: The role of optical sampling and spectral preprocessing on partial least squares errors." *Journal of Near Infrared Spectroscopy 25* (2):103–115. 10.1177/0967033516686653.

Pawar, Pallavi, Yifan Wang, Golshid Keyvan, Gerardo Callegari, Alberto Cuitino, and Fernando Muzzio. 2016. "Enabling real time release testing by NIR prediction of dissolution of tablets made by continuous direct compression (CDC)." *International Journal of Pharmaceutics 512* (1):96–107. 10.1016/j.ijpharm.2016.08.033.

Pell, R. J., M. B. Seasholtz, K. R. Beebe, and M. V. Koch. 2014. "Process analytical chemistry and chemometrics, Bruce Kowalski's legacy at the dow chemical company." *Journal of Chemometrics 28* (5):321–331. 10.1002/cem.2535.

Peng, D. Y., A. Zilian, J. Norton, M. G. Van Trieste, J. J. Orloff, P. Stojanovski, G. Millili, A. Viehmann, K. Iyer, and L. X. Yu. 2015. "Symposium summary report: Using process capability to enhance pharmaceutical product quality." *Pharmaceutical Engineering 35* (5):126–133.

Petersen, Lars, Pentti Minkkinen, and Kim H. Esbensen. 2005. "Representative sampling for reliable data analysis: Theory of Sampling." *Chemometrics and Intelligent Laboratory Systems 77* (1–2):261–277. 10.1016/j.chemolab.2004.09.013.

Pinzon de la Rosa, C., V Rodriguez, M. L. Hormaza, and R. J. Romañach 2017. "TOS MEETS THE NSF I-CORPS™ PROGRAM." *8th World Conference on Sampling and Blending*, Perth, Australia.

Ramirez, José L., Michael K. Bellamy, and Rodolfo J. Romañach. 2001. "A novel method for analyzing thick tablets by near infrared spectroscopy." *AAPS PharmSciTech 2* (3):15–24. 10.1208/pt020311.

Rantanen, Jukka, and Johannes Khinast. 2015. "The future of pharmaceutical manufacturing sciences." *Journal of Pharmaceutical Sciences 104* (11):3612–3638. 10.1002/jps.24594.

Razuc, M., A. Grafia, L. Gallo, M. V. Ramírez-Rigo, and R. J. Romañach. 2019. "Near-infrared spectroscopic applications in pharmaceutical particle technology." *Drug Development and Industrial Pharmacy 45* (10):1565–1589. 10.1080/03639045.2019.1641510.

Robertson, R. M., J. A. de Haseth, and R. F. Browner. 1988. "MAGIC-LC/FT-IR spectrometry." *Mikrochimica Acta 95* (1–6):199–202. 10.1007/BF01349752.

Romañach, R. J. 2008. "PAT- A team effort." *Pharmaceutical Technology Europe 20* (10):44–46.

Romañach, R. J. 2021. "Sampling in pharmaceutical manufacturing: a critical business case element." *Spectroscopy Europe 33* (7):67–69.

Romañach, R. J., and J. A. de Haseth. 1988. "Flow cell ccc/ft-ir spectrometry." *Journal of Liquid Chromatography 11* (1):133–152. 10.1080/01483919808068319.

Romañach, R. J., and K. H. Esbensen. 2015. "Sampling in pharmaceutical manufacturing – Many opportunities to improve today's practice through the Theory of Sampling (TOS)." *TOS Forum 4*:5–9.

Romañach, Rodolfo J., and Mendez, Rafael 2019. *Stream Sampler—Mass Reduction System for Flowing Powders. Awarded by United States Patent Office.* University of Puerto Rico.

Romañach, Rodolfo J., Eduardo Hernández Torres, Andres Roman Ospino, Isamar Pastrana, and Fabiola Semidei. 2014. "NIR and Raman spectroscopic measurements to train the next generation of PAT scientists." *American Pharmaceutical Review 17* (6):82–87.

Román-Ospino, Andrés D., Ravendra Singh, Marianthi Ierapetritou, Rohit Ramachandran, Rafael Méndez, Carlos Ortega-Zuñiga, Fernando J. Muzzio, and Rodolfo J. Romañach. 2016. "Near infrared spectroscopic calibration models for real time monitoring of powder density." *International Journal of Pharmaceutics 512* (1):61–74. 10.1016/j.ijpharm.2016.08.029.

Ropero, J., L. Beach, M. Alcala, R. Rentas, R. N. Dave, and R. J. Romanach. 2009. "Near-infrared spectroscopy for the in-line characterization of powder voiding part I: Development of the methodology." *Journal of Pharmaceutical Innovation 4* (4):187–197. 10.1007/s12247-009-9069-z.

Ropero, J., Y. Colon, B. Johnson-Restrepo, and R. J. Romanach. 2011. "Near-infrared chemical imaging slope as a new method to study tablet compaction and tablet relaxation." *Applied Spectroscopy 65* (4):459–465. 10.1366/410-06078.

Rosas, J. G., M. Blanco, F. Santamaria, and M. Alcala. 2013. "Assessment of chemo metric methods for the non-invasive monitoring of solid blending processes using wireless near infrared spectroscopy." *Journal of Near Infrared Spectroscopy 21* (2):97–106. 10.1255/jnirs.1041.

Sacher, Stephan, Johannes Poms, Jakob Rehrl, and Johannes G. Khinast. 2022. "PAT implementation for advanced process control in solid dosage manufacturing – A practical guide." *International Journal of Pharmaceutics 613*:121408. 10.1016/j.ijpharm.2021.121408.

Sánchez-Paternina, Adriluz, Pedro Martínez-Cartagena, Jingzhe Li, James Scicolone, Ravendra Singh, Yleana C. Lugo, Rodolfo J. Romañach, Fernando J. Muzzio, and Andrés D. Román-Ospino. 2022. "Residence time distribution as a traceability method for lot changes in a pharmaceutical continuous manufacturing system." *International Journal of Pharmaceutics 611*:121313. 10.1016/j.ijpharm.2021.121313.

Seasholtz, M. B. 1999. "Making money with chemometrics." *Chemometrics and Intelligent Laboratory Systems 45* (1–2):55–63. 10.1016/s0169-7439(98)00089-6.

Shi, Z. Q., B. Igne, R. W. Bondi, J. K. Drennen, and C. A. Anderson. 2012. "Calibration transfer from pharmaceutical powder mixtures to compacts using the prediction augmented classical least squares (PACLS) method." *Applied Spectroscopy 66* (9):1075–1081. 10.1366/11-06501.

Sierra-Vega, Nobel O., Krizia M. Karry, Rodolfo J. Romañach, and Rafael Méndez. 2021. "Monitoring of high-load dose formulations based on co-processed and non co-processed excipients." *International Journal of Pharmaceutics 606*:120910. 10.1016/j.ijpharm.2021.120910.

Sierra-Vega, Nobel O., Pedro A. Martínez-Cartagena, Bárbara B. Alvarado-Hernández, Rodolfo J. Romañach, and Rafael Méndez. 2020a. "In-line monitoring of low drug concentration of flowing powders in a new sampler device." *International Journal of Pharmaceutics 583*:119358. 10.1016/j.ijpharm.2020.119358.

Sierra-Vega, Nobel O., Rodolfo J. Romañach, and Rafael Méndez. 2019. "Feed frame: The last processing step before the tablet compaction in pharmaceutical manufacturing." *International Journal of Pharmaceutics 572*:118728. 10.1016/j.ijpharm.2019.118728.

Sierra-Vega, Nobel O., Rodolfo J. Romañach, and Rafael Méndez. 2020b. "Real-time quantification of low-dose cohesive formulations within a sampling interface for flowing powders." *International Journal of Pharmaceutics 588*:119726. 10.1016/j.ijpharm.2020.119726.

Singh, R., A. Sahay, K. M. Karry, F. Muzzio, M. Ierapetritou, and R. Ramachandran. 2014a. "Implementation of an advanced hybrid MPC-PID control system using PAT tools into a direct compaction continuous pharmaceutical tablet manufacturing pilot plant." *International Journal of Pharmaceutics 473* (1–2):38–54. 10.1016/j.ijpharm.2014.06.045.

Singh, Ravendra, Abhishek Sahay, Fernando Muzzio, Marianthi Ierapetritou, and Rohit Ramachandran. 2014b. "A systematic framework for onsite design and implementation of a control system in a continuous tablet manufacturing process." *Computers & Chemical Engineering 66*:186–200. 10.1016/j.compchemeng.2014.02.029.

Stratton, MJ. 2004. "Business case development guideline." *Crystal Ball User Conference.*

Taipale-Kovalainen, Krista, Anssi-Pekka Karttunen, Hannes Niinikoski, Jarkko Ketolainen, and Ossi Korhonen. 2019. "The effects of unintentional and intentional process disturbances on tablet quality during long continuous manufacturing runs." *European Journal of Pharmaceutical Sciences 129*:10–20. 10.1016/j.ejps.2018.11.030.

Thakur, G., P. Ghumade, and A. S. Rathore. 2021. "Process analytical technology in continuous processing: Model-based real time control of pH between capture chromatography and viral inactivation for monoclonal antibody production." *Journal of Chromatography A 1658.* 10.1016/j.chroma.2021.462614.

U.S. Department of Health and Human Services, Food & Drug Administration. 2002. *ANDA's: Blend Uniformity Analysis.* Withdrawal of Draft Guidance.

U.S. Department of Health and Human Services, Food & Drug Administration. 2004. *Guidance for Industry – PAT A Framework for Innovative Pharmaceutical Development, Manufacturing, and Quality Assurance.*

Van der Voort Maarschalk, K., K. Zuurman, H. Vromans, G. K. Bolhuis, and C. F. Lerk. 1997. "Stress relaxation of compacts produced from viscoelastic materials." *International Journal of Pharmaceutics 151* (1):27–34. 10.1016/S0378-5173(97)04889-8.

Vargas, Jenny M., Sarah Nielsen, Vanessa Cárdenas, Anthony Gonzalez, Efrain Y. Aymat, Elvin Almodovar, Gustavo Classe, Yleana Colón, Eric Sanchez, and Rodolfo J. Romañach. 2018. "Process analytical technology in continuous manufacturing of a commercial pharmaceutical product." *International Journal of Pharmaceutics 538* (1–2):167–178. 10.1016/j.ijpharm.2018.01.003.

Vargas, Jenny M., Andres D. Roman-Ospino, Eric Sanchez, and Rodolfo J. Romañach. 2017. "Evaluation of analytical and sampling errors in the prediction of the active pharmaceutical ingredient concentration in blends from a continuous manufacturing process." *Journal of Pharmaceutical Innovation 12* (2):155–167. 10.1007/s12247-017-9273-1.

Zhang, J., Y. Ying, B. Pielecha-Safira, E. Bilgili, R. Ramachandran, R. Romanach, R. N. Dave, and Z. Iqbal. 2014. "Raman spectroscopy for in-line and off-line quantification of poorly soluble drugs in strip films." *International Journal of Pharmaceutics 475* (1–2):428–437. 10.1016/j.ijpharm.2014.08.051.

Zuurman, K., K. Van der Voort Maarschalk, and G. K. Bolhuis. 1999. "Effect of magnesium stearate on bonding and porosity expansion of tablets produced from materials with different consolidation properties." *International Journal of Pharmaceutics 179* (1):107–115. 10.1016/S0378-5173(98)00389-5.

Part IV

Modeling, Design Space, and Future Outlook

13

End-to-End Design Space for Continuous Manufacturing of Pharmaceuticals: Understanding Interactions Across Integrated Continuous Operations

Sayantan Chattoraj
Pharmaceutical Development, GlaxoSmithKline Pharmaceuticals R&D, Collegeville, PA, USA

CONTENTS

13.1 Introduction

Modernizing pharmaceutical manufacturing through advanced manufacturing approaches, such as continuous manufacturing, is a key focus area in today's drug development [1–3]. The key advantages of continuous manufacturing include enhanced process consistency and process robustness, precise control of product quality, flexibility to create demand adaptive supply chains, the ability to leverage advanced process analytics for process monitoring and control, enhanced manufacturing efficiency and shortened manufacturing cycle times, as well as reduced manufacturing footprint [4, 5]. These benefits of continuous manufacturing can be realized for drug substances as well as drug products for both small and large molecules [6, 7].

The development of a robust continuous manufacturing process requires an in-depth product and process understanding. Continuous manufacturing is ideally suited to provide an enhanced level of process understanding guided by the Quality-by-Design (QbD) principles in alignment with ICH Q8 – 11 [8–11], since a significant level of process understanding can be generated in a material-sparing approach within a short timeframe for continuous processes. One important consideration for process development for continuous manufacturing is the need for understanding the potential interactions that may occur across integrated operations on a continuous manufacturing line, and establishing the resultant impact on product quality as well as process robustness [12]. In addition, the impact of input/in-process material attributes and their interactions with manufacturing process parameters is also an important aspect of continuous process development. Indeed, the integrated nature of continuous processes and the importance of understanding the system integration have been highlighted as a key consideration in the recent ICH Q13 guidance document [13].

DOI: 10.1201/9781003149835-17

The terminology of "integrated process" refers to two or more operations being connected, resulting in potential interactions across operations. In traditional batch manufacturing mode, unit operations are discrete and separated over space and time. On more complex continuous manufacturing lines, several operations may be integrated or connected, which significantly enhances the manufacturing efficiency and reduces the manufacturing cycle times. There are a number of examples of commercial integrated continuous lines in today's pharmaceutical development both for drug substances as well as drug products, across small and large molecules. While examples of fully integrated end-to-end continuous lines connecting drug substance and drug product are relatively few, there are longer-term aspirations to connect drug substance and drug product manufacture to fully glean the benefits of continuous processes. For drug substance manufacture in the traditional batch manufacturing mode, each reaction stage involves the purification and isolation of the intermediate output material. In contrast, in continuous flow chemistry, several reaction stages can be integrated circumventing the need to isolate and test intermediates, thereby shortening cycle times [14–17]. Based on the complexity of the reaction stages, drug substance synthesis may involve a combination of batch and continuous flow chemistry modes. In addition to continuous flow chemistry for chemical reactions, continuous technologies have also been successfully developed and implemented for the operations of crystallization, filtration, and drying for drug substance manufacture [18–20]. Similarly, drug products based on continuous manufacturing have been successfully commercialized based on integrated continuous manufacturing lines for direct compression, wet granulation, and dry granulation.

The purpose of this chapter is to provide a summary of the key considerations for understanding the interactions across integrated operations in the continuous manufacturing of pharmaceuticals, using small molecule drug products as an example, focusing on the continuous manufacturing of oral solid tablet dosage form. However, the fundamental principles outlined here regarding the integrated nature of continuous manufacturing would apply across modalities for both drug substances and drug products for small and large molecules. Such an in-depth process understanding also forms the basis of the development of end-to-end design space for continuous processes across integrated operations, which can provide significant lifecycle regulatory flexibility for products when the design space is registered as part of regulatory submissions. In addition, such fundamental product and process understanding are key for performing data-driven risk assessments to guide product development resulting in the design of robust and consistent continuous manufacturing processes.

13.2 Continuous Manufacturing of Tablets

The development paradigm of drug products is driven by the requirements outlined in the Quality Target Product Profile (QTPP) of a medicine. For small molecule oral solid dose products, tablets constitute the major proportion of products in the market as well as products in development. The attributes of the drug substance will significantly influence the design selection of the drug product manufacturing process for tablets, such as direct compression, wet granulation, and dry granulation (by roller compaction). All these manufacturing processes are readily amenable to continuous manufacturing applications. From a design simplicity viewpoint, continuous direct compression is attractive due to the small number of unit operations that need to be integrated. For most continuous direct compression lines, the integrated operations include powder feeding, continuous blending, lubricant blending, and compression. Film-coating operation for coated tablets may or may not be integrated as part of a continuous line. However, not all products may necessarily be suitable for continuous direct compression. For example, very poorly flowing drug substances may face challenges to achieve feeding consistency into a continuous line, which can result in variability during powder feeding resulting in a potential impact on tablet content and content uniformity. In such scenarios, continuous granulation may be an attractive alternate approach for drug product manufacture, where the flowability can be enhanced significantly by appropriately designing the intragranular matrix structure. Similarly, for highly potent very low dose products, content uniformity is expected to be the highest risk drug product critical quality attribute (DP CQA). For such highly potent products, granulation is again an attractive approach to lock in the uniformity upstream in the process.

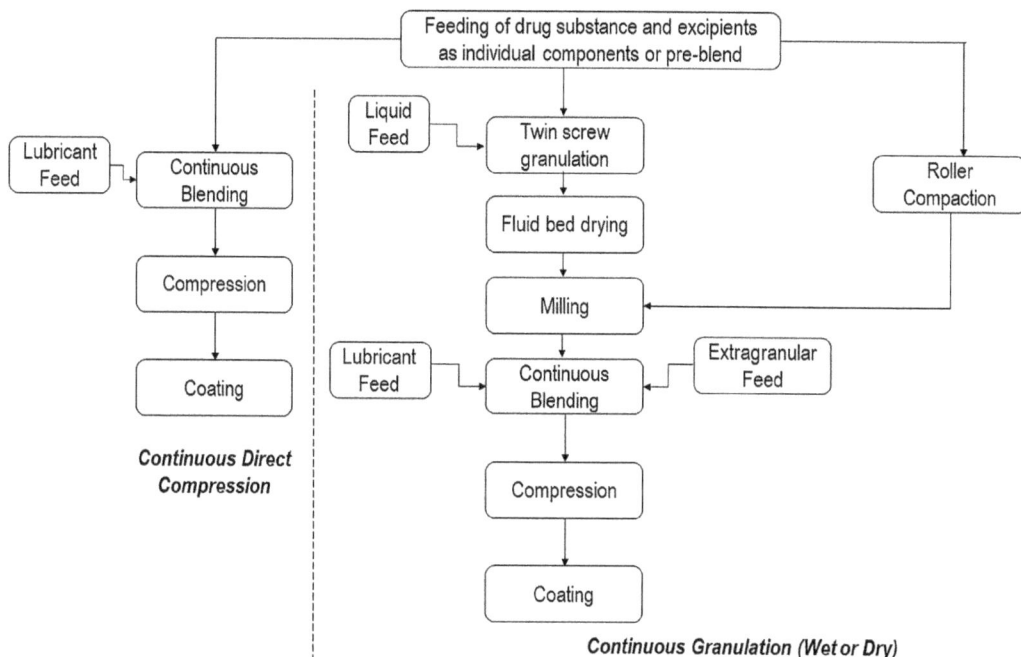

FIGURE 13.1 Integrated operations for continuous direct compression, continuous wet granulation and roller compaction for the manufacture of tablets.

There are examples of successful design of continuous granulation-based drug products with drug loading < 1%w/w in the tablet.

Figure 13.1 illustrates the integrated operations typically involved in continuous direct compression and continuous wet and dry granulation processes. Similar integrated systems also apply to drug substance continuous manufacture, where different reaction stages operating in flow (continuous) mode, continuous crystallization, and filter drying may be telescoped for drug substance synthesis.

Compared to continuous direct compression, which has inherent implementation simplicity due to the small number of operations (powder feeding, blending, and compression followed by coating), continuous wet or dry granulation process design is more complex due to the increased number of unit operations that need to be integrated. For example, for the continuous wet granulation process illustrated in the example shown in Figure 13.1, input materials are introduced into the continuous manufacturing line by powder feeding of either individual components (drug substance and granulation excipients fed individually) or premixed blends. Powder feeding is a key operation for continuous manufacturing of tablets, and understanding the gravimetric feeding operation by the Loss-in-Weight feeders is a key component for designing robust controls for continuous manufacturing. Following powder feeding, the powder is granulated using the granulation liquid (e.g., water) on a twin-screw granulator, following which the wet granules are dried in a continuous or semi-continuous fluid bed dryer. The dried granules are transferred through the continuous line for milling to normalize the granule size distribution. The dried milled granules are blended in a continuous blender with extragranular components and lubricant, and the lubricated compression blend is compressed into tablet cores. Similarly, for continuous dry granulation by roller compaction, the input materials are transformed into roller compacted ribbons using a roller compactor that can be readily integrated into a continuous manufacturing line. The roller compacted ribbons are dry milled to produce granules of appropriate granule attributes, which are blended with extragranular components and lubricant in a continuous blender, followed by compression of the lubricated blend. All these operations starting from powder feeding up to tablet compression can be integrated into a continuous manufacturing line for both continuous wet and dry granulation processes. Therefore, a key component of the process development for continuous granulation is to understand the potential interactions across operations from powder feeding to tablet compression to enable the development of a robust holistic drug product control strategy on the continuous manufacturing line.

13.3 Interactions Across Integrated Operations for Continuous Manufacturing of Tablets

A summary of the potential factors that can influence the product quality and process consistency for continuous direct compression, continuous wet granulation, and continuous dry granulation is presented in Table 13.1 for the operations of powder feeding to tablet compression. The actual list of manufacturing process parameters and input/in-process material attributes required for evaluation during a development program will be product and manufacturing line-specific and dictated by the equipment and process design features.

13.3.1 Potential Interaction Effects between Material Properties and Process Parameters

A holistic understanding of the impact of input/in-process material attributes and interaction effects with process parameters for continuous operations is important to design a robust continuous manufacturing process for both drug substances and drug products. For the continuous manufacturing of tablet dosage forms, the following material properties are routinely considered important during product design and development.

- Drug substance and excipient attributes, such as particle size distribution, density, specific surface area, flow, and compaction properties.
- In-process material attributes, such as granule size distribution, granule density, moisture content, etc.

Some illustrative examples of interaction effects between material attributes and process parameters for continuous operations are summarized below for the continuous manufacturing of tablets:

- Influence of drug substance and excipient particle sizes and flow properties on the consistency of the powder feeding operation, which can impact the content uniformity of the drug product. The impact is perhaps more pronounced for continuous direct compression, where further processing steps, such as granulation and drying, are not available to normalize potential disturbances in the upstream feeding operation.
- Influence of in-process material attributes, such as granule moisture content, on continuous line robustness: Overly wet granules can lead to clogging of filters in the dryers or can cause blockage of the continuous lines due to material adhesion. Likewise, overly dried granules can result in an increased proportion of fines, which can result in potential failure modes related to content uniformity and weight variation in the dosage units.
- Influence of in-process material attributes, such as granule size distribution and density, can impact the flow and compaction properties of compression blends, resulting in an impact on the product quality and compression process consistency (Table 13.1).

13.3.2 Potential Interaction Effects among Process Parameters Across Integrated Operations

On continuous lines, interaction effects can occur among process parameters between upstream and downstream continuous operations, and such effects can propagate across the continuous lines resulting in an impact on the final product quality. Some routinely observed interaction effects across integrated operations on continuous manufacturing lines for tablets are summarized below:

TABLE 13.1

Potential Interacting Factors Across Integrated Continuous Operations for Tablets

Continuous Process	Common Operations	Factors with Potential to Impact Product Quality and/or Process Consistency	
		Process Parameters	**Material Attributes**
Continuous Direct Compression	Powder Feeding	Feed rates of components or blends Feed factor Feeder screw type/speed Feeder refill strategy Hopper geometry/fill volume	Input material attributes of powders; e.g., particle size distribution, flow properties, cohesivity
	Continuous Blending	Blending speed Blending time Blender design and blender residence time	Particle size of excipients/extragranular components, specific surface area of lubricant Compression blend homogeneity
	Compression	Press speed (aligned with the throughput of the continuous process) Press feeder speed Pre-compression force or displacement Main-compression force or displacement	In-process material attributes of tablet cores, such as tablet weight, hardness, thickness
Continuous Wet Granulation and Compression	Powder Feeding	Feed rates of components or blend Feed factor Feeder screw type/speed Feeder refill strategy Hopper geometry/fill volume	Input material attributes of powders; e.g., particle size distribution, flow properties, cohesivity
	Wet Granulation (e.g., by twin screw granulation)	Liquid feed rate Granulation water level (or liquid to solid ratio) Granulator screw speed Granulator screw design (number of kneading and conveying elements) Granulator temperature Granulator residence time distribution (RTD)/mean residence time (MRT)	Granule attributes; e.g., wet/dried granule moisture content, dried granule size distribution, granule porosity/density, specific surface area, flowability, compressibility
	Fluid Bed Drying	Dryer air flow/fluidization volume Dryer air inlet temperature Dryer air dew point	
	Dry Milling	Mill screen size Mill impeller speed/geometry Mill hold up/residence time	Milled granule size distribution, granule porosity/density, specific surface area, flowability, compressibility
	Continuous blending	Blending speed Blending time Blender design and blender residence time	Particle size of excipients/extragranular components, specific surface area of lubricant Compression blend homogeneity
	Compression	Press speed (aligned with the throughput of the continuous process) Press feeder speed Pre-compression force or displacement Main-compression force or displacement	In-process material attributes of tablet cores, such as tablet weight, hardness, thickness

(Continued)

TABLE 13.1 (Continued)

Continuous Process	Common Operations	Factors with Potential to Impact Product Quality and/or Process Consistency	
		Process Parameters	**Material Attributes**
Continuous Dry Granulation (by Roller Compaction) and Compression	Powder Feeding	Feed rates of components or blend Feed factor Feeder screw type/speed Feeder refill strategy Hopper geometry/fill volume	Input material attributes of powders; e.g., particle size distribution, flow properties, cohesivity
	Roller Compaction	Roll force/pressure Roll speed Roll gap	Ribbon solid fraction, granule size distribution, granule porosity/density, specific surface area, flowability, compressibility
	Dry Milling	Mill screen size Mill impeller speed/geometry Mill hold up/residence time	Milled granule size distribution, granule porosity/density, specific surface area, flowability, compressibility
	Continuous Blending	Blending speed Blending time Blender design and blender residence time	Particle size of excipients/extragranular components, specific surface area of lubricant Compression blend homogeneity
	Compression	Press speed (aligned with the throughput of the continuous process) Press feeder speed Pre-compression force or displacement Main-compression force or displacement	In-process material attributes of tablet cores, such as tablet weight, hardness, thickness

- Impact of granulation operation on downstream processes, such as milling and compression. For example, the extent of granulation will influence the granule size distribution and density, which can impact the performance of downstream operations, such as granule milling and tablet compression. Overly granulated materials can be difficult to mill, as well as suffer from loss of compressibility. Similarly, under-granulated powders can generate a lot of fines during downstream continuous operations, resulting in tablet weight variability during compression, and potential variability in tablet content.

- Another frequently observed interaction effect in the continuous manufacturing of tablets is the interaction of wet granulation and drying operations. The water level used for wet granulation will have a direct impact on the downstream granule drying performance. During product development of a continuous wet granulation process, the interactions between granulation water level (hence the extent of granulation) and the drying parameters, such as dryer air volume and temperature, need to be carefully optimized through cross-operation DoEs to fully map out a robust region of the process that can consistently deliver an optimum granule drying performance.

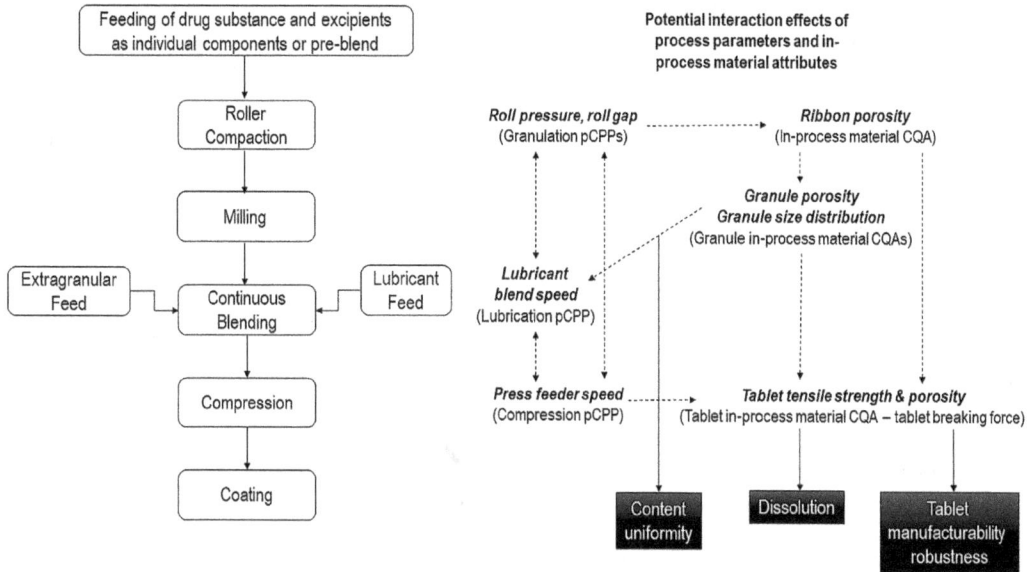

FIGURE 13.2 Illustration of a parameter-attribute interaction map across integrated continuous operations for a continuous dry granulation and compression line based on roller compaction process.

While some illustrative examples of potential interaction effects across continuous operations and input/in-process material attributes are presented above, a comprehensive risk assessment programme needs to be developed and implemented for every product under development, which will help guide the development of robust continuous manufacturing processes for pharmaceuticals.

To illustrate the interaction effects encountered across multiple integrated operations during continuous manufacturing of tablets, a case study for continuous dry granulation based on roller compaction is presented in Figure 13.2. The extent of granulation of the roller compacted ribbons is dependent on the potential critical process parameters (CPPs) of roll pressure and roll gap used during the roller compaction process, which influence the resultant in-process material CQA of ribbon porosity or ribbon solid fraction. The optimization of ribbon porosity as a function of roller compaction CPPs is a key development step during the design of a robust continuous dry granulation operation. The ribbon porosity impacts the granule attributes, such as granule porosity/density and granule size distribution. A non-optimum roller compacted ribbon porosity can lead to poor granule quality, which will directly impact downstream operations, such as tablet compression, as well as drug product CQAs, such as content uniformity and dissolution. Under-granulated ribbons can lead to the generation of fine particles during milling, which has the potential to impact tablet content uniformity, as well as lead to compression issues, such as tablet weight variability and compression sticking. Similarly, over-granulated material would impact the CQA of tablet dissolution and result in loss of tablet compressibility.

In a continuous dry granulation process, there is also the potential for a three-way interaction effect among the roller compaction, lubrication, and compression operations, which can impact tablet compression and dissolution. The extent of lubrication in a continuous dry granulation process can be impacted by a number of integrated operations, as summarized below:

- The roller compaction operation can impact the granule size distribution, which will have an impact on the lubricant blending efficiency downstream in the process. Fine versus coarse granules will blend differently under the same lubricant blending conditions.
- In the lubricant blending operation, the lubricant level, lubricant blend speed, and blend time are parameters that need to be optimized carefully during product development to avoid over/under-lubrication effects, which can negatively impact downstream processes, such as tablet compression, as well as product quality.

- Finally, there can be an interaction effect between the lubricant blending and compression feeding operations, where interactions have been frequently noted between the lubricant blend speed (in lubricant blending operation) and tablet press feeder speed (in tablet compression). On an integrated continuous line, the lubrication and the press feeder speed parameters need to be balanced properly to achieve optimum lubrication levels consistently during the continuous runs.

Inadequate lubrication can result in the potential risk of compression sticking and picking during extended continuous compression runs. The commercial run times for continuous processes for pharmaceutical drug products often last for several hours/days, where the risk of compression sticking is enhanced due to the long compression durations. Adequate lubrication is necessary to design out the compression sticking failure mode. Similarly, over-lubrication can also have a downstream impact on tablet compressibility and product performance (e.g., extended disintegration times and slow dissolution).

13.4 Holistic Control Strategy Elements for Continuous Manufacturing

Understanding the integrated nature of continuous manufacturing is essential to developing a robust, holistic control strategy that can ensure the consistency of product quality and process robustness. Figure 13.3 presents a summary of the various elements of the holistic control strategy for continuous manufacturing of drug substances and drug products, in alignment with ICH Q8(R2) [8] and ICH Q13 [13], and with the consideration of the regulatory and quality aspects of continuous manufacturing [21]. Fundamentally, the elements of the control strategy are the same for both batch and continuous manufacturing modes. However, the equipment design, the role of advanced process analytics (model-based and spectroscopic PAT) for process monitoring/control, the diversion strategy, and the management of transient process disturbances are further highlighted as key focus areas while developing the control strategies of pharmaceuticals based on continuous manufacturing.

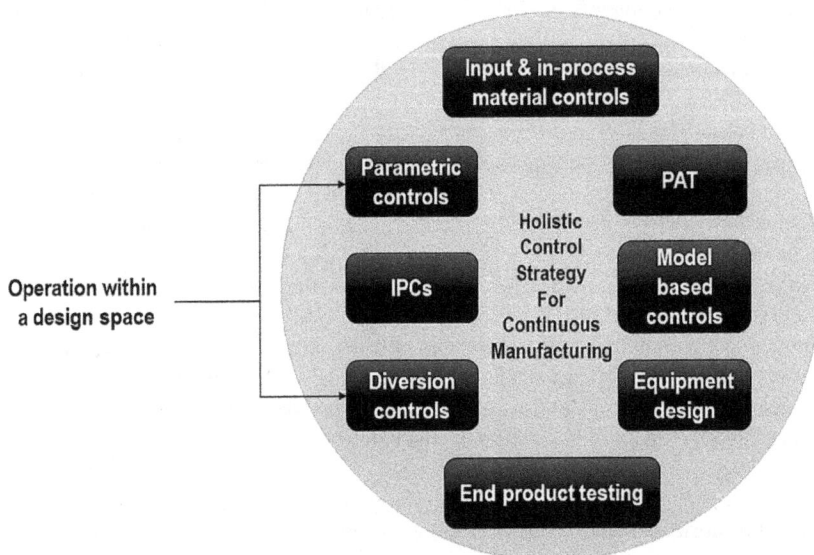

FIGURE 13.3 Holistic control strategy elements for continuous manufacturing of pharmaceuticals. Operation within an end-to-end design space across an integrated continuous line can form the basis of defining effective parametric controls, as well as designing meaningful diversion strategy to divert non-conforming materials produced outside the design space acceptable ranges.

There can be different approaches to designing robust control strategies for continuous processes, and the control strategy for a product will ultimately be dictated by the requirements of the product. Acceptable approaches for designing control strategies for continuous processes include the following:

- Parametric control strategy, where controls are based on established acceptable ranges and target values of process parameters across integrated operations on the continuous manufacturing line, underpinned by an enhanced level of process understanding aligned with QbD principles including operating within an established design space
- Control strategy with enhanced process monitoring /process controls based on advanced process analytics, which can be model-based (such as multivariate statistical process monitoring/control) or by leveraging spectroscopic PAT for real-time measurement of product attributes, guiding the decision-making on product disposition in real time on the continuous manufacturing line
- Control strategy dependent on end-product testing

Due to the integrated nature of the continuous manufacturing process and the potential for interaction effects among integrated process parameters as well as input/in-process material attributes, the development of a design space for the continuous process can be very beneficial during product development. Design space is defined as "the multidimensional combination and interaction of input variables (e.g., material attributes) and process parameters that have been demonstrated to provide assurance of quality" [8]. Establishing design space through multifactorial experiments has been common in pharmaceutical development over the last decade for batch processes both for an enhanced level of process understanding during product development, as well as to achieve greater regulatory flexibility during the product lifecycle. As opposed to univariate proven acceptable ranges (PARs) where one factor can be changed at a time, parameters within an established design space can be varied in a multifactorial manner within the acceptable ranges of parameters registered in regulatory submissions. Therefore, registered design space is attractive from product development and commercialization viewpoint.

In traditional batch manufacturing mode, design space is typically established for individual operations. While some interaction effects across unit operations may also occur for traditional batch manufacturing modes (e.g., batch granulation operation impacting downstream compression performance), there is limited benefit in establishing an integrated end-to-end design space in batch processing, since unit operations are separated over space and time and there is less likelihood of the propagation and/or amplification of variations from upstream operations to downstream processes. However, as the implementation of continuous manufacturing of pharmaceuticals is becoming more prevalent, the role of fully integrated end-to-end design space across the integrated continuous operations on a continuous manufacturing line is expected to become a key focus area as more pharmaceutical companies adopt continuous manufacturing for their products.

13.5 End-to-End Design Space Considerations for Continuous Manufacturing

End-to-end design space for continuous manufacturing, considering the impact of potential interactions among material attributes and parameters across integrated continuous operations, has several advantages while developing the control strategy for continuous manufacturing of pharmaceuticals. The key advantages of integrated end-to-end design space in continuous manufacturing are summarized below and illustrated in Figure 13.4:

- **Enhanced process understanding**: An end-to-end design space provides an enhanced level of product and process understanding for continuous manufacturing aligned with the QbD principles. Such an enhanced level of understanding is beneficial to demonstrate the robustness of the control strategy for commercial continuous products.
- **Establishing process control limits and maintaining State of Control**: For continuous processes, State of Control, which is defined in ICH Q10 as "a condition in which the set of controls

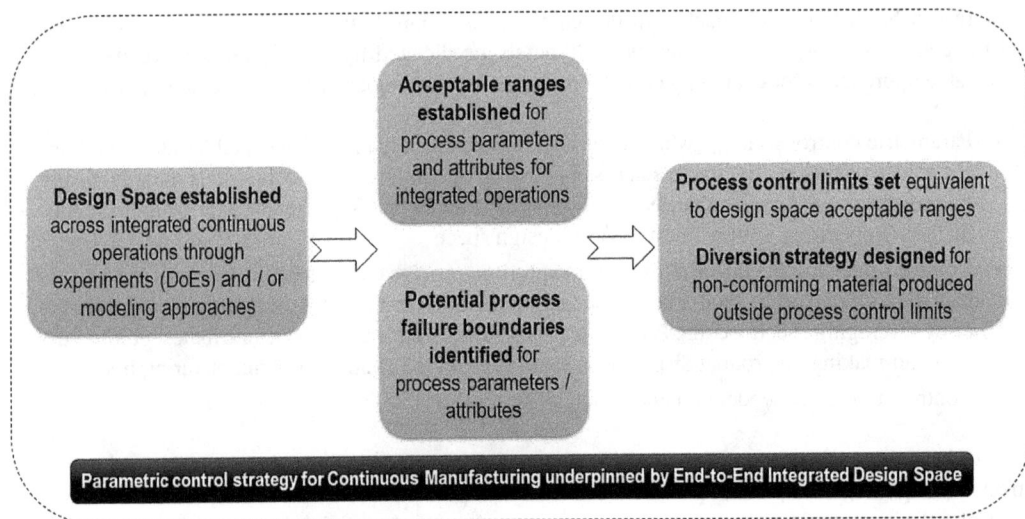

FIGURE 13.4 Role of an integrated end-to-end design space in the control strategy for continuous manufacturing of pharmaceuticals.

consistently provides assurance of continued process performance and product quality" [10], can be maintained by operating the process within the process control limits. The acceptable ranges and target values of parameters within the integrated design space for the continuous process can be used to establish the process control limits for a continuous process, and the maintenance of the State of Control can be ensured by operating within the design space acceptable ranges.

- **Inform the diversion strategy of non-conforming material**: The acceptable design space ranges can also guide product diversion strategy for a continuous process, where any material produced outside the process control limits can be diverted either to waste or for further evaluation.
- **Understanding of failure boundaries of the process**: Finally, an in-depth understanding of the interactions across parameters and material attributes can also help establish potential failure boundaries of the process. Identifying how the end-to-end integrated design space is separated from failure boundaries of the continuous process either from a manufacturability or product quality viewpoint can be highly beneficial to identify a robust manufacturing regime [22].

The approaches for establishing end-to-end design space for a continuous manufacturing line are illustrated in Figure 13.5, and summarized below:

- Approaches based on experimentation (such as, design of experiments or DoEs) are performed across integrated operations on a continuous line. Such a DoE will involve several parameters across the integrated operations, as well as material attributes, with the parameter and attribute selection for the DoE being guided by risk assessments. Continuous manufacturing can be uniquely suited for performing large DoEs with several factors, since the experiments can be performed by changing process conditions and dynamics within a short timeframe in a material-sparing approach, as opposed to batch manufacturing, where there is less flexibility to adjust process conditions within a batch.
- Design space approaches are guided by models [23], leveraging advanced process analytics [24], where the key benefit is a significant reduction in the level of experimentation required to establish the end-to-end design space. There are a number of modeling approaches that can help with design space development, such as data-driven modeling for design space [25] including response surface methodologies, Bayesian model-based approach for design space [26], and knowledge-based models. Model-informed design space development can significantly streamline and

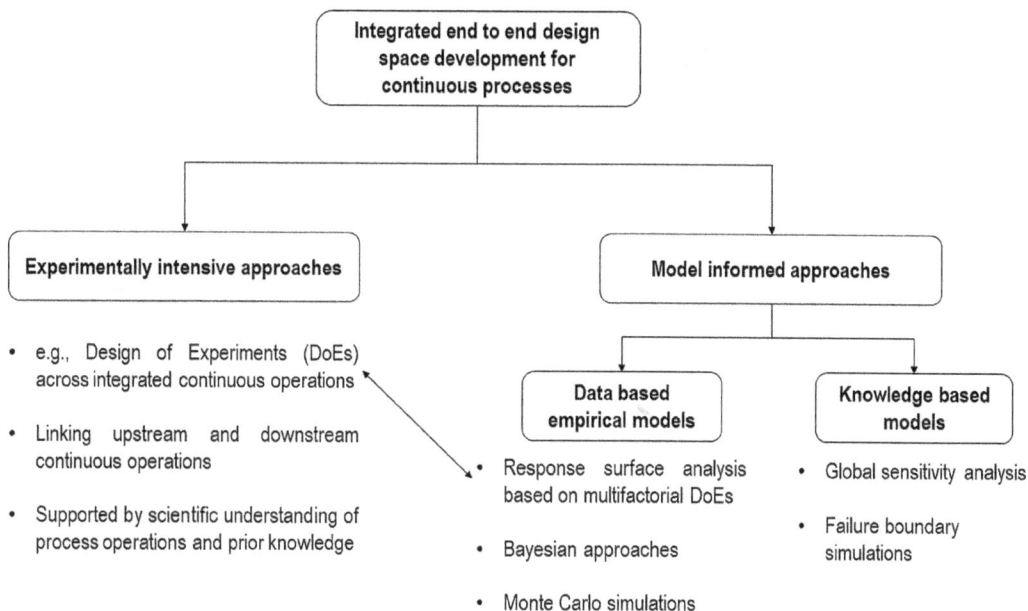

FIGURE 13.5 Approaches for establishing and describing end-to-end design space across integrated continuous operations for continuous manufacturing of pharmaceuticals.

accelerate continuous process development by reducing the need to perform extensive DoEs, as well as help with the simulation of the manufacturing process to determine potential failure boundaries of the process without the need to actually stretch the process to failure.

13.6 End-to-End Continuous Manufacturing Connecting Drug Substance and Drug Product

Until now, across the pharmaceutical industry, the application of continuous manufacturing for pharmaceuticals has largely focused on developing continuous technologies separately for drug substances and drug products. However, the implementation of a fully integrated end-to-end continuous manufacturing process connecting drug substances and drug products is also an emerging area of interest within the pharmaceutical community [27, 28]. One approach to designing a fully integrated end-to-end continuous manufacturing process connecting drug substance and drug product is to develop drug substances having optimum manufacturability attributes (e.g., powder flowability and compaction properties) that are appropriate for secondary drug product manufacturing processes, such as direct compression. Material engineering approaches leveraging crystal and particle engineering strategies can be beneficial here to enhance the powder flow and compaction attributes of drug substances to make them more suitable for downstream drug product processing through continuous direct compression [29]. In Figure 13.6, a schematic of an end-to-end integrated continuous manufacturing process connecting drug substance and drug product is illustrated. In this approach, the starting materials of the drug substance are transformed into the final tablet dosage form with no/minimal requirement of intermediate product isolation.

In this approach, the drug substance is manufactured semi-continuously/continuously by integrating flow chemistry reaction stages, continuous crystallization, and continuous/semi-continuous filtration and drying operations. There can be a number of material engineering approaches that can augment the manufacturability attributes of a drug substance to make it suitable for subsequent direct compression [29]. These may involve directly modifying the crystallization conditions using crystal engineering approaches to produce drug substances with better flow attributes, such as through spherical crystallization, or

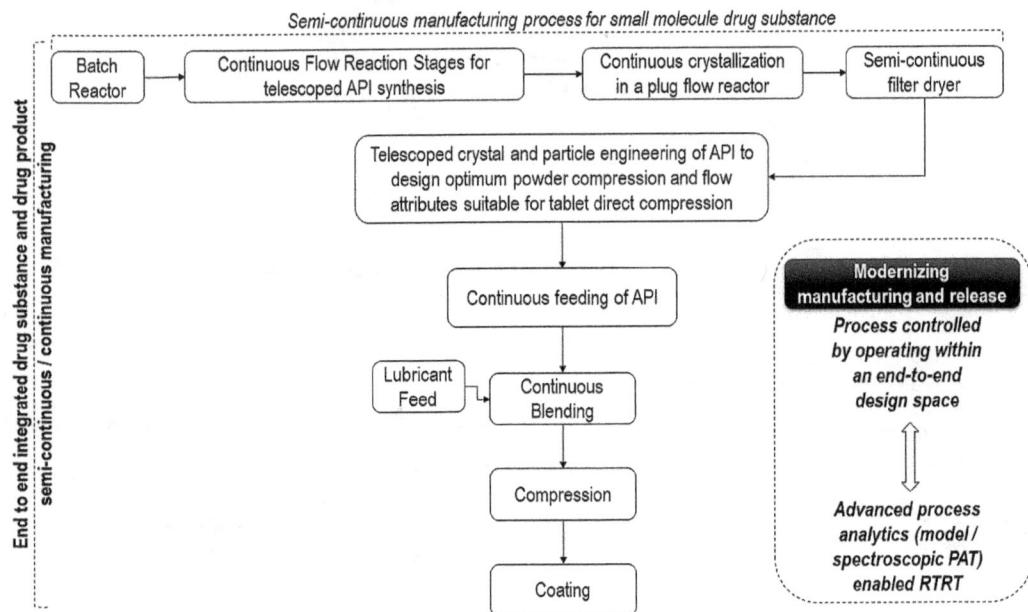

FIGURE 13.6 Vision for end-to-end integrated semi-continuous/continuous manufacturing of small molecule drug substance and drug product based on continuous direct compression, underpinned by crystal and particle engineering approaches to design optimum flow and compression attributes appropriate for direct compression. Advanced process analytics enable real time testing and release of the product.

telescoped particle engineering approaches after drying of the drug substance to enhance compression and powder flow properties of the drug substance. An attractive particle engineering approach that has shown promise in the pharmaceutical industry is nanocoating of drug substances or poorly flowing excipients using nanoscale materials, such as colloidal silicon dioxide, using dry milling operations that can enhance the powder flow properties significantly by reducing material cohesion [30]. Such a dry milling step can also be readily integrated into the continuous manufacturing line to connect the incoming drug substance and the powder feeding operation for direct compression, resulting in an integrated end-to-end continuous line connecting drug substance and drug product. Such materials with enhanced manufacturability attributes can be fed consistently for secondary drug product continuous manufacturing operations (e.g., by continuous direct compression).

A key open question for end-to-end continuous manufacturing connecting drug substance and drug product is the regulatory expectation around testing and release of drug substance leading to the final drug product. Since, such an integrated continuous process would involve minimal or no manual intervention or intermediate product isolation/purification and release testing, it will be important to design an appropriate analytical framework to support the testing and release of such products aligned with global regulatory expectations. Advanced process analytics including modeling and spectroscopic PAT approaches, underpinned by enhanced process understanding based on an end-to-end design space, is expected to play a key role here both for process monitoring/control, as well as to support real-time release testing (RTRT) of products. Such an approach will obviate the need to isolate and test intermediates and will be well suited to support the implementation of an end-to-end integrated continuous manufacturing line connecting drug substances and drug products.

Figure 13.7 shows an illustrative example of a fully integrated design space for an end-to-end continuous line connecting drug substance and drug product, considering potential interaction effects among material attributes and process parameters across integrated drug substance/drug product operations. In this example of the end-to-end design space, several parameters and material attributes are highlighted that may be important to consider for different integrated operations for the continuous line. While it is

**End-to-end integrated drug substance and drug product
semi-continuous / continuous manufacturing**

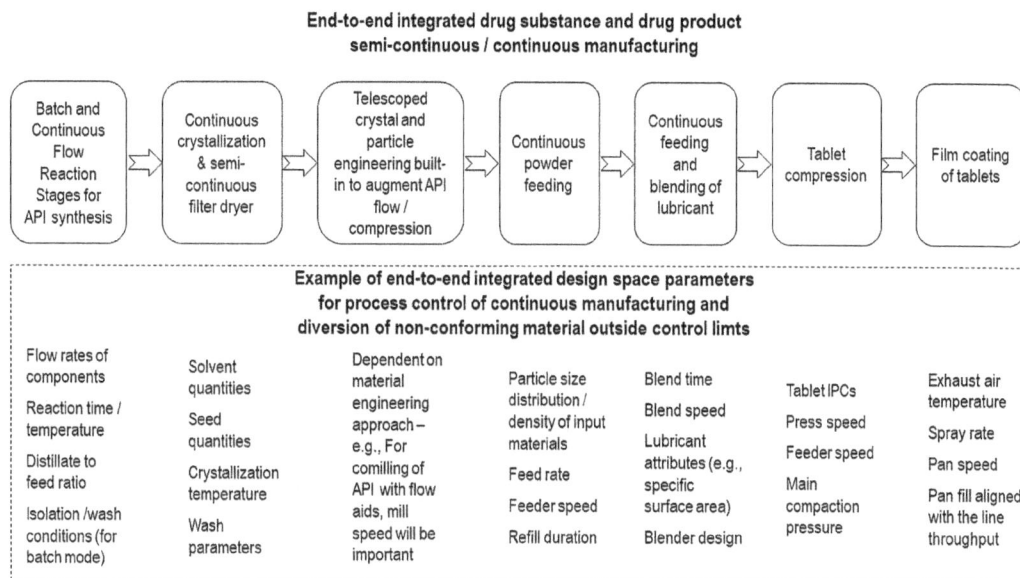

**Example of end-to-end integrated design space parameters
for process control of continuous manufacturing and
diversion of non-conforming material outside control limts**

Flow rates of components	Solvent quantities	Dependent on material engineering approach – e.g., For comilling of API with flow aids, mill speed will be important	Particle size distribution / density of input materials	Blend time	Tablet IPCs	Exhaust air temperature
Reaction time / temperature	Seed quantities			Blend speed	Press speed	Spray rate
Distillate to feed ratio	Crystallization temperature		Feed rate	Lubricant attributes (e.g., specific surface area)	Feeder speed	Pan speed
Isolation /wash conditions (for batch mode)	Wash parameters		Feeder speed		Main compaction pressure	Pan fill aligned with the line throughput
			Refill duration	Blender design		

FIGURE 13.7 Illustration of end-to-end integrated design space parameters across an end-to-end small molecule drug substance and drug product semi-continuous/continuous manufacturing process based on direct compression.

appreciated that establishing such a multifactorial end-to-end design space is aspirational and can be viewed as cumbersome, especially when adopting an experimentally intensive DoE approach for design space development, proper utilization of model-informed approaches described earlier can greatly mitigate the experimental burden and make such end-to-end design spaces more accessible to the pharmaceutical industry.

13.7 Conclusions

Continuous manufacturing is being actively adopted across the pharmaceutical industry to modernize pharmaceutical manufacturing. Due to the integrated nature of continuous manufacturing processes, there is significant potential for interaction effects among parameters across integrated continuous operations, as well as with material attributes. To design a robust continuous manufacturing process, it is important to develop a holistic understanding of such interactions across integrated continuous operations. Establishing an end-to-end design space for continuous processes can greatly enhance the level of product and process understanding to support the commercialization of continuously manufactured pharmaceuticals. While there is limited precedence in the pharmaceutical industry for establishing and registering end-to-end integrated design space, it is anticipated that such efforts will become more and more important with the increase in the adoption of continuous manufacturing by the pharmaceutical industry, potentially leading to the development of fully integrated end-to-end continuous manufacturing lines connecting the drug substance and drug product manufacturing operations.

REFERENCES

1. Srai, J. S.; Badman, C.; Krumme, M.; Futran, M.; Johnston, C., Future Supply Chains Enabled by Continuous Processing-Opportunities and Challenges May 20–21, 2014 Continuous Manufacturing Symposium. *J. Pharm. Sci.* 2015, *104* (3), 840–849.
2. Badman, C.; Trout, B. L., Achieving Continuous Manufacturing May 20–21 2014 Continuous Manufacturing Symposium. *J. Pharm. Sci.* 2015, *104* (3), 779–780.

3. Lee, S. L.; O'Connor, T. F.; Yang, X.; Cruz, C. N.; Chatterjee, S.; Madurawe, R. D.; Moore, C. M. V.; Yu, L.X.; Woodcock, J., Modernizing Pharmaceutical Manufacturing: From Batch to Continuous Production. *J. Pharm. Innov.* 2015, *10* (3), 191–199.

4. Plumb, K., Continuous Processing in the Pharmaceutical Industry: Changing the Mind Set. *Chem. Eng. Res. Des.* 2005, *83* (6), 730–738.

5. Badman, C.; Cooney, C. L.; Florence, A.; Konstantinov, K.; Krumme, M.; Mascia, S.; Nasr, M.; Trout, B. L., Why We Need Continuous Pharmaceutical Manufacturing and How to Make It Happen. *J. Pharm. Sci.* 2019, *108* (11), 3521–3523.

6. Byrn, S.; Futran, M.; Thomas, H.; Jayjock, E.; Maron, N.; Meyer, R. F.; Myerson, A. S.; Thien, M. P.; Trout, B. L., Achieving Continuous Manufacturing for Final Dosage Formation: Challenges and How to Meet Them May 20–21 2014 Continuous Manufacturing Symposium. *J. Pharm. Sci.* 2015, *104* (3), 792–802.

7. Baxendale, I. R.; Braatz, R. D.; Hodnett, B. K.; Jensen, K. F.; Johnson, M. D.; Sharratt, P.; Sherlock, J. P.; Florence, A. J., Achieving Continuous Manufacturing: Technologies and Approaches for Synthesis, Workup, and Isolation of Drug Substance May 20–21, 2014 Continuous Manufacturing Symposium. *J. Pharm. Sci.* 2015, *104* (3), 781–791.

8. International Council for Harmonization. *ICH Q8(R2): Pharmaceutical Development*. 2009.

9. International Council for Harmonization. *ICH Q9: Quality Risk Management*. 2005.

10. International Council for Harmonization. *ICH Q10: Pharmaceutical Quality System*. 2008.

11. International Council for Harmonization. *ICH Q11: Development and Manufacture of Drug Substances (Chemical Entities and Biotechnological/Biological Entities)*. 2012.

12. Domokos, A.; Nagy, B.; Szilágyi, B.; Marosi, G.; Nagy, Z. K., Integrated Continuous Pharmaceutical Technologies-A Review. *Org. Process Res. Dev.* 2021, *25* (4), 721–739.

13. International Council for Harmonization. *ICH Q13: Continuous Manufacturing of Drug Substances and Drug Products*. 2018.

14. Gutmann, B.; Cantillo, D.; Kappe, C. O., Continuous Flow Technology-A Tool for the Safe Manufacturing of Active Pharmaceutical Ingredients. *Angew. Chem., Int. Ed.* 2015, *54* (23), 6688–6728.

15. Ingham, R. J.; Battilocchio, C.; Fitzpatrick, D. E.; Sliwinski, E.; Hawkins, J. M.; Ley, S. V., A Systems Approach Towards an Intelligent and Self-Controlling Platform for Integrated Continuous Reaction Sequences. *Angew. Chem., Int. Ed.* 2015, *15* (1), 144–148.

16. Zhang, P.; Weeranoppanant, N.; Thomas, D. A.; Tahara, K.; Stelzer, T.; Russell, M. G.; O'Mahony, M.; Myerson, A. S.; Lin, H.; Kelly, L. P.; Jensen, K. F.; Jamison, T. F.; Dai, C.; Cui, Y.; Briggs, N.; Beingessner, R. L.; Adamo, A., Advanced Continuous Flow Platform for On-Demand Pharmaceutical Manufacturing. *Chem. Eur. J.* 2018, *24* (11), 2776–2784.

17. Hughes, D. L., Applications of Flow Chemistry in Drug Development: Highlights of Recent Patent Literature. *Org. Process Res. Dev.* 2018, *22* (1), 13–20.

18. Wong, S. Y.; Chen, J.; Forte, L. E.; Myerson, A. S., Compact Crystallization, Filtration, and Drying for the Production of Active Pharmaceutical Ingredients. *Org. Process Res. Dev.* 2013, *17* (4), 684–692.

19. Capellades, G.; Neurohr, C.; Azad, M.; Brancazio, D.; Rapp, K.; Hammersmith, G.; Myerson, A. S., A Compact Device for the Integrated Filtration, Drying, and Mechanical Processing of Active Pharmaceutical Ingredients. *J. Pharm. Sci.* 2020, *109* (3), 1365–1372.

20. Wood, B.; Girard, K. P.; Polster, C. S.; Croker, D. M., Progress to Date in the Design and Operation of Continuous Crystallization Processes for Pharmaceutical Applications. *Org. Process Res. Dev.* 2019, *23* (2), 122–144.

21. Allison, G.; Cain, Y. T.; Cooney, C.; Garcia, T.; Bizjak, T. G.; Holte, O.; Jagota, N.; Komas, B.; Korakianiti, E.; Kourti, D.; Madurawe, R.; Morefield, E.; Montgomery, F.; Nasr, M.; Randolph, W.; Robert, J. L.; Rudd, D.; Zezza, D., Regulatory and Quality Considerations for Continuous Manufacturing May 20–21, 2014 Continuous Manufacturing Symposium. *J. Pharm. Sci.* 2015, *104* (3), 803–812.

22. Facco, P.; Dal Pastro, F.; Meneghetti, N.; Bezzo, F.; Barolo, M., Bracketing the Design Space within the Knowledge Space in Pharmaceutical Product Development. *Ind. Eng. Chem. Res.* 2015, *54*, 5128–5138.

23. Burt, J. L.; Braem, A. D.; Ramirez, A.; Mudryk, B.; Rossano, L.; Tummala, S., Model-Guided Design Space Development for a Drug Substance Manufacturing Process. *J. Pharm. Innov.* 2011, *6*, 181–192.

24. Fonteyne, M.; Vercruysse, J.; De Leersnyder, F.; Van Snick, B.; Vervaet, C.; Remon, J. P.; De Beer, T., Process Analytical Technology for Continuous Manufacturing of Solid-Dosage Forms. *Trends Anal. Chem.* 2015, *67*, 159–166.

25. Boukouvala, F.; Muzzio, F. J.; Ierapetritou, M. G., Design Space of Pharmaceutical Processes Using Data-Driven-Based Methods. *J. Pharm. Innov.* 2010, *5*, 119–137.

26. Peterson, J. J., A Bayesian Approach to the ICH Q8 Definition of Design Space. *J.Biopharm. Stat.* 2008, *18*, 959–975.

27. Testa, C. J.; Hu, C.; Shvedova, K.; Wu, W.; Sayin, R.; Casati, F.; Halkude, B. S.; Hermant, P.; Shen, D. E.; Ramnath, A.; Su, Q., Design and Commercialization of an End-to-End Continuous Pharmaceutical Production Process: A Pilot Plant Case Study. *Org. Process Res. Dev.* 2020, *24*, 2874.

28. Domokos, A.; Nagy, B.; Gyürkés, M.; Farkas, A.; Tacsi, K.; Pataki, H.; Claire Liu, Y.; Balogh, A.; Firth, P.; Szilágyi, B.; Marosi, G.; Nagy, Z. K.; Kristóf Nagy, Z., End-to-End Continuous Manufacturing of Conventional Compressed Tablets: From Flow Synthesis to Tableting through Integrated Crystallization and Filtration. *Int. J. Pharm.* 2020, *581*, 119297.

29. Chattoraj, S.; Sun, C. C., Crystal and Particle Engineering Strategies for Improving Powder Compression and Flow Properties to Enable Continuous Tablet Manufacturing by Direct Compression. *J. Pharm. Sci.* 2018, *107* (4), 968–974.

30. Chattoraj, S.; Shi, L.; Sun, C. C., Profoundly Improving Flow Properties of a Cohesive Cellulose Powder by Surface Coating with Nano-silica Through Comilling. *J. Pharm. Sci.* 2011, *100*, 4943–4952.

14

Control Strategies in Continuous Direct Compression

Aditya Vanarase and Sherif Badawy
Bristol Myers Squibb Company, New Brunswick, NJ, USA

CONTENTS

14.1 Introduction

In recent years, continuous manufacturing (CM) has emerged as one of the ways to advance manufacturing technology in the pharmaceutical industry. One version of CM that is gaining popularity in oral solid dose (OSD) drug product manufacture is continuous direct compression (CDC). CDC is the simplest process among other continuous processes such as continuous dry and wet granulations, but it can accommodate formulations in a wide range of material properties. In batch manufacturing, direct compression process is often not selected when formulations have poor flow properties and high segregation tendency. In continuous blending, due to its process design, the risk of segregation is significantly lower than in batch (Oka et al., 2017; Jaspers et al., 2021). Continuous blenders negate the need for large bin blenders and hoppers where flow is often a challenge. Thus, CDC can enable certain formulations which otherwise would be difficult to manufacture using a batch direct compression process. This book chapter focuses on aspects of process design, in-process control (IPC), and material attributes that are critical in deciding the drug product control strategy for the CDC process.

DOI: 10.1201/9781003149835-18

Control strategy implementations in pharmaceutical manufacturing can be categorized into three levels (Lee et al., 2015; Rantanen & Khinast, 2015). In level 1 control strategy, process variables and quality attributes are controlled in real-time using active control systems without any need for offline testing of the attributes in the process intermediate or finished product. In level 2 control strategy, manufacturing is carried out within established ranges of process parameters and input material properties. In addition, the quality attributes are assured through testing or surrogate models. In level 3 control strategy, the operation is carried out within tightly constrained material attributes and process parameters. The risk of releasing poor-quality products is lowered through extensive end-product testing.

Continuous manufacturing (CM) lends itself well to Level 1 control (Figure 14.1). In this level of control, the process adjusts in real-time in response to measured variability, therefore assuring control of the desired quality attributes. Level 1 control is achieved via process analytics, process models and automation, all of which enable the implementation of advanced process control paradigms. These control strategies are broadly classified as open system or closed loop controls. In open control systems, no active controls are implemented but monitored signals may trigger external action. Clear rules of engagement with the process based on the measured signal should be established. Action limits should be developed and action details (e.g., separation of non-conforming material and/or operator adjustment) clearly defined. In closed loop controls, process variables are controlled using control strategies such as feedback, feedforward, or a combination of both. In CM, typically both the open and closed loop controls are implemented simultaneously. Due to the possibility of continuous monitoring and control of various attributes, CM processes inherently are more suitable for real-time-release (RTR).

In contrast, batch manufacturing typically has different unit operations that operate at fixed parameters, or parameters that vary within proven and acceptable ranges, and which are established upfront during product development according to level 2 or 3 controls. In these levels of control, quality attributes of process intermediates may or may not be monitored, but even if they are monitored, the purpose is usually limited to process verification rather than control and are not typically used to make batch decisions (Figure 14.2).

In a book chapter by Singh (2018), different types of advanced controls, the principles behind each of them and some examples of their applications for continuous pharmaceutical processes are described in detail. Proportional integral derivative (PID) controllers and model predictive controllers (MPC) are commonly used strategies for closed-loop dynamic control. In PID controls, corrective action requires minimal knowledge of the process and occurs as soon as the monitored variable deviates from the target point. MPC requires high fidelity process models (first principle or statistical models) which link critical process parameters, including manipulated variable(s), to the monitored parameter, or attribute. The MPC uses the model in conjunction with current and target values of the monitored parameter or attributes to calculate changes required in the manipulated variable(s). MPC is more capable of handling situations where multiple process variable interactions impact the monitored variable and is better at handling

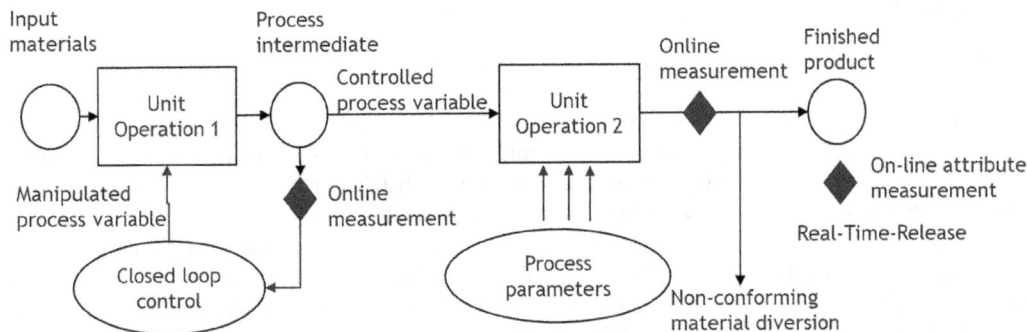

FIGURE 14.1 Advanced level of controls in continuous manufacturing.

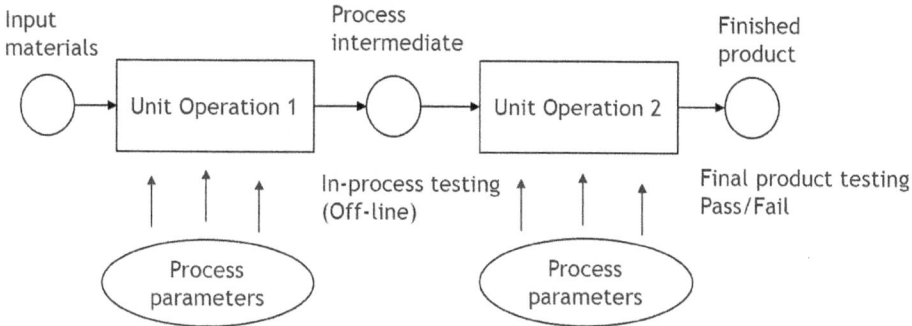

FIGURE 14.2 Low levels of controls in batch manufacturing.

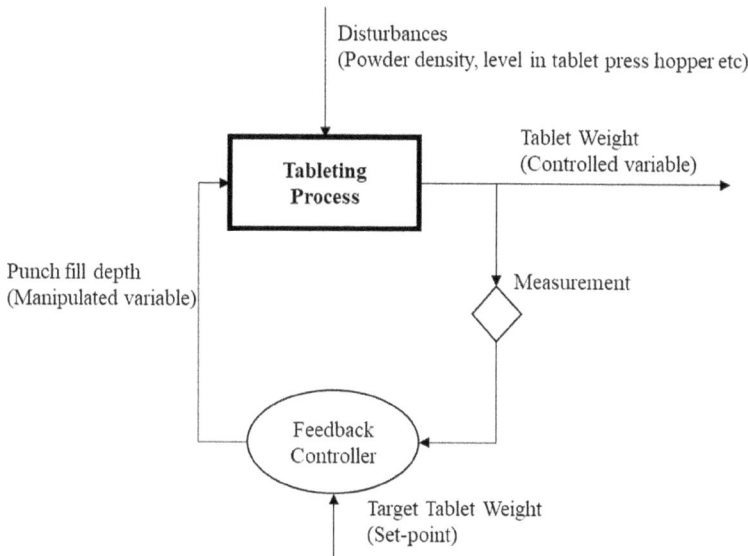

FIGURE 14.3 Feedback control of tablet weight.

process delays compared to PID controllers. Rigorous performance assessment and validation of the closed-loop system should be conducted prior to its implementation in manufacturing.

In the feedback closed-loop dynamic control, a process intermediate attribute is monitored, and the measurement is used to manipulate specific unit operation parameters to maintain the value of this intermediate attribute close to the target. An example of tablet weight control in tableting operation is shown in Figure 14.3. At the core of this method of process, control is the selection of the manipulated variable(s) which are varied to compensate for the effect of process disturbances on the monitored attribute and bring it closer to its target. Manipulated variable(s) should have a rapid and direct impact on the monitored variable with minimal process time delay.

In feedforward control (Figure 14.4), a specific attribute of the materials entering the process or any other information upstream of the process is used to adjust the manipulated variable based on a known relationship between the measured input attribute and the manipulated variable. In this type of control strategy, the impact of known disturbances on the process can be mitigated, and in an ideal scenario, it can be eliminated as well. However, in feedforward control, since the output (controlled variable) measurement is not fed back to the controller, there is always the risk of deviating from the set-point, especially

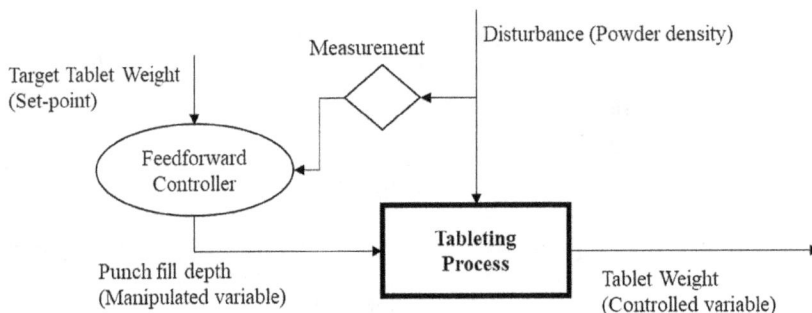

FIGURE 14.4 Feedforward control of tablet weight.

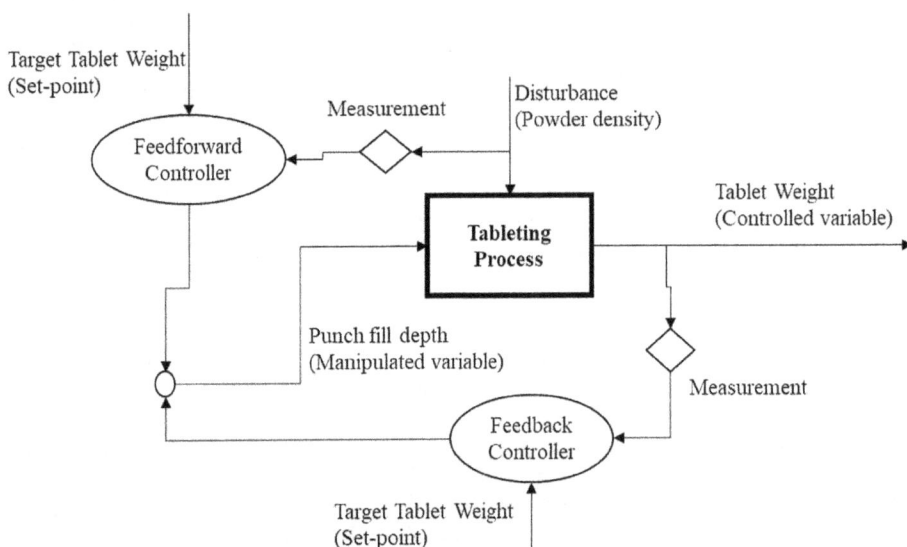

FIGURE 14.5 Combined feedback and feedforward control of tablet weight.

when the unmeasured process disturbances also influence the output. To overcome this challenge, a combined feedforward and feedback control strategy is often used to maximize the advantage of feedforward control. For example, in a continuous tablet manufacturing process, the changes in powder density of the blend can have a direct impact on tablet properties (Figure 14.5). If the powder density can be measured by a suitable method (such as near-infrared [NIR] spectroscopy), in a feedforward control system, an input can be provided to the control system to change the fill-depth of the punches. Simultaneously, a feedback control can also be exercised via continuous tablet weight monitoring and using that to manipulate fill depth.

In the CDC process, multiple loss-in-weight (LIW) feeders are used to feed the different components of the formulation. The relative feed rate of each component is determined by the ratio of the different components in the formulation. The LIW feeder has a feedback control loop that works to maintain the feed rate as close as possible to the target. Continuous blenders are used to blend the different components and feed the final blend to the tablet press feed frame. Process analytical technology (PAT) measurements can be used for both, blend uniformity of the blend prior to compression in the tablet press feed tube or in the feed frame and for content uniformity of tablets coming out of the tablet press. These PAT measurements are used to monitor product quality and possibly to make a determination on product acceptance or rejection. Non-conforming product rejection is accomplished automatically according to the algorithm established in the control system of the integrated CDC unit.

In the CDC, product content uniformity is tied to the consistency of material feed rate. If the active propagates in the system strictly in a plug flow pattern with no axial dispersion, any feed rate variability would directly manifest itself in the product content uniformity. However, some axial dispersion takes place as a result of blending and materials movement through the process which helps filter some of the variability in the feed rate, therefore allowing the process to tolerate some feed rate variation that otherwise would have resulted in the out-of-specification (OOS) product. Feeder variability that can be tolerated is dependent on the degree of axial mixing and mean residence time of the material, which are both captured in the residence distribution (RTD) model. The RTD models are therefore used to predict product uniformity based on feeder data and are valuable tools in support of process control strategy.

To implement a control strategy for the CDC process, knowledge of the impact of process parameters and material attributes on intermediate and finished product quality attributes is required. Further, to enable any process control strategies (open or closed loop), necessary methods to monitor desired quality attributes and process models need to be developed.

In this chapter, formulation considerations and process development strategies for unit operations in CDC, and development approaches for the in-process methods of blend concentration monitoring are described with relevant examples. In addition, control strategies from the perspective of the critical quality attributes of drug products are also presented.

14.2 Formulation Considerations and Development of Continuous Direct Compression Process

There are some key considerations that formulators need to be aware of while developing products using CDC technology. For CDC formulations, the material properties of the ingredients need to be suitable for feeding them through the LIW feeders. Feeding could be challenging when feed rates are extremely low and/or material properties of the ingredients are challenging (low bulk density, cohesive, etc.). Therefore, the composition should be designed with the expectation of having a good feeding performance for individual ingredients. Extreme low concentrations (e.g., < 0.5% w/w) should be avoided in the formulation.

In the current paradigm of batch manufacturing, formulations are typically developed using smaller scale equipment of any given process that is used in drug product manufacturing. While developing products using CDC technology, it is not advisable to follow the same philosophy. A smaller scale version of CDC equipment may not always be available and there may be limitations in using CDC equipment at a smaller batch size or throughput. Limitation on minimum batch size is due to the potential waste created during start-up/shut-down during manufacturing.

The very first step in developing a control strategy for any drug product manufacturing process is process development. During process development, process parameter ranges are identified for each unit operation such that the desired in-process and finished product attributes are met during manufacturing. Various approaches can be followed during process development including risk-based, design of experiment (DoE)-based, scientific/engineering principle-based, or a combination of all. One key aspect where process development in continuous manufacturing differs from the batch is that none of the unit operations can be fully developed as stand-alone operations; the inputs/outputs of each are always integrated with some other unit operation. While it is important to develop each unit operation in conjunction with others in the CDC line, batch process can be used to develop product understanding for attributes that are independent of the continuous aspect of the process. For example, for developing an understanding of dissolution or compaction behavior of the drug product, a smaller-scale batch process can be used during formulation development. Once the formulation composition is optimized, the sensitivity of process parameter ranges to the performance of these attributes is evaluated during CDC process development.

A schematic of the CDC equipment configuration is shown in Figure 14.6 In this example, two blenders in series are used where the first one is used to blend API and three other excipients. Lubricant and another excipient are blended in the second blender. The second blender provides lower shear, thus avoiding any possibility of over-lubrication. The blend from the second blender is continuously discharged in the tablet press. Blend concentration is monitored using PAT tools in the feed tube between the second blender and the tablet press.

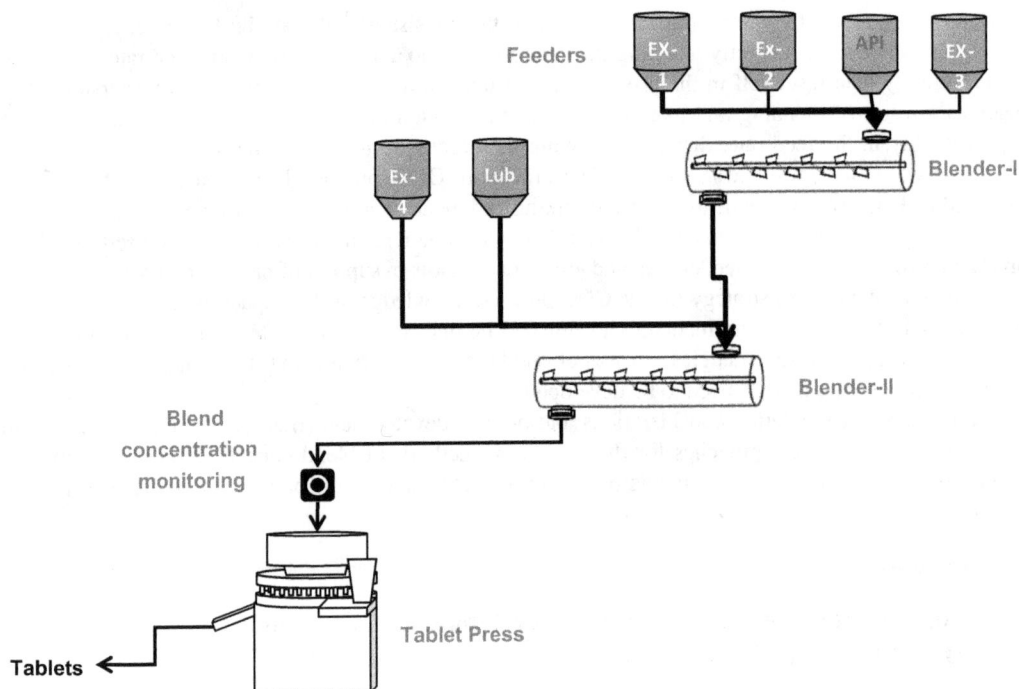

FIGURE 14.6   Continuous Direct Compression process schematic.

In this section, process development approaches for feeding and blending unit operations are described. Tableting operation is the same between batch or continuous manufacturing, thus not described in this chapter.

14.2.1 Feeding

Feeding is the first unit operation in any continuous manufacturing process. In a CDC process, feeding is preceded by refill operations of the feeder hopper and is followed by blending and tableting processes. The parameters of the feeding process need to be developed with the knowledge of their impact on refilling, blending and tableting operations.

The goal of feeding process development is to identify feeder equipment configuration and parameters where a consistent feed rate can be achieved. In this chapter, refill operation is considered a part of the feeding process and refill parameters are also identified during feeder process development. Feeder equipment configuration includes screw design, screen at nozzle discharge, hopper design and agitator design. Feeding process parameters are target feed rate, minimum refill volume and refill volume. The latter two parameters determine the frequency of hopper refilling and are based on knowledge of the dependence of feed rate and feed rate variability on the amount of material in the hopper.

To initiate feeder process development, an estimate of the total line throughput is required. Line throughput could be dependent on factors such as the achievable feed rate of individual ingredients, achievable throughput for blending and tableting and throughput of downstream unit operation such as film-coating and packaging if they are carried out continuously along with the CDC process. In the current example, the continuous process ends with tableting. Film-coating and packaging are carried out as stand-alone batch/continuous operations. The drug product formulation used in this example is a direct blend formulation with 2.0 % w/w drug load of API and tablet weight is 200 mg. Based on the knowledge of a typical range of tableting speeds (20–80 rpm) and the number of stations in the tablet press (38 stations), line throughput was estimated to be 9.1–36.5 kg/hr. Continuous blender typically does not limit throughput unless it is very high (> 200 kg/hr). Using this initial throughput estimate, target range of feed rate for every formulation ingredient can be calculated. For 2.0 % w/w drug loading, target range of feed rate for the API would be ~182–730 g/hr. Feeding process development would then focus on selecting appropriate equipment configuration and identifying a target feed rate where a consistent feed rate can be achieved.

Prior knowledge of the feeder with other materials can be used to select the initial equipment configuration. During this exercise, based on the available knowledge of feed factor (amount of material fed per single screw revolution) dependence on material properties, a screw configuration wherein the material is expected to achieve the desired feed factor consistently and a gear ratio where feeder can be operated within the allowable screw speed range is selected. Actual feeder runs are then conducted using the selected equipment configuration and a confirmation of the selection of screw design, screw size and the gear ratio is obtained. Wang et al. (2017) and Tahir et al. (2020) have provided examples where multivariate analysis was used to correlate feed factor and feeder variability with material flow properties. Such approaches greatly facilitate early process development when the availability of API material is limited. An example of feed factor correlation with material bulk density is provided in Figure 14.7.

After the initial selection of equipment configuration, refill parameters (minimum refill mass and refill size) need to be selected. Refill parameters influence feed rate variation during refills. Some examples of the extent of impact refills can have on feed rate deviations are presented in Engisch & Muzzio (2015). To decide the minimum mass in the hopper where a refill can be performed, feeder is run from the hopper full to empty and feed factor as a function of hopper net weight is obtained. An example of feed factor profile during hopper emptying process is shown in Figure 14.8.

In this example, the initial estimate of minimum refill mass in the hopper is ~200 g since the feed factor has less dependence on net weight above the minimum refill mass. Further, the measured mass flow RSD

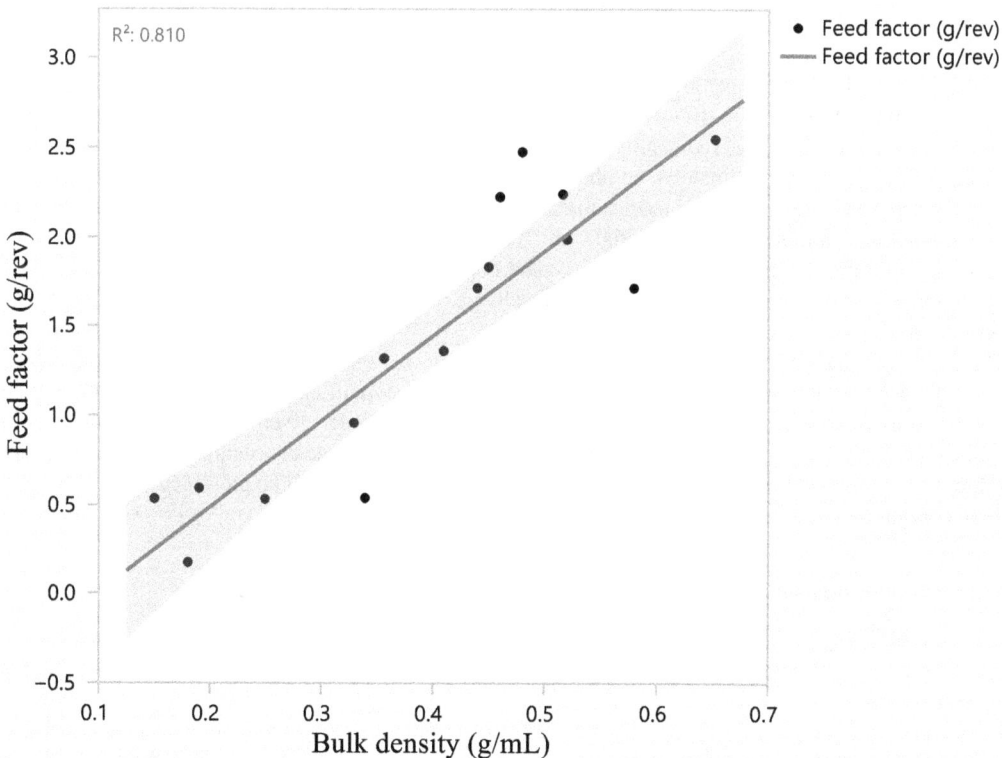

FIGURE 14.7 Feed factor correlation with bulk density.

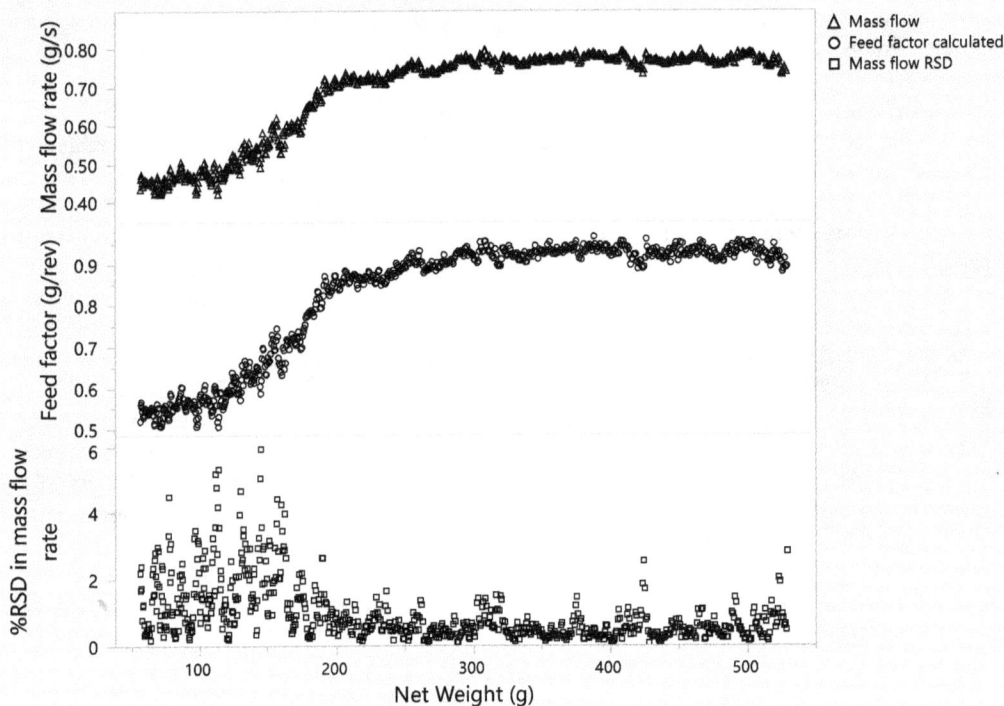

FIGURE 14.8 Feed factor profile during hopper emptying at a fixed screw speed of 50 rpm.

was also higher when the hopper level falls below the minimum refill mass. Once minimum refill mass in hopper is estimated, trials with different refill amounts are conducted and feed rate is monitored during refills. Depending on the observed results from these trials, minimum refill mass may need to be further optimized from the initial estimate. A combination of minimum refill mass in hopper and refill mass is selected where feed rate profiles are most stable. During these trials, material flow behavior in the hopper needs to be closely monitored. For materials which do not flow well in the hopper (causing issues such as arching, bridging, or sticking to side walls), modified impellers or modified hoppers can be used. If material tends to form large powder lumps at the discharge of feeder nozzle, a screen can be used to break up those lumps.

Once refill parameters are identified, feeder runs with periodic refills are conducted for extended periods and feeder data that mimics actual continuous processing conditions is obtained. The data is then analyzed to assess the acceptability of the feed rate variability under given conditions in the overall continuous process. For this assessment, knowledge of the residence time distribution of the downstream continuous blender and the continuous line is needed. This assessment will be presented in the next section on continuous blending.

14.2.2 Continuous Blending

Continuous blending process development follows feeding process development. While there are several approaches to process development for continuous blending, a mechanistic approach is presented in this book chapter.

In general, any powder mixing process is a result of convection, dispersion and shear mechanisms. The convective and dispersive mechanisms govern macromixing whereas shear governs the micromixing aspects of a blending process. The macromixing mechanism in a continuous blender can be characterized as a combination of axial mixing and cross-sectional mixing (Gao et al., 2011). Axial mixing is defined as the mixing along the direction of material transport, that is, from inlet to outlet of the blender, whereas cross-sectional mixing is orthogonal to the axial mixing direction. Axial mixing is required to compensate for the incoming variability in feed rate and cross-sectional mixing is required to mix the fed ingredients which are unmixed at the inlet. Depending on the formulation and material characteristics, the required degree of micromixing may be difficult to achieve in continuous blending. In those cases, additional blend processing methods such as de-lumping using conical screen milling may be required. During process development, blender process variables are chosen such that the required degree of macro- (axial and cross-sectional) and micromixing are achieved in the continuous blender.

14.2.2.1 Axial Mixing

Axial mixing component of continuous blending is governed by the residence time distribution of the blending system. Axial mixing is mathematically described using convolution as shown in Equation 14.1 where concentration at the outlet of the mixer $C_{out}(t)$ at time t is calculated as a function of concentration at the inlet of the mixer $C_{in}(t)$ and RTD of the blending process $E(\theta)$.

$$C_{out}(t) = \int_{0}^{\infty} C_{in}(t-\theta) \cdot E(\theta) \cdot d\theta \qquad (14.1)$$

To design axial mixing component of continuous blending, a set of blending conditions need to be identified where the RTD is adequate to filter the incoming variability in composition. Several studies have been reported in the literature (Vanarase & Muzzio, 2011; Vanarase et al., 2013; Palmer et al., 2020) where the impact of process variables, equipment configuration and material properties on RTDs is reported. In a typical scenario, the total flow rate of a continuous line is decided based on optimal performance and limitations of the feeding and/or tableting (die fill variation) unit operations. Process development of blending involves manipulating blender speed and/or impeller blade configuration to achieve the desired residence time distribution at the selected line throughput. Process performance is confirmed by monitoring the blend composition over time and demonstrating blend composition variability within certain limits. Blend composition can be monitored using an online spectroscopic method, a model-based approach, or via sampling from the continuous process.

In the example shown in Figure 14.9, axial mixing is considered not adequate since the measured concentration is often outside the acceptance limits (90–110%). Such temporal variation in composition is linked to the composition variation at the inlet and inadequate RTD of the blending system.

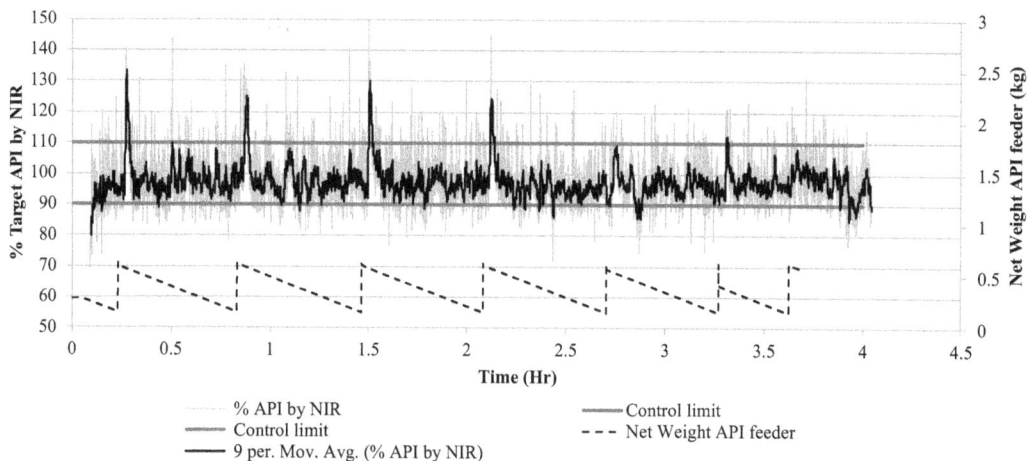

FIGURE 14.9 Blend concentration at the outlet of the blender.

In this case, feed rate variability was high due to sub-optimal choice of refill parameters and poor flow behavior of the material in the hopper due to its cohesive nature. To address this issue, the feeder performance was improved by optimizing refill parameters and using an improved agitator in the hopper. Further, the residence time in the continuous blender was increased by manipulating the blade configuration of the agitator. For the new set of feeder and blender parameters, the calculated input concentration of API based on feed rates and predicted output concentration using convolution are shown in Figure 14.10.

It is evident from the figure that the variation in input concentration is dampened in the continuous blending process, which is a result of axial mixing. Blend concentration is also monitored using a NIR spectroscopic method (Figure 14.11). Axial mixing performance was adequate considering the output API concentration is consistently maintained within the in-process acceptance limits of 90–100%.

Product performance was also monitored by sampling tablets from the CDC process and measuring their potency by NIR. As shown in Figure 14.12, product potency was maintained within 95–105% of the label claim.

14.2.2.2 Cross-Sectional Mixing

The second part of the macromixing aspect of continuous blending is the cross-sectional mixing. The degree of cross-sectional mixing is assessed by measuring variability in blend composition at a given time-point at any specific location within the continuous blender. Typically, the location is at the discharge of the continuous blender where sampling is possible. Relative to axial mixing, cross-sectional mixing is typically much faster and not a limiting factor in a continuous blending process. However, in a practical scenario, cross-sectional mixing is difficult to characterize experimentally when other factors such as agglomeration or segregation are also significant. Therefore, when variability in blend composition within a given time-point is assessed, it is a result of all possible mechanisms including cross-sectional mixing, agglomeration (micro-mixing) and segregation. To characterize blend composition variability within a time-point, sampling tablets is much more convenient than sampling and sub-dividing a blend. Instead of truly characterizing cross-sectional mixing (or within time-point variation) for the blender, it

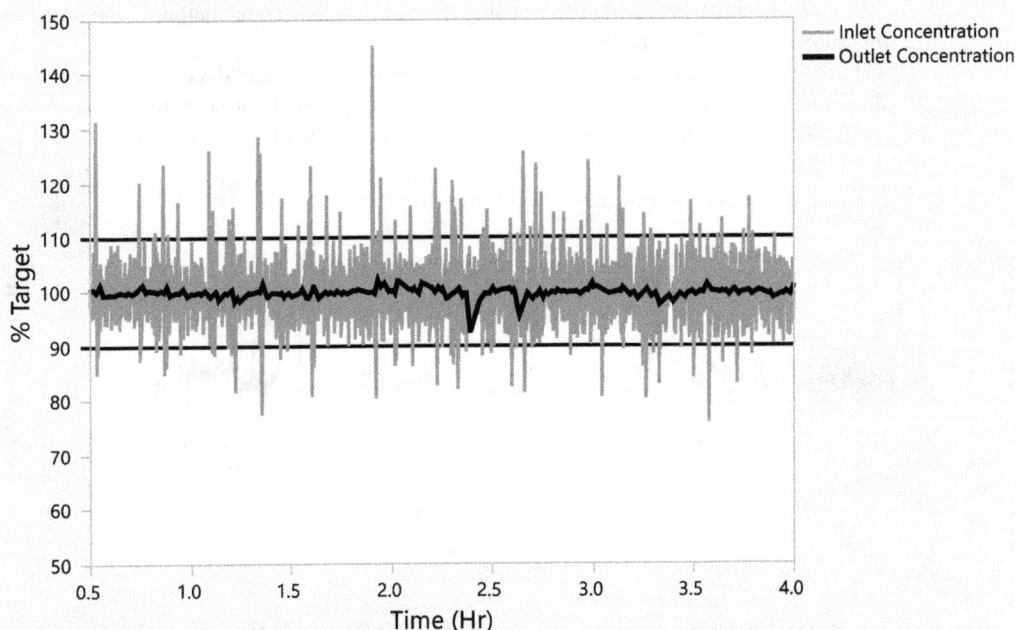

FIGURE 14.10 Overlay of fluctuations in input concentration and predicted output concentration at blender outlet demonstrating axial mixing.

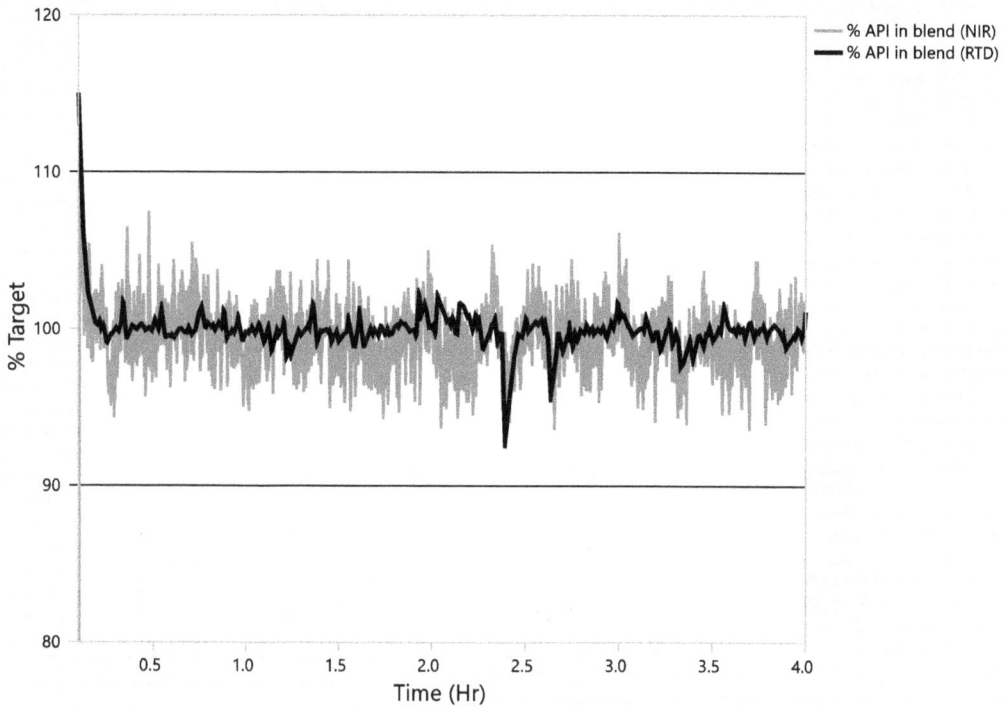

FIGURE 14.11 Overlay of output concentration monitored using NIR and RTD-based model.

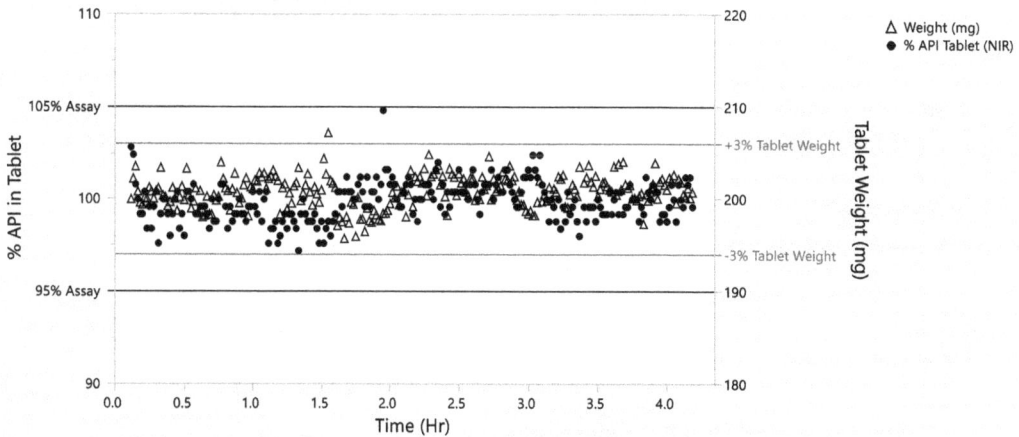

FIGURE 14.12 Tablet potency during continuous process.

can be defined for the full CM line and be characterized by sampling tablets. Using tablets, the sample size can also be controlled to the size of the unit dose.

In an example shown in Figure 14.13, within time-point variability was assessed by sampling tablets at the exit of a tablet press. Active concentration within a tablet was calculated by normalizing the tablet assay by its weight. In this case, uniformity within a time-point was good given that % RSD of blend concentration was <1%, and it was maintained at a similar level during the entire run.

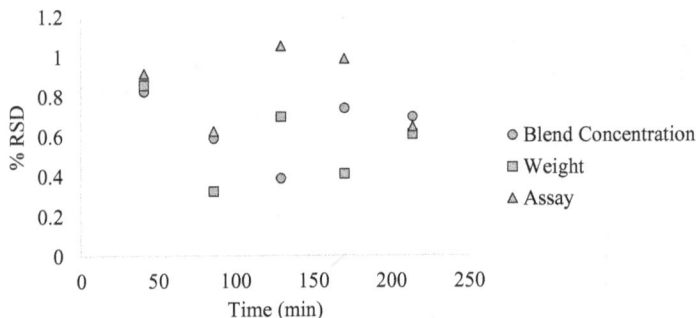

FIGURE 14.13   % RSD of tablet weight, assay and concentration at different time intervals during a continuous run (N = 10 per time-point).

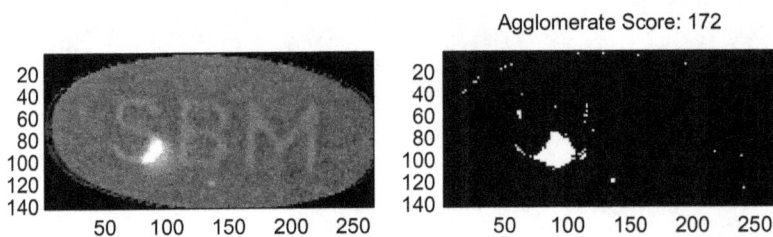

FIGURE 14.14   Chemical imaging of tablet surface.

As mentioned earlier, depending on the risk with a particular formulation, micromixing may be of importance in addition to macromixing. For example, for a low drug load formulation, the presence of large API agglomerates in the blend can lead to poor blend uniformity. In such cases, analysis of blend microstructure via NIR chemical imaging can help understand if blending conditions are providing the necessary shear forces to deagglomerate the API to produce a uniform blend. An example is shown in Figure 14.14 where the chemical imaging surface map revealed the presence of API agglomerates. To address such a risk, during process development, the use of a conical screen mill in the continuous process or appropriate selection of blending parameters (blade configuration, speed) becomes critical.

14.3 Process Control Strategies

The overall control strategy for drug products consists of controls on process parameters, in-process material attributes and input materials followed by finished product testing. In this section, key aspects involved in unit operation level control and associated IPC methods are described.

14.3.1 Control Strategies for Unit Operations

Control strategies used for drug product manufacturing unit operations can be broadly divided as parametric, attribute-based, or a combination of both. In a parametric control strategy, the process is operated within a set of parameter ranges that are validated during its development. For example, a batch blending process when operated within certain ranges of process parameters (impeller speed and blending time), the strategy would be called a parametric control strategy (Level 2 control in Section 1). In this strategy, within the validated ranges of process parameters, the desired attributes are expected to meet the quality criteria. In an attribute-based control strategy, process parameters are adjusted to meet the desired quality attributes. In an attribute-based control strategy for blending unit operation, blend uniformity is monitored using an online sensor and blending parameters (blending speed or blending time) are manipulated to meet the desired blend uniformity (Level 1 control in Section 1).

In continuous manufacturing, all unit operations are integrated with each other. Any deviation in any attribute has a cascading impact on downstream operations. In such a case, an attribute-based control strategy is the most flexible since parameters can be adjusted in response to potential deviations during manufacturing. CM is therefore more amenable to the Level 1 control strategy and the advanced feedback and feedforward control strategies described earlier. Typical control strategies used for the unit operations in CDC are described in the next section.

14.3.1.1 Feeding

In CDC, LIW or gravimetric feeders are used for feeding. Control of feed rate variability is critical to achieving product potency and content uniformity. In gravimetric feeders, the feed rate is continuously monitored using the weight of material in the feeder hopper and is controlled at the target by manipulating the screw speed. In a CDC operation, target feed rate set points are provided for each feeder and they are controlled using the above-mentioned feedback control strategy. For each feeder, refill parameters (refill volume and minimum refill mass in hopper) are provided in the recipe. Conveying of materials to the refill system, refill operation and gravimetric feeding are typically automated and driven by a set recipe. During certain periods such as refills, feeders may experience high feed rate variability that could make the feedback control difficult to operate. Under such circumstances, feeder temporarily operates under a fixed screw speed mode, called "volumetric" mode.

There can be two approaches to the feeding process control strategy. In the first approach, no control limits are placed on feed rate variability. Control of product potency and content uniformity is achieved using the IPCs used in blending and tableting processes. In the second approach, control limits can be provided for certain characteristics of feed variability and any deviation from those limits can be linked to diversion of the associated non-conforming product. As described previously, the RTD of the blending system filters feed rate variability to a certain extent. The output blend concentration variation is dependent on certain characteristics of feed rate variability (magnitude and duration of feed rate deviations). Deviations within shorter durations lead to a smaller impact on the output and those can be tolerated at higher levels. Disturbances within longer durations lead to a larger impact on output and those can be tolerated at lower levels. García-Muñoz et al. (2018) have shown the utility of a funnel plot in illustrating this concept. In a funnel plot, for a given disturbance, the maximum or minimum concentration at the output is calculated as a function of the extent of disturbance (i.e. feed rate deviation from target) and duration of the disturbance. A control strategy using this concept can be implemented by placing limits on feed rate deviation (magnitude) and its duration. This strategy is more conservative considering that the funnel plot is calculated using a one-sided disturbance. In actual runs, when there are both positive and negative deviations occurring simultaneously, the impact on output is less severe. In a practical scenario, the strategy of using controls on feed rate may not be advantageous considering the existing controls on blending and tableting processes.

14.3.1.2 Blending

As previously described, the target process parameters of feeding (feed rate, refill parameters) and blending (blender speed) are identified during process development. During CDC operation, most continuous blenders operate under a fixed impeller speed. The total flow rate or throughput is decided by the upstream feeders. The RTD of the blending system is dependent on total flow rate, impeller speed and formulation material properties. The powder hold-up in the blender is a result of the above-mentioned variables and is typically not a controlled variable. In some blender designs such as the portable continuous miniature module (PCMM) technology (Tonson et al., 2021), powder hold-up is controlled by measuring powder mass using load cells and controlling the flow rate using an outlet valve.

In blending, the quality attribute, that is, blend potency is monitored at the blender discharge using either a spectroscopic method or an RTD model or both. Since the blending operation is next to feeding, any deviation in the feed rate has a direct impact on blend potency. In a feedback control strategy, measured blend concentration can be used to control the blend potency by manipulating blender speed. However, this strategy is not practical due to several reasons. First, the blender speed may only have a limited ability to change the residence time and therefore limited ability to mitigate the impact of feed rate deviation. Feed rate deviations that are larger than the axial mixing ability of the blender would still generate an OOS blend which would need to be removed from the continuous process. Second, changing blender speed also changes the throughput which affects downstream tableting operation. In most practical scenarios, control strategy used for blending is the identification of blend with off-spec potency using the in-process blend concentration monitoring methods and subsequent removal of non-conforming material. There could be two strategies to remove OOS material from the CDC process. It could be removed after blending or after tableting. Almaya et al. (2017) have discussed the advantages and disadvantages of both approaches. In a case where the OOS blend is removed after blending, the strategy needs to account for its impact on downstream tableting operation. In a case where OOS material is removed after tableting, the amount of material to be rejected would depend on the residence time distribution of the tableting operation.

14.3.1.3 Tableting

For tableting, existent strategies used in batch manufacturing are also used in continuous manufacturing. Tablet weight and hardness are controlled by manipulating fill depth and compression force, respectively. In CM, the only constraint on the tableting operation is its throughput which needs to match with that of feeding and blending. Tableting speed is manipulated to match its throughput with blending. Required tableting speed in a continuous process is identified during the control of powder fill level in a tube or hopper between blending and tableting operations. Powder fill level is monitored using a level sensor and tablet press speed is continuously manipulated to maintain a constant fill level.

14.3.2 In-Process Methods for Monitoring Blend Concentration

Approaches for blend concentration monitoring include spectroscopic and RTD model-based methods. In this section, the working principle of each approach, common risks and mitigation strategies during their implementation and considerations for their control limits, are presented.

14.3.2.1 Spectroscopic Approach

14.3.2.1.1 Development of Spectroscopic Blend Concentration Monitoring Method

There are several spectroscopic or PAT methods available for blend concentration measurement including NIR, Raman and light-induced fluorescence (LIF) out of which NIR is most commonly used in continuous oral solid dose (OSD) manufacturing lines. In CDC lines, the spectroscopic sensor is typically in the discharge tube between blending and tableting or within the feed-frame of the tablet press. The spectroscopic sensors should be installed in a way that does not significantly interrupt the flow of materials. An example of NIR installation on side of the discharge tube is shown in Figure 14.15. In CM, one of the considerations for PAT systems is their ability to acquire spectra and process them through a prediction engine at a high speed and use the predictions in real-time in the control system of the continuous line.

During process development, the detectability of the active ingredient in the formulation using the spectroscopic method of choice is evaluated. If the spectroscopic method has the required sensitivity, a quantitative method needs to be built that can measure blend concentration within a pre-determined range. Partial least square (PLS) based models are commonly used for blend concentration monitoring (Vargas et al., 2018; Leersnyder et al., 2018). Typical approach of a PLS model development includes acquiring spectra of blends of reference compositions, identifying principal components (or latent variables) in the dataset and then building a regression vector that relates these latent variables to blend concentration. Spectroscopic methods are typically sensitive to chemical (composition), physical properties of blends (particle size, density) and nature of motion (moving vs. static) of the powder blend. Typically, while building the PLS models, pre-processing methods such as baseline correction, standard normal variate (SNV), multiple scattering correction (MSC) and first and second derivatives are evaluated to extract chemical composition-related information from the spectral data. Further, during the model

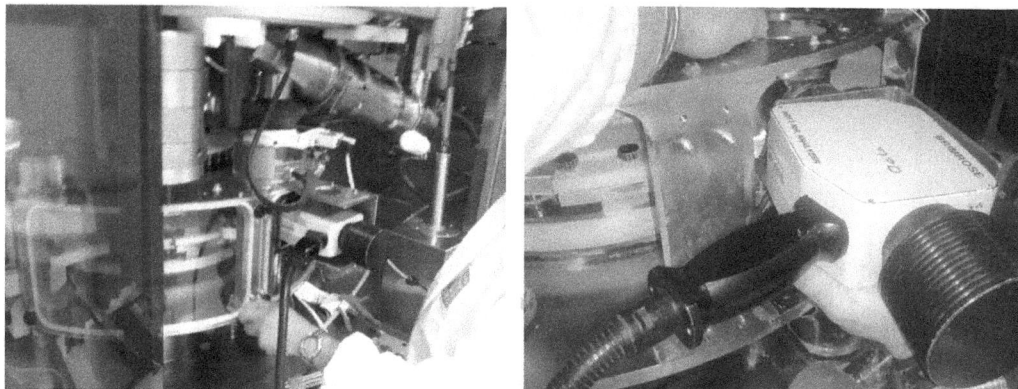

FIGURE 14.15 NIR sensor installation in a CDC line.

building stage, expected excipient and API variability is also included in the datasets. To ensure that the chemometric model is relevant and predictable in the actual continuous line, the calibration datasets are built accordingly with identical or similar experimental rigs. The measured spectra, depending on factors including spot size, speed of powder in front of the sensor and penetration depth represent a certain sample volume. The measured composition variability is dependent on this sample volume. Accordingly, a relevant number of spectra is usually averaged considering the volume sampled per scan and the tablet unit mass. Ideally, a few spectra equivalent to the tablet mass would be used for assessing blend uniformity; however, a long total scan time or large unit dose size may limit the number of scans used for this purpose.

14.3.2.1.2 Challenges, Risks and Mitigation Strategies

Some of the common challenges, risks and mitigation strategies associated with the spectroscopic approach are provided below:

1. The spectroscopic approach may not be feasible for certain formulations where either the drug load is very low (typically < 2%) or the API is not sufficiently distinguishable from the excipients. In such cases, the spectroscopic approach may not be a viable option.
2. The calibration models built during the development phase may not have captured all potential variability in the physicochemical properties of the formulation ingredients. Commercial life cycle of the drug product is typically much longer than development. During the commercial life cycle, if the properties of any of the ingredients vary significantly, predictions from the chemometric models may not be accurate. Such issues are typically addressed using a model maintenance plan. Deviations in model performance resulting from changes in excipient or API material properties must be closely monitored and the model needs to be updated accordingly.
3. Spectroscopic concentration measurements may show a bias or a drift even during steady state operation while the actual potency is not varying. An example of such an event is shown in Figure 14.16. In this example, the actual potency in tablets, measured by HPLC is close to target, but the in-line NIR measurements are lower than target. Such behavior could occur due to factors such as inherent calibration error, variation in the flow pattern around the sensor, sensor fouling due to material build-up, etc. In this case, product diversions were triggered at certain time points shown in the figure, which otherwise would not have been necessary if NIR measurements were not biased. Such issues may be difficult to address via a routine model maintenance plan. Simultaneous concentration measurement using a redundant approach such as RTD based model can address these issues. A hybrid approach (Section 3.2.3) can be implemented where both measurements can be used in the diversion.

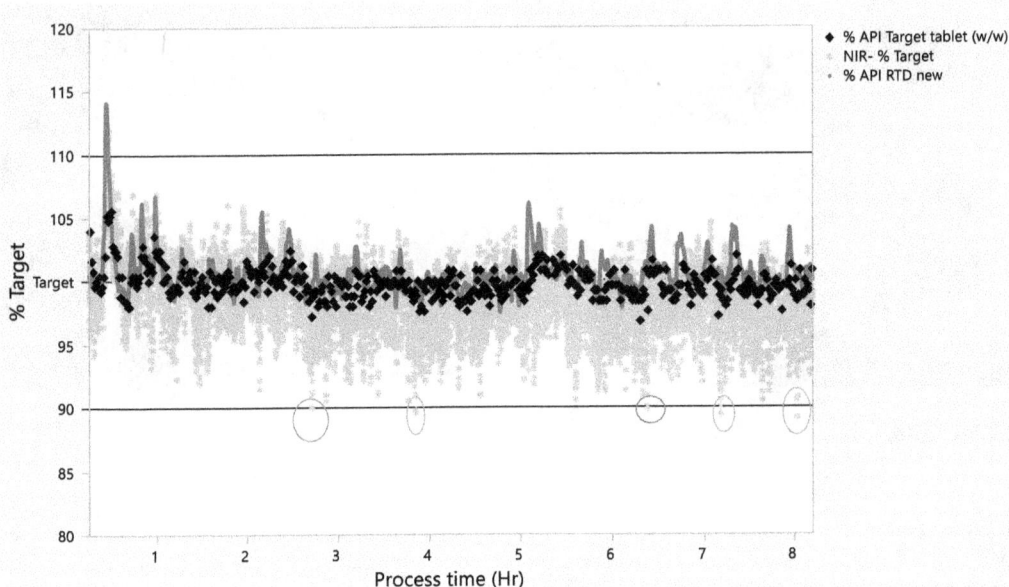

FIGURE 14.16 NIR measurements showing transient out-of-limit events (highlighted with circles).

While spectroscopic methods may not always be utilized in the control strategy for non-conforming product diversion decisions, they still have their role even under this scenario. If the RTD models described below are used for the product diversion decisions, NIR and other spectroscopic techniques would be instrumental to the development, validation and maintenance of the RTD models. Thus, regardless of their role in the control strategy, these tools are valuable (and one could argue even essential) for the continuous manufacturing program.

14.3.2.2 RTD Model-Based Approach

14.3.2.2.1 Development of RTD Model for Blend Concentration Monitoring

In recent years, an RTD-based modeling approach has become popular for monitoring blend concentration in continuous manufacturing lines. The genesis of this approach lies in the original convolution method proposed for liquid mixing in the article by Danckwerts (1953). For continuous flow systems, the output concentration is calculated using the convolution of input concentration and the RTD of the system as given in Equation (14.1). When continuous processes operate under a steady state, this approach can be used to predict blend concentration in real time. The RTD models can play a dual role in the continuous process. First, it can be used to predict concentration at a diverter location (e.g., using feeder data to determine active concentration in the tablets). Alternatively, it can be used to determine the propagation of non-conforming material identified by a PAT tool between a measurement location and the diverter location to support rejection start and stop decisions (e.g., NIR blend measurement in the press feed tube with diversion at the tablet press).

To implement this approach in real time, the concentration at the input and RTD model of the blending system are required. The input concentration is calculated using instantaneous feed rates of all the ingredients as they are measured by the LIW feeders (Equation 14.2).

$$C_{in}(t) = \frac{F_{in}(t)}{Total\ feed\ rate_{in}(t)} \tag{14.2}$$

The RTD model of the blending system is developed by fitting model equations to the experimental RTD data. Axial dispersion models (Gao et al., 2011) or stirred tanks and plug flow reactors in series

(Engisch & Muzzio, 2016; Escotet-Espinoza et al., 2019) are common approaches for the RTD models. Bhalode et al., (2021) in their review have provided detailed discussions on different approaches to RTD modeling. Experimental RTD data is generated by providing an impulse or a step input of a tracer and monitoring blend concentration at the outlet. Although both techniques can be used alternatively, there are a few considerations in solid mixing. One consideration is that the selected tracer material should not alter the flow behavior of material inside the blending system. A change in concentration of an ingredient may also change the flow behavior of the blend and thereby lead to a change in the RTD. Therefore, during step responses, one must assure that the selected step size does not lead to a significant change in the flow properties of the materials.

The predicted concentration in the case of granular mixing is an average concentration of the powder stream at any given time. There exists a variance around this concentration which depends on formulation properties such as drug load, particle size of ingredients, segregation, agglomeration, cross-sectional mixing, etc. This is different for liquids where mixing is ideal and the concentration of all material elements at any given time is the same. The variance in composition due to the granular nature of the material isn't captured by the convolution method. To account for granular mixing process, modifications to this equation were proposed by Weinekötter & Reh (1995) where the total variance in concentration at the output in a given continuous run was described as a sum of variance component from liquid-like mixing and a component of random variance due to granular nature of the materials. Gao et al. (2011) have presented a case study where this random variance was described as a sum of variance due to incomplete cross-sectional mixing of powders and variability in the RTDs. While implementing the convolution approach as an IPC method, consideration should be given to this variance while deciding the IPC limits for the predictions from the RTD model.

An example of RTD model fitting is provided below in Figure 14.17. In this example, an impulse of API material is provided at the inlet of the blender and samples are collected at the outlet of the tablet press. The RTD model therefore represents the entire system of blending and tableting. In this case, a model of two stirred tanks and one plug flow reactor in series was used. To estimate RTD model parameters, ordinary differential equations were set up and fitted to the experimental data using a non-linear data fitting algorithm.

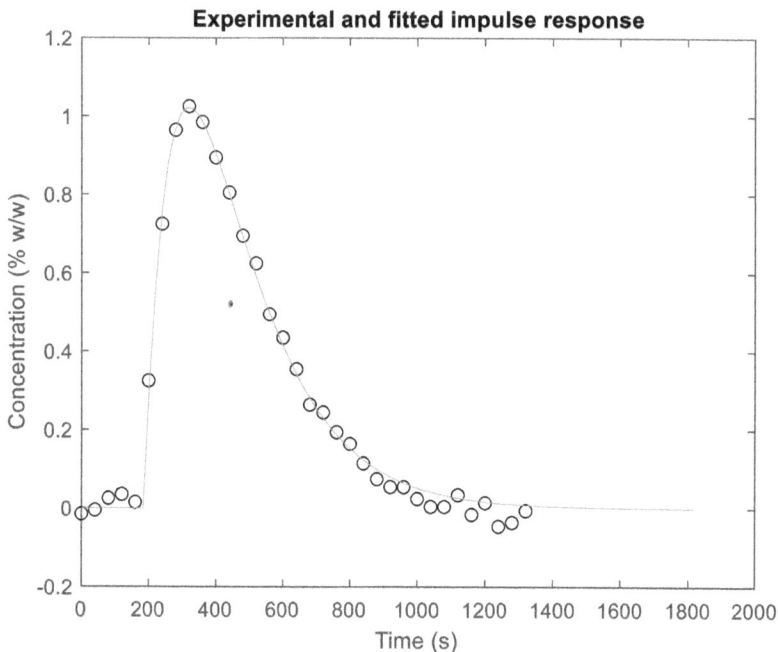

FIGURE 14.17 Example of fitting experimental RTD data to a model.

In this RTD model fitting example model, an error was 0.024% w/w (Equation 14.3). To get a better estimate of the model error, data from multiple RTDs need to be combined so that test-to-test variability, if any, is also captured in the model error.

$$Model\ error = \sqrt[2]{\frac{\sum_1^N (C_{pred} - C_{exp})^2}{N}} \tag{14.3}$$

Error of the RTD model depends on the measurement method. If online sensors such as NIR are used for measuring RTDs, model error is typically higher considering smaller sample volume interrogated in the measurement. One approach to overcome this challenge is to average NIR scans to assess blend uniformity at a relevant scale of scrutiny. However, total scan time per individual NIR prediction should be minimized as NIR measurement should be as "instantaneous" as possible to be congruent with the fast-sampling rate for the RTD prediction. An example of OOS blend identification via NIR and RTD model-based predictions in a CDC process is provided in Figure 14.18. Disturbances in feed rate during certain time periods led to deviations in blend potency which were detected by both NIR and RTD model-based predictions.

14.3.2.2.2 Challenges, Risks and Mitigation Strategies

Some of the common challenges, risks and mitigation strategies associated with the RTD model-based approach are provided below:

1. The RTD model is typically developed under steady-state conditions. During start-up/shutdown or any process interruptions, the steady state model is not applicable. The RTD-based predictions may not be accurate during these times. During such unsteady state times, alternate measurement from a spectroscopic approach, if available, can be used. If the process relies only on the RTD-based approach, product should be diverted until the process reaches a steady state.

2. RTD is expected to change if a new equipment configuration or process layout is used. Thus, RTD parameters from one equipment configuration are not applicable to others. On the contrary, spectroscopic approach would be able to measure concentration accurately despite such changes. The success of the RTD model-based approach as an in-process blend concentration

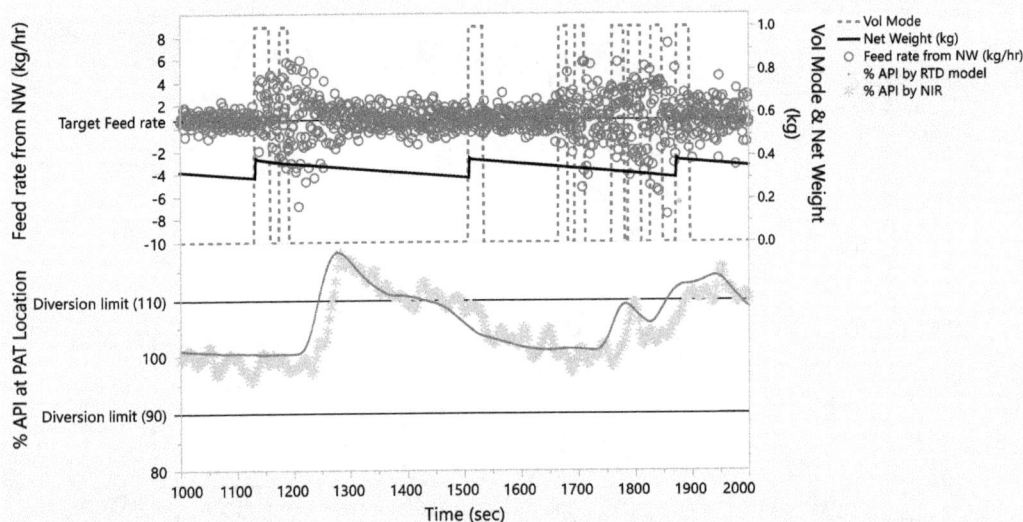

FIGURE 14.18 Example of out-of-specification blend identification by RTD-based prediction.

control method depends on several other aspects which must be ensured prior to its use. To avoid such risks, consistent equipment set-up from batch to batch should be ensured through the typical controls in the pharmaceutical GMP environment.

3. In the RTD model-based approach, blend concentration prediction depends on continuous measurement of feed rates. Feeders are refilled periodically during manufacturing. During the refill events, the feed rate is not measurable (also called blind time). To allow accurate model-based calculations during such periods, the estimated feed rate needs to be close to the actual feed rate. To address such issues, during development, the feeder refill parameters are selected such that any feed rate deviation due to refill itself is minimal. The feed rate during blind time is estimated using feed factor and screw speed. In addition, the refill time period itself can be minimized as much as possible.

4. One of the risks for the RTD model is that the model could be sensitive to variation in raw material properties. Previous studies by Vanarase et al., 2013 have shown that material properties such as bulk density and flowability could impact the RTDs. Raw material properties could vary from lot to lot or due to changes related to manufacturing processes, sites or vendors. Critical raw material properties should be monitored during development and commercial phases. If significant changes occur, the RTD model needs to be updated. A model maintenance plan needs to include these aspects.

5. As mentioned earlier, the RTD model-based prediction is the mean concentration of the material stream at any given time. Typically, the model does not predict concentration at unit dose scale and thus should not be used as an indicator of content uniformity. Further, the model does not take into account the material properties of the ingredients which may influence content uniformity. For example, if a particular lot of API is more cohesive than typical, the resulting blend may contain API agglomerates which can result in poor content uniformity.

Key differences between the spectroscopic and RTD model-based approaches are highlighted in Table 14.1

14.3.2.3 Hybrid Approach to In-Process Blend Concentration Monitoring

As described in the previous sections, there are some limitations with both approaches of blend concentration monitoring methods when either one is applied independently. In a practical scenario, if it is not feasible to overcome these limitations, a hybrid approach can be used where both approaches are

TABLE 14.1

Key Differences between Spectroscopic and RTD Model-Based Approaches for Blend Concentration Monitoring

	Spectroscopic Approach	RTD Model-Based Approach
Principle	Relies on prediction of a multivariate model built using spectral data of reference blends	Relies on prediction of a semi-empirical model of the blending system built using experimental RTD data
Measurement	Concentration is derived from direct measurement of blend spectra	Concentration is derived from direct measurement of feed rates
Scale of scrutiny	Function of speed of powder in front of the sensor, depth of penetration, sensor size and the number of averaged spectra	Function of the time scale of feed rate measurement
Key failure modes	-Sensor fouling -Bias and drift in the measurement from batch to batch or during process	-Blind times during volumetric operation of feeding -Unsteady state periods -Change in blend uniformity due to non-feeder-related aspects (e.g., API properties)
Key model maintenance triggers	-Change in excipient grades and raw material attributes relevant to measured spectra -Change in NIR/powder interface	-Change in excipient grades and raw material attributes relevant to material flow properties -Changes in equipment configuration, process layout

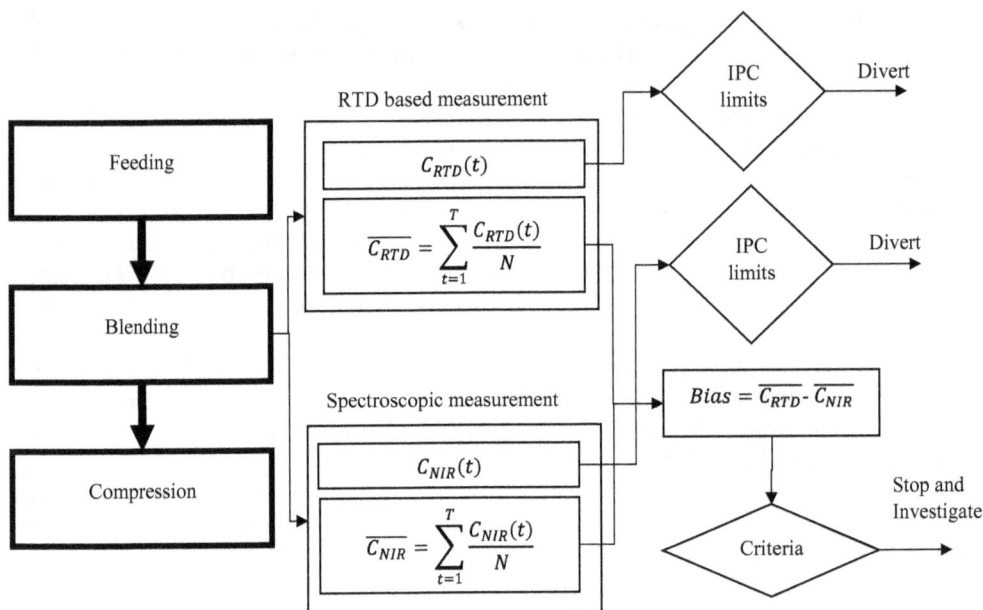

FIGURE 14.19   Hybrid strategy for in-process controls.

implemented simultaneously. In this approach, having redundant measurements of blend concentration also increases the overall robustness of the measurement system. An example of a hybrid strategy is provided in Figure 14.19.

In this strategy, a moving time average is calculated for the instantaneous signals of both RTD model-based and spectroscopic blend concentration measurements. In the diversion strategy, instantaneous as well as time-averaged signals are used. Diversion is triggered when either of the instantaneous measurements crosses the pre-defined thresholds of IPC limits. The moving averages between the RTD-based and spectroscopic concentration measurements are compared in real time and if the bias between the two is higher than a pre-defined criterion, the process is stopped and the reason for discrepancy is investigated.

Since both approaches of blend concentration measurements are used simultaneously, the chances of either one not being able to catch a transient disturbance due to any of the failure modes described previously are significantly reduced. Further, during times when either of them is not available for measurement, such as intermittent cleaning of the NIR sensor or RTD model predictions during unsteady periods (start-up/shut-down) during manufacturing, this approach of using both measurements avoids the need for excessive product diversion or finished product testing.

Cogoni et al. (2021) have demonstrated such a strategy where a hybrid NIR-soft sensor (RTD model-based) method for blend potency was used for real-time IPC of CDC manufacturing operations. They have reported improvement in overall estimation robustness and cross-site method transfer.

14.4 Control of Materials Attributes of Input Materials

Typically, during drug product development, an understanding of the impact of raw material attributes on process and product performance is developed. As a result of that exercise, critical material attributes are identified which then need to be monitored and maintained within certain specifications during the commercial life cycle of the drug product. The strategies used to identify and control these critical material attributes are mostly similar between products manufactured using either batch or continuous processes. One aspect where the CM differs is when the raw material attributes have an impact on the in-process measurement methods and process models. As described in previous sections, the spectroscopic and RTD models are critical to the identification and removal of non-conforming products in CM lines. Thus,

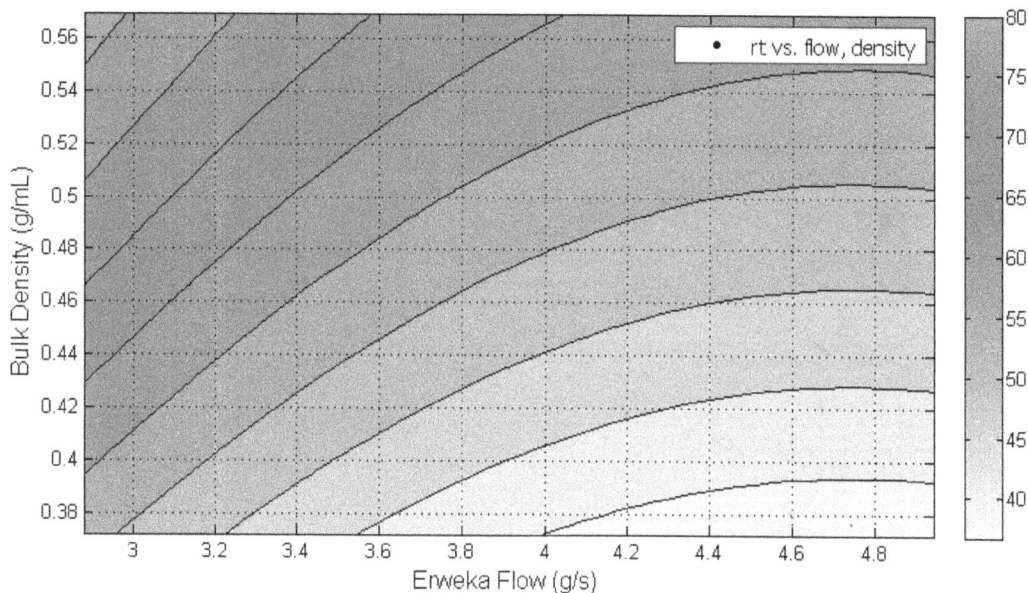

FIGURE 14.20 Effects of blend bulk density and flowability (Erweka flow (g/s)) on mean residence time.

knowledge of the impact of raw material variability on chemometric and process models is critical. For example, the mean residence time of RTD is dependent on the bulk density and flowability of the blend (Figure 14.20). During development, key formulation ingredients and their attributes that are likely to have an impact on bulk density and flowability of the blend need to be identified. Knowledge of the variability in excipient or API material properties needs to be built during development. The formulation, process parameters and non-conforming material diversion criteria should be selected such that normal lot-to-lot material variability is acceptable during routine manufacturing.

14.5 Control of Critical Quality Attributes in CDC

The ultimate objective of the control strategy is to ensure that final product attributes are adequately controlled. As described previously, the pillars of the control strategy are controls on input material, in-process attributes and process parameters combined with appropriate finished product release testing. Finished product release testing may be negated through robust controls by the other three pillars thus enabling an RTR strategy.

In continuous manufacturing, in-process attributes are continuously monitored to assess process stability and ensure the final product meets limits for its CQAs. Unlike a batch process where appropriate sampling of the final product can be used to assess product quality of the entire batch, in continuous processes, final product sampling only reflects the quality of product manufactured at a given time point. Traditional low-frequency sampling is therefore not adequate for the control of continuous processes. Sampling (monitoring) frequency should be therefore based on knowledge of system dynamics in order to detect transient disturbances and their potential impact on quality attributes. For attributes with high sampling frequency, final product testing may not be necessary thus enabling RTR strategies.

The control strategy for a CDC process is described below for typical tablet CQAs (Figure 14.21).

14.5.1 Tablet Content Uniformity and Potency

The control of tablet potency and content uniformity can be achieved as an RTR strategy or a combination of continuous monitoring and control of CQAs followed by finished product testing. Tablet potency and content uniformity are ensured through controls on blend potency, uniformity and tablet weight. As

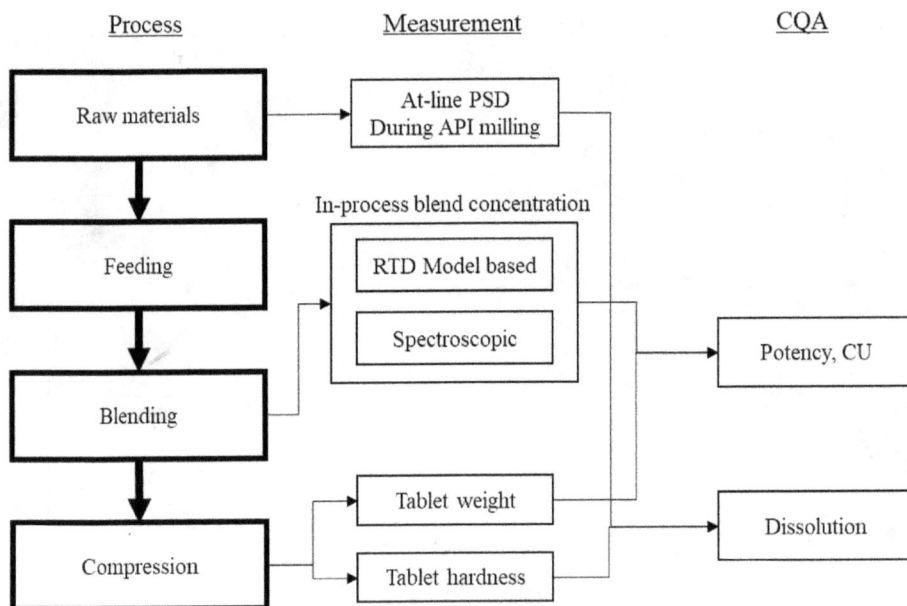

FIGURE 14.21   Real-time-release control strategy for potency, CU and dissolution.

described above, blend concentration (potency) in the CDC process is continuously monitored using PAT (e.g., NIR) and/or RTD models. The high frequency of blend potency measurement using these tools ensures that impactful disturbances are detected, and any resulting non-conforming product is rejected. NIR blend potency is evaluated either in the tablet press feed frame or in the feed tube to the press. RTD models can also be used to predict blend potency at the same measurement location as NIR and in the tablets thus providing a much higher assurance level of detecting transient disturbances. The limits on the in-process blend concentration measurement are drawn such that the finished product can be accepted as per the statistical criteria. In-process concentration limits can be decided based on limits on the potency of the finished product (individual unit doses), limits on the tablet weight variation and uncertainty (or error) associated with model prediction.

Advanced process controls in the tablet press ensure robust control of tablet weight in compression. The relationship between tablet weight and compression force at constant displacement (punch separation or in-die thickness) enables the advanced process control loop to reject tablets that demonstrate compression force outside of the acceptance limits. An alternative control strategy for the tablet weight is achieved through the established relationship between in-die thickness (punch displacement) and tablet weight at constant compression (or pre-compression) force.

An RTR control strategy for tablet potency requires continuous monitoring and control of blend concentration and tablet weight. An RTR control strategy for content uniformity, in addition to controlling the potency, requires continuous monitoring and control of blend uniformity. RTD model-based predicted concentrations are often not at the unit dose scale and also the approach itself does not take into account any attributes other than feed rates. Spectroscopic measurement of blend potency at the unit dose scale may be a challenge considering the limitations associated with sample volume analyzed in each measurement and the limitation with the number of individual measurements that can be averaged. RTR strategy for content uniformity can be achieved if these limitations can be addressed during process development.

To implement any RTR strategies, in addition to applying limits on individual measurements, application of statistical methods to PAT and RTD data enables continuous assessment of blend potency and uniformity. Statistical process control (SPC) approach using run charts, particularly *x-bar* and *s* charts, provides a comprehensive assessment of blend potency and uniformity, respectively. Sample size and acceptance limits on the mean and standard deviation for the SPC charts, in addition to acceptance limits on individual measurements of blend potency, are established for the control of tablet potency and content uniformity. The acceptance limits are selected to ensure with a high level of statistical confidence that tablet content uniformity would meet compendial requirements provided tablet weight controls are adequate.

In addition to acceptance limits, the SPC charts also have statistical limits that reflect common causes or expected variation in the process. The statistical limits should be tighter than the acceptance limit if the process has good capability. A process with statistical limits outside the acceptance limits is not a controlled process and should be re-designed to improve capability. Appropriate action should be taken if the statistical limits are exceeded. While exceeding acceptance limits trigger product diversion for rejection, exceeding statistical limits may indicate process disturbance or special cause variability. The process should therefore be stopped, and an investigation conducted if statistical limits are exceeded for pre-defined time period, even if acceptance limits are met.

The controls on blend concentration using redundant tools (PAT and RTD) and tablet weight control in compression provide a high level of assurance that tablet potency and content uniformity acceptance criteria are continuously met in the CDC process. This renders final tablet testing for these attributes superfluous and consequently provides a strong basis for an RTR strategy that does not include tablet testing. If tablet testing is still desired, traditional sampling and testing plans of the tablets (as used for a batch process) should be adequate. Tablet testing can be accomplished using traditional liquid chromatography methods or spectroscopic methods, if feasible. In contrast, if some of the elements of the control strategy described above are not met (particularly, if only RTD model is used for blend concentration prediction), more burden falls on tablet testing to demonstrate adequate control of potency and content uniformity in the continuous process. In this case, sampling plans that samples and tests a significantly larger number of tablets than traditional plans (large N plans) are usually necessary. While the sampling frequency in the Large N plans may not necessarily reflect the fast process dynamics and the potential frequency of impactful disturbances, such plans provide a more detailed characterization of process performance than the traditional plans and therefore complement existing IPC.

14.5.2 Dissolution

Dissolution control strategy may not be in essence different for the continuous process than the batch process. Traditional composite sampling plans of tablets throughout compression can be used in the CDC process for dissolution release testing similar to the batch process. However, the robustness of this strategy is contingent on the assumption that variation in functional excipient levels due to transient disturbances does not impact dissolution rate. The response of dissolution rate to variation in excipient levels, such as table disintegrant, should therefore be studied in development to demonstrate limited sensitivity. If this does not turn out to be the case, monitoring of the level of the critical excipient using RTD or NIR may be warranted using similar principles as described for the active. As for the active, tablets that do not meet the required content of the critical excipient can be rejected to ensure consistent dissolution behavior of the tablets throughout the batch.

While not necessary, RTR strategies are usually desirable for continuous manufacturing due to the inherent nature of the process and continuous monitoring associated with it. However, dissolution presents a challenge to the RTR strategy, particularly for low solubility compounds (BCS II or IV) for which final product testing is usually expected. Predictive tools for tablet dissolution have recently gained growing interest and can be used to support RTR strategy for a continuous process. The predictive tools can be broadly classified as spectroscopic tools or multivariate models of material and process parameters. NIR has been used to predict dissolution behavior of tablets (Pawar et al., 2016) and can be used as a surrogate of tablet dissolution testing in order to support RTR dissolution strategy for products manufactured by a continuous process. Predictive dissolution model can be illustrated through the example in Figure 14.21. In this example, development studies clearly demonstrated that tablet dissolution for this product was solely determined by the drug substance particle size and tablet hardness. All other material and process variables did not impact tablet dissolution. A bivariate model with drug substance particle size and tablet hardness as the independent variables can be implemented to predict dissolution for any given batch. For this model to be used as a surrogate for dissolution release testing, it will need to be appropriately validated to demonstrate that it is fit for this purpose. The predictive dissolution modeling approach requires exhaustive development studies to ensure that all relevant variables impacting dissolution are identified and captured in the model.

14.6 Conclusions

CM offers benefits to the development as well as the manufacturing organizations of the pharmaceutical industry. To bring forward new drug products using CM, efficient use of material characterization data in building predictive models that allow material optimization and asset selection early in development is required. In this chapter, key principles involved in the development of CDC processes and associated control strategies of critical drug product quality attributes were presented. As real-time monitoring of product quality is an integral part of the continuous process, development of robust in-process monitoring methods and process models is key to successful implementation of continuous processes. These models enable continuous assessment of product quality and real-time decisions on the diversion of product that does not meet the desired quality criteria. Further, advancing the development and implementation of performance indicating models in the commercial life cycle of drug products is needed to allow for the RTR of the drug product for CM to realize the promise of quality by design (QbD).

ACKNOWLEDGMENTS

The authors would like to acknowledge the BMS drug product pilot operations staff for facilitating the process development trials; Kevin Macias and Dongsheng Bu for developing PAT methods and providing the examples used in this chapter; Tim Stevens, Admassu Abebe and Anthony Tantuccio for their inputs on CDC control strategies; Olga Yee for the statistical analysis of input material properties; scientists from BMS analytical laboratories for supporting analytical testing and BMS management for their guidance and support.

REFERENCES

Almaya A, De Belder L, Meyer R, Nagapudi K, Homer Lin H, Leavesley I, Jayanth J, Bajwa G, DiNunzio J, Tantuccio A, Blackwood D, Admassu A. Control strategies for drug product continuous direct compression—State of control, product collection strategies, and startup/shutdown operations for the production of clinical trial materials and commercial products. *Journal of Pharmaceutical Sciences.* 2017;*106*(4):930–943.

Bhalode P, Tian H, Gupta S, Razavi SM, Roman-Ospino AR, Talebian S, Singh R, Scicolone JV, Muzzio FJ, Ierapetritou M. Using residence time distribution in pharmaceutical solid dose manufacturing – A critical review. *International journal of Pharmaceutics.* 2021;*610*:121248.

Cogoni G, Liu YA, Husain A, Alam MA, Kamyar R. A hybrid NIR-soft sensor method for real time in-process control during continuous direct compression manufacturing operations. *International Journal of Pharmaceutics.* 2021;*602*:120620.

Pawar P, Wang Y, Keyvan G, Callegari G, Cuitino A, Muzzio F. Enabling real time release testing by NIR prediction of dissolution of tablets made by continuous direct compression (CDC). *International Journal of Pharmaceutics* 2016;*512*:96–107.

Danckwerts PV. Continuous flow systems. Distribution of residence times. *Chemical Engineering Science.* 1953;*2*:1–13.

Engisch W, Muzzio F. Using residence time distributions (RTDs) to address the traceability of raw materials in continuous pharmaceutical manufacturing. *Journal of Pharmaceutical Innovation.* 2016;*11*:64–81.

Engisch W, Muzzio FJ. Feed rate deviations caused by hopper refill of loss-in-weight feeders, *Powder Technology* 2015;*283*:389–400.

Escotet-Espinoza MS, Moghtadernejad S, Oka S, Wang Z, Wang Y, Roman-Ospino A, Schäfer E, Cappuyns P, Assche IV, Futran M, Muzzio F, Ierapetritou M. Effect of material properties on the residence time distribution (RTD) characterization of powder blending unit operations. Part II of II: Application of models. *Powder Technology.* 2019;*344*:525–544.

Gao Y, Vanarase A, Muzzio F, Ierapetritou M. Characterizing continuous powder mixing using residence time distribution. *Chemical Engineering Science* 2011;*66*(3):417–425.

García-Muñoz S, Butterbaugh A, Leavesley I, Manley LF, Slade D, Bermingham S. A flowsheet model for the development of a continuous process for pharmaceutical tablets: An industrial perspective. *AICHE Journal.* 2018;*64*(2):511–525.

Jaspers M, de Wit MTW, Kulkarni SS, Meir B, Janssen PHM, van Haandel MMW, Dickhoff BHJ. Impact of excipients on batch and continuous powder blending. *Powder Technology.* 2021;*384*:195–199.

Lee SL, O'Connor TF, Yang X, Cruz CN, Chatterjee S, Madurawe RD, Moore CMV, Yu LX, Woodcock J. Modernizing pharmaceutical manufacturing: From batch to continuous production. *Journal of Pharmaceutical Innovation* 2015;*10*:191–199.

Leersnyder FD, Peeters E, Djalabi H, Vanhoorne B, Van Snick B, Hong K, Hammond S, Liu AY, Ziemons E, Vervaet C, De Beer T. Development and validation of an in-line NIR spectroscopic method for continuous blend potency determination in the feed frame of a tablet press. *Journal of Pharmaceutical and Biomedical Analysis.* 2018;*151*:274–283.

Oka S, Sahay A, Meng W, Muzzio F. Dimished segregation in continuous powder mixing. *Powder Technology.* 2017;*309*:79–88.

Palmer J, Reynolds GK, Tahir F, Yadav IK, Meehan E, Homan J, Bajwa G. Mapping key process parameters to the performance of a continuous dry powder blender in a continuous direct compression system. *Powder Technology.* 2020;*362*:659–670.

Rantanen J, Khinast J. The future of pharmaceutical manufacturing sciences. *Journal of Pharmaceutical Sciences* 2015;*104* (11):3612–3638.

Singh R. Chapter 13 – Model-based control system design and evaluation for continuous tablet manufacturing processes (via direct compaction, via roller compaction, via wet granulation). *Computer Aided Chemical Engineering.* 2018;*41*:317–351.

Tahir F, Palmer J, Khoo J, Homan J, Yadav IK, Reynolds GK, Meehan E, Mitchell A, Bajwa G, Development of feed factor prediction models for loss-in-weight powder feeders. *Powder Technology* 2020;*364*:1025–1038.

Tonson P, Doshi P, Matic M, Siegmann E, Blackwood D, Jain A, Brandon J, Wilsdon D, Kimber J, Verrier H, Khinast J, Jajcevic D. Continuous mixing technology: Validation of a DEM model. *International Journal of Pharmaceutics.* 2021;*608*:121065.

Vanarase AU, Muzzio FJ. Effect of operating conditions and design parameters in a continuous powder mixer. *Powder Technology.* 2011;*208*:26–36.

Vanarase AU, Osorio JG, Muzzio FJ. Effects of powder flow properties and shear environment on the performance of continuous mixing of pharmaceutical powders. *Powder Technology* 2013;*246*:63–72.

Vargas JM, Nielsen S, Cárdenas V, Gonzalez A, Aymat EY, Almodovar E, Classe G, Colón Y, Sanchez E, Romañach RJ. Process analytical technology in continuous manufacturing of a commercial pharmaceutical product. *International Journal of Pharmaceutics* 2018;*538*:167–178.

Wang Y, Li T, Muzzio FJ, Glasser BJ. Predicting feeder performance based on material flow properties. *Powder Technology.* 2017;*308*:134–148.

Weinekötter R and Reh L. Continuous mixing of fine particles. *Particle and Particle Systems Characterization* 1995;*12*(1):46–53.

15

Framework for the Validation of Mechanistic and Hybrid Models as Process Analytical Tools in the Pharmaceutical Industry

Pedro Valente
Research & Development, Hovione FarmaCiência, Lisbon, Portugal

Nuno Matos
Corporate Quality, Hovione FarmaCiência, Lisbon, Portugal

Luís Eça
Instituto, FarmaCiência, Lisbon, Portugal

CONTENTS

15.1 Introduction

15.1.1 PAT Journey from Hard Sensors to Soft Sensors and Modeling

The technological ability to monitor quality attributes of products during their manufacturing process has enabled various industries to design and control processes to meet desired quality standards leading to enhancements in efficiency and efficacy. Technological advancements have broadened the process analytical technologies (PAT) applications with tools that can effectively measure analytes (quantities) of a variety or at levels previously inaccessible.

There are, however, complex quality attributes that are not possible to measure with PAT "hard sensors". "Hard-sensor" is meant as a sensor that directly measures the attribute of interest as opposed to a "soft-sensor" which indirectly infers the attribute based on a combination of process data and "hard-sensor" data. Such challenges surface, for example, on continuous tableting where a "soft-sensor" is needed for the *in-process* quantification of the dissolution "performance" of a pharmaceutical tablet, which is a common critical quality attribute due to its impact on the bioavailability and consequent efficacy of the delivered dose. This quality attribute is commonly assessed by destructively testing a set of representative tablets dissolving them individually in an appropriate medium and profiling the API release at predetermined points in time. It is possible, nonetheless, to combine multiple attributes measured with hard

DOI: 10.1201/9781003149835-19

sensors with process parameter data into a model that predicts the dissolution profile, which is commonly denoted as a PAT "soft-sensor" due to its indirect measurement of the quality attribute (Zaborenko et al., 2019 [1]; for a more general introduction to soft-sensors refer to Fortuna et al., 2007 [2]).

Even when it is possible to directly measure a quality attribute with a "hard-sensor" it is often advantageous to independently predict the same attribute with a model or "soft-sensor". In those situations, the reconciliation of the two data "measurements", also denoted as "sensor fusion", can be leveraged to reduce the uncertainty of the combined prediction. The field of sensor fusion has a wide variety of applications, some of which are familiar to the reader, for example, our stereoscopic vision and sense of depth or smartphone location using a fusion of, for example, GPS data and inertial navigation systems (accelerometers and gyroscopes) to provide an accuracy far greater than would normally be achieved by the relatively low fidelity instruments alone (Grewal & Andrews, 2014 [3], Bar-Shalom et al., 2004 [4]).

As the reader might appreciate, managing measurement or prediction uncertainty plays a central role in ascertaining the adequacy of a PAT implementation for a given application. For the standard "hard sensor" applications, the *Uncertainty Quantification* is a central part of method qualification and follows well-established pharmaceutical guidelines. For the "soft-sensor" applications where a purely statistical multivariate model is used, the qualification procedures for "hard sensors" is typically directly applicable. However, when mechanistic models are used in the "soft-sensor" applications or for sensor fusion applications, the method qualification guidelines are not as comprehensive and had their first contact in the ASME V&V40 standard (ASME V&V40, 2018 [5]) directed at the qualification of numerical solutions of mathematical/computational models (in silico simulations) used for medical devices.

Finally note that although statistical models are, by definition, non-extrapolatable and are used within their calibration ranges, mechanistic models embody theoretical first principles and can in principle be used beyond the calibration range – the example provided below presents an illustration of this capability.

15.1.2 The ASME Verification and Validation Approach

Nowadays, the use of modeling and simulation is common practice in industry and pharmaceutical manufacturing is not an exception. There are several stages for the development and application of a simulation tool in practice, which affect the results obtained from in-silico experiments. In the last 20 years, several organizations, for example, the ASME, have made an effort to identify the different sources of uncertainty in modeling and simulation and provide technical guidance to quantify these uncertainties. The goal of this endeavor is to establish the credibility of modeling and simulation and increase the trust in its use.

In the ASME standards (ASME V&V10, 2019 [6], ASME V&V20, 2009 [7]), several errors/uncertainties are identified in the quantities of interest of a simulation performed with a given mathematical/computational model. In general, errors cannot be evaluated because they require the unknown true value of the quantity of interest and so uncertainties must be estimated.

Mathematical/computational models include assumptions and approximations, for example, the perfect gas law, that generates the modeling error/uncertainty. Physics-based models require boundary conditions, initial conditions, material properties, and possibly heat transfer coefficients that are not known exactly, which leads to the input parameters error/uncertainties. Last but not the least, most models require the use of a numerical solution that leads to numerical error/uncertainty. All these contributions appear combined in the simulation error/uncertainty.

Assessment of the credibility of modeling and simulation is established by comparing simulation results with experiments, which are also affected by experimental error/uncertainties. Therefore, the simple comparison of quantities of interest obtained from simulations and experiments without the quantification of all the uncertainties involved is prone to misleading conclusions.

In the ASME nomenclature, verification corresponds to the check of the correctness (*Code Verification*) and numerical accuracy (*Solution Verification*) of in silico simulations. *Code Verification* guarantees that the computational model is a faithful representation of the mathematical model, whereas *Solution Verification* estimates the numerical uncertainty of a given simulation.

The goal of validation is the estimation of the modeling error/uncertainty of the selected quantities of interest for a given mathematical/computational model. This requires the results of an experiment and of a simulation. As mentioned above, simulation results are also affected by input parameter uncertainties which require *Uncertainty Quantification* techniques to estimate its magnitude. In complex applications, input parameters may be hard-wired to the mathematical/computation model and so the input parameter uncertainty is absorbed in the modeling error/uncertainty.

ASME V&V20 (ASME V&V20, 2009 [7]) provides techniques to estimate experimental, numerical, input, and modeling uncertainties. These techniques allow the estimation of intervals that should contain with a selected degree of confidence the modeling error of the selected quantities of interest obtained with a given mathematical/computational model.

ASME V&V10 (ASME V&V10, 2019 [6]) also addresses two other aspects of the validation assessment: the definition of the acceptance criteria and the validation comparison that decides the acceptance or rejection of the mathematical model for the specified context of use (COU).

ASME V&V40 (ASME V&V40, 2018 [5]) describes a risk-based approach for decision-making regarding model use and is described in more detail in Section 1.3.

15.1.3 Potential Interface of V&V40 with Pharmaceutical Guidelines

The ASME V&V40 standard was developed by and for the medical devices' community, including device manufacturers, regulators, academy, and software developers. It provides a risk-based framework to support the decision on the level of verification and validation required for a computational model that will be used to evaluate the safety and/or efficacy of a medical device. In other words, it provides the organization with a methodology to determine the appropriate level of credibility required for the computational model. Credibility is defined by ASME as the trust in the predictive capability of a computational model for a COU. The standard defines a set of credibility factors to be considered for verification, validation, and applicability assessment.

The principles and concepts that are part of or support the ASME V&V40 standard may also have an expression in the Pharmaceutical Manufacturing realm and are well within the expectations driven by ICH Q8, Q9, and Q10 guidelines [8–10] (later, ICH Q11 [11] would be endorsed to articulate these guidelines to drug substance development and manufacture). These documents result from a new vision for quality agreed upon in 2003 that emphasized risk and science-based approach to pharmaceuticals [ICH Q8, Q9, Q10 Final Concept Paper, 12], and a pharmaceutical quality system model based on International Standards Organization (ISO) quality concepts [ICH Q10, 10]. This set of guidelines was mostly silent on the development and usage of models to support development and/or manufacturing of drug products (or drug substances). This was partially mitigated with the later issuance of "Points to Consider" (PtC), an endorsement document to complement the implementation of ICH Q8, Q9, and Q10 guidelines [ICH PtC, 13].

The use of models for the development of pharmaceutical products and processes is considered in ICH Q8 [8] namely, to help prioritize the factors to be studied from a list of potential parameters, provide in-silico experimental capacity to achieve a higher level of process understanding, help describe and deploy a Design Space, support process scaling-up, and be part of the process control strategy to monitor ongoing performance. The use of these models can thus be extended to pharmaceutical commercial manufacturing, articulating knowledge gained during development, supporting decision-making, and contributing to continued process verification.

Models used in pharmaceutical development and manufacture are expected to undergo proper validation and verification. The ICH PtC document brings forward an impact-based approach to advice on the level of validation and documentation required. Parallel aspects between the ICH PtC document and the ASME V&V40 can be found, as shown in Table 15.1.

While there are many parallel concepts/elements between the two documents, it is worthwhile to acknowledge that they are not equivalent documents. While ICH PtC document is a complement to a set of guidelines that are translated to many regional regulatory requirements, the ASME V&V40 document is a standard practice thus having much more detail for an applicational framework.

Importantly, two distinctions between these documents should also be highlighted: the definition of verification and considerations about lifecycle management. The ASME V&V body of guidance and documents from the GMP landscape will differ regarding the definition of "verification". For ASME

TABLE 15.1

Listing of Parallel Aspects between ICH PtC and V&V40 Documents

ICH PtC	ASME V&V40
Impact is related to model's contribution to assuring the quality of the product.	Uses a risk-informed credibility assessment framework, where the foundational element is model risk, related to the consequence to the patient in case of a wrong decision driven by model utilization.
Level of oversight is commensurate with the level of risk associated with the model.	Model risk is used to establish the required extension of credibility activities required to ensure model validity.
First step in model development is to define the purpose of the model.	Requires the definition of the question of interest as being the specific question, decision, or concern that is being addressed.
Variables' selection during model calibration to be based on a risk-based approach and considering the underlying phenomena and baseline knowledge.	Participants should have appropriate knowledge and experience to assess computational model credibility; also, a tool (Phenomena Identification and Ranking Table) is suggested to help identify and provide rationale for setting the goal of each credibility factor.
Collection of experimental data required to support model development and in such a way that ensures variable ranges targeted during model development are covered.	Quantity and Range of Test Samples and Test Conditions are credibility factors that are part of validation assessment.
Model development to include impact evaluation of prediction uncertainty on model's purpose.	Quantification of uncertainties is included in several credibility factors within validation assessment.
Model validation includes testing predictions against an external independent dataset to assess accuracy of prediction.	Addresses/discusses validation demonstrated by comparing the computational model predictions with the results of reference solutions taken from experiments.
Level of detail for describing a model is dependent on the impact	Relevant aspects of verification, validation, and applicability assessment activities should be documented.

V&V standards, "verification" aims to ensure that the mathematical models are implemented correctly and then accurately solved thus being a pre-validation activity, as mentioned in Section 1.2.1. For ICH PtC, "verification" happens as post-validation activities to ensure the ongoing validity of the model. The "verification" in ASME V&V standards may find a parallel in the GMP world as the *documented* sum of activities undertaken to develop a model to fit its intended purpose. From this derives a significant contribution from ASME V&V standards to GMP models application by filling the gap of providing a standard framework to model development stage.

Following the previous paragraph, the ASME V&V documents do not scope the post-validation activities. In other words, the ASME V&V standards do not address the whole model lifecycle management. While it may be implicit, there are no considerations on maintaining the validation state or addressing required updates to keep being relevant for the Question of Interest or the Context of Use adjusted. However, there are available standards used for GMP applications [USP <1039>, 14; EP 5.21, 15; ASTM E2891, 16; ASTM E2898, 17] whose principles on models' lifecycle management can complement the use of ASME V&V standards.

It should also be noted that the application of the different credibility factors as per ASME V&V40 will occur at different stages of an application in a GMP environment. Table 15.2 provides a brief discussion of typical applicability of the different credibility factors in a GMP context.

While ASME V&V standards bring new concepts and a distinct framework, it also has several parallel aspects with other GMP standards or guidelines, namely ICH PtC document. In fact, the framework established in the ASME V&V40 standard should not be seen as a departure from GMP requirements. It provides a validation approach that is science and risk-based for models also to be used in the GMP space, allowing the articulation of the impact-based classification suggested in the ICH PtC document with defining the extension of validation activities that should be performed.

TABLE 15.2

Possible Point of Application of ASME V&V40 Credibility Factors in a GMP Application

ASME V&V40 Activities	ASME V&V40 Credibility Factors	GMP Environment
Verification of Code	Software quality assurance Numerical *Code Verification*	These activities will mostly occur as part of software validation/qualification, following [ISPE GAMP 5, 18]
Verification of Calculation	Discretization error Numerical solver error Use error	ASME V&V40 is particularly applicable to models that make use of a solver for converging to a solution. Different modeling approaches may warrant different credibility factors. In cases the verification of calculation can be done regardless of specific applications (e.g., modeling approaches not requiring solver), it can be performed as part of software validation/qualification, following [ISPE GAMP 5, 18]
Validation of Computational Model	Model form Model inputs	The discussion of the applicability of a certain modeling approach to a specific application is often documented as part of model development. It includes, for a given intended purpose, the justification to use a certain model, the assumptions made, and the scope of applicability. The requirements of a specific application are often translated into an analytical target profile (ATP), describing performance criteria for key characteristics of the model output and/or decision risk probabilities expected in routine use of the analytical procedure [USP <1039>, 14].
Validation of Comparator	Test samples Test conditions	Relatable with the justification of the model validation approach and the definition of a validation protocol, namely type and number of samples to use, tests to be performed, ranges to be tested, and criteria to be met.
Validation of Assessment	Equivalency of input parameters Output comparison	The execution of the validation protocol to obtain the figures of merit for the model performance.
Applicability	Relevance of the quantities of interest	The definition of quantities of interest is typically done as part of the ATP.
	Relevance of the validation activities to the Context of Use	The evaluation of the validation activities output with the validation criteria as per the validation protocol and final decision about model validity for the intended purpose.

15.2 Case-Study on the Use of ASME V&V40 on a Pharmaceutical Application

15.2.1 Application Description

To illustrate the concepts included in ASME V&V standards with a practical application, consider an application case study of drying a slab of material in a vacuum contact dryer illustrated in Figure 15.1. This is a common process to remove residual content of process solvents from pharmaceutical powders, whereby the slab of material is subjected to low absolute pressure – below the solvents vapor pressure (henceforth denoted as process pressure or $P_{process}$). Due to the low pressure, the convection heat transfer is negligible and instead the powder slab is heated from contact with a heated base (henceforth denoted at process temperature or $T_{process}$).

To continuously monitor the content of given residual process solvent in the slab, a PAT "hard sensor" and a "soft-sensor" are used and two applications benefiting from their synergies are exploited. The overall flow chart is illustrated in Figure 15.2.

The PAT "hard-sensor" is a near-infrared (NIR) probe installed at the base of the slab and in direct contact with the powder bed. The PAT method also requires a multivariate statistical model (also denoted

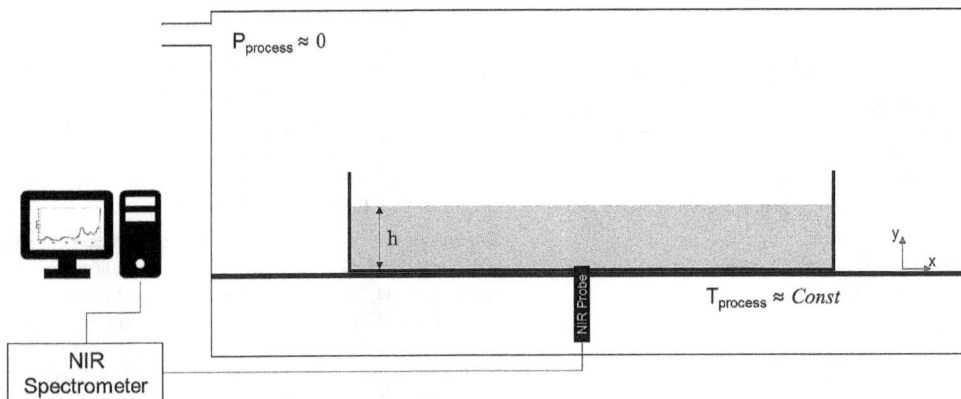

FIGURE 15.1 Idealized drying process with PAT for real-time monitoring of water and residual solvent content.

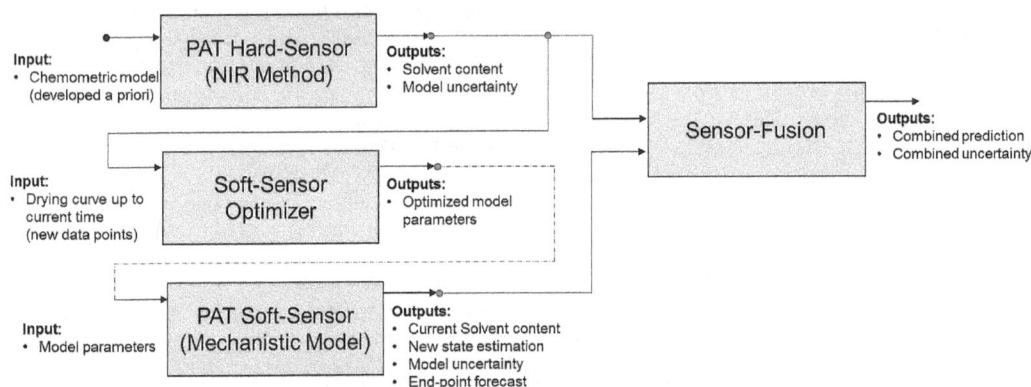

FIGURE 15.2 Flow chart of interplay between hard and soft PAT sensors and sensor fusion.

as a chemometric model) to calculate the specific residual solvents from the complex absorbance spectra. These represent the quantities of interest of the model used in the PAT "hard-sensor" that needs to be verified and validated previously. These two activities will ensure the correct implementation of the multivariate statistical model (verification) and the information about the uncertainty obtained from the "hard-sensor" (validation). For the readers less familiar with NIR implementations, refer to (Bakeev, 2010 [19]). For the purpose of this case study, the PAT "hard-sensor" data are generated synthetically from the drying model but retain physically relevant features such as the noise in the predictions and the decreased drying kinetics when the intra-particle diffusion becomes the rate-limiting phenomenon as discussed in (Hsieh et al., 2015 [20]).

The PAT "soft-sensor" is a mechanistic model of drying which predicts the residual solvent content throughout the slab in time. There are several approaches possible to model the drying kinetics, which in general require the solution of a coupled heat and mass transfer partial differential equation with appropriate initial and boundary conditions. For simplicity's sake, the model used in (Hsieh et al., 2015 [20]) is considered which involves solving the one-dimension transient diffusion equation,

$$\frac{\partial C}{\partial t} = D\frac{\partial^2 C}{\partial y^2},$$

(15.1)

where C is the concentration of the process solvent D is the effective diffusivity of the solvent in the powder bed of height h (assumed to be approximately constant and independent of the temperature and residual solvent content) and y is the direction perpendicular to the heated base. The initial condition is a uniform initial concentration C_o in the slab and the space boundary conditions assume that at the surface of the powder bed the concentration is zero and at the base, the wall is impermeable, which means derivative of C with respect to y equal to zero. This constitutes a mechanistic model with a single adjustable parameter (the diffusivity parameter) which has a first principles basis. Equation (15.1) can be solved numerically by discretization with a Backward-Euler integration scheme in time and a central differences scheme for the spatial diffusion term. The computational/discrete model is implemented in Scilab™ 5.5.2.

Note that the model itself is a crude approximation, since it assumes that the powder bed can be treated as a continuous medium with a single diffusivity parameter characterizing the mass transfer of powder bed when in fact the physical mechanisms are more complex and depend on intra-particle mass transfer and inter-particle mass transfer through the contact points as well as through the voids between the powder particles (Tsotsas et al. 2007 [21]). Nonetheless, after a calibration of the effective diffusivity parameter, one can get a reasonable prediction of the drying curve as shown in (Hsieh et al., 2015 [20]). This simple model has an analytic solution that is not adopted in this example since most mechanistic models require a numerical solution. As for the "hard-sensor", the mechanist model also requires verification and validation activities performed a priori. *Code Verification* guarantees that the computational model (discretized version of Equation (15.1)) is a correct representation of Equation (15.1), which is easy to do in this example due to the existence of an analytical solution. *Solution Verification* is required to quantify the numerical uncertainty of the solution as a function of time step and grid spacing. Finally, the comparison with experimental data will produce a quantification of the modeling error/uncertainty. Note that this modeling error/uncertainty evaluation is influenced by the uncertainty in the specification of D that needs to be propagated through Equation (15.1) to obtain the input uncertainty. Usually, this estimation is performed with a sampling technique. However, in the present example, its determination is straightforward due to the existence of an analytic solution. It is noteworthy to mention that the soft-sensor has a significant advantage relative to the "hard-sensor" since the former allows to determine solvent content along the thickness of the powder bed as well as in different time instants, which can be used to, for example, forecast the process end-point.

With both a "hard-sensor" and a "soft-sensor" available it is possible to use a sensor-fusion technique to minimize the uncertainty in the prediction of the residual solvent content by using an optimal estimator (Gelb, 1974 [22]). This uncertainty depends on the uncertainties of the two sensors that determine the input quantities of the sensor-fusion technique. As illustrated in Figure 15.2, the uncertainty of the output of the "soft-sensor" can be minimized using an optimization routine that receives the "hard-sensor" PAT data to continuously improve the input parameters of the "soft-sensor".

15.2.2 Sources of Error and Uncertainty

As described in the previous section, the different components of the system illustrated in Figure 15.2 are affected by uncertainties that affect the accuracy of the predicted quantities of interest. Therefore, it is important to identify and quantify the uncertainties that affect each of the system components and how they propagate through the system.

The PAT "hard-sensor" method development and qualification requirements are well established in guidelines as they are routinely used in pharmaceutical manufacturing. The uncertainty of the method prediction is bound by the independent external validation data set and typically characterized by the root mean square error of prediction (RMSEP) within a pre-defined range of model validity that is within the calibration range. The total uncertainty is explicitly measured prior to model qualification and includes all uncertainty sources, both those intrinsic to the PAT implementation (from instrument noise and error to sample variability unrelated to the measured analyte and to statistical modeling error) as well as the experimental error of the reference data upon which the model calibration and validation are based. From the authors' experience, it is often the case that the latter outweighs the former. Note that, in addition to method *Uncertainty Quantification*, there are other potential sources of error that are mitigated during development and monitored throughout the deployed PAT methods lifecycle to avoid inadvertent application outside their development boundaries which could lead to erroneous results or out-of-bound uncertainties.

The PAT soft-sensor requires a different approach to map the potential sources of error and uncertainty. For simplicity's sake these are broadly grouped by, (i) model implementation error (*Code Verification*); (ii) model input parameters uncertainty sources (*Uncertainty Quantification*); and (iii) model solution uncertainty sources (*Solution Verification*). *Code Verification* ensures that the model implementation is a faithful representation of the mathematical model, whereas *Uncertainty Quantification* and *Solution Verification* quantify the uncertainty of the model outputs which are key in establishing whether the "soft-sensor" is fit-for-purpose. This decision is based on the quantification of the modeling accuracy provided by the validation exercises.

The *Code Verification* activities include:

a. **Model implementation errors**: inaccuracies in translating the intended mathematical model into a computable algorithm,

b. **Coding errors**: coder-induced programming mistakes (popularly referred to as "programming bugs"),

c. **Numerical solution errors**: faulty numerical solution algorithms that do not adequately reproduce or converge to the intended mathematical model for the range of inputs.

   Note that *Code Verification* must be performed *a priori* to *Solution Verification* and input *Uncertainty Quantification* to avoid common pitfalls. For example, erroneous model calibration (e.g., determining the diffusivity parameter by benchmarking the output against experimental data) by factoring in and cancelling out numerical solution errors and uncertainties. This will lead to erroneous model predictions for model input parameters outside those used in the model calibration.

   The *Uncertainty Quantification* activities aim at identifying and quantifying the influence of model input parameters on the quantities of interest, which includes:

d. **Model input uncertainty**: identification of uncertainty in model parameters (e.g., the diffusivity parameter) and other model inputs (e.g., the initial solvent content of the powder),

e. **Uncertainty propagation**: quantify the propagation of uncertainty from the model inputs into its outputs and predictions.

   The goal of *Solution Verification* activities is to determine the numerical accuracy of the simulations,

f. **Numerical solution uncertainties**: differences between the exact solutions of the mathematical models and their practical numerical computation (which decreases with increased numerical resolution and thus increased numerical effort).

The estimation of the modeling accuracy of the "soft-sensor" model requires the comparison of the quantities of interest obtained from simulations and experiments. Therefore, besides *Uncertainty Quantification* and *Solution Verification*, **experimental uncertainty** is also part of the *Validation* exercises that quantify the modeling accuracy of the soft-sensor model.

The information collected from the *Validation* exercises leads to the outcome of the V&V study of the "soft-sensor" model:

• **Model adequacy**: adequacy of assumptions that went into establishing the mathematical model and their validity in the intended application.

It should be mentioned that ideally numerical, input parameters, and experimental uncertainties should be reduced to negligible levels to obtain a reliable estimation of the modeling error.

Lastly, the "soft-sensor optimizer" and the "sensor-fusion" method illustrated in Figure 15.2 are algorithms which require similar *Code Verification* activities and *Uncertainty Quantification* should be considered. *Solution Verification* activities for "soft-sensor optimizer" are not applicable whereas the sensor-fusion methods can be thought of as a weighted average prediction based on the input PAT measurements/predictions (in our case a PAT hard sensor and a soft-sensor) and their respective uncertainty distributions. The combined uncertainty can be theoretically estimated and shown to be generally lower than the uncertainty of the individual inputs. However, these sensor-fusion methods often assume that the uncertainty is Gaussian distributed and thus the adequacy of this assumption must be assessed.

15.2.3 Applying ASME V&V20 to Assess Model Uncertainty

In this section, the techniques presented in the ASME V&V20 standard (ASME V&V20, 2009 [7]) are applied to the case study to illustrate the execution of the activities necessary to quantify the uncertainty and establish the validity of the soft-sensor model.

To quantify numerical solution errors (*Code verification* activity listed above as activity "c") one can benchmark the numerical solution of Equation (15.1) against the exact explicit solution given by (Crank, 1975 [23]):

$$C(y,t) = \frac{4C_o}{\pi} \sum_{n=0}^{\infty} \frac{1}{2n+1} \exp\left(-\frac{D(2n+1)^2 \pi^2 t}{4h^2}\right) \sin\left(\frac{(2n+1)\pi(y+h)}{2h}\right) \tag{15.2}$$

with $0 \leq y \leq h$ and $t > 0$. The total solvent content $M(t)$ at time t may be obtained integrating Equation (15.2) in space to obtain

$$\frac{M(t)}{M(0)} = \sum_{n=0}^{\infty} \frac{8}{(2n+1)^2 \pi^2} \exp\left(-\frac{D(2n+1)^2 \pi^2 t}{4h^2}\right), \tag{15.3}$$

where $M(0) = C_o h$. Equations (15.2) and (15.3) are convergent infinite series and so only a finite number of terms needs to be computed. In the present example, 13 terms were used to calculate the reference solutions, which guarantees the accuracy of machine precision (14 digits).

The numerical solution should converge to the exact solution as the numerical resolution increases, that is, as the integration time step (Δt) and grid spacing (Δy) decrease. For sufficiently refined grids and sufficiently small time steps, the discretization error of any quantity of interest ϕ should be given by (Eça et al. 2019 [24])

$$e(\phi) = \phi_i - \phi_{\text{exact}} = \alpha_y (\Delta y)^{p_y} + \alpha_t (\Delta t)^{p_t} \tag{15.4}$$

where α_y and α_t are constants and p_y and p_t are the orders of grid and time convergence, respectively. In the present example, the expected values of p_y and p_t are equal to 1 and so Equation (15.4) may be re-written as,

$$e(\phi) = \phi_i - \phi_{\text{exact}} = \alpha (\Delta \lambda)^p. \tag{15.5}$$

For a correctly implemented computational model, a plot of $e(\phi)$ as a function of $\Delta \lambda$ should exhibit a straight line with a slope $p = 1$.

To demonstrate the correctness of the code, three different variables have been selected:

1. The maximum error of $C(x,t)$ after 0.4 time units of simulation,

$$L_\infty[e(C(x_i, 0.4))] = [C(x_i, 0.4) - C(x_i, 0.4)_{\text{exact}}]_{\max};$$

2. The root mean square of the error of $C(x,t)$ after 0.4 time units of simulation,

$$L_{RMS}[e(C(x_i, 0.4))] = \sqrt{\frac{\sum_{i=1}^{N_x - 1} (C(x_i, 0.4) - C(x_i, 0.4)_{\text{exact}})^2}{N_x - 1}};$$

3. The drying time to evaporate 50% of initial solvent content,

$$t_{50} \Rightarrow M\left(t_{50}\right) = \frac{1}{2}M(0).$$

The exact value of t_{50} is obtained from Equation (15.3) and for $D = 0.5\,\text{m}^2/\text{s}$ and $h = 1\,\text{m}$ is $t_{50} = 0.3935$ s. The numerical determination of t_{50} requires the numerical integration of $C(x,t)$ in space and an interpolation in time to determine t_{50} from the discrete results. A second-order trapezoidal rule is used to determine $M(t)$ and a cubic interpolation is performed to determine t_{50}. This choice guarantees that all post-processing is performed with an accuracy larger than that used to obtain the numerical solution. Furthermore, the use of the quantity of interest relevant to the application includes the post-processing in the *Code Verification* activities.

Figure 15.3 presents the error of the three selected variables as a function of $\Delta\lambda = \Delta t = r\Delta x$, for $r = 10$ and $r = 1$. All variables exhibit the expected linear behavior in the log-log scales with $p = 1$. The errors obtained with the smallest Δy for the same Δt ($r = 1$) are one order of magnitude smaller than those calculated with $r = \Delta y/\Delta t = 10$. On the other hand, reducing Δt for the same value of Δy has a smaller influence on the discretization error, which means than α_y is larger than α_t. Naturally, the results presented in Figure 15.3 could be used to determine these two constants, but that is not the goal of *Code Verification*.

After establishing the correctness of the discretized version of the mathematical model, it is necessary to select the quantities of interest, which in the present example are related to the total solvent content at a given time instant $M(t)$. The assessment of the model adequacy is based on the validation evidence that requires the evaluation of the modeling uncertainty from the outcome of simulations and experiments. As mentioned above, simulations also involve input and numerical uncertainties, whereas experiments are affected by experimental uncertainties.

The simplest approach to propagate the uncertainty in the model inputs (*Uncertainty Quantification* activity listed above as activity "e") is the determination of sensitivity coefficients. To a first approximation, the sensitivity coefficients are estimated by the corresponding first-order partial derivatives of the quantities of interest with respect to each of the three inputs, D, h, and C_o. For example, for the determination of $M(t)$ the sensitivity coefficients correspond to $\partial M/\partial D$, $\partial M/\partial h$, and $\partial M/\partial C_o$. Based on Equation (15.3), $M(t)$ is proportional to the initial solvent content and thus $\partial M/\partial C_o = M/C_o$, for example, a 5% error in C_o will propagate to a 5% of error in $M(t)$. On the other hand, Equation (15.3) shows that $M(t)/M(0)$ is independent of C_o and so t_{50} is not affected by the uncertainty in C_o.

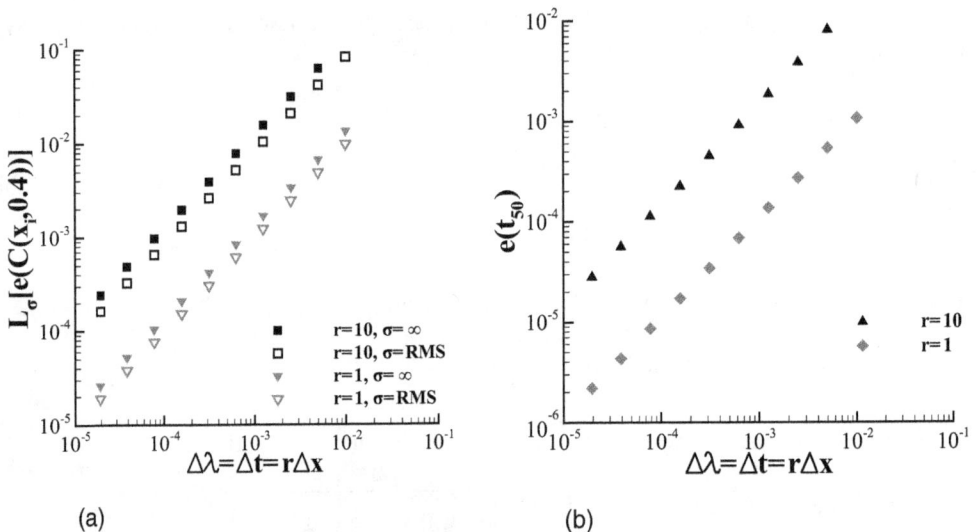

(a)   (b)

FIGURE 15.3 Numerical solution convergence.

One can also evaluate the sensitivity coefficients numerically by applying a finite-difference scheme. For example, to estimate the sensitivity coefficient of t_{50} corresponding to the diffusivity coefficient D, one can calculate $\partial t_{50} / \partial D \approx (t_{50}(D^+) - t_{50}(D^-))/(D^+ - D^-)$. $t_{50}(D^+)$ and $t_{50}(D^-)$ can be evaluated from Equation (15.3) or from the numerical solution of the discrete model. In the latter case, grid and time step should guarantee that the refinement level is sufficient to attain $p_y = p_t = 1$. Using the data of the example ($D = 0.5\,\text{m}^2/\text{s}$ and $h = 1\text{m}$), $D^+ = 0.51\,\text{m}^2/\text{s}$ and $D^- = 0.49\,\text{m}^2/\text{s}$, Equation (15.3) leads to $\partial t_{50}/\partial D \approx t_{50}/D$.

When more than one parameter is uncertain and their contributions are independent, the total input uncertainty can be determined from the root mean squared sum of the different components. For example, the input uncertainty of t_{50} depends on D and h and so it is obtained from $\sqrt{(\partial t_{50}/\partial D)^2 \delta D^2 + (\partial t_{50}/\partial h)^2 \delta h^2}$ (ASME V&V20).

Numerical uncertainty is quantified by *Solution Verification* (activity listed above as activity "f"), which is generally performed without the knowledge of the exact solution. It is desirable to have a numerical uncertainty that can be considered negligible when compared to the modeling error. The typical rule of thumb is to guarantee a numerical uncertainty two orders of magnitude below the other sources of uncertainty in the estimation of the modeling error (validation). In the present example, the data presented in Figure 15.3 can be used to tune Δy and Δt for the desired numerical uncertainty. As illustrated in the right plot of Figure 15.3 for t_{50}, the choice of Δt depends on Δy and so there is more than one choice that can meet the selected threshold. Therefore, simulation efficiency can help to make the best option.

To quantify modeling errors the "soft-sensor" model predictions are compared against experimental measurements or against the PAT "hard-sensor" data, which is the approach exemplified in this case study (Figure 15.4). The soft-sensor prediction generally describes the drying process throughout the entire drying process. However, for low contents of solvent (below 10% of the initial solvent content) it overpredicts the drying rate and thus underestimates the actual solvent content (cf. insert of Figure 15.4).

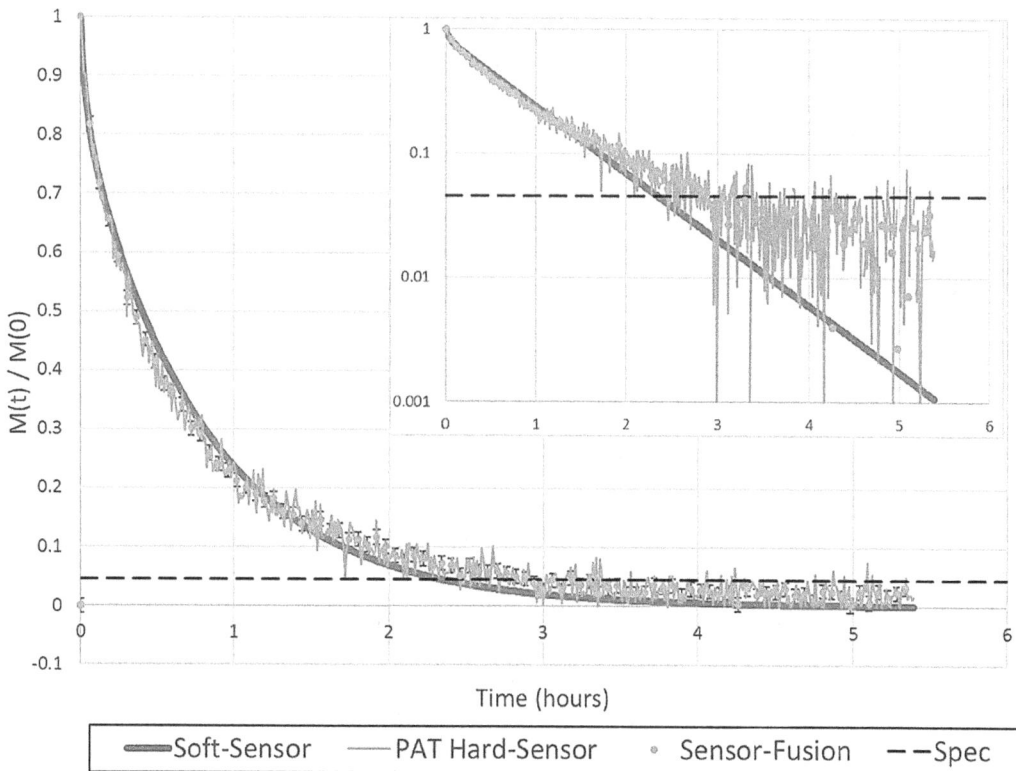

FIGURE 15.4 Drying curve of the case study as measured by the PAT hard-sensor, soft-sensor, and sensor fusion. In the inset, the same data are plotted with logarithmic ordinates.

As discussed in (Hsieh et al., 2015 [20]), the soft-sensor model is not adequate when the intra-particle diffusion becomes the rate-limiting phenomenon. Regardless of the bias, a model error can be quantified by using the RMSEP

$$RMSEP = \sqrt{(y_{pred} - y_{obs})^2 / N},$$

which for this case study can be calculated to be 1.27×10^{-2} or 1.27% of $M(0)$. This value represents the expected value of the modeling accuracy of the "soft-sensor". The uncertainty in its determination is quantified by the validation uncertainty, which is a combination of experimental, input parameters, and numerical uncertainties. For comparison, the PAT "hard-sensor" synthetic data were generated with a $RMSEP_{Hard-sensor}$ of 2×10^{-2} or 2% of $M(0)$ and for low solvent contents this measurement "noise" leads to a measured solvent content above specification even after 5 hours of drying (cf. Figure 15.4). Note that the "hard-sensor" error in this case study is larger than the error of the "soft-sensor" even though the latter fails to adequately predict the low solvent contents below the specification limit. This is an example where uncertainty analysis is a necessary, but not sufficient, step in establishing model adequacy which is further discussed in the following section.

Finally, the sensor-fusion in this case study is an optimal state estimator and the error of the combined prediction can be approximated as $(1/RMSEP_{Soft-sensor}^2 + 1/RMSEP_{Hard-sensor}^2)^{-1/2}$, assuming that both "hard-sensor" and "soft-sensor" measurement errors are random, unbiased, independent, and Gaussian distributed (Gelb et al. 1974 [22]). Optimal estimation is a powerful technique since it uses complementary sources of information alongside their uncertainties to provide a combined measurement/prediction with lower uncertainty than the uncertainty of each of the individual sensors. This is illustrated in Figure 15.4 where the combined sensor-fusion measurement of the solvent content has a lower noise which is consistent with the lower signal uncertainty. As noted above, the error of the soft-sensor is biased as the underlying model does not adequately capture the drying kinetics for low solvent content and thus the error of the sensor-fusion would require a more comprehensive analysis which is beyond the scope of this example, but a more detailed exposition can be found in (Gelb, 1975 [22], Bar-Shalom et al. 2004 [4], Grewal, 2014 [3]). For the reader proficient in PAT "hard-sensors", a signal smoothing operation such as a moving average could also be used to reduce measurement noise instead of the exemplified sensor fusion. However, note that there are at least two important advantages of sensor fusion over a signal smoothing operation:

- Signal smoothing operation cannot improve the Limit of Detection of the PAT "hard-sensor" whereas a sensor-fusion methodology, in certain applications, enables the possibility to do so;
- The use of sensor-fusion methodology accomplishes the reduction of measurement noise without imparting the added latency of response or the dampening of cyclical patterns from the typical signal smoothing operation.

15.2.4 Applying ASME V&V40 to Assess Model Credibility

In this section, the principles of ASME V&V40 are applied to this case study to discuss how to establish model credibility in the context of a pharmaceutical analytical method qualification, and based on the verification and validation exercises described in the previous section. The presentation of this case study is thus completed and concluded by showing how the different activities come together to establish credibility and whether the PAT sensor based on sensor-fusion is "fit for the intended use". This is different from the chronological sequence of activities where one would start by establishing the intended purpose (related to the *Question of Interest* in the ASME V&V40) and the ATP for the PAT method (related to the *Context of Use*, COU, in the ASME V&V40 as discussed in Section 1.3) prior to establishing the adequate level of *Credibility Activities* suitable to a given *Model Risk*, which typically encompass the V&V activities discussed in the previous section. The ASME V&V40 workflow is adapted to the current PAT sensor-fusion application as illustrated in Figure 15.5.

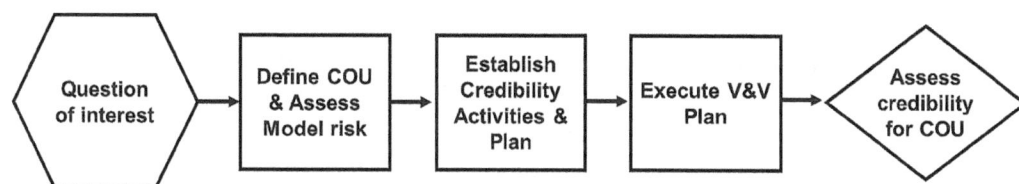

FIGURE 15.5 Risk-based approach to soft-sensor qualification by assessing the model credibility for the context of use.

For the current illustrative case study, the *intended purpose* is to have an *in-process* quantification method of the content of a residual process solvent to identify the drying end-point (process end-point where the solvent content is below a pre-defined specification limit). The product quality is assured during released testing based on a composite sample. The related *Question of Interest* within the context of ASME V&V40 would be "when is the solvent content below a target specification limit to determine the drying end-point?". The *Analytical Target Profile* of the method should include that it needs, for example, to be specific/selective (it must not confound the output with quantification of other process solvents) and with a Limit of Quantification below, for example, half the specification limit or 2.5% of $M(0)$ to be adequate for the application.

Following the defined *Question of Interest* and COU, one can evaluate the *Model Risk* following the ASME V&V40 risk assessment which factors *Model Influence* in the decision and *Decision Consequence*. Concerning *Model Influence*, it would arguably be considered high risk since the PAT sensor plays a determinant role in determining the end-point of the process. Regarding the *Decision Consequence*, it would be considered low risk since the final testing of the product would detect any faulty decision; however, to account for the business risk of the need for reprocessing or rejection of the batch in case the fault is only detected at release, the *Decision Consequence* is considered to be medium risk. The product of these two risk factors would lead to a model with a risk score of 6 out of 9 points and thus would be, overall, medium-high risk. This analysis is consistent with the ICH PtC document where *medium-impact models* are described as "(...) models [that] can be useful in assuring quality of the product but are not the sole indicators of product quality (e.g., most design space models, many in-process controls)".

The ASME V&V40 guides in planning the adequate level of *Credibility Activities* based on the risk assessment of the PAT soft-sensor/sensor-fusion application. These are broadly summarized in Tables 15.3–15.7 alongside a discussion on how they may be addressed by the V&V activities illustrated in the previous section.

By diligently performing the above credibility activities, model adequateness could be established. However, as the reader proficient in the development and validation of analytical and process analytical methods for pharmaceutical manufacturing applications may attest, there is a level of subjective interpretation and differences in terminology in the ASME V&V40 that require further consideration and standardization. This is discussed in the next and final section of this book chapter.

TABLE 15.3

Verification of Code – Credibility Activities Based on the Risk Assessment

Credibility Factors	ASME V&V40 Suggested Activities	Discussion
Verification of Code		
Software quality assurance	"Procedures were specified and documented"	Software Quality Assurance for pharmaceutical applications is well established
Numerical *Code Verification*	"Discretization error quantified by comparison to an exact solution, and a grid convergence study demonstrated (…)"	The execution of this activity following the guidelines of ASME V&V20 was illustrated for the present case study in Section 2.3

TABLE 15.4

Verification of Calculation – Credibility Activities Based on the Risk Assessment

Credibility Factors	ASME V&V40 Suggested Activities	Discussion
Verification of Calculation		
Discretization error	"Applicable grid or time-step convergence analyses were performed (…)"	Addressed in present application during Numerical *Code Verification*.
Numerical solver error	"No solver parameter sensitivity was performed. Solver parameters were established based on (…) verified computation model"	Not applicable for the current application. As noted in the discretization error, this activity is directed to CFD/FEM.
Use error	"Key inputs and outputs were verified by the practitioner"	Not applicable for the current application as the inputs are fixed during application development

TABLE 15.5

Computational Model Validation – Credibility Activities Based on the Risk Assessment

Credibility Factors	ASME V&V40 Suggested Activities	Discussion
Computational Model Validation		
Model form	"Influence of expected key model form assumptions was explored"	In Sections 2.1 and 2.3, the key model assumptions were presented alongside a discussion of the model limitations, particularly on the lower part of the solvent contents range
Model inputs	Quantification of Sensitivities: "Sensitivity analysis on expected key parameters was performed" Quantification of Uncertainties: "Uncertainties on expected key inputs were identified/quantified, but were not propagated (…)"	Both were illustrated at a high level in Section 2.3 where the uncertainty propagation analysis was also discussed.

TABLE 15.6

Comparator Validation – Credibility Activities Based on the Risk Assessment

Credibility Factors	ASME V&V40 Suggested Activities	Discussion
Comparator Validation		
Test samples	Test Samples/Quantity: "Multiple samples were used, but not enough to be statistically relevant" Test Samples/Range: "Samples representing the expected extreme values of the parameters (…)" Test Samples / Measurement: "One of more key characteristics of the test samples were measured" Test Samples / Uncertainty: "Uncertainty analysis incorporated instrument accuracy/repeatability"	In Section 2.3 the soft-sensor is benchmarked against the PAT hard-sensor (independently validated) for one simulated process which broadly illustrates the purpose of this exercise. In an actual application, multiple process conditions would need to be used.
Test conditions	Test Conditions/Range: "Test conditions representing the expected extreme conditions (…)" Test Conditions/Measurements: "One or more key characteristics of the test conditions (…)" Test Conditions/Uncertainty: "Uncertainty analysis incorporated (…)"	For the PAT Sensor fusion, considering that it is an optimal estimator that includes PAT hard-sensor data, an independent set of measurements would be required.

TABLE 15.7

Credibility Assessment – Credibility Activities Based on the Risk Assessment

Credibility Factors	ASME V&V40 Suggested Activities	Discussion
Credibility Assessment		
Equivalency of input parameters	"The types of inputs were similar, but the ranges were not equivalent"	This is not directly applicable to this application. This activity is pertinent to complex simulations where initial and boundary conditions are often simplified
Output comparison	Output Comparison Quantity: "Multiple outputs were compared"	The intent of this criterion is meant for complex CFD/DEM simulations and is not directly applicable to the present case.
	Output Comparison Equivalency: "Types of outputs were similar"	In section 2.3 the benchmark of the Soft-sensor against the Hard-sensor considering the uncertainty analysis would arguably address the scope of these credibility activities if performed and documented in detail.
	Output Comparison Rigor: "Uncertainty in the output of the computational model or the comparator were used (…)"	
	Output Comparison Agreement: "The level of agreement of the output comparison was satisfactory for key comparisons (…)"	

15.3 Conclusions and Recommendations

Establishing credibility of simulations and model-based applications such as PAT soft-sensors and sensor-fusion is of paramount importance to enable their use in a pharmaceutical setting, particularly for high-risk applications. It is the authors' opinion that there is a wealth of opportunities that have yet to be explored and will be strongly enabled by reliable and regulated workflow in establishing credibility and qualifying model-based applications for pharmaceutical manufacturing.

The principles behind ASME V&V40 are science and risk-based and embody many of the concepts already present in pharmaceutical guidelines. These concepts provide an opportunity to complement the principles outlined in the ICH PtC document regarding model application in the pharmaceutical industry.

Nevertheless, the simple case study presented here may help evidence some limitations which inhibit ASME V&V40 to be directly applicable to guide the qualification of model-based pharmaceutical manufacturing applications. This may be expected since it is an *ASME standard* pertaining to medical device development.

In the authors' opinion, to guide qualification of model-based pharmaceutical manufacturing applications the following gaps should be bridged.

ASME V&V40 is essentially conceptual using broader concepts, definitions, and recommendations which are subject to interpretation, which is understandable owing to the wide scope encompassing the class of "Medical devices". Pharmaceutical manufacturing guidelines avoid subjective interpretation by standardizing concepts and terminology which differ from those used in ASME V&V40. For example, COU which is a key definition in ASME V&V40 could be interpreted as the analogue for ATP (discussed in Section 1.3), but it directly encompasses other considerations such as application within the context of the control strategy which in pharmaceutical manufacturing is typically considered separately. This poses significant challenges as it can lead to workflows based on ASME V&V40 that challenge pharmaceutical manufacturing guidelines. Specifically, within the framework of ASME V&V40, when the model credibility assessment does not meet the requirement for the COU one possible outcome may be redefining the COU (cf. Figure 15.4-1 of ASME V&V40), whereas the expectation in the Pharmaceutical Manufacturing guidelines is that the method qualification effort (regardless of being model-based or not) should only occur when all the development supports that the method will be fit-for-purpose and the validation is a formal demonstration of the claim.

ASME V&V40 focuses on complex computational simulations that are executed as standalone efforts to support medical device development. This contrasts with pharmaceutical manufacturing applications where the models developed are intended to be used in routine manufacturing and therefore require a lifecycle management strategy which is not considered in ASME V&V40; nonetheless, the techniques presented in ASME V&V20 can be adapted for this purpose. The pharmaceutical manufacturing model-based applications are also typically less complex than the computational fluid dynamics (CFD) and finite element analysis (FEM) methodologies but, in contrast, show an increasing use of hybrid models (e.g., where a statistical module based on a PLS works together with a mechanistic or first principles model) which is not addressed by ASME V&V40.

Nevertheless, it should be reinforced that the ASME V&V standards contain key principles that need to be considered to qualify the increasing number of model-based applications containing mechanistic or first principles models and thus contain solvers for ordinary or partial differential equations (ODE/PDE) and for which the current treatment for statistical or multivariate models in the pharmaceutical manufacturing guidelines is insufficient. For example, multivariate model development and validation heavily rely on calibration and validating against experimental data and tracking the associated statistical uncertainties. As discussed in this chapter, when ODE/PDE solvers are in-built into the model, an artificially low error can be due to fortuitous cancelling out of errors if these are not addressed in a systematic methodology. On the opposite end, one can also reject valid models due to uncertainty sources that are due to coding errors or non-nominal causes of errors due to poor numerical convergence.

It is the authors' recommendation that a guideline is developed to bridge the gap in the body of pharmaceutical guidelines for model-based method qualification and lifecycle management. Such a guideline would converge with the principles of ASME V&V40 but adopt workflows and activities more in line with the pharmaceutical applications. This new guideline should be read together and augment the current body of ICH quality guidelines for the development and validation of models – mechanistic, statistical, or hybrid – used in pharmaceutical development and manufacturing.

REFERENCES

1. Zaborenko, N., Shi, Z., Corredor, C.C., Smith-Goettler, B.M., Zhang, L., Hermans, A., Neu, C.M., Alam, M.A., Cohen, M.J., Lu, X., and Xiong, L., First-Principles and Empirical Approaches to Predicting In Vitro Dissolution for Pharmaceutical Formulation and Process Development and for Product Release Testing, *The AAPS Journal 21*: 32, 2019.
2. Fortuna L., Graziani S., Rizzo A., and Xibilia M.G., *Soft Sensors for Monitoring and Control of Industrial Processes*, Springer-Verlag, London, 2007.
3. Grewal, M. S., and Andrews, A. P., *Kalman Filtering: Theory and Practice with Matlab*, John Wiley & Sons, 2014.
4. Bar-Shalom, Y., Li, X. R., and Kirubarajan, T., *Estimation with Applications to Tracking and Navigation: Theory Algorithms and Software*, John Wiley & Sons, 2004.
5. ASME V&V 40-2018, *Assessing Credibility of Computational Modeling Through Verification and Validation: Application to Medical Devices*, The American Society of Mechanical Engineers (ASME), New York.
6. ASME V&V 10-2019, *Standard for Verification & Validation in Computational Solid Mechanics*, The American Society of Mechanical Engineers (ASME), New York.
7. ASME V&V 20-2009 (R2016), *Standard for Verification and Validation in Computational Fluid Dynamics and Heat Transfer*, The American Society of Mechanical Engineers (ASME), New York.
8. ICH Q8(R2), *Pharmaceutical Development*, 2009.
9. ICH Q9, *Quality Risk Management*, 2005.
10. ICH Q10, *Pharmaceutical Quality System*, 2008.
11. ICH Q11, *Development and Manufacture of Drug Substances (Chemical Entities and Biotechnological/Biological Entities)*, 2012.
12. ICH Implementation Working Group on ICH Q8, Q9, and Q10, *Final Concept Paper*, 2007.
13. ICH Implementation Working Group on ICH Q8, Q9, and Q10, *ICH-Endorsed Guide for ICH Q8/Q9/Q10 Implementation, Points to Consider*, 2011.

14. United States Pharmacopeia and National Formulary (USP41-NF36), *<1039> Chemometrics*.

15. Ph. Eur, *5.21 Chemometric Methods Applied to Analytical Data*.

16. ASTM E2891, *Standard Guide for Multivariate Data Analysis in Pharmaceutical Development and Manufacturing Applications*, 2020.

17. ASTM E2898, *Standard Guide for Risk-Based Validation of Analytical Methods for PAT Applications*, 2020.

18. ISPE GAMP 5 Guide, *Compliant GxP Computerized Systems*, 2008.

19. Bakeev, K. A., *Process Analytical Technology: Spectroscopic Tools and Implementation Strategies for the Chemical and Pharmaceutical Industries*, John Wiley & Sons, 2010.

20. Hsieh, D. S., Yue, H., Nicholson, S. J., Roberts, D., Schild, R., Gamble, J. F., and Lindrud M., The Secondary Drying and the Fate of Organic Solvents for Spray Dried Dispersion Drug Product, *Pharm Res. 32*: 1804–1816, 2015.

21. Tsotsas, E., Kwapinska, M., and Saage, G., Modeling of Contact Dryers, *Drying Tech. 25*: 1377–1391, 2007.

22. Gelb, A., *Applied Optimal Estimation*, MIT Press, 1974.

23. Crank, J., *The Mathematics of Diffusion*, Oxford University Press, 1975.

24. Eça, L., Vaz, G., Toxopeus, S. L., and Hoekstra, M., Numerical Errors in Unsteady Flow Simulations, *ASME. J. Verif. Valid. Uncert. 4*(2): 021001, 2019.

16

Understanding the History of Continuous Manufacturing in Other Industries to Guide Future Development in Pharmaceuticals

Ian M. Leavesley
Modern Pharma Consulting LLC

CONTENTS

16.1 Introduction – What Is Continuous Manufacturing and Why Is It Used?

Continuous manufacturing is a technology that has been used for over 2000 years to make almost every product imaginable – from foodstuffs to consumer products, plastics, building materials and most recently pharmaceuticals.

This chapter will trace the evolution of continuous manufacturing in three dimensions: time, industry and degree of complexity. The objective of the chapter is to enable the pharmaceutical engineer to better understand where continuous manufacturing came from to be able to inform future adoption and continuous improvement within the pharmaceutical industry.

The examples will illustrate common themes that show the advantages of continuous manufacturing over batch manufacturing:

1. Higher quality of product
2. More product produced in the same space
3. More product produced per person

Continuous manufacturing is conceptually very simple. It is the constant feeding of material into a system and subsequent continuous discharge of material out of the system. This results in the production of a product whose quality is time-invariant and whose batch size can vary from run to run to meet customer demand. Batch manufacturing on the other hand has: (i) process parameters (and potentially quality) that vary over time and (ii) fixed batch sizes which are determined by the physical size of the equipment. Continuous manufacturing is governed by the same equation as batch processing. The equation is the

DOI: 10.1201/9781003149835-20

mass balance equation which is the first equation taught to an undergraduate chemical engineer. For batch manufacturing, the units are mass while for continuous manufacturing the units are mass flow rate.

$$\text{Input} + \text{Generation} = \text{Output} + \text{Accumulation} + \text{Consumption} \qquad (16.1)$$

The equation can be applied to any chemical process either dry, liquid, solid or a combination thereof, and can be applied to any industry and at any scale. This is why it will be so useful to pharmaceutical engineers in understanding and learning both the history of continuous manufacturing and how it is used today in other industries.

This chapter will build progressively:

1. Most simple examples of first-century Roman food production with a single unit operation to increase manufacturing capacity to meet the growing demands for food in Roman cities.
2. Advanced systems for the same task which integrate multiple unit operations together and leverage water power to increase capacity and improve quality and therefore value.
3. Invention of the critical unit operation for modern continuous manufacturing processes and how various industries have contributed to its continuous evolution over an almost 50-year period. This takes advantage of what was at the time a recently developed new technology – the microprocessor.
4. Integration of multiple unit operations together with new technologies of process analytical technology (PAT) to provide computer control of the entire system of unit operation. This again yields higher capacity and quality, and therefore lower cost. This is enabled by the development of the computer.

With this understanding it will be possible to understand how the pharmaceutical industry fits into the broader historical and technical context. This will then enable the industry to evolve in its own way to meet the same objectives: quality, capacity and efficiency. For the purposes of the chapter, quality will be defined as the way every industry except pharmaceuticals uses the word. That is, minimum variation over time that is significantly less than the acceptance limits and an average value that is as close to the target as possible. Using this definition, quality can be continuously improved until the variation over time from the target for each data point is 0 and the standard deviation of the set of data points is 0. This is different from the traditional "within the specification limits" definition of quality where being exactly on target or barely within acceptance limits is the same "quality." Most other industries abandoned this approach to definition of quality in the 1960s to 1980s.

A reasonable starting point to discuss continuous manufacturing is foodstuffs since this was, and continues to be, the most important product produced by man. This pattern will play out throughout this section that the most vital products of human life are the first to receive innovation with regard to their manufacture.

16.2 A Very Early Example of Continuous Processing – Milling Grain in Pompeii 79 AD

Grains such as corn and wheat were originally milled by hand. Hand milling is an example of a batch process. The same amount of material is added into a container each time and then processed from an unmilled state to a milled state. Then the container is emptied and the process is repeated. There is no steady-state operation. (The pharmaceutical industry uses the term "state of control" rather than the term "steady state" which is used outside the pharmaceutical industry.) As the Roman Empire grew and cities with high population density appeared it became necessary to mill grains more efficiently and hence a very early version of continuous manufacturing was employed. While continuous mills likely existed earlier than the period immediately before 79 A.D., there are very well-preserved examples in the ruins of the city of Pompeii which was buried by volcanic ash in 79 A.D. There are 72 mills of two different

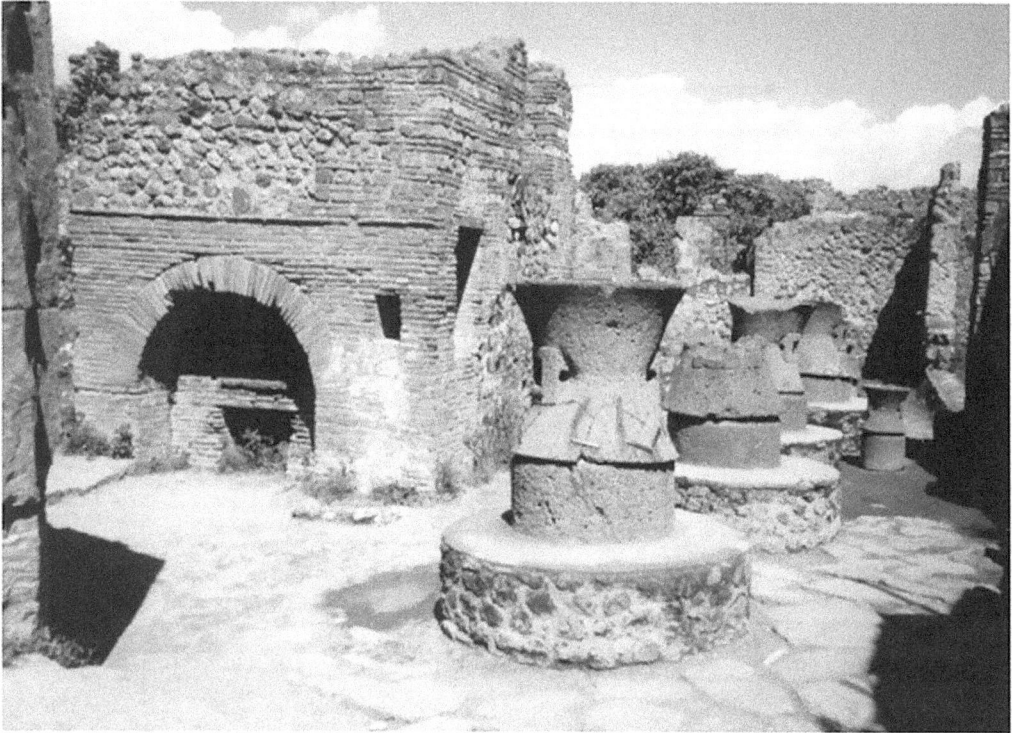

FIGURE 16.1 Bakery with Multiple Millstones in Pompeii (Photography courtesy Sue and Martin Watts, The Mill Archive Trust).

styles found in the ruins. Of these 47 "hourglass" designs are animal driven and 25 smaller "rotary hand type" mills are human-driven [1]. Figure 16.1 shows a typical bakery in Pompeii with larger animal-driven hourglass-style mills. From an engineering perspective, there are two unit operations visible in this "plant." The first unit operation are the mills, which are operated continuously and milled material collected in a basin resting on the ledge below the mill. This is decoupled from the baking oven unit operation with a design that has changed little in the last 2000 years. The oven is an example of batch manufacturing. This decoupling of batch from continuous unit operations is a configuration that is still seen today in many processes across all industries including pharmaceuticals.

Figure 16.2 shows a diagram of an "hourglass" type mill (Buffone et. al.). Part D is the rotating *catillus* which holds the unmilled grain. Part A is the non-moving *meta*. The gap between part A and part D is where the grinding occurs.

The reason this is a continuous process is that the flow rate between the hopper formed by A through the milling section is operating at a constant rate which is controlled by (i) the RPM of the upper section and (ii) the gap between the *meta* and *cattilus*. Furthermore, as long as the hopper is kept fed, the mill can run continuously. There is no limit to how much grain can be milled except perhaps the ability of the animal to keep moving at a constant speed or if accumulation (see Equation 16.1) within the mill changes the milling characteristics. The hopper that is formed above the mill would always have powder in it. The level would raise and lower during operation as the level is being drawn down and then refilled, likely from a sack manually unloaded by a person. Again, this is a style of operation that continues to this day in every hopper in every industry. During correct operation, there is always some powder in the hopper and this is referred to as "flood feeding." The level rises and lowers between refills, but as long as there is some material in the hopper the process works as intended. We will see flood feeding and refilling in every example in this chapter.

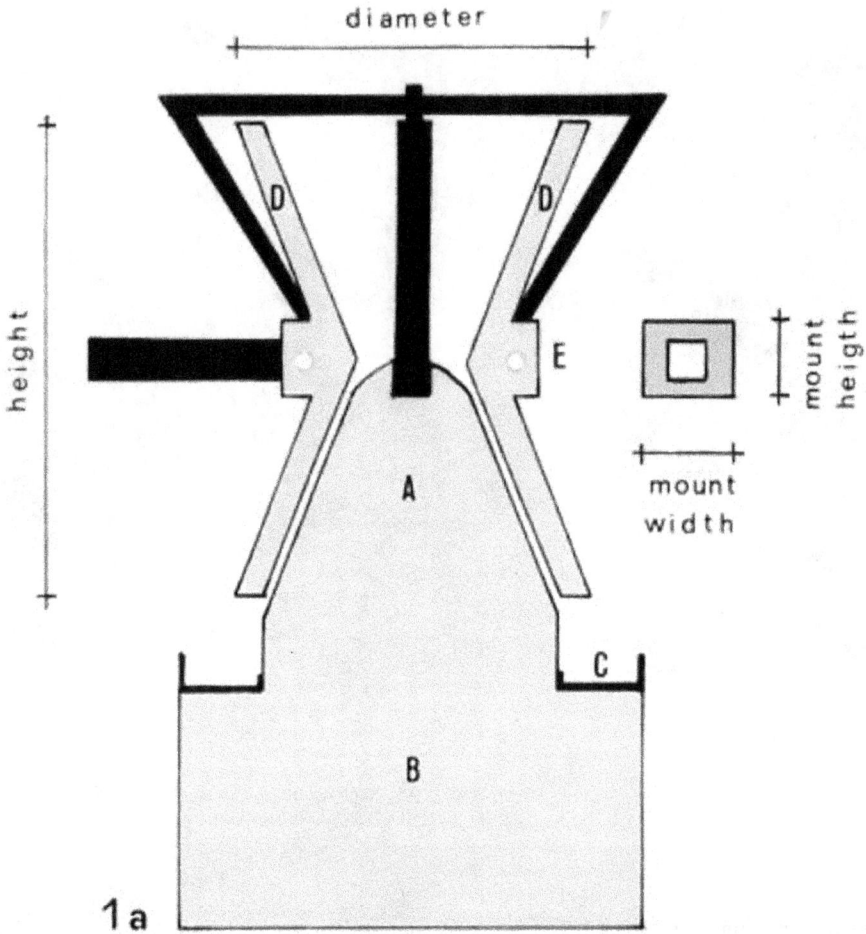

FIGURE 16.2 Design of an Hourglass Style Mill I Pompeii. (*Source*: Buffone, Luigi, Sergio Lorenzoni, Mauro Pallara and Eleonara Zanettin. The Millstones of Ancient Pompeii: A Petro-Archaeometric Study. *European Journal of Mineralogy* 15:1 (2003) pp. 207–15.)

    This fulfills the objectives of continuous manufacturing. It is a high capacity, highly efficient process compared to batch milling that can run indefinitely to make small or large batches as desired. It also has time-invariant quality.

    As technology in other fields developed, it was quickly adopted in the powder process engineering field. This is seen in the water-powered mills which are common all over the world starting even in Roman times and truly flourishing and expanding in the Industrial Revolution. This is followed by the electric-powered energy of the late 19th century. However, the principle remains the same today and can be seen throughout most industries. That is to pass the material between two closely spaced rough surfaces. This type of milling is often found in pharmaceutical manufacturing today in the form of cone mills.

16.3   Moving From Single Unit Operation to Multiple Integrated Unit Operations

A more advanced version of a method for milling flour is presented next. Again, it shares the traits of continuous manufacturing of higher quality, higher capacity and greater efficiency and the ability to run for a variable period of time to meet customer needs. In this case, multiple unit operations are linked together and the motive power is now water instead of human or animal power. This example is a powder mill patented by Oliver Evans granted on December 19, 1790. One author refers to this as "one of the first examples of the modern factory." [2]

There are four interesting aspects to this example:

1. Integration of multiple unit operations into a single plant.
2. One of the very earliest examples of a US Patent. Specifically, it is US patent X3, the third US patent ever granted.
3. Application of this technology was licensed by the first US President – George Washington – for use in his personal business.
4. Production of higher quality, and therefore higher value, products. These were of suitable quality that the flour was exported from the US overseas because of its high quality.

Figure 16.3 shows a diagram of this system. Note that it is not a small system, it is approximately 60 feet wide. This is a much larger process than seen in Pompeii in Figure 16.1 and therefore much higher throughput.

This brings together many of the unit operations that are still found in manufacturing processes today. There are multiple hoppers such as the unloading hopper #2 on the far right, inclined chutes which feed the powder down out of the hopper, and two vertical bucket elevators in the center and far left to raise the powder vertically to a higher level. Bucket elevators are a very common unit operation today except in the food and pharmaceutical systems. They are not used in those industries because of their inability to be

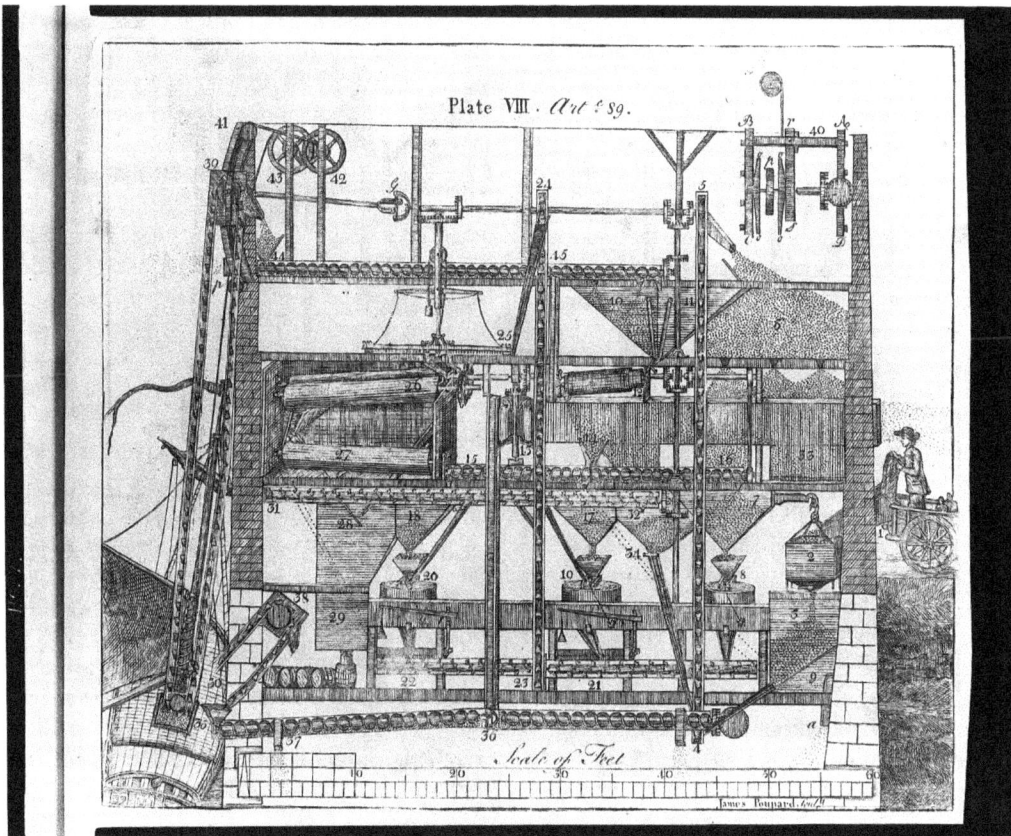

FIGURE 16.3 Diagram of grain mill licensed by George Washington from US Patent X3 by Oliver Evans [3]. (*Source*: US Library of Congress, Poupard, James, Engraver. *Automated mill, designed by Oliver Evans, for processing grain/James Poupard, scult*, 1795. Photograph.)

easily cleaned. In food plants and some pharmaceutical plants and more modern non-food plants bucket elevators have been replaced by pneumatic conveyors which are both more reliable and easier to clean. Either system, bucket elevators, screws or pneumatic conveyors are essential to an integrated continuous plant in that they are able to continuous move material long distances either horizontally or vertically. Figure 16.3 also shows three horizontal transfer screws. They use the same technology principles as those used in loss-in-weight (LIW) powder feeders that are so ubiquitous today in modern continuous pharmaceutical systems (the LIW feeder itself will be discussed extensively in Section 16.4). This entire facility is a mill and so obviously the process contains a mill unit operation to grind the flour or corn. There is also a screen #26 & #27 (known as a bolter in this design since it is made from a bolt of fabric) which separates the milled product into superfine flour, fine flour and bran. This separation of milled material by one or more screens into different particle sizes is a very common unit operation outside of pharmaceuticals and was the technique used in pharmaceuticals to measure particle size prior to the laser particle size analyzer. Raw material suppliers use the method of screens to separate material into different particle size grades of material (e.g., lactose or microcrystalline cellulose grades). Even today raw material specifications in pharmaceuticals will be reported as "on 60 mesh" or "through 250 mesh" where mesh size is the number of openings per inch in the screen. So, the concept of the bolter exists today in pharmaceuticals with a name change and a change from fabric to metal screens. The only place where this is seen in pharmaceutical milling processes is in the screen sizes of a cone mill. Patent X3 was a high-volume operation and again highlights the productive capacity of a facility with a relatively small footprint and low staffing. In 1797 it milled 275,000 pounds of flour and 178,000 pounds of corn [4].

From this, we see at least one early example of a highly integrated continuous manufacturing facility using many of the unit operations that are still in use today in a facility operating in the 18th century to produce high volumes of high-quality products. We see the use of hoppers, vertical conveyors, screw conveyors, mills, screens for sizing and drums as intermediate containers for storing material and transporting, domestically and internationally, to where they are ultimately converted into the product that consumers need. This is more than 100 years before the widespread adoption of the electric motor enabled each unit op to be individually powered rather than be powered by a single water wheel.

In this example, the controls and inline process monitoring are performed by skilled individuals rather than by PAT. This manual inspection technique is a feature that still exists in the pharmaceutical industry. In subsequent examples, we see how the adoption of enabling new technologies from other fields such as electric motors, microprocessors, PAT measurement and computers further advance the field of continuous manufacturing to enable continuous improvement toward the goals of quality, capacity and efficiency.

16.4 Loss-in-Weight Feeder

The breakthrough in formulating products to a tightly controlled formula on a continuous basis is the LIW feeder. This represents a major breakthrough in powder processing with the ability to accurately meter ingredients together in the correct ratio by feeding each one individually. Within a few years of the first commercialization of LIW feeders, these had spread to use in every industry that required accurate control of a formulated powder. Figure 16.4 is the drawing from US patent 4,054,784 showing the invention of the LIW feeder. While the individual elements are difficult to read, the entire drawing is presented to understand the complexity of this equipment at the time it was developed.

The physical aspect of the feeder itself is easily recognizable today in every industry including pharmaceutical continuous manufacturing. It is located in the upper left corner. The physical feeder system itself is the system comprises items 10–24 with a hopper (item 124) above it and the powder flow stream exiting labeled as 14. Note that the feed screw (item 16) is exactly the same principle as seen in Figure 16.3. Note also the presence of a flood feed hopper (item 12) showing a continuity in this approach to powder handling. The output stream from the feeder may pass into another hopper in which case it would be flood-feeding the unit operation below the hopper. In pharmaceuticals, this is the case in the feed frame above the tablet press.

While most of remaining numbered elements in the patent are difficult to read, the important thing is that they are not physical elements but rather electronics and logic flows. Here we see for the first time a

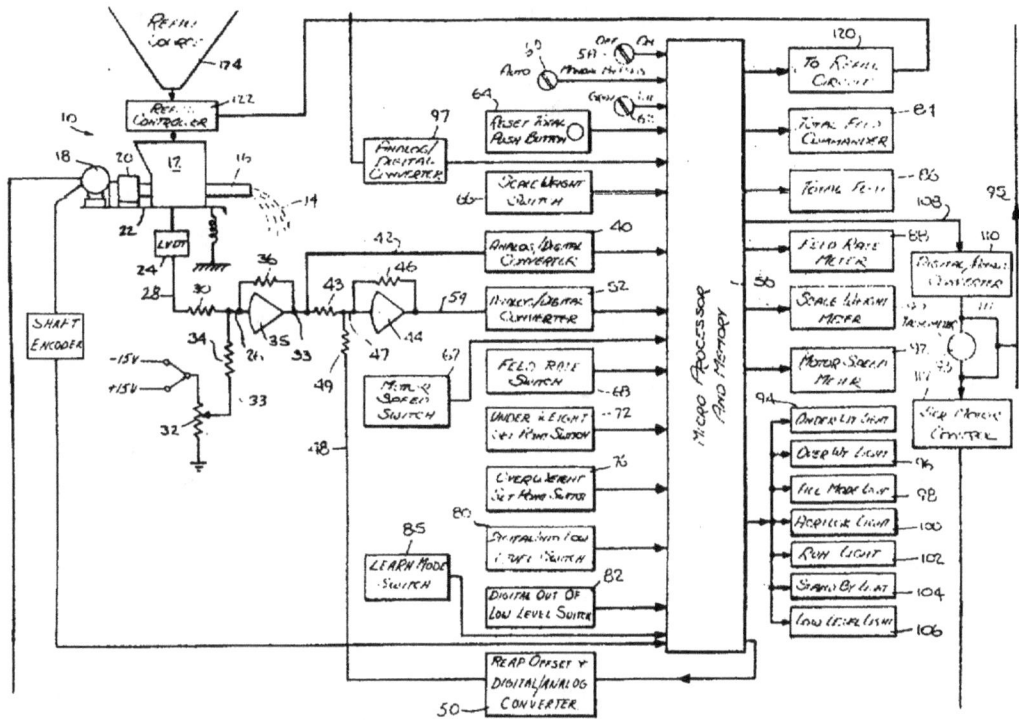

FIGURE 16.4   Loss-in-Weight Feeder System. US Patent 4,054,784. (*Source*: United States Patent and Trademark Office.)

piece of equipment in powder processing that is inseparably mechanical and electronic. The tall rectangle (item 50) that runs from the top to bottom of Figure 16.4 is labeled "microprocessor and memory" and is absolutely essential to this equipment. Without the microprocessor the equipment would not exist. Again, we see the role of rapid adoption of novel enabling technologies from one technology field enabling the powder processing field. Microprocessors were a very novel technology in 1976. To put it in historical perspective, this was prior to the personal computer and about the time of the handheld calculator. Specifically, the first low cost widely available microprocessor, the Intel 4004, was introduced only five years before this patent was granted [5].

Conceptually, a LIW feeder is very simple. A hopper holds an excess of powder above a screw and the mass flow rate out of the screw is proportional to the RPM of the screw. If the mass flow rate is not critical and only needs to be approximately right to supply the next step then a simple hopper and screw, without feedback control, will suffice. This is known as a volumetric feeder. An early example can be seen in Figure 16.3 near the top of the mill where a long screw (item 45) conveys material horizontally from a small hopper (item 44).

The real challenge to accurate feeding is that powder does not flow uniformly from a hopper and powders are compressible. Therefore, an internal process control loop is necessary. From a control theory perspective, this equipment initially used proportional controllers in a feedback loop. This approach calculates the difference between the actual (present value or PV) change in weight per unit time and the desired change in weight per unit time (set point or SP). If there is no difference between the PV and the SP, there is no need to change the speed of the conveying screw/auger. The screw speed is corrected faster or slower in proportion to the difference between SP and PV. However, as in all good control loops, the proportionality constant (k) is less than 1, so for example a 2% low PV might be corrected with a 1% higher speed if $k = 0.5$. Some initially think this counter-intuitive and ask "why not use k = 1?" The answer is that all measurements have measurement error and responding to all the discrepancy between SP and PV means responding to error. This error is "averaged out" by repeating the correction at a high frequency. Basically, lots of small corrections are more accurate than a few large corrections. This is the complete opposite of the way weight control is traditionally executed in the pharmaceutical industry with a tablet press which uses low-frequency measurement with large corrections.

Despite this novelty of microprocessors, feeders became widespread in industries from plastics to foods to consumer goods within a few years. This is typical of breakthrough enabling technologies that are readily adopted within a few years. The pharmaceutical process engineers' challenge is to be constantly looking for new enabling technologies.

The fundamental technical challenge, then and now, is accurately weighing in very small time increments (therefore small weight differences) in an environment hostile to precision weighing. For this reason, the earliest uses were in applications where the throughput is measured in hundreds of kilograms to tons per hour so that a robust weight difference existed between the one-time sample point and the next time sample point. Many, but not all, applications in plastics, foods and consumer goods fall into this category.

The evolution of this technology to meet the needs of other industries led to a continuous series of improvements by equipment vendors to control lower flow rates. Different industries have contributed different improvements to LIW feeders and today's feeders represent the sum total of all these improvements from all these different industries. This low flow rate feeding opened the door to their use in pharmaceuticals with feed rates of grams per hour. This ability to control low flow rates is the result of two trends: (i) Weigh cells have evolved to have higher and higher precision and (ii) the electronic components of the control have been continually evolving and continue to evolve.

These evolutions and improvements in feeders and controls have been driven by the needs of the users. Some industries need the ability to feed at low feed rates, such as adding nutritional supplements to foods, and so solutions to address these needs were developed. Other industries such as foods and consumer goods work with poorly flowing materials and solutions were developed by vendors to address these needs. The plastics industry needs very high precision to ensure consistent performance of their polymers. Because of the inclusion of solutions to these needs by the vendors, modern feeders are a wonder in control engineering and signal processing. The control parameters such as sampling time and proportionality constants themselves adapt to changes in conditions during a run. Put another way, the parameters that govern how the screw speed is adjusted are themselves constantly changing through a run. An important concept is noise. This is the variation from one measurement to another that is not due to actual feeding. Someone walking by or touching a feeder or a forklift truck driving by a feeder will generate random noise. A vibrating source such as a poorly balanced motor can cause constant frequency noise. In modern feeders, the feeder itself will automatically adjust the control parameters which are then used to control the feed screw. The approach to how these control parameters can change is defined when the process is developed and scaled up. For instance, a process developer may choose to have the feeder ignore all data while the weight signal to noise value is below a defined threshold. In this case, the system may operate in constant RPM mode until the noise dies down. Operation in constant, or near constant, RPM mode is what is used during refill of the hopper since in that case a LIW cannot be determined since the overall system is actually gaining weight. Another alternative is the process developer may choose to adjust k to a lower value so the corrections are not as dramatic as they would be if the system had less noise. Some systems have real-time Fast Fourier Transform (FFT) filters and can filter out the low-frequency and/or high-frequency noise with a high pass or low pass filters, respectively. A different alternative is for the process developer to have the system adjust the time interval between measurements from as low as 80 msec up to close to a second or more. This results in a greater absolute change in weight between measurements, which reduces the contribution of the noise relative to the actual change in weight itself. All these different options represent the cumulative solutions to the needs of all customers over the years. This is an excellent example of how close cooperation between the end user and the equipment manufacturer has led to continuous improvement in the capability of the equipment.

The pharmaceutical industry identified the need to feed in the grams per hour range, to meet pharmaceutical grade cleaning standards and to deal with extremely poor flowing materials such as active pharmaceutical ingredients (APIs). The ability to feed at lower and lower feed rates has been developed over the last decade based on the needs of the pharmaceutical industry. Collaboration with equipment manufacturers and process developers will be essential to keep this evolution of technologies.

It is critical that the people developing the feeder recipe and the people maintaining the feeders understand all these options and how best to program the feeders to respond. Feeders are much more complicated than other pharmaceutical unit operations with the possible exception of tablet presses. Given this constant evolution over the last 45 years and the complexity of the control structure described above, it is not hard to imagine that advanced techniques such as multivariate statistical process control, artificial intelligence and machine learning will likely become prominent components of powder feeders sooner rather than later.

The next step in the complexity of feeding is to realize that formulated products are made up of multiple ingredients and therefore multiple feeders. The obvious first step would be to calculate the desired total feed rate and the percent for a given ingredient and use that as the set point for each feeder. This should result in a very constant overall feed rate but with some slight variation in percent of each ingredient. The next step from that is to recognize that the desired attribute of the product is the percent of each ingredient rather than the total feed rate. This approach treats multiple feeders as a single system. An option that was developed by the feeder manufacturers for the food industry is called a ratio controller. It defines one feeder as the master feeder and lets the system use the percent of each ingredient to calculate the setpoint of the other feeders. As the master-feeder varies, the other feeders will increase or decrease their setpoints to maintain the correct ratio of each ingredient. If done correctly, this can result in even tighter control of the formula. It is up to the process developer to determine how complex a solution is required.

16.5 Integration of Automated Control Across Multiple Unit Operations with Multiple Sensors – Laundry Industry 2001

Now that we have introduced the integration of mechanical equipment and electronic control within a single unit operation such as a LIW feeder, we can see how this can be expanded to a system of multiple unit operations and multiple sensors.

This example from the seemingly mundane laundry detergent industry represents an integrated system of approximately ten unit operations and two real-time sensors to control two product attributes. While this system operates in units of tons/hour rather than the kg/hour of pharmaceuticals, the approach is directly applicable to the pharmaceutical industry and many of the unit ops are easily recognizable to pharmaceutical engineers.

- Approximately four LIW feeders each feeding raw powder ingredients. Note that the individual feeders are not shown but they all feed into the point labeled "Raw powders" at the top of the process flow diagram.
- Mixer 1 Horizontal paddle mixer – This equipment would be recognizable to a pharmaceutical continuous manufacturer as a horizontal shaft mixer such as is available from Gericke, Lödige and others.
- Binder liquid and diluent liquid (water) added by four computer-controlled pumps into mixer 1 and mixer 2.
- Mixer 2 (similar to mixer 1) combines the fine agglomerates formed in mixer 1 with the two liquids from the upper right.
- A fluid bed dryer utilizing the same principles as found in pharmaceutical continuous drying processes such as GEA, Glatt and others. Because of the tons/hour flow rates involved it is oriented horizontally instead of vertically and operated in a true continuous manner rather than the semi-continuous manner currently found in the pharmaceutical industry.

Importantly, there are two real-time sensors in this process. The pharmaceutical industry refers to these as PAT sensors. The first sensor, in the lower right of Figure 16.5, is a "PSD camera" which measures particle size, particle size distribution and particle shape factors of the discharge from mixer 2 before entering the dryer. The second sensor, at the end of this process flow diagram, measures bulk density. Neither of these measurements would be considered release criteria but are rather in-process controls.

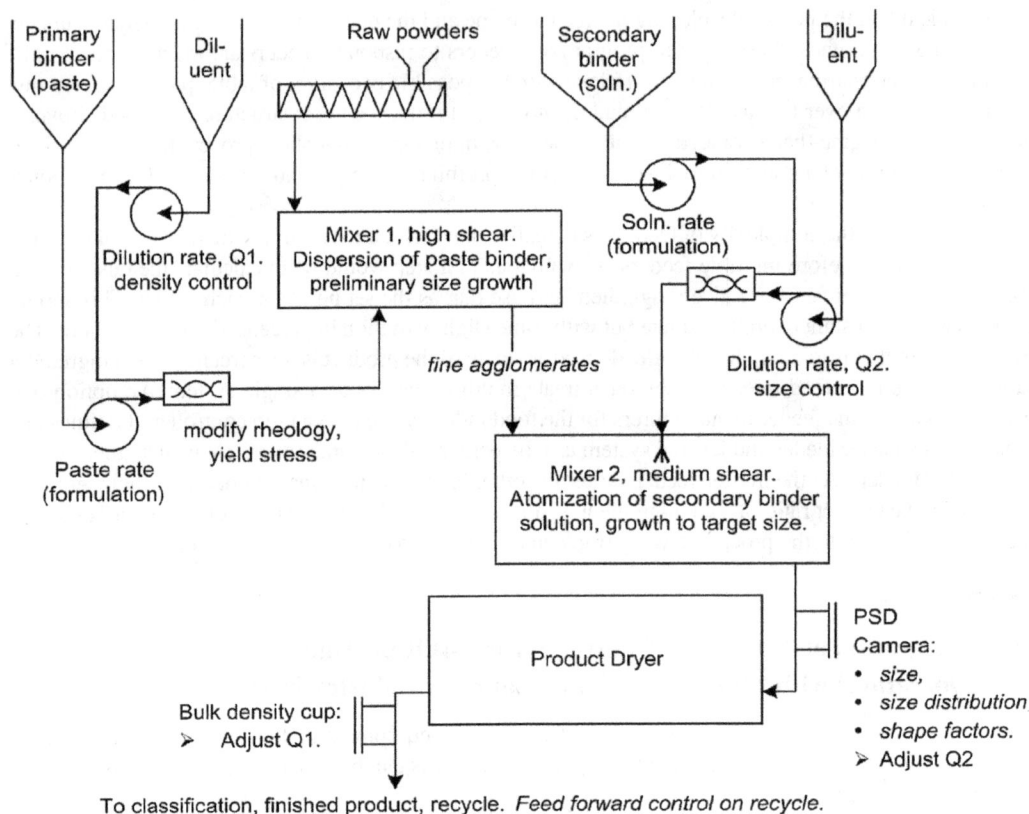

FIGURE 16.5 Process Flow Diagram of Laundry Detergent Manufacturing with Multiple Sensors and Multiple Unit Operations Controlling Multiple Product Attributes. (*Source*: Mort et. al., 2001.) [6]

What is most informative for the pharmaceutical industry is how these sensors are used. Both are used to provide feedback to adjust an earlier unit operation. The PSD Camera adjusts the dilution rate of the secondary binder, which is fed at a constant flow rate, diluted by the diluent which is fed at a variable feed rate based on the PAT sensor signal. The change in dilution rate changes the final particle size of the granules. In both cases, the diluent is water which is subsequently evaporated. Therefore, this example is directly transferrable to pharmaceuticals since these dilution steps have no impact on the unit formula. The other feedback loop is from the bulk density measurement at the exit of the dryer back to Q1, the dilution rate of the primary binder. Similar to the other controller, the primary binder flow rate is constant and the diluent fed into it is variable. This change affects the preliminary size growth of the agglomerates. To further complicate things, these two feedback loops are nested within each other. This results in a system of ten unit operations and two sensors, operating at flow rates of tons/hour, yielding the consistent size and density that customers expect when they open a box of detergent. Note that this process flow only obliquely mentions a control approach that is very rarely used in pharmaceutical manufacturing. This is the feedforward control loop mentioned at the very bottom of Figure 16.5. Pharmaceutical engineers should be aware of this capability if the need arises.

Unlike the LIW feeders which are purchased from the vendor as an integrated unit operation with self-contained signal generators (weight, screw RPM) and control logic, this example spans multiple unit operations and sensors. The unit operations are all purchased from separate vendors and the integration is done by the manufacturer of the product rather than by the equipment vendor. The control logic is completely in the control of the company operating the process since the integration of the unit operations and the automation is performed by the company that operates the process, not by a vendor. These types of operations are typically outside of pharmaceuticals where the controls and automation run on a dedicated, independently integrated automation system such as a distributed control system (DCS) or a program-mable logic controller (PLC). This control system would be developed by the process and automation development team and extensively tested in the scale-up and validation phases of the project.

16.6 Contemporary Pharmaceutical Applications of Continuous Manufacturing

It should first be noted that the pharmaceutical industry has been practicing continuous manufacturing for some unit operations for a very long time. Tablet compression and capsule filling are both examples of unit operations being operated in a continuous mode where the desired operation is in a state of control. Similarly, roller compaction and the associated milling of the ribbons are continuous processes. The filling of tablets or capsules into bottles or blisters is also a continuous operation.

The biggest change between traditional batch processes and continuous pharmaceutical processes is in dispensing and blending. This difference has the most profound impact on a batch process train versus a continuous process train. The ability to continuous dispense and mix is the enabler of the ability to vary the lot (also referred to as batch) size at the manufacturing site [7]. It has the ability to change which allows the manufacturer to vary the lot size to meet business and patient requirements. This is contrasted with batch mixing where the batch size is determined by the physical size of the mixer which is speci-fied in the common technical document (CTD) and therefore very difficult to change. This can result in capacity limitations due to the mixer being too small for actual demand or conversely a high percentage of expiring products because the batch size is too large for actual demand.

Moving away from the typical tumble bin blender or V-blender used in batch processes also greatly reduces the risk of both inadequate blending and also "poor powder flow." This is because batch blender designs are a compromise between a hopper and a mixer. The design principle for a non-segregating, fully discharging hopper is referred to as a "mass flow hopper." The wall angles and opening sizes be calculated for a given material using the Jenike equations [8]. For optimal blending, there should be no dead spots. Obviously, this is a design trade-off because the steeper the hopper section is, the larger the dead spot in the mixer is. For this reason, batch blenders typically have shallower wall angles than a mass flow hopper. This results in "funnel flow" out of a hopper which leads to segregation of the mixture during discharge. Batch mixing is such a concern for the pharmaceutical industry there is an FDA draft guidance for the industry on the topic [9]. Powder mixing is a topic of concern across all industries. One paper alone has been cited over 1000 times [10]. These tend to focus on batch mixing. Because of the excellent mixing of continuous mixers, due to the absence of design trade-offs, the focus of recent papers on continuous mixing in pharmaceuticals tends to be on residence time distribution (RTD) more than on the quality of mixing. Unlike batch mixing, there is no regulatory guidance for continuous mixing because the need is dramatically less.

Two unit operations in continuous manufacturing processes could be argued to be microbatch processes even though they are marketed by the equipment vendors as continuous processes. One is coating and applies to most tablets. The other is drying which applies only to wet granulated products. In both cases, wet material is loaded in finite quantities which are much smaller than the overall lot, then heat is applied to drive off the water. The unit operation is then emptied, refilled without a cleaning step, and repeated multiple times over the course of the lot. Whether these unit operations are batch or continuous is aca-demic. They result in a process that overall is continuous in nature. They successfully meet the desired product quality and do not impede the operation of the continuous unit operations. They do require a surge between the preceding continuous step to accumulate product while they are processing, but for processes currently on the market, this surge is negligible and does not affect the operation of the line.

A pharmaceutical manufacturer has two options for pursuing continuous manufacturing – contract manufacture or in-house manufacture. There are two contract manufacturers actively marketing their con-tinuous manufacturing development and manufacturing skills and equipment. There are three equipment manufacturers actively selling their equipment for use in in-house manufacture. There are at least five pharmaceutical manufacturers that have explicitly announced they have approved products utilizing con-tinuous manufacturing as of 2022. These encompass three platforms: direct compression, wet granulation and direct compression. There are no major differences between vendors for a given platform. Notably absent is roller compaction which would seem to be a logical transition from batch to continuous since the compaction unit operation is already continuous. Direct compression has been the most common platform implemented for continuous manufacturing. This is likely due to the resolution of the "powder flow" issue which was an area of concern for batch direct compression. Elimination of the sub-optimally designed hopper function of a traditional batch mixer and minimization of the consolidation of powder above the feed frame has enabled direct compression to be a more viable process in continuous mode than in batch mode. Some products require wet granulation and at least two equipment suppliers provide equipment to meet those needs. Again, these are functionally similar in operation. It should be noted that the integrated wet granulation lines of the pharmaceutical equipment manufacturers are only just beginning to approach this level of sophistication, integration and level of complexity that the laundry detergent industry example in Section 16.5 which was published over 20 years ago. It can therefore be inferred that continuous manufacturing in pharmaceuticals is still in the early stages of development.

16.7 Challenges and Future Opportunities for Pharmaceutical Continuous Manufacturing

Future direction will be dictated by what is necessary for the product, producer and patient. Specific pharmaceutical advances will likely occur in the ability to accurate feed smaller and smaller feed rates. The second decade of the 21st century has seen progress on this front from the LIW feeder manufacturers making smaller feed rate equipment to meet the needs of the pharmaceutical industry. This trend will likely continue. Current pharmaceutical systems, while much smaller than their non-pharmaceutical counterparts, still have an opportunity to require smaller total quantities of material required to enable earlier clinical phase development and material sparing development. Improvements in modeling will be helpful but there is an opportunity for equipment that requires less total material while maintaining scalability. The integration of drug substance manufacture and drug product manufacture has been installed by one company [11]. Development of continuous capsule filling process has been developed by another company. Bilayer tablets is a product that is very difficult for continuous manufacturing. This might be an example of a product type best left to batch manufacture.

Technology opportunity areas likely will focus on control automation. Examples include more PAT sensing, the incorporation of artificial intelligence into process control [12] and advanced statistical process control (SPC) [13].

It is incumbent on future process development engineers to be aware of what other industries are doing and continue to push technology innovation forward to enable higher quality at a lower cost with improved environmental impact.

16.8 Summary

While continuous manufacturing is relatively new to the pharmaceutical industry, it has been practiced for at least 2000 years in other industries and extensively in some pharmaceutical unit operations. There have also been continuous improvements such as the evolution of human and animal power in Pompeii to water power in the Evans mill to electric power in the LIW feeder and the modern detergent manufacturing facility. Integration has increased from a single unit operation in Pompeii to a physically integrated system to a system of physical and automation integration in the 20th century. The movement from batch mixing to continuous mixing is the most significant change and has changed the tone of the research from blend quality, segregation and powder flow to residence time distribution and modeling of dilute powder flows rather than consolidated powder flows. The automation has advanced from a single unit operation in the LIW feeder example to a system of unit operations in the detergent manufacturing example. The driving forces have been quality and quantity and value. The pharmaceutical industry is still at the beginning of its journey into what is possible and what is needed to meet the needs of all the stakeholders in the industry. Advances in other industries with regard to the use of artificial intelligence, advanced process control and advanced statistical process control may provide inspiration for further advances in the field of pharmaceuticals.

REFERENCES

1. Buffone, L., S. Lorenzoni, M. Pallara, E. Zanettin. 2003. The Millstones of Ancient Pompei: A Petro-Archaeometric Study. *European Journal of Mineralogy 15*(1): 207–15.
2. Vono, C. T. Oliver Evans' Flour Mill and Tomorrow's Orbital Factory Floor. *Paper presented at AIAA Scitech 2020 Forum, AIAA 2020–1363 Session: History of Aerospace II: Astronautics.*
3. US Library of Congress, Reproduction #LC-USZ62-110379, Illus. in TS2145 .E8 Am Imp [Rare Book RR])
4. Pogue, D. J., E. C. White. 2005. *George Washington's Gristmill at Mount Vernon.* Mount Vernon, Virgina: Mount Vernon Ladies' Association.
5. Aspray, W. 1997. The Intel 4004 microprocessor: what constituted invention? *IEEE Annals of the History of Computing 19*(3): 4–15.
6. Mort, P. R., S. W. Capeci, J. W. Holder. 2001. Control of Agglomerate Attributes in a Continuous Binder-Agglomeration Process. *Powder Technology 117*(1–2): 173–176.
7. *Continuous Manufacturing of Drug Substances and Drug Products Q13 (Currently under Public Consultation), International Council for Harmonisation of Technical Requirements for Pharmaceuticals for Human Use.* Endorsed on 27 July 2021.
8. Jenike, A. W. 1964. *Storage and Flow of Solids.* Bulletin 123; 53, no. 26, Utah Engineering Research Station.
9. *Draft Guidance for Industry – Powder Blends and Finished Dosage Units – Stratified In-Process Dosage Unit Sampling and Assessment.* US Department of Health and Human Services, Food and Drug Administration, Center for Drug Evaluation and Research (CDER). October 2003.
10. Zhu, H. P., Z. Y. Zhou, R. Y. Yang, A. B. Yu. 2008. Discrete Particle Simulation of Particulate Systems: A Review of Major Applications and Findings. *Chemical Engineering Science 63*(23): 5728–5770.
11. Testa, C. J., C. Hu, K. Shvedova, et al. 2020. Design and Commercialization of an End-to-End Continuous Pharmaceutical Production Process: A Pilot Plant Case Study. *Organic Process Research & Development 24*(12): 2874–2889
12. Kurahara, S. S. 2021. Artificial Intelligence and the Control of Continuous Manufacturing. In *Process Control, Intensification, and Digitalisation in Continuous Biomanufacturing*, ed. G. Subramanian. Wiley.
13. Anwar, S. M., Muhammad Aslam, Muhammad Riaz, Babar Zaman. 2020. On mixed Memory Control Charts Based on Auxiliary Information for Efficient Process Monitoring. *Quality and Reliability Engineering International 36*(6): 1949–1968.

17

Process Systems Engineering Tools toward Digital Twins of Pharmaceutical Continuous Manufacturing Processes

---

Yingjie Chen and Marianthi Ierapetritou
University of Delaware, Newark, DE, USA

Pooja Bhalode
Rutgers, The State University of New Jersey, Piscataway, NJ, USA

CONTENTS

17.1 Introduction

Driven by the competitive market and increased regulatory scrutiny for better quality control, the pharmaceutical industry has been focused on improving manufacturing processes over the past decade (Rogers and Ierapetritou 2014a). Among other advances, the transition from batch to continuous manufacturing has attracted much attention from academia, industry, and regulatory agencies (O'Connor, Yu, and Lee 2016). With clearly identified benefits, including but not limited to smaller footprint, increased controllability, reduced human intervention, and shortened time-to-market, continuous manufacturing has been considered as an emerging technology that can facilitate the development of flexible, agile, and robust processes to produce high-quality drug products at lower costs (Fisher et al. 2022; Ierapetritou, Muzzio, and Reklaitis 2016; Lee et al. 2015).

Following the development of Industry 4.0, also known as the fourth revolution of manufacturing, enterprises are moving forward to attain a fully digitalized manufacturing (Liao et al. 2017; Zhong et al. 2017). The key pillar technologies enabling the development of an Industry 4.0 framework are the Internet of Things, data collection and processing, big data analytics, and cloud computing (Haag and Anderl 2018; Tao et al. 2019; Tourlomousis and Chang 2017). According to Glaessgen and Stargel (Glaessgen and Stargel 2012), a digital twin is an integrated multi-physics, multiscale, probabilistic simulation of a complex process that uses the best available data, sensors, and models to mirror the behavior of its corresponding physical twin. The establishment of digital twins allows for the integration of manufacturing practices, physical and cyber infrastructures, process information, and computational tools across the enterprise to build an integrated, autonomous, and self-organizing manufacturing system (Qi et al. 2018). Such a system can be used to better understand, predict, analyze, and optimize the process performance to improve overall design and operation efficiency (Chen et al. 2020b).

With the recent studies on Industry 4.0 framework and digital twin applications, their potentials in facilitating remote sensing, data acquisition, information flow, process visualization, and process knowledge extraction has been demonstrated (Damiani et al. 2018; Li, X. et al. 2015; Uhlemann et al. 2017; Zühlke 2014). Pharmaceutical industry is embracing this new digitalization concept in research and development, supply chain management, quality control laboratories, as well as manufacturing practices (Arden et al. 2021; Beke et al. 2021; Ding 2018; Gerogiorgis and Castro-Rodriguez 2021; Kumar et al. 2020; Rantanen and Khinast 2015; Reinhardt, Oliveira, and Ring 2020; Steinwandter, Borchert, and Herwig 2019; Wang et al. 2021). In the design stage, a digital twin platform can accelerate the selection of appropriate manufacturing routes. An in-depth understanding of process variations can be obtained from a digital twin, allowing for the prediction of key quality attributes, and subsequently reducing the efforts in conducting time-intensive physical experiments. In the operation phase, real-time process monitoring and visualization allow for implementation of process control and optimization. In addition, digital twins can also be used as a training platform by simulating different process scenarios and provide real-time feedback to operators and process engineers.

For digital twins of continuous pharmaceutical manufacturing, research efforts are focused on improving process models at a unit operation level as well as building models for entire process flowsheet (Arden et al. 2021; Onaji et al. 2022; Szilágyi et al. 2022). Models are needed to maintain precise representations of processes and conduct detailed analyses. However, digital twin development tasks for continuous pharmaceutical manufacturing are challenging. Firstly, multiscale information of the process, ranging from powder properties to bulk flow behaviors, needs to be integrated (Bhalode, Chen and Ierapetritou 2022; Sarkis et al. 2021). Among all the information, some relationships between process variables or powder flow characteristics remain unknown, limiting the capability of predictive modeling (Wang and Ierapetritou 2018a). In addition, as models have different capability in capturing and considering process variations, there are concerns on model robustness and adaptability (Bhalode, Chen and Ierapetritou 2022). The large number of variables involved in process analysis is challenging for developing appropriate control schemes (Wang, Escotet-Espinoza, and Ierapetritou 2017b). Also, a company's management team often needs solid evidence from cost analysis and/or environmental sustainability information to make business decisions. Finally, with complex processes, challenges with efficient optimization need to be addressed (Boukouvala and Ierapetritou 2013).

To facilitate the development of digital twins in continuous pharmaceutical manufacturing and to address the aforementioned challenges, process systems engineering (PSE) tools focusing on modeling and analysis approaches are developed to provide *in silico* insights to process development and operations. From a modeling perspective, predictive unit operation models, process analytical technology (PAT) models, flowsheet models, and control system models can be developed to incorporate different levels of information to provide process understanding and integration. For process analyses, efficient tools in sensitivity analysis, feasibility analysis, techno-economic analysis (TEA), life cycle assessment (LCA), and optimization are established to be incorporated into digital twin platforms, serving different objectives as listed in Table 17.1. Utilizing these PSE tools, an integrated, model-centric digital twin with comprehensive analyses can be realized for continuous pharmaceutical manufacturing.

TABLE 17.1

Process Systems Engineering Tools and their Objectives in Process Development

PSE Tools	Objectives
Unit operation models	Process understanding/Prediction
PAT chemometric models	Process understanding/Information extraction
Adaptive models	Process update
Flowsheet models	Process integration/Process simulation
Sensitivity analysis	Process understanding
Feasibility analysis	Process understanding
Techno-economic analysis	Business decision
Life cycle assessment	Process sustainability
Optimization	Process improvement

This chapter reviews the recent advancements of PSE tools for the development of digital twins for downstream, solid-based continuous pharmaceutical processes for drug product manufacturing. Section 17.2 introduces various PSE modeling tools for digital twin development. Due to the extensive availability of control models in literature, they are not discussed here, and readers are recommended to consult other sources on process control of continuous pharmaceutical manufacturing such as the papers by Singh et al. 2014 and Su et al. 2017. Section 17.3 covers the tools for process analyses, with conclusion and future directions covered in Section 17.4.

17.2 Process Modeling Tools

Process modeling translates process knowledge into mathematical representations and is an essential tool to support engineering activities (Chen and Ierapetritou 2020). Generally, the models can be categorized as unit operation models that describe process behavior, flowsheet models that integrate the entire process flow, PAT-based chemometric models that extract in-process critical quality attributes (CQA) for continuous monitoring, and control system models to provide control actions. In this chapter, discussions are focused on unit operation and flowsheet models with a brief introduction of PAT model-related topics.

In continuous pharmaceutical manufacturing processes, different unit operations can be governed by different physical phenomena, which can be characterized using models with varying levels of accuracy and complexity. The model selection highly depends on modeling objective, availability of data, and process knowledge. Based on these criteria, unit operation models can be categorized into first-principles models, phenomenological models, surrogate models, and hybrid models, as shown in Figure 17.1. Detailed description of each type can be found in subsequent sections of this chapter.

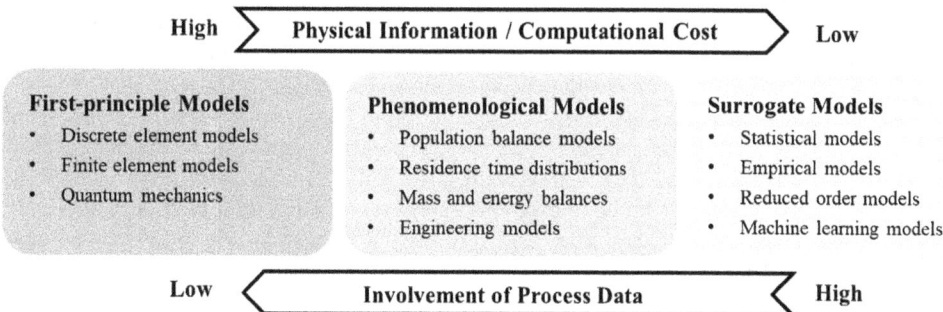

FIGURE 17.1 Different types of unit operation models.

With the development of PAT and the guidance from the U.S. Food and Drug Administration (FDA) (CDER 2017; Vargas et al. 2018), PAT tools that can extract process and product information in-line or at-line have gradually substituted the traditional sampling methods as product quality assurance metrics (Pauli et al. 2019; Rehrl et al. 2018). Different spectroscopy methods such as Near Infra-Red (NIR) and Raman spectroscopy have become popular PAT options (Roman-Ospino et al. 2021; Vargas et al. 2018). To translate spectra information to quality attributes, completely data-driven chemometric models are often developed and integrated with unit operation models (Ortega-Zuniga et al. 2018; Roman-Ospino et al. 2016).

PAT and process models can be integrated together to form a flowsheet model, which contributes to combining knowledge of various units and results in a thorough understanding of the entire production line. The integration is key to further process analyses.

17.2.1 First-Principles Modeling

A solid-based pharmaceutical manufacturing process mainly involves particulate systems. Unlike fluid-based flows, behaviors of powders are not always well understood (Rogers, Hashemi, and Ierapetritou 2013a). To improve macroscopic understanding of particulate behaviors in solid-based systems, particle–particle and particle–environment interactions can be examined with first-principles models derived from fundamental laws of motion (Rogers, Hashemi, and Ierapetritou 2013a; Rogers and Ierapetritou 2014a). In continuous pharmaceutical manufacturing, high-fidelity modeling strategies such as discrete element modeling (DEM) have been widely used as first-principles models (Bhalode and Ierapetritou 2020a; Escotet-Espinoza, Foster, and Ierapetritou 2018a; Rogers and Ierapetritou 2014b; Toson et al. 2018).

DEM is a numerical technique that has been used to simulate granular systems and hence widely applied in the predictive modeling of powder flow in pharmaceutical unit operations and manufacturing flowsheets (Hancock and Ketterhagen 2011). Based on Newton's laws of motion, DEM involves quantification of particle forces acting on particles in contact which dictate the particle trajectories during the subsequent time step (Cundall and Strack 1980). The DEM workflow involves detection of particle contacts, calculation of particle forces, and evaluation of particle trajectories, which is replicated at each time step until the end of the simulation period. The details of DEM workflow are outlined in Bhalode and Ierapetritou and briefly described in the following paragraphs (Bhalode and Ierapetritou 2020a, 2020b).

The main steps in developing a DEM simulation for a granular system are as follows. First, a desired computer-aided design (CAD) geometry is developed in the simulation environment and particles of desired shape and size are added to the system using virtual particle factories, placed within the geometry. Particles can then be added to the system, and a soft-sphere approach is used, allowing particles to deform based on the forces acting on them. Particle shape is also an important consideration especially for pharmaceutical applications. Pharmaceutical powders being in the range of few microns are normally scaled up to be in the range of 1000 microns to achieve reasonable computational times (Bhalode and Ierapetritou 2020a; Dubey et al. 2011; Marigo and Stitt 2015; Yan et al. 2016). Following the selection of particles, different contact models are utilized in DEM ranging from elastic linear and non-linear models to inelastic models. Other non-contact models are also developed to simulate electrostatics, liquid forces and Van der Waal forces (Coetzee, Corne 2020; Coetzee 2017; Yeom et al. 2019). The normal and tangential contact forces are evaluated based on Hertzian contact theory (Hertz 1882; Mindlin and Deresiewicz 1953). These forces direct particle trajectories in the subsequent time steps. A standard rolling friction model is also implemented in conjunction with the contact model to account for the rotational motion of particles in contact. Other contact models such as Edinburgh Elasto Plastic Adhesion (EEPA) model and Johnson-Kendall Roberts (JKR) model can further be added to the DEM simulation for simulating cohesive systems (Bhejani et al. 2020; Gao 2018; Karkala et al. 2019; Wilkinson et al. 2017; Yeom et al. 2019).

DEM has been widely applied for simulating various unit operations and equipment such as powder feeder (Bhalode and Ierapetritou 2020a; Cleary 2007; Toson and Khinast 2019), continuous horizontal blender (Bhalode and Ierapetritou 2021; Portillo, Muzzio, and Ierapetritou 2008b;), vertical blender (Toson et al. 2018), feed frame (Siegmann et al. 2020), compaction (Jerier et al. 2011), granulator (Sampat, Baranwal, et al. 2018b; Zheng et al. 2021), mill (Deng et al. 2015), screws (Hou, Dong, and Yu 2014; Kretz et al. 2016; Patinge and Prasad 2016), and hopper (Hancock and Ketterhagen 2011).

17.2.2 Surrogate Modeling

In contrast to first-principles models that require detailed powder-level information and process knowledge, surrogate models, also known as data-driven or black-box models, allow for the representation of high-dimensional, computationally expensive models in a lower-dimensional space using a large amount of process data (Boukouvala, Muzzio, and Ierapetritou 2011). The idea of using a surrogate to represent a complex phenomenon or to substitute a complex model has become increasingly popular in recent years (Baraldi et al. 2013; Boukouvala, Muzzio, and Ierapetritou 2011; Ge 2017; Qin 2009; Solomatine and Ostfeld 2008; Tao et al. 2017; Xie et al. 2018). Commonly implemented approaches in continuous pharmaceutical manufacturing include the statistical techniques like multivariate analyses (especially for PAT chemometric models), response surface, empirical/semi-empirical modeling, Kriging, artificial neural network (ANN), high-dimensional model representation (HDMR), support vector regression (SVR), and Monte Carlo (Barasso and Ramachandran 2012; Gantt and Gatzke 2006; Jia et al. 2009; Rogers, Hashemi, and Ierapetritou 2013a; Roman-Ospino et al. 2021; Shirazian et al. 2017; Vargas et al. 2018; Xie et al. 2018). To train these models, data from experiments or from simulating higher-order models need to be supplied, resulting in models that are data dependent. Although these methods may be computationally less intensive, due to the lack of physical understanding in the developed models, the prediction outside of the space of the datasets is often ineffective.

Due to different characteristics of surrogate models, sometimes the use of a single surrogate model cannot meet the modeling objective. In such cases, multiple surrogate models may be used to serve different purposes. For unit operation models in continuous pharmaceutical manufacturing, Ismail et al. 2019 used ANN as a surrogate to predict the mean residence time of granules in twin-screw wet granulation. Since ANN had a poor prediction performance outside the range of training data, Kriging interpolation was used to interpolate the mean residence time on new points. These new interpolated points were further used to update the ANN model.

17.2.3 Phenomenological Modeling

Based on first principles and process data, phenomenological models are derived by applying underlying assumptions or computing average system behaviors to reduce their dimensionality and complexity (Escotet-Espinoza 2018; Ramkrishna and Singh 2014). These models with lower complexity can involve macroscopic material and energy balances, system force balance, and bulk transport phenomena (Barrasso, El Hagrasy, et al. 2015b; Rantanen and Khinast 2015). These models often assume spatial homogeneity or consider average spatial gradients, and they involve different parameters that are used to calibrate the model for different conditions. Even if the spatial information on process characteristics is missing, the development of phenomenological models can still represent the bulk behavior of the system as a function of time with simplified statements (Rogers, Hashemi, and Ierapetritou 2013a). Due to their relatively low computational complexity, and the fact that they are mainly based on fundamental principles, phenomenological models have been a popular tool in formulating a variety of continuous pharmaceutical manufacturing units, such as feeder, blender, granulator, dryer, mill, and tablet press (Escotet-Espinoza 2018; Escotet-Espinoza et al. 2018b; Gao et al. 2011; Gao, Muzzio, and Ierapetritou 2012b; Metta, N. et al. 2018; Reynolds et al. 2010; Wang, Escotet-Espinoza, Singh, and Ierapetritou 2017a).

Population balance model (PBM) also belongs to this class of models, which describes the development of properties in populations of variables over a period of time (Rogers, Hashemi, and Ierapetritou 2013a). In continuous pharmaceutical manufacturing, PBMs are used for the characterization of particle states with respect to internal and external coordinates (Barrasso et al. 2013). The modeling method is often applicable to processes with changing particle size and to processes in which particles in a specific region of the unit have similar properties. As compared to the first-principles models, PBM has lower dimensionality as the powders are grouped so only their average states are tracked.

17.2.4 Hybrid Modeling

First-principles modeling, phenomenological modeling and surrogate modeling have different levels of requirements in terms of the degree of process knowledge and amount of data needed. Although the development of a first-principles or phenomenological model is cumbersome and requires detailed process knowledge, the resulting model is generalizable with interpretable variables (von Stosch et al. 2014). In contrast, surrogate-based approaches are quickly applicable, more computationally efficient, and require less amount of knowledge, but the poor generalizability, low interpretability, and the demand on data present a major drawback (Zendehboudi, Rezaei, and Lohi 2018). Hybrid modeling strategy is therefore introduced to balance the advantages and disadvantages of the three approaches (Bhutani, Rangaiah, and Ray 2006). With different structures to combine data with process knowledge, hybrid models offer more flexibility in modeling.

There are three main types of hybrid model structures, namely serial, parallel, and combined structure, as shown in Figure 17.2(a), with the structure selection being problem specific (von Stosch et al. 2014). Serial structures are appropriate when part of the original model is not available, too complex, or inappropriate. Under this structure, the higher-order sub-model usually includes the conservation laws or fundamental relationship equations, and the lower-order or the surrogate part substitutes for the unknown or complex mechanism, such as reaction kinetics, material correlations, mass transfer isotherm, and transfer coefficients (Chen and Ierapetritou 2020).

In the parallel structure, the higher-order first-principles or phenomenological sub-models and the surrogate models are developed in parallel, as demonstrated in Figure 17.2(b). It is common for the higher-order models to have large residuals between model prediction and plant data, which might be attributed to the lack of model generalizability, unreasonable assumptions, and oversimplifications (Zendehboudi, Rezaei, and Lohi 2018). A surrogate sub-model is therefore introduced to compensate for the discrepancy between model and process. This structure is usually suitable when different effects in the model can be uncoupled.

There are several ways to combine higher-order and lower-order models to fit different problem needs, as shown in Figure 17.2(c). For complex problems, one can translate process knowledge into pieces of higher-order models and couple them with different low-order models to achieve the best performance. Though the combined structure can be more flexible, it comes with higher complexity, indicating a potentially higher computational cost and an increased risk of overfitting.

In continuous pharmaceutical manufacturing, given the multiscale nature of modeling and complex flow behavior, different hybrid model constructions, such as PBM-DEM hybrid, Surrogate-PBM hybrid, multi-zonal DEM, and phenomenological-surrogate hybrid are commonly implemented (2014; Barrasso, Eppinger, et al. 2015b; Barrasso and Ramachandran 2015; Barrasso, Tamrakar, and Ramachandran 2015a; Bhalode, Chen, and Ierapetritou 2022; Sampat, Baranwal, et al. 2018b; Sampat, Bettencourt, et al. 2018a; Sen et al. 2013b). These hybrid model applications are discussed in the subsequent sections.

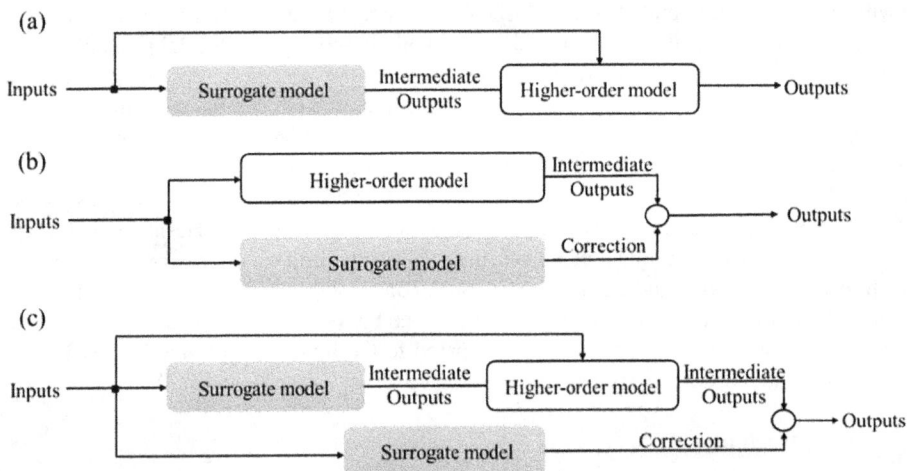

FIGURE 17.2 Hybrid model in (a) Serial structure; (b) Parallel structure; (c) Combined structure.

17.2.4.1 PBM-DEM and Multi-Zonal DEM

Given the high computational requirement associated with DEM simulation, it is challenging to use the method when real-time process dynamics need to be captured. To address this gap, some innovative approaches of developing reduced order models that combine DEM with other modeling strategies such as PBM and multi-zonal compartment models have been developed (Barrasso, Eppinger, et al. 2015c; Barrasso and Ramachandran 2015; Barrasso, Tamrakar, and Ramachandran 2015a; Bhalode and Ierapetritou 2021). PBM models have been widely used to capture changes in particle size over time, as observed in modeling particle breakage and are preferable due to lower computational expense compared to DEM. PBM is thus combined with DEM (PBM-DEM) in a serial approach to obtain faster simulations with good prediction of particle size along time. In the combined approach (PBM-DEM), the parameters for breakage distribution function and kernels are obtained from DEM and the equations corresponding to PBM are solved (Barrasso, Eppinger, et al. 2015c). This approach has been demonstrated for unit operations such as co-mill and granulator (Barrasso and Ramachandran 2015; Barrasso, Tamrakar, and Ramachandran 2015a).

To move one step further, a computationally efficient approach of integrating PBM, DEM and surrogate models has been developed for co-mill (Metta, Ramachandran, and Ierapetritou 2019a), for which a surrogate-PBM hybrid in serial structure is used and compared with PBM-DEM approach. In this case, the surrogate model is used to map the mechanistic knowledge obtained from DEM as a function of process parameters and the proposed hybrid approach shows good predictions as compared to the intensive PBM-DEM approach along with faster simulation time. Similar work has also been performed for the simulation of continuous granulation.

Alternatively, multi-zonal compartment models have also been explored to integrate mechanistic knowledge obtained from DEM within a computationally efficient framework that can be incorporated within process flowsheets. Multi-zonal compartment model focuses on combining systemic and local process knowledge to simulate complex systems, by developing multiscale models (Bhalode and Ierapetritou 2021; Jourdan et al. 2019; Tajsoleiman et al. 2019). In this approach, systemic information (using mechanistic equations) is combined with the local particle information (using high fidelity simulations such as DEM). The local information obtained from DEM is reduced by dividing the unit into various compartments based on local particle properties such as particle velocity. The inter-connection flowrates between these compartments are obtained to simulate the systemic profile of the unit under study. This approach has been recently demonstrated for continuous powder blenders, wherein the authors divide the blender into periodic sections to further reduce the computational expense required for simulation (Bhalode and Ierapetritou 2021). The authors compare the multi-zonal compartment modeling approach with the original DEM model by assessing the values of a mixing index (relative standard deviation) at the system outlet for evaluating mixing along the radial direction and by characterizing residence time distributions for capturing the overall powder flow. Multi-zonal compartment modeling approach essentially reduces the computational time of the system from the order of hours to minutes, thus providing significant time savings.

17.2.4.2 Phenomenological-Surrogate Model

As mentioned earlier in the chapter, phenomenological models are derived from first principles with assumptions to capture average behaviors. With a large number of phenomenological models being used in continuous pharmaceutical manufacturing, disagreements between model predictions and plant data are often observed due to limited process knowledge and inappropriate development of models.

To resolve this issue, research has been focused on combining phenomenological understandings and process data. One approach is to identify the mismatch terms in the phenomenological models by utilizing various correlation analysis like partial correlation or mutual information, followed by a substitution in serial structure using surrogate models trained with process data (Meneghetti et al. 2014). Another approach is to directly train a surrogate model with residual data and append the surrogate to the original phenomenological model in a parallel structure. The method has been applied to feeding and blending unit operations in a continuous direct compaction process (Chen and Ierapetritou 2020) and can be expanded to other unit operations.

Alternatively, one can develop this type of hybrid model by re-considering the physics involved and building a new mathematical formulation. In a twin screw feeder case study, vertical stress distribution in the hopper was considered as a critical parameter in determining the dynamic mass flow rate out (Bascone et al. 2020). The authors used a phenomenological model for computing the vertical stress distribution and substituted the results into an empirical surrogate in a serial manner. With the further incorporation of geometric details of the equipment, the model can be made robust so as to apply to various feeder geometries.

This hybrid model construction can also be found in the development of PAT chemometric models. Often times, PAT models are subject to high degree of noise in the collected data, and in order to address this issue, Gallo-Molina et al. introduced an adaptive Kalman filter algorithm to the PAT surrogate model and incorporated the predictions with a phenomenological RTD model to improve accuracy (Gallo-Molina et al. 2022). The typical online Partial Least Square (PLS) regression model can also be augmented with estimations from another soft sensor in parallel to compare the results from different sources and to ensure the product is within specification. To demonstrate this, a hybrid NIR-soft sensor method that integrates the NIR PLS model with a phenomenological based process model (soft sensor) to predict tablet potency was developed. The PLS estimation based on calibrated models may deviate from the blend potency mean, but this offset can be detected by comparing the mean potency trajectory obtained by both models and can be corrected (Cogoni et al. 2021).

17.2.4.3 Physics Informed Neural Networks

Physics informed neural networks (PINN) have been a popular research topic in recent years, under the overall 'scientific machine learning' scheme (Eugene, Gao, and Dowling 2019; Rackauckas et al. 2021). It can be considered as a special case of the serial hybrid structure, but instead of constructing the black-box model first and sending results to higher-fidelity models, PINN approach reverses the sequence by bringing in phenomenological knowledge into the surrogate training process. An early application of PINN was shown on fluid systems (Raissi, Perdikaris, and Karniadakis 2019), but its application in pharmaceutical manufacturing is still at its infancy.

In continuous pharmaceutical manufacturing, the PINN framework is used by Sampat and Ramachandran (2021) in modeling granulation. Using ANN as a surrogate model, the cumulative particle size distribution, granule density, and the growth regime that characterizes the granule growth profile can be predicted. To improve model accuracy, information of the desired granule growth regime, characterized by the Stokes deformation number being less than 0.1, is added to the loss function of the surrogate model training process, for which data points out of the steady growth region are penalized. The resulting PINN model performs better in predicting the growth regime, and it can identify points that are out of the growth regime more accurately than the original ANN model, with an error rate of less than 1%.

17.2.5 Adaptive Modeling

The development of surrogate and hybrid models has a challenge related to model update. These models are trained on historical data, resulting in a static model that can only reflect the system at the time of training. However, shifts in manufacturing processes can happen over time with the changes in environment, equipment, material properties, operating conditions (Gama et al. 2014). Often times, these changes are not captured in training datasets, leading to deteriorating prediction performance and the need for model update.

Adaptive modeling strategies are therefore developed to serve as a model update tool for non-linear time-varying changes in process. For unit operation models, a model update framework for continuous pharmaceutical manufacturing processes has been proposed (Bhalode, Chen and Ierapetritou 2022). Using historical data, an initial surrogate model can be built and can be integrated into hybrid model structures (optional). Model predictions are compared with actual outputs continuously. Based on certain user-defined criteria, the adaptive algorithm checks if an update on the model is required and retrains the model. The workflow is summarized in Figure 17.3.

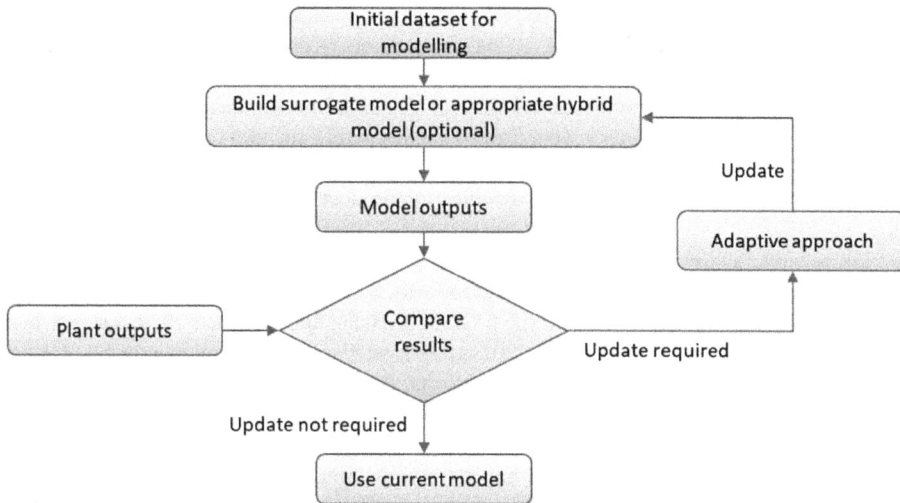

FIGURE 17.3 General adaptive modeling framework.

Many different adaptive algorithms have been proposed, which can mainly be categorized as blind adaptation and informed adaptation method (Gama et al. 2004; Gama et al. 2014; Grbic, Sliskovic, and Kadlec 2012). A blind adaptation is where the model is adapted regardless of whether a process change is observed, whereas an informed technique includes a change detection mechanism and adapts only when the defined criteria are triggered (Bifet and Gavaldà 2006).

Both the moving window method (blind adaptation) and adaptive windowing (informed adaptation) method are applied to continuous feeder and blender (Bhalode, Chen and Ierapetritou 2022). For the moving window method, as new samples come into the data lake, the window slides to include a set number of the newest samples and forgets the older ones. For the adaptive windowing method, points included in a window grow until a change is detected. The algorithm then splits the overall window into two sub-windows and checks if the difference in means is greater than set tolerance. If so, the points before such change are discarded.

In terms of the PAT models, a detailed review of the adaptive algorithms can be found in (Kadlec, Grbić, and Gabrys 2011), where different just-in-time adaptation methods, recursive adaptation methods, and ensemble methods are all discussed. With the increasing adoption of NIR spectroscopy in continuous pharmaceutical manufacturing, the use of adaptive PAT models has been seen with the use of NIR to monitor blend uniformity (Gallo-Molina et al. 2022).

17.2.6 RTD Models

In addition to the different types of models discussed previously, residence time distribution (RTD) based unit operation models represent a special type. It is a phenomenological-based reduced-order model that provides quick predictions of the overall flow dynamics in the unit operations or in a complete manufacturing line. RTD corresponds to the probability distribution of time that the material spends in the unit operation. The distribution of time it takes to traverse the length of the unit operation describes the overall flow dynamics of the unit operation. RTD has been widely used for characterizing powder flow in various unit operations including powder feeders (Blackshields and Crean 2018; Engisch and Muzzio 2016; Li et al. 2020; Van Snick et al. 2019), continuous blenders (Gao et al. 2011; Gao, Muzzio, and Ierapetritou 2012b; Gao, Muzzio, and Ierapetritou 2012a; Portillo, Ierapetritou, and Muzzio 2008a; Escotet-Espinoza, Moghtadernejad, Oka, Wang, Roman-Ospino, et al. 2019a; Oka et al. 2017), feed frames (Dülle, Özcoban, and Leopold 2019; Furukawa, Singh, and Ierapetritou 2020; Mateo-Ortiz and Méndez 2015; Mateo-Ortiz, Muzzio, and Méndez 2014; Puckhaber et al. 2020; Sasic et al. 2015; Ward et al. 2013), dryers (Chen, Diep, et al. 2020a), granulators (Kumar et al. 2016; Kumar et al. 2015), extruders (Reitz et al. 2013; Wesholowski, Berghaus, and Thommes 2018b; Wesholowski, Jens, Berghaus, and Thommes 2018a) and roller compactors (Kruisz et al. 2017; Mangal and Kleinebudde 2017). Along with its application for characterizing powder flow dynamics within any unit operation, RTD models have been demonstrated to be useful for quality assurance as they can provide information essential for process control, material traceability, diversion of off-specification product, and overall system health monitoring (Bhalode et al. 2021).

To develop accurate analysis for these applications, it is imperative to develop accurate RTDs of the unit operations. Towards this end, a lot of attention is focused on identifying sources of error during experimentation and finding ways to avoid them (Bérard, Blais, and Patience 2020; Escotet-Espinoza, Moghtadernejad, Oka, Wang, Wang, et al. 2019a; Escotet-Espinoza, Moghtadernejad, Oka, Wang, Roman-Ospino, et al. 2019b). Despite numerous efforts, the RTD profiles still retain some aspects of variability. This variability leads to uncertainty concerning the true profile of RTD, which further gets propagated in RTD applications.

To address the above-mentioned concerns, uncertainty quantification, denoising, and truncation have been recently investigated (Bhalode et al. 2021). A study by Tian, H. et al. (2022) focuses on characterizing RTD uncertainty and its propagation using a data-based and a model-based approach. The data-based approach incorporates the RTD uncertainty as observed in the experimentally obtained data itself whereas, model-based approach quantifies the RTD uncertainty based on RTD model parameters. RTD denoising focuses on separating the true underlying signal from the noisy RTD profile using smoothing techniques applied across time and frequency domains. Different techniques have been compared in literature to identify the most appropriate denoising strategy for RTD profiles, along with appropriate RTD truncation methods for optimizing the time and efforts required to obtain RTD experimentally. Case studies of RTD truncation have also highlighted the potential avenues for recording RTD profiles focusing on the peak without any effects on the Out of Specification (OOS) product determination (Bhalode 2022).

17.2.7 Flowsheet Modeling

The developed individual unit operation models of all types can be integrated into flowsheets by establishing an information flow between the different unit operation in the continuous line. The resulting flowsheet models replicate the flow and transformation of materials in physical plants and can be used to simulate the entire continuous pharmaceutical manufacturing processes (Kamyar et al. 2021; Nagy et al. 2021).

In continuous pharmaceutical manufacturing, flowsheet models have been developed to describe production using direct compaction, wet granulation, and dry granulation (Bhalode et al. 2020; Boukouvala et al. 2012; Galbraith et al. 2020; García-Muñoz et al. 2018; Metta et al. 2019b; Sen, Chaudhury, et al. 2013a; Wang, Escotet-Espinoza, and Ierapetritou 2017b). Multiple simulation software platforms exist for developing flowsheets of continuous pharmaceutical manufacturing processes, and some representative ones used by pharmaceutical industry are gPROMS (PSE 2020), ASPEN Plus (aspentech 2020), MATLAB (MathWorks 2020), and PharmaPy (Casas-Orozco et al. 2021). These platforms offer a library of process models and tools, allowing users to integrate unit operations into flowsheet models. Most of these platforms, however, do not support the incorporation of first-principles models (Rogers and Ierapetritou 2015), and the computational costs for simulations are often high since the flowsheet models are complex. Therefore, when establishing a flowsheet, lower-fidelity and reduced order models are often used.

In addition to hosting the flowsheet models, the platforms need to have the capability to integrate with data management systems, and cloud services so that information can be communicated to and from the physical process. Many of the simulation platforms have been developing their own cloud services (e.g., gPROMS Digital Applications Platform (PSE 2020), Mindsphere (Siemens 2020)) and integration channels with common commercial service platforms (e.g., TIBCO Cloud (TIBCO 2020), SEEQ (SEEQ 2020), Amazon Web Services (Amazon 2020), Microsoft Azure (Microsoft 2020)).

17.3 System Analyses Tools

Following the Quality-by-Design (QbD) paradigm, a flowsheet model allows for the use of sensitivity analysis to investigate the influence of process parameters to intermediate and final quality attributes (Wang, Escotet-Espinoza, and Ierapetritou 2017b; Yu et al. 2014). Feasibility analysis can also be performed to establish the design space of process variables and guide the development of control schemes (Rogers and Ierapetritou 2015). Moreover, TEA can be performed dynamically with respect to time and market demand to assist with the decision-making process (Schaber et al. 2011). Environmental impacts can be assessed systematically to support sustainability (Luo and Ierapetritou 2020). Finally, process optimization can be performed so that unit operation performance can be optimized as a part of the whole line (Castle and Forbes 2013; Wang, Escotet-Espinoza, and Ierapetritou 2017b).

17.3.1 Sensitivity Analysis

Sensitivity analysis is a critical PSE tool for risk assessment through identification of critical process parameters (CPPs) and investigation of how variability in the model inputs contributes to that in the model outputs. It is an effective tool for ranking and prioritizing the most important process inputs. Since the less important factors can be screened out, the overall dimensionality of the flowsheet model can be reduced, lowering the computational burden (Wang, Escotet-Espinoza, and Ierapetritou 2017b). In process development stage, sensitivity analysis can also help researchers to identify areas of focus, reducing experimental and modeling efforts. In this section, selected global methods are the focus as they are more relevant to continuous pharmaceutical manufacturing processes, and the readers are encouraged to check (Saltelli et al. 2008) for detailed calculation and review.

The commonly used global sensitivity analysis methods can be characterized into screening methods, regression-based methods, and variance-based methods (Iooss and Lemaître 2015). The method selection depends on the modeling objective, sampling budget, computational cost. In models with a large number of parameters and with high computational costs, screening methods, as methods with low computational costs and qualitative information only, are often used to identify the subset of parameters that contributes the most to output variability. The Morris method, as one of the most commonly used and most effective screening methods, uses mean and standard deviation of local sensitivity measures to provide global sensitivity information of input parameters. Regression-based methods stems from linear regression models, which they explain each output variable with a linear regression model of input variables (Metta et al. 2019a; Wang, Escotet-Espinoza, and Ierapetritou 2017b). A typical method is the Partial Rank Correlation Coefficient (PRCC), which is an extension of the Partial Correlation Coefficient (PCC) (Wang, Escotet-Espinoza, and Ierapetritou 2017b). Variance-based methods decompose the variance of the output into components, including individual inputs and the interactions between inputs. One of the most well-known variance-based methods is the Sobol method, which uses Monte Carlo techniques to quantitatively determine the interaction between variables (Wan et al. 2015).

Sensitivity analysis methods have been applied to different routes of the continuous pharmaceutical manufacturing processes and have become a critical tool in risk-based quality assessment. Boukouvala et al. (Boukouvala et al. 2012) and Rogers et al. (Rogers, Inamdar, and Ierapetritou 2013b) applied the analysis to continuous direct compaction and roller compaction process back in 2012 and 2013. Rehrl et al. (Rehrl et al. 2017) then utilized the methods to a blender-tablet press system to check the sensitivity of six inputs. Wang et al. (Wang, Escotet-Espinoza, and Ierapetritou 2017b) further applied the approach to continuous direct compaction to screen 22 input variables of the process. Matsunami et al. (Matsunami et al. 2018) integrated the methodology into a decision support process to decide if transition from batch to continuous manufacturing should take place. Metta et al. (Metta et al. 2019a) then adopted a similar framework to continuous wet granulation, examining the effects of 5 inputs variables onto 20 outputs. Tian et al. (Tian et al. 2019) from the Center for Drug Evaluation Research of FDA has also presented a case study with 28 variables. Peterwitz et al. (Peterwitz et al. 2022) recently reported their sensitivity analysis results on continuous direct compaction flowsheet based on the use of RTD models.

17.3.2 Feasibility Analysis

After applying sensitivity analysis to identify the subset of influential input factors, feasibility analysis can be conducted to characterize the feasible region (or design space) of the process. For continuous pharmaceutical manufacturing process, the analysis can indicate the range in which the operating conditions and/or the material properties need to be controlled in order to ensure product quality (Yang et al. 2022).

Exhaustive sampling can be performed with process models that have low computational costs, and the results can be used to directly identify the feasible region. Huang et al. (Huang et al. 2009), Prpich et al. (Prpich et al. 2010), and Brueggemeier et al. (Brueggemeier et al. 2012) all established the design space of pharmaceutical manufacturing processes. However, for models with high computational costs, it can become computationally infeasible to use exhaustive sampling, and efficient methods such as surrogate-based adaptive sampling approaches (Rogers and Ierapetritou 2016; Wang and Ierapetritou 2017) are more desirable for predicting the design space.

A surrogate-based adaptive approach depends on the development of a surrogate model to approximate the feasibility function of the original computationally costly simulation efficiently and accurately. This surrogate model starts with a low sampling budget and can then be gradually updated and improved with adaptive sampling, during which new sample points that satisfy the infill criteria are selected (Wang, Escotet-Espinoza, and Ierapetritou 2017b). These new points can help the surrogate to quickly get to the feasible boundary of the original function. The general workflow can be found in Figure 17.4.

Boukouvala and Ierapetritou (Boukouvala and Ierapetritou 2012) started developing and using this framework for continuous direct compaction applications with a Kriging surrogate and a modified expected improvement function. Rogers and Ierapetritou (Rogers and Ierapetritou 2016) then extended the algorithm for feasibility analysis of continuous roller compaction. With the successful implementations, Boukouvala et al. (Boukouvala 2013; Boukouvala, Muzzio, and Ierapetritou 2010) provided a systematic comparison on the prediction performance of the design space of continuous mixing and roller compaction process of the framework with the use of response surface, Kriging, and HDMR as surrogates. Wang and Ierapetritou (Wang, Escotet-Espinoza, Singh, and Ierapetritou 2017a) then adopted the approach to continuous direct compaction with radial-basis function as the surrogate. Metta et al. (Metta, Ramachandran, and Ierapetritou 2020) further applied the framework with ANN to continuous direct compaction and wet granulation. Bano et al. (Bano et al. 2018) also extends the framework by using PLS to reduce the dimensionality of input space, followed by using the adaptive sampling framework with RBF surrogate. The resulting algorithm was applied to continuous direct compaction. To further incorporate model maintenance ideas, Bano et al. (Bano et al. 2019) coupled dynamic state estimation with the surrogate-based feasibility analysis to provide design space update through online model adaptation.

17.3.3 Techno-Economic Analysis

TEA has been widely used across various domains of engineering to evaluate the industrial process from the perspective of economic viability. It involves consideration of process efficiency using process models, equipment, and design along with process economics including equipment cost, capital and operating cost, profitability analysis, and cashflow analysis. TEA has been previously applied for pharmaceutical applications to evaluate the transition from batch to continuous mode of operation (Schaber et al. 2011). For these applications, TEA is used to compare the process economics while ensuring consistent product quality.

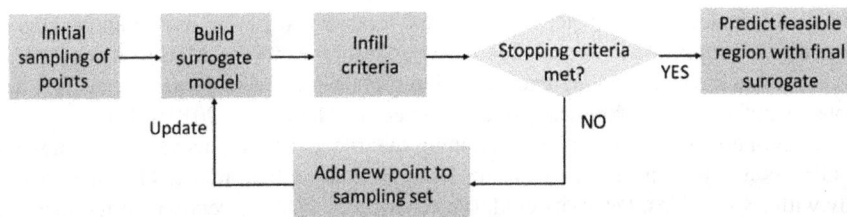

FIGURE 17.4   General surrogate-based feasibility analysis framework with adaptive sampling.

Moreover, TEA can be used to reduce energy consumption. The pharmaceutical industry can spend more than $1 billion USD annually for energy (Christina et al. 2006), with manufacturing processes accounting for over 50%. Increasing energy efficiency and utilization of the manufacturing process can reduce environmental impact and improve profits.

Sampat et al. (Sampat et al. 2022) illustrates TEA for comparison of tablet production costs manufactured using batch and continuous modes of production. The authors consider wet granulation route of manufacturing and include granulator, dryer, and mill as unit operations. The results indicate a 26% saving in energy and 44% saving in tablet manufacturing cost when converting from batch to continuous process.

17.3.4 Life Cycle Assessment

LCA is a recognized system-wide methodology to estimate the potential environmental impact of products or processes (Emara et al. 2018). The assessment can quantify the metrics like resource consumption and emission throughout the supply chain and identify opportunities to reduce environmental impact. Depending on the modeling objectives, the LCA evaluation can have different boundaries, as it can consider the entire product life cycle from cradle to grave, a single plant from gate to gate, or a partial life cycle from resource extraction to factory gate (cradle to gate) (Jiménez-González and Overcash 2014). To conduct the most common LCA inventory analysis, process LCA and economic input-output LCA (EIO-LCA) are the conventional tools introduced in this section. Interested readers are referred to Luo and Ierapetritou for a detailed review (Luo and Ierapetritou 2020).

Despite growing interest and concerns over the environmental impacts across the globe, the use of LCA in the pharmaceutical industry is still limited (Peake et al. 2016). Challenges are mainly associated with the lack of life cycle inventory data as most APIs and excipients are not in common databases (Parvatker et al. 2019), the inhomogeneity of existing LCA practices in the pharmaceutical industry as the selections of system boundaries, functional units, data quality, and assessment methods are different because of the distinctive goals (Emara et al. 2018; Siegert et al. 2019).

The industry and academic community have begun to gear their focus in tackling these challenges. Studies in emission data of APIs have been reported from both the industry and the academia (Lee, Khoo, and Tan 2016; Parvatker et al. 2019). Multiple teams are developing specialized databases for pharmaceutical ingredients. One example is the development of *EstiMol*, a neural network model that can predict emission data by analyzing molecular structure from a team in ETH Zurich (Wernet et al. 2009). Some companies are also adopting LCA-based tools for internal use, such as the Fast LCA of Synthetic Chemistry tool by GlaxoSmithKline (Curzons et al. 2007). Standard methods, assessment metrics, and product category rules have also been proposed and studied (Siegert et al. 2019).

In terms of LCA analysis for pharmaceutical manufacturing processes, most of the work focuses on process intensification of API manufacturing (Ott et al. 2014; Poechlauer et al. 2010), and the analysis of emission profiles between batch and continuous API manufacturing (Bennett, Campbell, and Abolhasani 2019; Dallinger and Kappe 2017; Hartman 2020; Newman and Jensen 2013; Poechlauer et al. 2013; Rogers and Jensen 2019). A recent paper from Eli Lilly also reported a comparison of sustainability performance between batch and continuous manufacturing in six different cases, where continuous synthesis or continuous flow chemistry is in general more beneficial (Kerr and Cole 2022).

For downstream tableting process, Sharma et al. (Sharma, Sarkar, and Singh 2020) assessed the cradle-to-gate LCA profiles from material preparation to packaging and identified three hotspots of environmental impacts. Chen and Ierapetritou (Chen and Ierapetritou 2022) computed global warming potential metric for the continuous wet granulation process using both process LCA and EIO-LCA. The sustainability metric is further incorporated into an optimization process.

17.3.5 Optimization

With flowsheet models, optimization of continuous pharmaceutical manufacturing processes can be performed to identify the best operating conditions to meet different objectives such as minimizing the cost or maximizing process yield while maintaining product quality. With the guidance from *in silico* simulations, number of experiments needed to search for optimal conditions can be reduced greatly, saving money and time in the process development stage and allowing researchers to focus on process conditions close to the identified optimal values (Rogers, Inamdar, and Ierapetritou 2013b).

In continuous pharmaceutical manufacturing applications, only limited optimization cases based on original flowsheets are reported in literature as the computational cost can be extremely high. Sen et al. (Sen, Rogers, et al. 2013b) used optimization for an integrated continuous pharmaceutical manufacturing process consisting of a crystallizer, filter, dryer, and a blender unit. Wang et al. (Wang, Escotet-Espinoza, and Ierapetritou 2017b) also used a gradient-based method to optimize a continuous direct compaction process, minimizing its total operating cost of a 24-hour continuous operation. Moving to end-to-end continuous pharmaceutical manufacturing system that consists of both upstream API crystallization and downstream tableting process, Patrascu and Barton (Patrascu and Barton 2018, 2019) applied the method in a dynamic setting to maximize the overall yield under constraints.

A more common optimization framework in continuous pharmaceutical processes is surrogate-based optimization, also known as derivative-free optimization (Bhosekar and Ierapetritou 2018). In this framework, an initial surrogate is built to substitute the complicated functions describing the process behavior, followed by an iteration of optimization. The next sampling location for improving the surrogate is identified by an infill criterion, which locates the point with promising objective value or high degree of uncertainty (Boukouvala and Ierapetritou 2014). With the new sampling location and the simulation result, the surrogate model is updated to be used for optimization. This workflow is performed iteratively until a user-defined criterion is met, and the near-optimal solution is attained with the final surrogate model.

This strategy has been widely used in continuous pharmaceutical manufacturing. Jia et al. (Jia et al. 2009) used both response surface methodology (RSM) and Kriging for the optimization on continuous direct compaction. A similar study was conducted by Boukouvala et al. (Boukouvala and Ierapetritou 2013) on continuous mixing and roller compaction process to compare the performance of different surrogates. Furthermore, Boukouvala et al. (Boukouvala and Ierapetritou 2013, 2014) also reported different approaches for implementing Kriging and other RSMs as surrogate-based methods in two case studies to minimize product variability. In more recent applications, Wang and Ierapetritou (Wang et al. 2017b; Wang and Ierapetritou 2018a) expanded the surrogate-based optimization framework with Kriging to both deterministic systems and stochastic systems with feasibility enhanced infill criterion and applied this method to continuous direct compaction process. The resulting framework is more reliable and accurate in getting a feasible optimal solution. They applied a similar framework in solving problems with heteroscedastic noise, and the algorithm was demonstrated in a continuous direct compaction system (Wang, and Ierapetritou 2018b). Chen and Ierapetritou (Chen and Ierapetritou 2022) extended the surrogate-based optimization framework into multi-objective space, where a Kriging model is constructed for each different objective. Such framework was applied to continuous wet granulation process to determine Pareto solutions between cost and carbon dioxide emissions, allowing for a better decision-making strategy.

17.4 Conclusions

The development and implementation of digital twin has attracted significant attention from the pharmaceutical industry. A complete digital twin consists of a physical component that involves all the process included in the production of the final product, a virtual component that represents the exact digital replica of the physical component and enables system analysis and an automated bi-directional communication between the two components (Kritzinger et al. 2018). The virtual component is indispensable, but the development of a digital twin with such accurate virtual representation in continuous pharmaceutical manufacturing remains challenging due to the complexity of the processes involved. This chapter reviews various process systems engineering tools as building blocks for developing the virtual component of the digital twin, with a focus on continuous pharmaceutical manufacturing systems. Specifically, models of different levels of complexity and rigor have been described, as they are vital for the accurate depiction of physical processes. With the incorporation of multiscale, multi-physics, and probabilistic process knowledge (e.g., unit geometry, physical characteristic, dynamic behavior), the developed models can be used together with sensor information and input data to build and run the virtual component of the digital twin and enable functional services such as mirroring the physical entity and predicting its performance (Tao et al. 2022; Wright and Davidson 2020). Analyses tools that empower the assessments of process risks, economics, sustainability, and optimization have also been reviewed. These tools can serve as additional applications of the virtual component to complement the time-consuming, cost-intensive experimental work and to guide the overall pharmaceutical development process (Moreno-Benito et al. 2022). Facilitated by the application of these PSE tools, an accurate virtual component of a digital twin can be built with efficient and insightful systems-based analytic capabilities. Incorporating the virtual part with appropriate physical components and bi-directional information transfer can then support the realization of a fully integrated digital twin, accelerating the intensification process of pharmaceutical industry.

Acknowledgements

The authors would like to acknowledge financial support from the U.S. Food and Drug Administration through grant DHHS-FDA-1U01FD006487-01 and FDABAA-20-00123.

REFERENCES

Amazon. 2020. "Start building on AWS today." Accessed 6/19/2020. https://aws.amazon.com/.

Arden, N. S., A. C. Fisher, K. Tyner, L. X. Yu, S. L. Lee, and M. Kopcha. 2021. "Industry 4.0 for pharmaceutical manufacturing: Preparing for the smart factories of the future." *International Journal of Pharmaceutics 602*: 120554. https://doi.org/10.1016/j.ijpharm.2021.120554.

aspentech. 2020. "aspenONE product portfolio." Accessed 6/19/2020. https://www.aspentech.com/en/products/full-product-listing.

Bano, G., P. Facco, M. Ierapetritou, F. Bezzo, and M. Barolo. 2019. "Design space maintenance by online model adaptation in pharmaceutical manufacturing." *Computers & Chemical Engineering 127*: 254–271. https://doi.org/10.1016/j.compchemeng.2019.05.019.

Bano, G., Z. Wang, P. Facco, F. Bezzo, M. Barolo, and M. Ierapetritou. 2018. "A novel and systematic approach to identify the design space of pharmaceutical processes." *Computers & Chemical Engineering 115*: 309–322. https://doi.org/10.1016/j.compchemeng.2018.04.021.

Baraldi, P., F. Cadini, F. Mangili, and E. Zio. 2013. "Model-based and data-driven prognostics under different available information." *Probabilistic Engineering Mechanics 32*: 66–79. https://doi.org/10.1016/j.probengmech.2013.01.003.

Barasso, D., and R. Ramachandran. 2012. "A comparison of model order reduction techniques for a four-dimensional population balance model describing multi-component wet granulation process." *Chemical Engineering Science 80*: 380–392.

Barrasso, D., A. El Hagrasy, J. D. Litster, and R. Ramachandran. 2015b. "Multi-dimensional population balance model development and validation for a twin screw granulation process." *Powder Technology 270*: 612–621. https://doi.org/10.1016/j.powtec.2014.06.035.

Barrasso, D., T. Eppinger, F. E. Pereira, R. Aglave, K. Debus, S. K. Bermingham, and R. Ramachandran. 2015c. "A multi-scale, mechanistic model of a wet granulation process using a novel bi-directional PBM–DEM coupling algorithm." *Chemical Engineering Science 123*: 500–513. https://doi.org/10.1016/j.ces.2014.11.011.

Barrasso, D., S. Oka, A. Muliadi, J. Litster, C. Wassgren, and R. Ramachandran. 2013. "Population balance model validation and prediction of CQAs for continuous milling processes: Toward QbDin pharmaceutical drug product manufacturing." *Journal of Pharmaceutical Innovation 8* (3): 147–162. https://doi.org/10.1007/s12247-013-9155-0.

Barrasso, D., and R. Ramachandran. 2015. "Multi-scale modeling of granulation processes: Bi-directional coupling of PBM with DEM via collision frequencies." *Chemical Engineering Research and Design 93*: 304–317. https://doi.org/10.1016/j.cherd.2014.04.016.

Barrasso, D., A. Tamrakar, and R. Ramachandran. 2014. "A reduced order PBM–ANN model of a multi-scale PBM–DEM description of a wet granulation process." *Chemical Engineering Science 119*: 319–329. https://doi.org/10.1016/j.ces.2014.08.005.

Barrasso, D., A. Tamrakar, and R. Ramachandran. 2015a. "Model order reduction of a multi-scale PBM-DEM description of a wet granulation process via ANN." *Procedia Engineering 102*: 1295–1304. https://doi.org/10.1016/j.proeng.2015.01.260.

Bascone, D., F. Galvanin, N. Shah, and S. Garcia-Munoz. 2020. "Hybrid mechanistic-empirical approach to the modeling of twin screw feeders for continuous tablet manufacturing." *Industrial & Engineering Chemistry Research 59* (14): 6650–6661. https://doi.org/10.1021/acs.iecr.0c00420.

Beke, Á. K., M. Gyürkés, Z. K. Nagy, G. Marosi, and A. Farkas. 2021. "Digital twin of low dosage continuous powder blending – Artificial neural networks and residence time distribution models." *European Journal of Pharmaceutics and Biopharmaceutics 169*: 64–77. https://doi.org/10.1016/j.ejpb.2021.09.006.

Bennett, J. A., Z. S. Campbell, and M. Abolhasani. 2019. "Role of continuous flow processes in green manufacturing of pharmaceuticals and specialty chemicals." *Current Opinion in Chemical Engineering 26*: 9–19. https://doi.org/10.1016/j.coche.2019.07.007.

Bérard, A., B. Blais, and G. S. Patience. 2020. "Experimental methods in chemical engineering: Residence time distribution—RTD." *The Canadian Journal of Chemical Engineering 98* (4): 848–867. https://doi.org/10.1002/cjce.23711.

Bhalode, P. 2022. "Multi-scale modeling and analysis for continuous pharmaceutical manufacturing" Ph.D. Thesis, Department of Chemical and Biochemical Engineering, Rutgers - The State University of New Jersey

Bhalode, P., Y. Chen, and M. Ierapetritou. 2022. "Hybrid modelling strategies for continuous pharmaceutical manufacturing within digital twin framework." *Computer Aided Chemical Engineering 49*:2125–2130. https://doi.org/10.1016/B978-0-323-85159-6.50354-7

Bhalode, P., and M. Ierapetritou. 2020a. "Discrete element modeling for continuous powder feeding operation: Calibration and system analysis." *International Journal of Pharmaceutics 585*: 119427. https://doi.org/10.1016/j.ijpharm.2020.119427.

Bhalode, P., and M. Ierapetritou. 2020b. "A review of existing mixing indices in solid-based continuous blending operations." *Powder Technology 373*: 195–209. https://doi.org/10.1016/j.powtec.2020.06.043.

Bhalode, P., and M. Ierapetritou. 2021. "Hybrid multi-zonal compartment modeling for continuous powder blending processes." *International Journal of Pharmaceutics 602*: 120643. https://doi.org/10.1016/j.ijpharm.2021.120643. https://www.ncbi.nlm.nih.gov/pubmed/33901598.

Bhalode, P., N. Metta, Y. Chen, and M. Ierapetritou. 2020. "Efficient data-based methodology for model enhancement and flowsheet analyses for continuous pharmaceutical manufacturing." In *30th European Symposium on Computer Aided Process Engineering*, In Computer Aided Chemical Engineering, 127–132.

Bhalode, P., H. Tian, S. Gupta, S. M. Razavi, A. Roman-Ospino, S. Talebian, R. Singh, J. V. Scicolone, F. J. Muzzio, and M. Ierapetritou. 2021. "Using residence time distribution in pharmaceutical solid dose manufacturing – A critical review." *International Journal of Pharmaceutics 610*: 121248. https://doi.org/10.1016/j.ijpharm.2021.121248.

Bhejani, M. A., Y. G. Motlagh, A. E. Bayly, and A. Hassanpour. 2020. "Assessment of blending performance of pharmaceutical powder mixtures in a continuous mixer using Discrete Element Method (DEM)." *Powder Technology 366*: 73–81. https://doi.org/10.1016/j.powtec.2019.10.102.

Bhosekar, A., and M. Ierapetritou. 2018. "Advances in surrogate based modeling, feasibility analysis, and optimization: A review." *Computers & Chemical Engineering 108*: 250–267. https://doi.org/10.1016/j.compchemeng.2017.09.017.

Bhutani, N., G. P. Rangaiah, and A. K. Ray. 2006. "First-principles, data-based, and hybrid modeling and optimization of an industrial hydrocracking unit." *Industrial & Engineering Chemistry Research 45* (23): 7807–7816. https://doi.org/10.1021/ie060247q.

Bifet, A., and R. Gavaldà. 2006. *Kalman Filters and Adaptive Windows for Learning in Data Streams*. Berlin: Heidelberg.

Blackshields, C. A., and A. M. Crean. 2018. "Continuous powder feeding for pharmaceutical solid dosage form manufacture: A short review." *Pharmaceutical Development and Technology 23* (6): 554–560. https://doi.org/10.1080/10837450.2017.1339197.

Boukouvala, F. 2013. "Integrated Simulation and Optimization of Continuous Pharmaceutical Manufacturing." Doctor of Philosophy, Chemical and Biochemical Engineering, Rutgers, The State University of New Jersey.

Boukouvala, F., and M. G. Ierapetritou. 2012. "Feasibility analysis of black-box processes using an adaptive sampling Kriging-based method." *Computers & Chemical Engineering 36*: 358–368. https://doi.org/10.1016/j.compchemeng.2011.06.005.

Boukouvala, F., and M. G. Ierapetritou. 2013. "Surrogate-based optimization of expensive flowsheet modeling for continuous pharmaceutical manufacturing." *Journal of Pharmaceutical Innovation 8* (2): 131–145. https://doi.org/10.1007/s12247-013-9154-1.

Boukouvala, F., and M. G. Ierapetritou. 2014. "Derivative-free optimization for expensive constrained problems using a novel expected improvement objective function." *AIChE Journal 60* (7): 2462–2474. https://doi.org/10.1002/aic.14442.

Boukouvala, F., F. J. Muzzio, and M. G. Ierapetritou. 2010. "Design space of pharmaceutical processes using data-driven-based methods." *Journal of Pharmaceutical Innovation 5* (3): 119–137. https://doi.org/10.1007/s12247-010-9086-y.

Boukouvala, F., F. J. Muzzio, and M. G. Ierapetritou. 2011. "Dynamic data-driven modeling of pharmaceutical processes." *Industrial & Engineering Chemistry Research 50* (11): 6743–6754. https://doi.org/10.1021/ie102305a.

Boukouvala, F., V. Niotis, R. Ramachandran, F. J. Muzzio, and M. G. Ierapetritou. 2012. "An integrated approach for dynamic flowsheet modeling and sensitivity analysis of a continuous tablet manufacturing process." *Computers & Chemical Engineering 42*: 30–47. https://doi.org/10.1016/j.compchemeng.2012.02.015.

Brueggemeier, S. B., E. A. Reiff, O. K. Lyngberg, L. A. Hobson, and J. E. Tabora. 2012. "Modeling-based approach towards quality by design for the ibipinabant API step." *Organic Process Research & Development 16* (4): 567–576. https://doi.org/10.1021/op2003024.

Casas-Orozco, D., D. Laky, V. Wang, M. Abdi, X. Feng, E. Wood, C. Laird, G. V. Reklaitis, and Z. K. Nagy. 2021. "PharmaPy: An object-oriented tool for the development of hybrid pharmaceutical flowsheets." *Computers & Chemical Engineering 153*: 107408. https://doi.org/10.1016/j.compchemeng.2021.107408.

Castle, B. C., and R. A. Forbes. 2013. "Impact of quality by design in process development on the analytical control strategy for a small-molecule drug substance." *Journal of Pharmaceutical Innovation 8* (4): 247–264. https://doi.org/10.1007/s12247-013-9165-y.

Cder, F. 2017. "Advancement of emerging technology applications for pharmaceutical innovation and modernization guidance for industry."

Chen, H., E. Diep, T. A. Langrish, and B. J. Glasser. 2020a. "Continuous fluidized bed drying: Residence time distribution characterization and effluent moisture content prediction." *AIChE Journal 66* (5): e16902.

Chen, Y., and M. Ierapetritou. 2020. "A framework of hybrid model development with identification of plant-model mismatch." *AIChE Journal 66* (10): e16996. https://doi.org/10.1002/aic.16996.

Chen, Y., and M. Ierapetritou. 2022. "A surrogate-based multi-objective optimization with adaptive sampling for advanced pharmaceutical manufacturing." *AIChE Annual Meeting* Paper 138g.

Chen, Y., O. Yang, C. Sampat, P. Bhalode, R. Ramachandran, and M. Ierapetritou. 2020b. "Digital twins in pharmaceutical and biopharmaceutical manufacturing: A literature review." *Processes 8* (9). https://doi.org/10.3390/pr8091088.

Christina, G., C. Sheng-Chieh, W. Ernst, and R. M. Eric. 2006. *Improving Energy Efficiency in Pharmaceutical Manufacturing Operations*. California, USA: Lawrence Berkeley National Laboratory. https://eta.lbl.gov/publications/improving-energy-efficiency

Cleary, P. W. 2007. "DEM modelling of particulate flow in a screw feeder model description." *Progress in Computational Fluid Dynamics, an International Journal 7* (2): 128–138. http://inderscience.metapress.com/content/J555136884771031.

Coetzee, C. 2017. "Review: Calibration of the discrete element method." *Powder Technology 310*: 104–142. https://doi.org/10.1016/j.powtec.2017.01.015.

Coetzee, C. 2020. "Calibration of the discrete element method: Strategies for spherical and non-spherical particles." *Powder Technology 364*: 851–878. https://doi.org/10.1016/j.powtec.2020.01.076.

Cogoni, G., Y. A. Liu, A. Husain, M. A. Alam, and R. Kamyar. 2021. "A hybrid NIR-soft sensor method for real time in-process control during continuous direct compression manufacturing operations." *International Journal of Pharmaceutics 602*: 120620. https://doi.org/10.1016/j.ijpharm.2021.120620.

Cundall, P. A., and O. D. L. Strack. 1980. "Discussion: A discrete numerical model for granular assemblies." *Géotechnique 30* (3): 331–336. https://doi.org/10.1680/geot.1980.30.3.331.

Curzons, A. D., C. Jiménez-González, A. L. Duncan, D. J. C. Constable, and V. L. Cunningham. 2007. "Fast life cycle assessment of synthetic chemistry (FLASC™) tool." *The International Journal of Life Cycle Assessment 12* (4): 272. https://doi.org/10.1065/lca2007.03.315.

Dallinger, D., and C. O. Kappe. 2017. "Why flow means green – Evaluating the merits of continuous processing in the context of sustainability." *Current Opinion in Green and Sustainable Chemistry 7*: 6–12. https://doi.org/10.1016/j.cogsc.2017.06.003.

Damiani, L., M. Demartini, G. Guizzi, R. Revetria, and F. Tonelli. 2018. "Augmented and virtual reality applications in industrial systems: A qualitative review towards the industry 4.0 era." *IFAC-PapersOnLine 51* (11): 624–630. https://doi.org/10.1016/j.ifacol.2018.08.388.

Deng, X., J. Scicolone, X. Han, and R. N. Davé. 2015. "Discrete element method simulation of a conical screen mill: A continuous dry coating device." *Chemical Engineering Science 125*: 58–74. http://dx.doi.org/10.1016/j.ces.2014.08.051.

Ding, B. 2018. "Pharma Industry 4.0: Literature review and research opportunities in sustainable pharmaceutical supply chains." *Process Safety and Environmental Protection 119*: 115–130. https://doi.org/10.1016/j.psep.2018.06.031.

Dubey, A., A. Sarkar, M. Ierapetritou, C. R. Wassgren, and F. J. Muzzio. 2011. "Computational approaches for studying the granular dynamics of continuous blending processes, 1 – DEM based methods." *Macromolecular Materials and Engineering 296* (3–4): 290–307. https://doi.org/10.1002/mame.201000389.

Dülle, M., H. Özcoban, and C. S. Leopold. 2019. "Influence of the feed frame design on the powder behavior and the residence time distribution." *International Journal of Pharmaceutics 565*: 523–532. https://doi.org/10.1016/j.ijpharm.2019.05.026.

Emara, Y., M.-W. Siegert, A. Lehmann, and M. Finkbeiner. 2018. "Life cycle management in the pharmaceutical industry using an applicable and robust LCA-based environmental sustainability assessment approach." In *Designing Sustainable Technologies, Products and Policies: From Science to Innovation*, edited by Enrico Benetto, Kilian Gericke and Mélanie Guiton, 79–88. Cham: Springer International Publishing.

Engisch, W., and F. Muzzio. 2016. "Using residence time distributions (RTDs) to address the traceability of raw materials in continuous pharmaceutical manufacturing." *Journal of Pharmaceutical Innovation 11* (1): 64–81. https://doi.org/10.1007/s12247-015-9238-1.

Escotet-Espinoza, M. S. 2018. "Phenomenological and residence time distribution models for unit operations in a continuous pharmaceutical manufacturing process." Ph.D. Thesis, Department of Chemical and Biochemical Engineering, Rutgers, The State University of New Jersey.

Escotet-Espinoza, M. S., C. J. Foster, and M. Ierapetritou. 2018a. "Discrete Element Modeling (DEM) for mixing of cohesive solids in rotating cylinders." *Powder Technology 335*: 124–136. https://doi.org/10.1016/j.powtec.2018.05.024.

Escotet-Espinoza, M. S., S. Moghtadernejad, S. Oka, Y. Wang, A. Roman-Ospino, E. Schäfer, P. Cappuyns, I. Van Assche, M. Futran, M. Ierapetritou, and F. Muzzio. 2019a. "Effect of tracer material properties on the residence time distribution (RTD) of continuous powder blending operations. Part I of II: Experimental evaluation." *Powder Technology 342*: 744–763. https://doi.org/10.1016/j.powtec.2018.10.040.

Escotet-Espinoza, M. S., S. Moghtadernejad, S. Oka, Z. Wang, Y. Wang, A. Roman-Ospino, E. Schäfer, P. Cappuyns, I. Van Assche, M. Futran, F. Muzzio, and M. Ierapetritou. 2019b. "Effect of material properties on the residence time distribution (RTD) characterization of powder blending unit operations. Part II of II: Application of models." *Powder Technology 344*: 525–544. https://doi.org/10.1016/j.powtec.2018.12.051.

Escotet-Espinoza, M. S., S. Vadodaria, R. Singh, F. J. Muzzio, and M. G. Ierapetritou. 2018b. "Modeling the effects of material properties on tablet compaction: A building block for controlling both batch and continuous pharmaceutical manufacturing processes." *International Journal of Pharmaceutics 543* (1–2): 274–287. https://doi.org/10.1016/j.ijpharm.2018.03.036.

Eugene, E. A., X. Gao, and A. W. Dowling. 2019. Learning and optimization with Bayesian hybrid models. *arXiv e-prints*: arXiv:1912.06269. Accessed April 11, 2020.

Fisher, A., W. Liu, A. Schick, M. Ramanadham, S. Chatterjee, R. Brykman, S. Lee, S. Kozlowski, A. Boam, S. Tsinontides, and M. Kopcha. 2022. "An audit of pharmaceutical continuous manufacturing regulatory submissions and outcomes in the US." *International Journal of Pharmaceutics 622*:121778. https://doi.org/10.1016/j.ijpharm.2022.121778.

Furukawa, R., R. Singh, and M. Ierapetritou. 2020. "Effect of material properties on the residence time distribution (RTD) of a tablet press feed frame." *International Journal of Pharmaceutics 591*: 119961. https://doi.org/10.1016/j.ijpharm.2020.119961.

Galbraith, S. C., S. Park, Z. Huang, H. Liu, R. F. Meyer, M. Metzger, M. H. Flamm, S. Hurley, and S. Yoon. 2020. "Linking process variables to residence time distribution in a hybrid flowsheet model for continuous direct compression." *Chemical Engineering Research and Design 153*: 85–95. https://doi.org/10.1016/j.cherd.2019.10.026.

Gallo-Molina, J. P., G. Cogoni, E. Peeters, S. Rao Ambati, and I. Nopens. 2022. "A hybrid model for multipoint real time potency observation in continuous direct compression manufacturing operations." *International Journal of Pharmaceutics 613*: 121385. https://doi.org/10.1016/j.ijpharm.2021.121385.

Gama, J., P. Medas, G. Castillo, and P. Rodrigues. 2004. *Learning with Drift Detection*. Berlin: Heidelberg.

Gama, J., I. Žliobaitė, A. Bifet, M. Pechenizkiy, and A. Bouchachia. 2014. "A survey on concept drift adaptation." *ACM Computing Surveys 46* (4): 1–37. https://doi.org/10.1145/2523813.

Gantt, J. A., and E. P. Gatzke. 2006. "A stochastic technique for multidimensional granulation modeling." *AIChE Journal 52* (9): 3067–3077. https://doi.org/10.1002/Aic.10911.

Gao, Y. 2018. "Quantitative simulation on powder shear flow using discrete element method." *Journal of Pharmaceutical Innovation 13* (4): 330–340. https://doi.org/10.1007/s12247-018-9324-2.

Gao, Y., F. J. Muzzio, and M. G. Ierapetritou. 2012a. "Optimizing continuous powder mixing processes using periodic section modeling." *Chemical Engineering Science 80*: 70–80.

Gao, Y., F. J. Muzzio, and M. G. Ierapetritou. 2012b. "A review of the Residence Time Distribution (RTD) applications in solid unit operations." *Powder Technology 228* (0): 416–423. https://doi.org/10.1016/j.powtec.2012.05.060.

Gao, Y., A. Vanarase, F. Muzzio, and M. Ierapetritou. 2011. "Characterizing continuous powder mixing using residence time distribution." *Chemical Engineering Science 66* (3): 417–425. https://doi.org/10.1016/j.ces.2010.10.045.

García-Muñoz, S., A. Butterbaugh, I. Leavesley, L. F. Manley, D. Slade, and S. Bermingham. 2018. "A flowsheet model for the development of a continuous process for pharmaceutical tablets: An industrial perspective." *AIChE Journal 64* (2): 511–525. https://doi.org/10.1002/aic.15967.

Ge, Z. 2017. "Review on data-driven modeling and monitoring for plant-wide industrial processes." *Chemometrics and Intelligent Laboratory Systems 171*: 16–25. https://doi.org/10.1016/j.chemolab.2017.09.021.

Gerogiorgis, D. I., and D. Castro-Rodriguez. 2021. "A digital twin for process optimisation in pharmaceutical manufacturing." In *Computer Aided Chemical Engineering*, edited by Metin Türkay and Rafiqul Gani, 253–258. Amsterdam, Netherlands: Elsevier.

Glaessgen, E. H., and D. S. Stargel. 2012. "The digital twin paradigm for future NASA and U.S. Air Force vehicles." *53rd AIAA/ASME/ASCE/AHS/ASC Structures, Structural Dynamics and Materials Conference - Special Session on the Digital Twin*, Honolulu, HI; United States.

Grbic, R., D. Sliskovic, and P. Kadlec. 2012. "Adaptive soft sensor for online prediction based on moving window Gaussian process regression." *2012 11th International Conference on Machine Learning and Applications*.

Haag, S., and R. Anderl. 2018. "Digital twin – Proof of concept." *Manufacturing Letters 15*: 64–66. https://doi.org/10.1016/j.mfglet.2018.02.006.

Hancock, B. C., and W. R. Ketterhagen. 2011. "Discrete element method (DEM) simulations of stratified sampling during solid dosage form manufacturing." *International Journal of Pharmaceutics 418* (2): 265–272. https://doi.org/10.1016/j.ijpharm.2011.05.042.

Hartman, R. L. 2020. "Flow chemistry remains an opportunity for chemists and chemical engineers." *Current Opinion in Chemical Engineering 29*: 42–50. https://doi.org/10.1016/j.coche.2020.05.002.

Hertz, H. 1882. "On the contact of rigid elastic solids." *Journal fur die Reine und Angewandte Mathematik*: 156–171.

Hou, Q. F., K. J. Dong, and A. B. Yu. 2014. "DEM study of the flow of cohesive particles in a screw feeder." *Powder Technology 256*: 529–539. https://doi.org/10.1016/j.powtec.2014.01.062.

Huang, J., G. Kaul, C. Cai, R. Chatlapalli, P. Hernandez-Abad, K. Ghosh, and A. Nagi. 2009. "Quality by design case study: An integrated multivariate approach to drug product and process development." *International Journal of Pharmaceutics 382* (1): 23–32. https://doi.org/10.1016/j.ijpharm.2009.07.031.

Ierapetritou, M., F. Muzzio, and G. Reklaitis. 2016. "Perspectives on the continuous manufacturing of powder-based pharmaceutical processes." *AIChE Journal 62* (6): 1846–1862. https://doi.org/10.1002/aic.15210.

Iooss, B., and P. Lemaître. 2015. "A review on global sensitivity analysis methods." In *Uncertainty Management in Simulation-Optimization of Complex Systems*, In Operations Research/Computer Science Interfaces Series, 101–122.

Ismail, H. Y., M. Singh, S. Darwish, M. Kuhs, S. Shirazian, D. M. Croker, M. Khraisheh, A. B. Albadarin, and G. M. Walker. 2019. "Developing ANN-Kriging hybrid model based on process parameters for prediction of mean residence time distribution in twin-screw wet granulation." *Powder Technology 343*: 568–577. https://doi.org/10.1016/j.powtec.2018.11.060.

Jerier, J. F., B. Hathong, V. Richefeu, B. Chareyre, D. Imbault, F. V. Donze, and P. Doremus. 2011. "Study of cold powder compaction by using the discrete element method." *Powder Technology 208* (2): 537–541. https://doi.org/:10.1016/j.powtec.2010.08.056.

Jia, Z., E. Davis, F. Muzzio, and M. Ierapetritou. 2009. "Predictive modeling for pharmaceutical processes using kriging and response surface." *Journal of Pharmaceutical Innovation 4* (4): 174–186. https://doi.org/10.1007/s12247-009-9070-6.

Jiménez-González, C., and M. R. Overcash. 2014. "The evolution of life cycle assessment in pharmaceutical and chemical applications – a perspective." *Green Chemistry 16* (7): 3392–3400. https://doi.org/10.1039/c4gc00790e.

Jourdan, N., T. Neveux, O. Potier, M. Kanniche, J. Wicks, I. Nopens, U. Rehman, and Y. Le Moullec. 2019. "Compartmental Modelling in chemical engineering: A critical review." *Chemical Engineering Science 210*. https://doi.org/10.1016/j.ces.2019.115196.

Kadlec, P., R. Grbić, and B. Gabrys. 2011. "Review of adaptation mechanisms for data-driven soft sensors." *Computers & Chemical Engineering 35* (1): 1–24. https://doi.org/10.1016/j.compchemeng.2010.07.034.

Kamyar, R., D. Lauri Pla, A. Husain, G. Cogoni, and Z. Wang. 2021. "Soft sensor for real-time estimation of tablet potency in continuous direct compression manufacturing operation." *International Journal of Pharmaceutics 602*: 120624. https://doi.org/10.1016/j.ijpharm.2021.120624.

Karkala, S., N. Davis, C. Wassgren, Y. Shi, X. Liu, C. Riemann, G. Yacobian, and R. Ramachandran. 2019. "Calibration of discrete-element-method parameters for cohesive materials using dynamic-yield-strength and shear-cell experiments." *Processes 7* (5): 278. https://doi.org/10.3390/pr7050278.

Kerr, M. S., and K. P. Cole. 2022. "Sustainability case studies on the use of continuous manufacturing in pharmaceutical production." *Current Research in Green and Sustainable Chemistry 5*: 100279. https://doi.org/10.1016/j.crgsc.2022.100279.

Kretz, D., S. Callau-Monje, M. Hitschler, A. Hien, M. Raedle, and J. Hesser. 2016. "Discrete element method (DEM) simulation and validation of a screw feeder system." *287*: 131–138. https://doi.org/10.1016/j.powtec.2015.09.038.

Kritzinger, W., M. Karner, G. Traar, J. Henjes, and W. Sihn. 2018. "Digital Twin in manufacturing: A categorical literature review and classification." *16th IFAC Symposium on Information Control Problems in Manufacturing. IFAC-PapersOnLine 55*(37):1016–1022. https://doi.org/10.1016/j.ifacol.2018.08.474.

Kruisz, J., J. Rehrl, S. Sacher, I. Aigner, M. Horn, and J. G. Khinast. 2017. "RTD modeling of a continuous dry granulation process for process control and materials diversion." *International Journal of Pharmaceutics 528* (1–2): 334–344.

Kumar, A., M. Alakarjula, V. Vanhoorne, M. Toiviainen, F. De Leersnyder, J. Vercruysse, M. Juuti, J. Ketolainen, C. Vervaet, J. P. Remon, K. V. Gernaey, T. De Beer, and I. Nopens. 2016. "Linking granulation performance with residence time and granulation liquid distributions in twin-screw granulation: An experimental investigation." *European Journal of Pharmaceutical Sciences 90*: 25–37. https://doi.org/10.1016/j.ejps.2015.12.021.

Kumar, A., J. Vercruysse, V. Vanhoorne, M. Toiviainen, P.-E. Panouillot, M. Juuti, C. Vervaet, J. P. Remon, K. V. Gernaey, T. D. Beer, and I. Nopens. 2015. "Conceptual framework for model-based analysis of residence time distribution in twin-screw granulation." *European Journal of Pharmaceutical Sciences 71*: 25–34. https://doi.org/10.1016/j.ejps.2015.02.004.

Kumar, S., D. Talasila, M. Gowrav, and H. Gangadharappa. 2020. "Adaptations of pharma 4.0 from industry 4.0." *Drug Invention Today 14* (3): 405–415.

Lee, C. K., H. H. Khoo, and R. B. H. Tan. 2016. "Life cyle assessment based environmental performance comparison of batch and continuous processing: A case of 4-d-erythronolactone synthesis." *Organic Process Research & Development 20* (11): 1937–1948. https://doi.org/10.1021/acs.oprd.6b00275.

Lee, S. L., T. F. O'Connor, X. Yang, C. N. Cruz, S. Chatterjee, R. D. Madurawe, C. M. V. Moore, L. X. Yu, and J. Woodcock. 2015. "Modernizing pharmaceutical manufacturing: From batch to continuous production." *Journal of Pharmaceutical Innovation 10* (3): 191–199. https://doi.org/10.1007/s12247-015-9215-8.

Li, T., J. V. Scicolone, E. Sanchez, and F. J. Muzzio. 2020. "Identifying a loss-in-weight feeder design space based on performance and material properties." *Journal of Pharmaceutical Innovation 15* (3): 482–495. https://doi.org/10.1007/s12247-019-09394-4.

Li, X., D. Li, J. Wan, A. V. Vasilakos, C.-F. Lai, and S. Wang. 2015. "A review of industrial wireless networks in the context of Industry 4.0." *Wireless Networks 23* (1): 23–41. https://doi.org/10.1007/s11276-015-1133-7.

Liao, Y., F. Deschamps, E. d. F. R. Loures, and L. F. P. Ramos. 2017. "Past, present and future of Industry 4.0 – a systematic literature review and research agenda proposal." *International Journal of Production Research 55* (12): 3609–3629. https://doi.org/10.1080/00207543.2017.1308576.

Luo, Y., and M. Ierapetritou. 2020. "Comparison between different hybrid life cycle assessment methodologies: A review and case study of biomass-based p-xylene production." *Industrial & Engineering Chemistry Research 59* (52): 22313–22329. https://doi.org/10.1021/acs.iecr.0c04709.

Mangal, H., and P. Kleinebudde. 2017. "Experimental determination of residence time distribution in continuous dry granulation." *International Journal of Pharmaceutics 524* (1): 91–100. https://doi.org/10.1016/j.ijpharm.2017.03.085.

Marigo, M., and E. H. Stitt. 2015. "Discrete Element Method (DEM) for industrial applications: Comments on calibration and validation for the modelling of cylindrical pellets." *Kona Powder and Particle Journal 32* (0): 236–252. https://doi.org/10.14356/kona.2015016.

Mateo-Ortiz, D., and R. Méndez. 2015. "Relationship between residence time distribution and forces applied by paddles on powder attrition during the die filling process." *Powder Technology 278*: 111–117. https://doi.org/10.1016/j.powtec.2015.03.015.

Mateo-Ortiz, D., F. J. Muzzio, and R. Méndez. 2014. "Particle size segregation promoted by powder flow in confined space: The die filling process case." *Powder Technology 262*: 215–222. https://doi.org/10.1016/j.powtec.2014.04.023.

MathWorks. 2020. "Simulation and model-based design." Accessed 6/19/2020. https://www.mathworks.com/products/simulink.html.

Matsunami, K., T. Miyano, H. Arai, H. Nakagawa, M. Hirao, and H. Sugiyama. 2018. "Decision support method for the choice between batch and continuous technologies in solid drug product manufacturing." *Industrial & Engineering Chemistry Research 57* (30): 9798–9809. https://doi.org/10.1021/acs.iecr.7b05230.

Meneghetti, N., P. Facco, F. Bezzo, and M. Barolo. 2014. "A methodology to diagnose process/model mismatch in first-principles models." *Industrial & Engineering Chemistry Research 53* (36): 14002–14013. https://doi.org/10.1021/ie501812c.

Metta, N., M. Ghijs, E. Schäfer, A. Kumar, P. Cappuyns, I. V. Assche, R. Singh, R. Ramachandran, T. D. Beer, M. Ierapetritou, and I. Nopens. 2019b. "Dynamic flowsheet model development and sensitivity analysis of a continuous pharmaceutical tablet manufacturing process using the wet granulation route." *Processes 7* (4). https://doi.org/10.3390/pr7040234.

Metta, N., R. Ramachandran, and M. Ierapetritou. 2019a. "A computationally efficient surrogate-based reduction of a multiscale comill process model." *Journal of Pharmaceutical Innovation* https://doi.org/10.1007/s12247-019-09388-2.

Metta, N., R. Ramachandran, and M. Ierapetritou. 2020. "A novel adaptive sampling based methodology for feasible region identification of compute intensive models using artificial neural network." *AIChE Journal 67* (2). https://doi.org/10.1002/aic.17095.

Metta, N., M. Verstraeten, M. Ghijs, A. Kumar, E. Schafer, R. Singh, T. De Beer, I. Nopens, P. Cappuyns, I. Van Assche, M. Ierapetritou, and R. Ramachandran. 2018. "Model development and prediction of particle size distribution, density and friability of a comilling operation in a continuous pharmaceutical manufacturing process." *International Journal of Pharmaceutics 549* (1–2): 271–282. https://doi.org/10.1016/j.ijpharm.2018.07.056.

Microsoft. 2020. "Create solutions today that adapt for tomorrow. Invent with purpose." Accessed 6/19/2020. https://azure.microsoft.com/en-us/.

Mindlin, R. D., and H. Deresiewicz. 1953. "Elastic spheres in contact under varying oblique force." *ASME Journal of Applied Mechanics 20*: 327–344.

Moreno-Benito, M., K. Lee, D. Kaydanov, H. Verrier, D. Blackwood, and P. Doshi. 2022. "Digital twin of a continuous direct compaction line for drug product and process design using a hybrid flowsheet modelling approach." *International Journal of Pharmaceutics 628*: 122336. https://doi.org/10.1016/j.ijpharm.2022.122336

Nagy, B., B. Szilágyi, A. Domokos, B. Vészi, K. Tacsi, Z. Rapi, H. Pataki, G. Marosi, Z. K. Nagy, and Z. K. Nagy. 2021. "Dynamic flowsheet model development and digital design of continuous pharmaceutical manufacturing with dissolution modeling of the final product." *Chemical Engineering Journal 419*: 129947. https://doi.org/10.1016/j.cej.2021.129947.

Newman, S. G., and K. F. Jensen. 2013. "The role of flow in green chemistry and engineering." *Green Chemistry 15* (6): 1456–1472. https://doi.org/10.1039/C3GC40374B.

O'Connor, T. F., L. X. Yu, and S. L. Lee. 2016. "Emerging technology: A key enabler for modernizing pharmaceutical manufacturing and advancing product quality." *International Journal of Pharmaceutics 509* (1–2): 492–498. https://doi.org/10.1016/j.ijpharm.2016.05.058.

Oka, S., A. Sahay, W. Meng, and F. Muzzio. 2017. "Diminished segregation in continuous powder mixing." *Powder Technology 309*: 79–88. https://doi.org/10.1016/j.powtec.2016.11.038.

Onaji, I., D. Tiwari, P. Soulatiantork, B. Song, and A. Tiwari. 2022. "Digital twin in manufacturing: Conceptual framework and case studies." *International Journal of Computer Integrated Manufacturing*: 1–28. https://doi.org/10.1080/0951192X.2022.2027014.

Ortega-Zuniga, C., C. P. la Rosa, A. D. Roman-Ospino, A. Serrano-Vargas, R. J. Romanach, and R. Mendez. 2018. "Development of near infrared spectroscopic calibration models for in-line determination of low drug concentration, bulk density, and relative specific void volume within a feed frame." *Journal of Pharmaceutical and Biomedical Analysis 164*: 211–222. https://doi.org/10.1016/j.jpba.2018.10.046.

Ott, D., D. Kralisch, I. Denčić, V. Hessel, Y. Laribi, P. D. Perrichon, C. Berguerand, L. Kiwi-Minsker, and P. Loeb. 2014. "Life cycle analysis within pharmaceutical process optimization and intensification: Case study of active pharmaceutical ingredient production." *ChemSusChem 7* (12): 3521–3533. https://doi.org/10.1002/cssc.201402313.

Parvatker, A. G., H. Tunceroglu, J. D. Sherman, P. Coish, P. Anastas, J. B. Zimmerman, and M. J. Eckelman. 2019. "Cradle-to-gate greenhouse gas emissions for twenty anesthetic active pharmaceutical ingredients based on process scale-up and process design calculations." *ACS Sustainable Chemistry & Engineering 7* (7): 6580–6591. https://doi.org/10.1021/acssuschemeng.8b05473.

Patinge, S., and K. Prasad. 2016. "Effect of parameters on the screw feeder performance using discrete element method." *Journal for Convergence In Technology (AJCT) 2* (2): 1–4.

Patrascu, M., and P. I. Barton. 2018. "Optimal campaigns in end-to-end continuous pharmaceuticals manufacturing. Part 2: Dynamic optimization." *Chemical Engineering and Processing Process Intensification 125*: 124–132. https://doi.org/10.1016/j.cep.2018.01.015.

Patrascu, M., and P. I. Barton. 2019. "Optimal dynamic continuous manufacturing of pharmaceuticals with recycle." *Industrial & Engineering Chemistry Research 58* (30): 13423–13436. https://doi.org/10.1021/acs.iecr.9b00646.

Pauli, V., Y. Roggo, L. Pellegatti, N. Q. Nguyen Trung, F. Elbaz, S. Ensslin, P. Kleinebudde, and M. Krumme. 2019. "Process analytical technology for continuous manufacturing tableting processing: A case study." *Journal of Pharmaceutical and Biomedical Analysis 162*: 101–111. https://doi.org/10.1016/j.jpba.2018.09.016.

Peake, B. M., R. Braund, A. Y. C. Tong, and L. A. Tremblay. 2016. "8 - Green chemistry, green pharmacy, and life-cycle assessments." In *The Life-Cycle of Pharmaceuticals in the Environment*, edited by Barrie M. Peake, Rhiannon Braund, Alfred Y. C. Tong and Louis A. Tremblay, 229–242. Cambridge, UK: Woodhead Publishing.

Peterwitz, M., J. Jodwirschat, R. Loll, and G. Schembecker. 2022. "Tracking raw material flow through a continuous direct compression line Part I of II: Residence time distribution modeling and sensitivity analysis enabling increased process yield." *International Journal of Pharmaceutics 614*: 121467. https://doi.org/10.1016/j.ijpharm.2022.121467.

Poechlauer, P., S. Braune, A. H. M. d. Vries, and O. S. May. 2010. "Sustainable route design for pharmaceuticals why, how and when." *Chimica Oggi / Chemistry Today 28*: 14–17.

Poechlauer, P., J. Colberg, E. Fisher, M. Jansen, M. D. Johnson, S. G. Koenig, M. Lawler, T. Laporte, J. Manley, B. Martin, and A. O'Kearney-McMullan. 2013. "Pharmaceutical roundtable study demonstrates the value of continuous manufacturing in the design of greener processes." *Organic Process Research & Development 17* (12): 1472–1478. https://doi.org/10.1021/op400245s.

Portillo, P., M. Ierapetritou, and F. Muzzio. 2008a. "Characterization of continuous convective powder mixing processes." *Powder Technology 182* (3): 368–378. https://doi.org/10.1016/j.powtec.2007.06.024.

Portillo, P., F. Muzzio, and M. Ierapetritou. 2008b. "Using compartment modeling to investigate mixing behavior of a conituous mixer." *Journal of Pharmaceutical Innovation 3*: 161–174.

Prpich, A., M. T. am Ende, T. Katzschner, V. Lubczyk, H. Weyhers, and G. Bernhard. 2010. "Drug product modeling predictions for scale-up of tablet film coating—A quality by design approach." *Computers & Chemical Engineering 34* (7): 1092–1097. https://doi.org/10.1016/j.compchemeng.2010.03.006.

PSE. 2020. "gPROMS formulated products." Accessed 6/19/2020. https://www.psenterprise.com/products/gproms/formulatedproducts.

Puckhaber, D., S. Eichler, A. Kwade, and J. H. Finke. 2020. "Impact of particle and equipment properties on residence time distribution of pharmaceutical excipients in rotary tablet presses." *Pharmaceutics 12* (3). https://doi.org/10.3390/pharmaceutics12030283.

Qi, Q., F. Tao, Y. Zuo, and D. Zhao. 2018. "Digital twin service towards smart manufacturing." *Procedia CIRP 72*: 237–242. https://doi.org/10.1016/j.procir.2018.03.103.

Qin, S. J. 2009. "Data-driven fault detection and diagnosis for complex industrial processes." *IFAC Proceedings Volumes 42* (8): 1115–1125. https://doi.org/10.3182/20090630-4-es-2003.00184.

Rackauckas, C., Y. Ma, J. Martensend, C. Warnera, K. Zubove, R. Supekara, D. Skinnera, A. Ramadhan, and A. Ramadhana. 2021. "Universal differential equations for scientific machine learning." *arXiv e-prints*: arXiv:2001.04385.

Raissi, M., P. Perdikaris, and G. E. Karniadakis. 2019. "Physics-informed neural networks: A deep learning framework for solving forward and inverse problems involving nonlinear partial differential equations." *Journal of Computational Physics 378*: 686–707. https://doi.org/10.1016/j.jcp.2018.10.045.

Ramkrishna, D., and M. R. Singh. 2014. "Population balance modeling: Current status and future prospects." *Annual Review of Chemical and Biomolecular Engineering 5*: 123–146. https://doi.org/10.1146/annurev-chembioeng-060713-040241. https://www.ncbi.nlm.nih.gov/pubmed/24606333.

Rantanen, J., and J. Khinast. 2015. "The future of pharmaceutical manufacturing sciences." *Journal of Pharmaceutical Sciences 104* (11): 3612–3638. https://doi.org/10.1002/jps.24594.

Rehrl, J., A. Gruber, J. G. Khinast, and M. Horn. 2017. "Sensitivity analysis of a pharmaceutical tablet production process from the control engineering perspective." *International Journal of Pharmaceutics 517* (1–2): 373–382.

Rehrl, J., A. P. Karttunen, N. Nicolai, T. Hormann, M. Horn, O. Korhonen, I. Nopens, T. De Beer, and J. G. Khinast. 2018. "Control of three different continuous pharmaceutical manufacturing processes: Use of soft sensors." *International Journal of Pharmaceutics 543* (1–2): 60–72. https://doi.org/10.1016/j.ijpharm.2018.03.027.

Reinhardt, I. C., D. J. C. Oliveira, and D. D. T. Ring. 2020. "Current perspectives on the development of industry 4.0 in the pharmaceutical sector." *Journal of Industrial Information Integration 18*. https://doi.org/10.1016/j.jii.2020.100131.

Reitz, E., H. Podhaisky, D. Ely, and M. Thommes. 2013. "Residence time modeling of hot melt extrusion processes." *European Journal of Pharmaceutics and Biopharmaceutics 85* (3, Part B): 1200–1205. https://doi.org/10.1016/j.ejpb.2013.07.019.

Reynolds, G., R. Ingale, R. Roberts, S. Kothari, and B. Gururajan. 2010. "Practical application of roller compaction process modeling." *Computers & Chemical Engineering 34* (7): 1049–1057. https://doi.org/10.1016/j.compchemeng.2010.03.004.

Rogers, A., A. Hashemi, and M. Ierapetritou. 2013a. "Modeling of particulate processes for the continuous manufacture of solid-based pharmaceutical dosage forms." *Processes 1* (2): 67–127. https://doi.org/10.3390/pr1020067.

Rogers, A., and M. Ierapetritou. 2014a. "Challenges and opportunities in pharmaceutical manufacturing modeling and optimization." In *Proceedings of the 8th International Conference on Foundations of Computer-Aided Process Design*, In Computer Aided Chemical Engineering, 144–149.

Rogers, A., and M. Ierapetritou. 2015. "Challenges and opportunities in modeling pharmaceutical manufacturing processes." *Computers & Chemical Engineering 81*: 32–39. https://doi.org/10.1016/j.compchemeng.2015.03.018.

Rogers, A., and M. Ierapetritou. 2016. "Mathematical tools for the quantitative definition of a design space." In *Process Simulation and Data Modeling in Solid Oral Drug Development and Manufacture*, edited by Marianthi G. Ierapetritou and Rohit Ramachandran, In Methods in Pharmacology and Toxicology, 225–279. New York: Springer.

Rogers, A., and M. G. Ierapetritou. 2014b. "Discrete element reduced-order modeling of dynamic particulate systems." *AIChE Journal 60* (9): 3184–3194. https://doi.org/10.1002/aic.14505.

Rogers, A. J., C. Inamdar, and M. G. Ierapetritou. 2013b. "An integrated approach to simulation of pharmaceutical processes for solid drug manufacture." *Industrial & Engineering Chemistry Research 53* (13): 5128–5147. https://doi.org/10.1021/ie401344a.

Rogers, L., and K. F. Jensen. 2019. "Continuous manufacturing – the Green Chemistry promise?" *Green Chemistry 21* (13): 3481–3498. https://doi.org/10.1039/C9GC00773C.

Roman-Ospino, A. D., Y. Baranwal, J. Li, J. Vargas, B. Igne, S. Bate, D. Brouckaert, F. Chauchard, D. Hausner, R. Ramachandran, R. Singh, and F. J. Muzzio. 2021. "Sampling optimization for blend monitoring of a low dose formulation in a tablet press feed frame using spatially resolved near-infrared spectroscopy." *International Journal of Pharmaceutics 602*: 120594. https://doi.org/10.1016/j.ijpharm.2021.120594.

Roman-Ospino, A. D., R. Singh, M. Ierapetritou, R. Ramachandran, R. Mendez, C. Ortega-Zuniga, F. J. Muzzio, and R. J. Romanach. 2016. "Near infrared spectroscopic calibration models for real time monitoring of powder density." *International Journal of Pharmaceutics 512* (1): 61–74. https://doi.org/10.1016/j.ijpharm.2016.08.029.

Saltelli, A., M. Ratto, T. Andres, F. Campolongo, J. Cariboni, D. Gatelli, M. Saisana, and S. Tarantola. 2008. *Global Sensitivity Analysis. The Primer.* Vol. *304*. West Sussex, England: John Wiley & Sons.

Sampat, C., Y. Baranwal, I. Paraskevakos, S. Jha, M. Ierapetritou, and R. Ramachandran. 2018b. "HPC enabled parallel, multi-scale & mechanistic model for high shear granulation using a coupled DEM-PBM framework." In *13th International Symposium on Process Systems Engineering (PSE 2018)*, In Computer Aided Chemical Engineering, 1459–1464.

Sampat, C., F. Bettencourt, Y. Baranwal, I. Paraskevakos, A. Chaturbedi, S. Karkala, S. Jha, R. Ramachandran, and M. Ierapetritou. 2018a. "A parallel unidirectional coupled DEM-PBM model for the efficient simulation of computationally intensive particulate process systems." *Computers & Chemical Engineering 119*: 128–142. https://doi.org/10.1016/j.compchemeng.2018.08.006.

Sampat, C., L. Kotamarthy, P. Bhalode, Y. Chen, A. Dan, S. Parvani, Z. Dholakia, R. Singh, B. J. Glasser, M. Ierapetritou, and R. Ramachandran. 2022. "Enabling energy-efficient manufacturing of pharmaceutical solid oral dosage forms via integrated techno-economic analysis and advanced process modeling." *Journal of Advanced Manufacturing and Processing 4*(4): e10136.

Sampat, C., and R. Ramachandran. 2021. "Identification of granule growth regimes in high shear wet granulation processes using a physics-constrained neural network." *Processes 9* (5). https://doi.org/10.3390/pr9050737.

Sarkis, M., A. Bernardi, N. Shah, and M. M. Papathanasiou. 2021. "Emerging challenges and opportunities in pharmaceutical manufacturing and distribution." *Processes 9* (3): 457. https://www.mdpi.com/2227-9717/9/3/457.

Sasic, S., D. Blackwood, A. Liu, H. W. Ward, and H. Clarke. 2015. "Detailed analysis of the online near-infrared spectra of pharmaceutical blend in a rotary tablet press feed frame." *Journal of Pharmaceutical and Biomedical Analysis 103*: 73–79. https://doi.org/10.1016/j.jpba.2014.11.008.

Schaber, S. D., D. I. Gerogiorgis, R. Ramachandran, J. M. B. Evans, P. I. Barton, and B. L. Trout. 2011. "Economic analysis of integrated continuous and batch pharmaceutical manufacturing: A case study." *Industrial & Engineering Chemistry Research 50* (17): 10083–10092. https://doi.org/10.1021/ie2006752.

SEEQ. 2020. "SEEQ product overview." Accessed 6/19/2020.

Sen, M., A. Chaudhury, R. Singh, J. John, and R. Ramachandran. 2013a. "Multi-scale flowsheet simulation of an integrated continuous purification-downstream pharmaceutical manufacturing process." *International Journal of Pharmaceutics 445* (1–2): 29–38. https://doi.org/10.1016/j.ijpharm.2013.01.054.

Sen, M., A. Dubey, R. Singh, and R. Ramachandran. 2013c. "Mathematical development and comparison of a hybrid PBM-DEM description of a continuous powder mixing process." *Journal of Powder Technology 2013*: 11. https://doi.org/10.1155/2013/843784.

Sen, M., A. Rogers, R. Singh, A. Chaudhury, J. John, M. G. Ierapetritou, and R. Ramachandran. 2013b. "Flowsheet optimization of an integrated continuous purification-processing pharmaceutical manufacturing operation." *Chemical Engineering Science 102*: 56–66. https://doi.org/10.1016/j.ces.2013.07.035.

Sharma, R. K., P. Sarkar, and H. Singh. 2020. "Assessing the sustainability of a manufacturing process using life cycle assessment technique—a case of an Indian pharmaceutical company." *Clean Technologies and Environmental Policy 22* (6): 1269–1284. https://doi.org/10.1007/s10098-020-01865-4.

Shirazian, S., M. Kuhs, S. Darwish, D. Croker, and G. M. Walker. 2017. "Artificial neural network modelling of continuous wet granulation using a twin-screw extruder." *International Journal of Pharmaceutics 521* (1): 102–109. https://doi.org/10.1016/j.ijpharm.2017.02.009.

Siegert, M.-W., A. Lehmann, Y. Emara, and M. Finkbeiner. 2019. "Harmonized rules for future LCAs on pharmaceutical products and processes." *The International Journal of Life Cycle Assessment 24* (6): 1040–1057. https://doi.org/10.1007/s11367-018-1549-2.

Siegmann, E., T. Forgber, P. Toson, M. C. Martinetz, H. Kureck, T. Brinz, S. Manz, T. Grass, and J. G. Khinast. 2020. "Powder flow and mixing in different tablet press feed frames." *Advanced Powder Technology 31* (2): 770–781. https://doi.org/10.1016/j.apt.2019.11.031.

Siemens. 2020. "Engineer innovation with CFD- focused multiphysics simulation." Accessed 6/19/2020. https://www.plm.automation.siemens.com/global/en/products/simcenter/STAR-CCM.html.

Singh, R., A. Sahay, F. Muzzio, M. Ierapetritou, and R. Ramachandran. 2014. "A systematic framework for onsite design and implementation of a control system in a continuous tablet manufacturing process." *Computers & Chemical Engineering 66*: 186–200. https://doi.org/10.1016/j.compchemeng.2014.02.029.

Solomatine, D. P., and A. Ostfeld. 2008. "Data-driven modelling: Some past experiences and new approaches." *Journal of Hydroinformatics 10* (1): 3–22. https://doi.org/10.2166/hydro.2008.015.

Steinwandter, V., D. Borchert, and C. Herwig. 2019. "Data science tools and applications on the way to Pharma 4.0." *Drug Discovery Today 24* (9): 1795–1805. https://doi.org/10.1016/j.drudis.2019.06.005.

Su, Q., M. Moreno, A. Giridhar, G. Reklaitis, and Z. Nagy. 2017. "A systematic framework for process control design and risk analysis in continuous pharmaceutical solid-dosage manufacturing." *Journal of Pharmaceutical Innovation 12*: 327–346. https://doi.org/10.1007/s12247-017-9297-6.

Szilágyi, B., A. Eren, J. L. Quon, C. D. Papageorgiou, and Z. K. Nagy. 2022. "Digital design of the crystallization of an active pharmaceutical ingredient using a population balance model with a novel size dependent growth rate expression. From development of a digital twin to in silico optimization and experimental validation." *Crystal Growth & Design 22* (1): 497–512. https://doi.org/10.1021/acs.cgd.1c01108.

Tajsoleiman, T., R. Spann, C. Bach, K. V. Gernaey, J. Kruisz, and U. Kruhne. 2019. "A CFD based automatic method for compartment model development." *Journal of Energy Storage 123*: 236–245. https://doi.org/papers3://publication/doi/10.1016/j.compchemeng.2018.12.015.

Tao, F., J. Cheng, Q. Qi, M. Zhang, H. Zhang, and F. Sui. 2017. "Digital twin-driven product design, manufacturing and service with big data." *The International Journal of Advanced Manufacturing Technology 94* (9–12): 3563–3576. https://doi.org/10.1007/s00170-017-0233-1.

Tao, F., Q. Qi, L. Wang, and A. Y. C. Nee. 2019. "Digital twins and cyber–physical systems toward smart manufacturing and industry 4.0: Correlation and comparison." *Engineering 5* (4): 653–661. https://doi.org/10.1016/j.eng.2019.01.014.

Tao, F., B. Xiao, Q. Qi, J. Cheng, and P. Ji. 2022. "Digital twin modeling." *Journal of Manufacturing Systems 64*: 372–389. https://doi.org/10.1016/j.jmsy.2022.06.015.

Tian, G., A. Koolivand, N. S. Arden, S. Lee, and T. F. O'Connor. 2019. "Quality risk assessment and mitigation of pharmaceutical continuous manufacturing using flowsheet modeling approach." *Computers & Chemical Engineering 129*. https://doi.org/10.1016/j.compchemeng.2019.06.033.

Tian, H., P. Bhalode, S. Razavi, and M. Ierapetritou. 2022. "Characterization and propagation of RTD uncertainty for continuous solid-based drug manufacturing process." [In Preparation].

TIBCO. 2020. "TIBCO cloud: Connected intelligence, delivered." Accessed 6/19/2020. https://cloud.tibco.com/.

Toson, P., and J. Khinast. 2019. "Particle-level residence time data in a twin-screw feeder." *Data in Brief 27*: 104672. https://doi.org/10.1016/j.dib.2019.104672.

Toson, P., E. Siegmann, M. Trogrlic, H. Kureck, J. Khinast, D. Jajcevic, P. Doshi, D. Blackwood, A. Bonnassieux, P. D. Daugherity, and M. T. Am Ende. 2018. "Detailed modeling and process design of an advanced continuous powder mixer." *International Journal of Pharmaceutics 552* (1–2): 288–300. https://doi.org/10.1016/j.ijpharm.2018.09.032.

Tourlomousis, F., and R. C. Chang. 2017. "Dimensional metrology of cell-matrix interactions in 3D microscale fibrous substrates." *Procedia CIRP 65*: 32–37. https://doi.org/10.1016/j.procir.2017.04.009.

Uhlemann, T. H. J., C. Schock, C. Lehmann, S. Freiberger, and R. Steinhilper. 2017. "The digital twin: Demonstrating the potential of real time data acquisition in production systems." *Procedia Manufacturing 9*: 113–120. https://doi.org/10.1016/j.promfg.2017.04.043.

Van Snick, B., A. Kumar, M. Verstraeten, K. Pandelaere, J. Dhondt, G. Di Pretoro, T. De Beer, C. Vervaet, and V. Vanhoorne. 2019. "Impact of material properties and process variables on the residence time distribution in twin screw feeding equipment." *International Journal of Pharmaceutics 556*: 200–216. https://doi.org/10.1016/j.ijpharm.2018.11.076.

Vargas, J. M., S. Nielsen, V. Cardenas, A. Gonzalez, E. Y. Aymat, E. Almodovar, G. Classe, Y. Colon, E. Sanchez, and R. J. Romanach. 2018. "Process analytical technology in continuous manufacturing of a commercial pharmaceutical product." *International Journal of Pharmaceutics 538* (1–2): 167–178. https://doi.org/10.1016/j.ijpharm.2018.01.003.

von Stosch, M., R. Oliveira, J. Peres, and S. Feyo de Azevedo. 2014. "Hybrid semi-parametric modeling in process systems engineering: Past, present and future." *Computers & Chemical Engineering 60*: 86–101. https://doi.org/10.1016/j.compchemeng.2013.08.008.

Wan, H., J. Xia, L. Zhang, D. She, Y. Xiao, and L. Zou. 2015. "Sensitivity and interaction analysis based on Sobol' method and its application in a distributed flood forecasting model." *Water 7* (12): 2924–2951. https://doi.org/10.3390/w7062924.

Wang, L. G., R. Ge, X. Chen, R. Zhou, and H.-M. Chen. 2021. "Multiscale digital twin for particle breakage in milling: From nanoindentation to population balance model." *Powder Technology 386*: 247–261. https://doi.org/10.1016/j.powtec.2021.03.005.

Wang, Z., M. S. Escotet-Espinoza, and M. Ierapetritou. 2017b. "Process analysis and optimization of continuous pharmaceutical manufacturing using flowsheet models." *Computers & Chemical Engineering 107*: 77–91. https://doi.org/10.1016/j.compchemeng.2017.02.030.

Wang, Z., M. S. Escotet-Espinoza, R. Singh, and M. Ierapetritou. 2017a. "Surrogate-based optimization for pharmaceutical manufacturing processes." In *Computer Aided Chemical Engineering*, edited by Antonio Espuña, Moisès Graells and Luis Puigjaner, 2797–2802. Amsterdam, Netherlands: Elsevier.

Wang, Z., and M. Ierapetritou. 2017. "A novel feasibility analysis method for black-box processes using a radial basis function adaptive sampling approach." *AIChE Journal 63* (2): 532–550. https://doi.org/10.1002/aic.15362.

Wang, Z., and M. Ierapetritou. 2018a. "Constrained optimization of black-box stochastic systems using a novel feasibility enhanced Kriging-based method." *Computers & Chemical Engineering 118*: 210–223. https://doi.org/10.1016/j.compchemeng.2018.07.016.

Wang, Z., and M. Ierapetritou. 2018b. "Surrogate-based feasibility analysis for black-box stochastic simulations with heteroscedastic noise." *Journal of Global Optimization*. https://doi.org/10.1007/s10898-018-0615-4.

Ward, H. W., D. O. Blackwood, M. Polizzi, and H. Clarke. 2013. "Monitoring blend potency in a tablet press feed frame using near infrared spectroscopy." *Journal of Pharmaceutical and Biomedical Analysis 80*: 18–23. https://doi.org/10.1016/j.jpba.2013.02.008.

Wernet, G., S. Papadokonstantakis, S. Hellweg, and K. Hungerbühler. 2009. "Bridging data gaps in environmental assessments: Modeling impacts of fine and basic chemical production." *Green Chemistry 11* (11). https://doi.org/10.1039/b905558d.

Wesholowski, J., A. Berghaus, and M. Thommes. 2018a. "Inline determination of residence time distribution in hot-melt-extrusion." *Pharmaceutics 10* (2). https://doi.org/10.3390/pharmaceutics10020049.

Wesholowski, J., A. Berghaus, and M. Thommes. 2018b. "Investigations concerning the residence time distribution of twin-screw-extrusion processes as indicator for inherent mixing." *Pharmaceutics 10* (4). https://doi.org/10.3390/pharmaceutics10040207.

Wilkinson, S. K., S. A. Turnbull, Z. Yan, E. H. Stitt, and M. Marigo. 2017. "A parametric evaluation of powder flowability using a Freeman rheometer through statistical and sensitivity analysis: A discrete element method (DEM) study." *Computers and Chemical Engineering 97*: 161–174. https://doi.org/10.1016/j.compchemeng.2016.11.034.

Wright, L., and S. Davidson. 2020. "How to tell the difference between a model and a digital twin." *Advanced Modeling and Simulation in Engineering Sciences 7*, 13. https://doi.org/10.1186/s40323-020-00147-4

Xie, Q., H. Liu, D. Bo, C. He, and M. Pan. 2018. "Data-driven modeling and optimization of complex chemical processes using a novel HDMR methodology." In *13th International Symposium on Process Systems Engineering (PSE 2018)*, In Computer Aided Chemical Engineering, 835–840.

Yan, Z., S. K. Wilkinson, E. H. Stitt, and M. Marigo. 2016. "Investigating mixing and segregation using discrete element modelling (DEM) in the Freeman FT4 rheometer." *International Journal of Pharmaceutics 513* (1–2): 38–48. https://doi.org/10.1016/j.ijpharm.2016.08.065.

Yang, W., W. Qian, Z. Yuan, and B. Chen. 2022. "Perspectives on the flexibility analysis for continuous pharmaceutical manufacturing processes." *Chinese Journal of Chemical Engineering 41*: 29–41. https://doi.org/10.1016/j.cjche.2021.12.005.

Yeom, S. B., E.-S. Ha, M.-S. Kim, S. H. Jeong, S.-J. Hwang, and D. H. Choi. 2019. "Application of the discrete element method for manufacturing process simulation in the pharmaceutical industry." *Pharmaceutics 11* (8): 414. https://doi.org/10.3390/pharmaceutics11080414.

Yu, L. X., G. Amidon, M. A. Khan, S. W. Hoag, J. Polli, G. K. Raju, and J. Woodcock. 2014. "Understanding pharmaceutical quality by design." *The AAPS Journal 16* (4): 771–783. https://doi.org/10.1208/s12248-014-9598-3.

Zendehboudi, S., N. Rezaei, and A. Lohi. 2018. "Applications of hybrid models in chemical, petroleum, and energy systems: A systematic review." *Applied Energy 228*: 2539–2566. https://doi.org/10.1016/j.apenergy.2018.06.051.

Zheng, C., L. Zhang, N. Govender, and C.-Y. Wu. 2021. "DEM analysis of residence time distribution during twin screw granulation." *Powder Technology 377*: 924–938. https://doi.org/10.1016/j.powtec.2020.09.049.

Zhong, R. Y., X. Xu, E. Klotz, and S. T. Newman. 2017. "Intelligent manufacturing in the context of industry 4.0: A review." *Engineering 3* (5): 616–630. https://doi.org/10.1016/j.Eng.2017.05.015.

Zühlke, D. 2014. "Human-machine-interaction in the industry 4.0 era." *2014 12th IEEE International Conference on Industrial Informatics (INDIN)*, Porto Alegre, Brazil.

Index

For Product Safety Concerns and Information please contact our EU
representative GPSR@taylorandfrancis.com
Taylor & Francis Verlag GmbH, Kaufingerstraße 24, 80331 München, Germany